D1167713

# Illustrated
# Medical Dictionary

# The
# Medical
# Adviser Series

Medical
Adviser
Series

Parr/
C. Murphy Combs, M.D.

# Illustrated
# Medical
# Dictionary

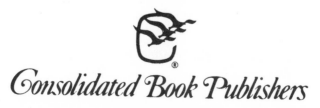

*Consolidated Book Publishers*

NEW YORK • CHICAGO

Copyright ©1976 by Consolidated Book Publishers, 420 Lexington
Avenue, New York, New York 10017
Based on *Parr's Medical Encyclopedia* copyright ©1971 by Elsevier
Publishing Co., Ltd., Barking, Essex, England. Previously published
under the title, *Illustrated Family Medical Encyclopedia,* by Consolidated
Book Publishers. All rights reserved under the International and
Pan-American Copyright Conventions. Manufactured in the United
States of America and published simultaneously in Canada by George J.
McLeod Limited, Toronto, Ontario.

Library of Congress Catalog Card Number: 76-16457
ISBN: 0-8326-2237-0

# Contents

# A

**abacterial.** Free from bacteria.

**abalienation.** An old term for mental deterioration or insanity.

**abarognosis.** Inability to estimate weight.

**abarticular.** 1. Unconnected with a joint. 2. Not near a joint.

**abasia.** 1. A reeling gait. 2. An abnormal method of walking.

**abdomen.** The region of the trunk between the lower end of the breastbone and the pelvis. It contains the liver, gall bladder, spleen, kidneys, stomach, and the intestinal tract. Also called *abdominal cavity, belly.*

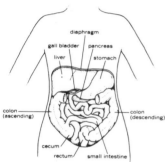

ABDOMEN (organs of the abdomen)

**acute abdomen.** A term indicating that the patient has a condition within the abdomen requiring urgent operation—acute appendicitis, for example.

**pendulous abdomen.** An abdomen that sags and may hang down below the level of the groins.

**scaphoid abdomen.** A caved-in, hollow abdomen, which may be caused by starvation or severe disease.

**abdominal areas.** Anatomically, the abdomen is divided into nine areas.

The top right area is the right hypochondrium, the top middle is the epigastrium, and the top left is the left hypochondrium. The central region containing the umbilicus is called the umbilical area, on either side of which lie the right and left lumbar areas. The lowest areas are the hypogastrium, in the center, flanked by the right and left inguinal areas.

**abdominalgia.** Pain arising within the abdomen.

**abdominal pain.** Any persistent pain in the abdomen, whether continuous or intermittent, requires medical advice. Such pain should never be treated by purgatives, even mild ones like milk of magnesia, for they seldom relieve abdominal pain and may make the condition worse. Neither is the taking of proprietary indigestion remedies a safe procedure, for they cannot cure disease and, by masking symptoms, may allow a disease to progress before an accurate diagnosis is obtained—perhaps too late. This advice is especially important to mothers who give children medicine for all abdominal pain.

**abdomino-.** A combining form relating to involvement of the abdomen with another part, or describing an operation performed on the abdomen, for example, abdominocentesis.

**abdominocentesis.** The operation of draining the abdomen of fluid which may be due to a liver disease or a growth.

**abdominoscopy.** Examination of the interior of the abdomen by means of an instrument inserted through its wall.

**abducens.** The sixth cranial nerve. It supplies the external rectus muscle of the eye. Paralysis of this nerve and muscle causes squinting. The muscle is also known as the abducens.

**abduct.** To draw away from the middle line of the body. If the arm is moved sideways from the body, it is said to have been abducted. The reverse movement is called adduction.

**abductor.** A muscle producing the movement of abduction.

**aberrant.** A departure from the normal course. If, for example, an artery is found in a position different from that expected, it is referred to as being aberrant.

**aberration.** A departure from the normal. It often refers to a mental disorder or to an error of refraction in a lens.

**ablate.** To get rid of, to cut away, or to remove surgically.

**abocclusion.** A condition in which the mandibular teeth are not in contact with the maxillary teeth.

**abort.** 1. To miscarry, as in abortion. 2. To cut short the course of a disease by prompt treatment.

**abortion.** The expulsion of a baby from the uterus before the 28th week of pregnancy. It is not expected that a baby born before this time would survive, but after the 28th week a baby has a slender chance which increases with every week before birth. A baby born between the 28th and the 40th weeks of pregnancy is referred to as premature.

**accidental abortion.** A pregnant woman who starts to bleed and experiences womb contractions should go to bed, keep quite still, and send for the doctor.

**artificial abortion.** Intentional termination of pregnancy.

**habitual abortion.** Recurrent abortion with each pregnancy. It may be due to a disease of the womb, such as fibroids; to an immature womb that refuses to enlarge; to a defect in hormone production; or to a constitutional disease.

**incomplete abortion.** An abortion in which some of the fetal tissue is retained in the womb. It leads to heavy bleeding and it is necessary to have the womb scraped in a hospital. Also called *partial abortion.*

**induced abortion.** See ARTIFICIAL ABORTION, above.

---

**To facilitate use of the Medical Encyclopedia, the editors have observed certain stylistic conventions:**

Entry Terms: Main-entry terms are in **boldface type** and extend into the left margin. They are lowercase unless standard usage dictates otherwise.

Subentry Terms: These are also in boldface type but are flush with the text of the definition.

Definitions: Different meanings for entry terms are preceded by a boldface number.

Editorial Notes: Information which is of historical or medical interest, but not an essential part of a definition, follows some entries. These notes are in *italic type.*

Cross References: Direct cross references to another main entry are preceded by "See" and are printed in small roman

capitals (See COLOR BLINDNESS.). Cross references to a subentry are preceded by "See" and name both the main entry and the subentry (See TUBE: FALLOPIAN TUBE.). Cross references from one subentry to another in the same definition are followed by "above" or "below," depending on the alphabetical place of the subentry (**induced abortion.** See ARTIFICIAL ABORTION, above.). Comparisons, which are not strictly cross references but which indicate related topics, are preceded by "See also" (See also CASTLE'S FACTORS.).

Synonyms: Alternate names for an entry or subentry term follow the definition, are preceded by "also called," and are printed in italic type (Also called *dystopia.*).

**inevitable abortion.** An abortion in which the neck of the womb is already open so that the pregnancy cannot be saved.

**missed abortion.** An abortion in which the fetus has died but has not been expelled within two weeks.

**partial abortion. 1.** See INCOMPLETE ABORTION. above. **2.** An abortion in which one fetus has been expelled leaving behind a twin that survives.

**psychiatric abortion.** An abortion induced surgically because of the mental state of the mother.

**spontaneous abortion.** Any abortion not induced by artificial means.

**therapeutic abortion.** Termination of pregnancy for a reason vital to a mother's health.

**tubal abortion.** Extrusion of the embryo from the oviduct into the abdominal cavity occurring in ectopic pregnancy.

**abortionist.** One who unlawfully produces an abortion. In most states this is a serious crime punishable in the courts. The term does not usually refer to the gynecologist who terminates a pregnancy because of danger to the mother's health or other legally accepted reasons.

**abortus fever.** A feverish illness with a remittent temperature caused by bacteria of the genus *Brucella.* In man the disease leads to general weakness, loss of weight, and anemia. It is rarely transmitted from person to person but spreads regularly from animal to animal and then from animals to man, sometimes by means of unpasteurized milk from an infected animal. Cattle, goats, and pigs are the chief sources of infection. Also called *brucellosis, Malta fever, Mediterranean fever, undulant fever.*

**abrachia.** A developmental anomaly characterized by complete absence of the arms.

**abrade.** To remove the skin's surface by friction. When pieces of skin are torn off by being rubbed against a rough surface, the resulting shallow injury is called an abrasion. Abrasion, sometimes called dermabrasion, is now employed medically, using sterilized sandpaper rolls and wire brushes driven by a motor working at high velocity, to take off scars and such marks as acne pits from areas of the skin's surface that are too extensive to be excised surgically.

**abreaction.** A treatment used by psychiatrists to obtain a patient's emotional release. By administering various drugs or by carbon dioxide inhalation, the doctor causes the patient to relive the incident that caused his fear. As a sequel to his emotional discharge, which may resemble a hysterical attack, the patient experiences relief.

**abscess.** A localized collection of pus. When germs such as bacteria invade the body their presence sets up a reaction whereby white blood cells migrate to the spot to try to devour the bacteria. In doing so, the white blood cells die. When millions of these cells containing dead germs collect together, they form the yellow substance called pus. There is, of course, no limit to the number of sites in the body where abscesses can develop.

dead leucocytes and dead bacteria (pus)
capillaries containing leucocytes
wound
leucocytes fighting bacteria
bacteria

ABSCESS

**absolute.** Complete or pure.

**absolute alcohol.** Alcohol containing less than 1 percent of water.

**absorb.** To soak up. The body can absorb heat, light, liquids, and gases.

**absorbefacient. 1.** Any agent which promotes absorption. **2.** Causing or producing absorption.

**acalculia.** Inability to do even the simplest arithmetical calculation.

**acanthoma.** A cancerous skin growth.

**acanthoma verrucosa seborrhoeica.** Warts occurring in old people.

**acanthosis.** Any skin disease which causes thickening of the prickle cell or lower layer of the epidermis, with or without thickening of the outer layer.

**acanthosis nigricans.** A skin disorder leading to the appearance of pigmented warty growths, especially in the armpits, breasts, genital areas, mouth, and anus. When the disorder appears after middle age it is often associated with cancer of the intestines. If it occurs before middle age it is sometimes associated with diabetes or an endocrine gland disturbance.

**acariasis.** Any disease caused by a mite. See also SCABIES.

**acarophobia.** A morbid mental state characterized by a fear of catching scabies. In its more advanced state it may involve a fear of small insects, spiders, or even small inanimate objects.

**accentuation. 1.** Increased emphasis. **2.** Intensification of a disease.

**accessory. 1.** Auxiliary to. **2.** Assisting.

**accessory nerve.** The eleventh cranial nerve. It supplies the sternocleidomastoid and trapezius muscles.

**accessory organ.** A subsidiary organ which contributes to the function of a main organ. For example, the eyelid, eyebrow, and conjunctival membrane are accessory organs for the eye.

**accidental.** Due to an accident or to an unknown cause.

**accidental hemorrhage.** Bleeding from the afterbirth before the child is born, due to premature separation of the afterbirth from the wall of the womb.

**accidents in the home.** These are accidents usually caused by negligence. For instance, a child may pull the cloth off a table and with it a pot of boiling tea; or he may reach up to a saucepan handle on the stove and upset boiling stew all over himself. Worn mats and mats with holes in them are often responsible for falls; a person may catch his toe in a hole or on a loose strand, stumble, and fracture a bone. Or someone may stand on something insecure, slip, fall, and injure himself. Many accidents are due to failure to repair something that has long been in need of attention: frayed insulation on a wire connected to an electrical appliance, which sooner or later wears through causing the person using the appliance to be either burned or electrocuted; or badly maintained gas fittings that leak. Keeping medicines or drugs within reach of children is asking for trouble. Children know that these articles are consumed by their parents and instinctively feel that they are perfectly safe for them to take. They then swallow them and are removed to the hospital poisoned with an excessive dose of a drug. Many dangerous chemicals, such as floor polish, bleaching agents, detergents, and soap powders are kept under the kitchen sink in easy reach of small children. Lemonade and milk bottles containing gasoline, kerosene, or other chemicals are sometimes left in the kitchen, garage, or garden shed, and a child, reassured by the familiar bottle, drinks from it and is poisoned.

**accommodation.** Alteration in shape of the eye lens in focusing to bring a clear image onto the retina.

**accoucheur.** See OBSTETRICIAN.

**acetabulum.** The cup-shaped socket in the side of the pelvis into which the head of the femur bone of the thigh is fitted, thus forming the hip joint.

**acetic acid.** The pungent chemical which produces the acid taste in vinegar.

**acetylsalicylic acid.** See ASPIRIN.

**achalasia.** Failure of a muscular valve, such as in the esophagus or in the anus, to relax to allow the gastrointestinal contents to pass on.

**Achard-Thiers syndrome.** Diabetes that occurs in bearded women.

**ache.** A dull, nagging pain which is persistent but not severe.

**acheiria.** 1. The condition of having been born without hands. 2. A hysterical condition in which the patient alleges he has lost all sensation in his hands or denies that he possesses hands.

**Achilles tendon.** The powerful tendon connecting the muscles in the calf with the heel bone.

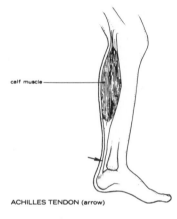

calf muscle

ACHILLES TENDON (arrow)

**acholuria.** Absence of bile pigment in the urine.

**achondroplasia.** An inherited condition which begins before birth and is due to malformation of cartilage and the growing bones in the limbs. The growing ends of the bone join with the bone shaft and prevent it from developing, so that the child becomes a dwarf. The trunk, however, develops almost normally. These children, although extremely small, are of normal intelligence, strong, and very agile. Most of the little men seen in circuses are achondroplastic dwarfs. Also called *fetal rickets*.

**achromia.** 1. Nonpigmented. 2. The state of being an albino. Also called *achroma.*

**achromatopsia.** See COLOR BLINDNESS.

**acid.** A compound containing hydrogen as an essential constituent and that possesses a sour taste, changes blue vegetable colors to red, neutralizes alkalis, and combines with bases to form salts.

**acid-fast.** A term applied to bacteria that are not easily stained for microscopic examination, but when once stained resist the removal of stain even by acids. The commonest example is the tubercle bacillus.

**acid-forming.** A term applied to foods which leave an acid residue. The popular belief that such foods make acid in the blood or joints is a fallacy, for because of a complicated mechanism, acid cannot form in the blood and so cannot be deposited in the joints or anywhere else in the body.

**acidity.** Sourness or the excessive production of acid. The only region in the body where acid can be formed is the stomach, which has acid-producing glands. These glands can be irritated to produce an excess of gastric acid, which rises up in the gullet. The patient then complains of "heartburn."

**acidosis.** The body is a vast mass of chemicals which normally are in complete equilibrium, acid balancing alkali. If too much alkali is lost to the body or there is a build-up of incompletely oxidized acid base then the condition is called acidosis. It is met with in children after severe vomiting attacks, and occurs in badly controlled cases of diabetes, in which it may become so severe that they develop air hunger (gasping breathing) which may even progress to coma. See also KETOSIS. The cause of this excess acid may be an overindulgence in food or liquor or even anxiety that keys up the nervous system and the nerves of the stomach. Relief can be quickly obtained by using an acid-neutralizing powder or medicine. The use of bicarbonate of soda for this purpose is to be condemned because it not only initiates further production of acid but, at the same time, produces stomach gas, which is difficult for the patient to get rid of. Medicines in use for neutralizing excess gastric acid include aluminum hydroxide, the various trisilicates, and magnesium hydroxide. Preparations of bismuth do not neutralize the acid but coat the stomach with an opaque powder that allays irritation of the lining and lessens the output of acid. Chalk preparations and bland food, such as milk, will also neutralize and soak up excess acid, and it is for this reason that many people suffering from acidity find that frequent small meals of bland foods bring relief. If gastric acidity and indigestion persist beyond two or three days, a doctor should be consulted, as important investigations may be necessary and the continued use of antacid preparations may merely conceal a condition in urgent need of medical attention.

**acne.** An inflammatory disease of the sebaceous glands of the skin, which secrete the greasy material called sebum. The condition occurs in those whose skin is excessively greasy so that the glands become plugged with sebum. The glands may become infected and turn into small pustules. The pustules should never be squeezed, for this, together with the infection, may leave the skin scarred and pitted, which can be most distressing for young people. Much of this scarring, however, can now be removed by a dermatologist using a high-speed abrasive drill. There are many types of acne, the most common being acne vulgaris, which usually begins in puberty and rarely lasts beyond the 25th year. See also ACNE ROSACEA, ROSACEA; SEBORRHEA DERMATITIS.

**acne rosacea.** Acne of the cheek and nose areas characterized by red coloration due to dilated blood vessels, flushing, and the presence of pustules. Also called *rosacea.*

**acolous.** Limbless.

**acoustics.** 1. The sense of hearing. 2. The science of sound.

**acquired.** A condition, disorder, or disease acquired after birth, as opposed to a condition present at birth, which is referred to as congenital.

**acrid.** Pungent to the smell or taste.

**acriflavine.** An orange-colored chemical with a pronounced nonirritant antiseptic action. Mixed in the proportion of one in a thousand in pure glycerine, it is used to clean infected wounds and to treat boils. The antiseptic action of acriflavine kills the germs and the glycerine acts as a drawing agent, sucking to the surface body fluids, which wash out the wound from its very depths.

**acrocephaly.** A congenital abnormality in which the head is cone-shaped. Also called *oxycephaly.*

**acrocyanosis.** A condition in which there is interference with the blood circulation in the distant parts of the limbs, such as the feet and hands. The fingers and toes look blue and are painful.

**acrodynia.** See PINK DISEASE.

**acromegaly.** A disease of the pituitary gland resulting in excessive growth of bones and enlargement of the chin, hands, and feet. This, together with complaints of headaches and a characteristic facial appearance, make the condition easily recognizable. Success in arresting the disease has been obtained by directing deep x-rays at the pituitary gland.

**acromion.** A bony process on the spine of the scapula forming the highest point on the shoulder.

3

**acroparaesthesia.** See ACROPARESTHESIA.

**acroparesthesia.** A disease manifested by tingling or crawling sensations in the hands or feet plus hypersensitivity of the parts to pain. There may be pallor or blueness of the fingers, which may feel cold when touched. The disease is caused by spasms of the blood vessels and is commonly found in middle-aged women suffering from anxiety conditions. Also called *paresthesia.*

**acrophobia.** Fear of being at a great height.

**acrosclerosis.** Hardening of the skin in the distal parts of the extremities.

**ACTH.** The abbreviation of the adrenocorticotrophic hormone, which is produced by the anterior lobe of the pituitary gland and controls the suprarenal glands.

**actinic.** Relating to light rays beyond the violet portion of the spectrum that produce chemical effects.

**actinodermatitis.** The extreme reaction of the skin to excessive sunlight or ultraviolet light. See also SUNBURN.

**actinomycosis.** A disease caused by a fungus, which results in the infected area, often the jaw region, suppurating and discharging through multiple holes a yellow discharge containing granules. At one time an incurable disease, it now responds to penicillin in heavy dosage.

**actinotherapy.** Treatment by rays of light, especially ultraviolet light.

**action tremor.** Rhythmical tremors or incoordination of the limbs; usually the result of a disturbance in the brain.

**acuity.** Clearness or acuteness.

**acupuncture.** An ancient Chinese treatment in which silver or gold needles are inserted into various areas to produce counterirritation and relief of pain. Recently revived, it is now used primarily as an anesthetic, using stainless steel needles.

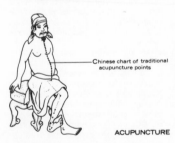

Chinese chart of traditional acupuncture points

ACUPUNCTURE

**acute.** Refers to the severity of an illness. An acute illness is one of short, sharp, rapid onset.

**adactylia.** Congenital absence of either fingers or toes, or of both.

**Adair-Dighton syndrome.** Also called *fragilitas ossum.* See OSTEOGENESIS IMPERFECTA.

**Adam's apple.** The prominence in the front of the neck, which moves up and down with swallowing and is, in effect, the larynx. It is more noticeable in men and thin-necked people.

**Adams-Stokes disease.** People with this complaint have an extremely slow heartbeat as a result of interference with the action of the heart. When the heart action becomes too slow to push enough blood into the brain, the patient faints. It is in fact a fainting attack with or without convulsions. Also called *Stokes-Adams disease.* See also HEART ATTACK.

**adaptation.** The ability of an organ or organism to adjust itself to its environment.

**addict.** A person who has an addiction.

**addiction.** A condition in which the individual has an uncontrollable craving for a drug and becomes physically dependent on it. This is accompanied by an increasing tolerance to the drug along with harmful effects both to the individual and to society. See also HABITUATION.

**Addison's disease.** A disease caused by destruction of the cortex of the suprarenal glands located above the kidneys. It is characterized by pigmentation of the skin, weakness, loss of muscular power, wasting, loss of appetite, and low blood pressure. It may be due to tuberculosis of the suprarenal gland, syphilis, amyloid disease, bleeding into the gland, infarction, and malignant growths. In many cases there is just a wasting of the cortex of the gland, the cause being entirely unknown.

**additive.** Something that has been added, such as a drug added to a medicine.

**adduct.** To draw a limb towards the central line of the body. The reverse movement is called abduction.

**adduction.** The movement towards the central line of the body.

**adductor.** A muscle effecting the movement of adduction.

**adenalgia.** Pain arising from a gland.

**adenectomy.** Surgical removal of a gland.

**Aden fever.** A feverish illness caused by a virus transmitted by mosquitoes; it is both infectious and contagious and may be endemic or epidemic. The incubation period is from three to five days and the onset is sudden. The disease is characterized by paroxysms of fever, severe pains in bones and muscles, swelling, reddening and pain of the joints, with sometimes a skin rash.

The temperature may be as high as 106° F. The fever lasts for three or four days, and then subsides for an interval, after which the cycle recurs. Complications are rare but the disease is very debilitating and convalescence is slow. Also called *breakbone fever, dandy fever, dengue.*

**adenitis.** Inflammation of a gland.

**adeno-.** A combining form relating to a gland in the body.

**adenocarcinoma.** Cancer of a gland. In this connection "adeno" may be used as a prefix to indicate the type of cancer, for instance, adenosarcoma or adenochondrosarcoma.

**adenocyst.** An epithelial tumor with a glandlike structure associated with cysts. Also called *adenocystoma.*

**adenofibroma.** A harmless growth composed of glandular and fibrous tissue. It is not a cancer and is frequently found in the breasts of young women. These growths are not fixed and can be moved freely in the breast tissue by the fingers.

**adenoid.** Glandlike. The word is generally associated with adenoids or adenoid vegetations, the enlargements of the glandular tissue at the back of the nasal cavity. Similar tissue at the back of the throat is called the tonsils. In effect, the tonsils are adenoids of the throat and adenoids are the tonsils of the nasal cavity. Adenoids frequently enlarge in children, causing nasal obstruction. This in turn blocks the drainage tube serving the ear, resulting in frequent attacks of inflamed eardrums and ultimately, if untreated, in deafness. The presence of nasal obstruction can be seen not only by the fact that the child breathes through the mouth instead of the nose, and frequently snores at night, but also because, in severe cases, there seems to be a slight mental deterioration and a facial appearance that can only be described as fishlike. Removal of the adenoids produces a dramatic change—the face alters in appearance, the child appears to be intellectually brighter, and the recurrent attacks of earache, discharging ears, and nasal obstruction disappear.

**adenoidectomy.** Removal of the adenoids by surgical operation.

**adenoma.** An enlarged gland which is not malignant and only causes trouble by the size to which it enlarges and the fears it engenders in the patient. Adenoma of the thyroid gland can be troublesome because it may irritate the thyroid until it becomes overactive and causes hyperthyroidism or Graves' disease. See also GOITER.

**adenomatosis.** A generalized enlargement of the glands.

**adenomyoma.** A growth composed of both muscular and glandular tissue.

**adenopathy.** A disease of a gland. Also called *adenosis*.

**adenosarcoma.** A malignant growth arising in glandular tissue. Also called *sarcoadenoma*.

**adenosclerosis.** Hardening of a gland.

**adenosis.** Any disease of a gland.

**adhesion.** An abnormal joining together of two adjacent parts of the body. On occasion adhesions form following an operation or inflammation within the abdominal cavity, and they can become so taut as to cause interference with the normal working of the bowels and even, in severe cases, to cause intestinal obstruction.

**adipocere.** A waxlike degeneration of the fatty tissues of the body after death. It is especially noticeable in bodies that have been buried in moist ground.

**adiposis.** The state of being fat or obese. See OBESITY.

**adiposis dolorosa.** A condition characterized by the presence of painful, tender lumps of fat in the body. The condition usually affects females. Also called *Dercum's disease*.

**adjustment.** The changes an organ or organism makes to adapt itself to changing conditions.

**adjuvant.** A second drug added to a medicine that has an action which will assist and enhance the action of the principal drug.

**Adler's theory.** The theory that a person develops a neurosis to overcome an inferiority complex.

**ad lib.** 1. To do something at will for as long as one likes. 2. Spontaneous.

**ad nauseam.** To the point of making one feel sick.

**adnexa.** Literally means adjoining parts, but is frequently used to refer to the parts adjacent to the womb, such as the ovaries and Fallopian tubes.

**adnexopexy.** An operation to stitch a dropped ovary back into its proper position. Should an ovary drop out of position it interferes with sexual intercourse and causes the woman pain.

**adnexitis.** Inflammation of the ovaries and Fallopian tubes.

**adolescence.** The period between childhood and adulthood. The period of life beginning with puberty, when the appearance of secondary sexual characteristics commence, to the development of full sexual maturity.

**adrenal glands.** Two ductless glands, one situated on top of each kidney, which produce the hormone adrena-

line. Each gland is about 2½ inches long by 1½ inches wide and weighs ¼ ounce. Also called *suprarenal glands*.

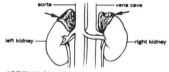

ADRENAL GLANDS (arrows)

**adrenaline.** The hormone secreted by the adrenal glands. Its function is to release for immediate use the glucose stored in the liver as glycogen. This is one of the body's protective mechanisms, and faced with a crisis, a disaster, or threat of attack, the brain signals the adrenals to release adrenaline; this in turn releases glucose into the bloodstream to nourish the muscles for impending violent activity—either to fight or run away. Simultaneously, and in order to increase the blood supply to the limbs, adrenaline contracts the abdominal blood vessels, causing a tumbling feeling described by some people as "the tummy turning over." Since its discovery and introduction into medicine there are few medicaments more versatile than adrenaline. It is used as a vasoconstrictor and cardiac stimulant; is incorporated in local anesthetics to enhance their action, localize their spread, and restrict bleeding; it is injected to relax the lungs in asthma attacks; it is used on swabs to pack the nose in cases of severe nose bleeding; it is used as an emergency injection for severe allergic or anaphylactic reactions; and it is dabbed on boxers' cuts to stop bleeding during rests between rounds. Also called *epinephrine*.

**adrenogenital syndrome.** A condition caused by oversecretion of hormones by the adrenal cortex. Some of the symptoms are excessive growth of hair, obesity, menstrual disorders, and other incomplete features similar to Cushing's syndrome in women. In the baby this hormonal oversecretion may produce precocious sexual development such as virilism and hirsutism. It may also produce Achard-Thiers syndrome.

**adrenosympathetic syndrome.** Paroxysms of high blood pressure, sugar in the urine, rapid pulse, pallor, flushing, headache, nausea, and vomiting; caused by tumors of the adrenal medulla.

**adsorbent.** A substance which is capable of adsorption.

**adsorption.** The concentration of a substance on or near the surface of any solid or liquid. This is entirely different from absorption, which is the soaking up of a substance into the texture of a material. See also ABSORB.

**ADT.** An abbreviation sometimes used on a placebo prescription to indicate to the pharmacist that he can flavor the medicine with what he likes: *A* for "any," *D* for "what you desire," and *T* for "thing."

**adulteration.** 1. Pollution. 2. The fraudulent addition of a cheap substitute to food or medicine.

**adventitia.** The outer layer of the three layers that compose the wall of a blood vessel.

**aegophony.** See EGOPHONY.

**aeremia.** The presence of air in the blood. This is usually a fatal condition and sometimes the cause of death in criminal abortion.

**aero-anaerobic.** See FACULTATIVE.

**aerobe.** Bacteria which must have oxygen in order to live. Also called *aerobium*.

**aeroneurosis.** A nervous disorder encountered among aircrews and pilots of aircraft. It was first noted during the Second World War in pilots who had undertaken so many battle missions that they were showing evidence of nervous breakdowns and were overdue for rests. The disease was also noticed in exceptionally nervous individuals who could not take the nervous stress involved in either bombing missions or air battle.

**aerophagia.** Air swallowing. People with indigestion sometimes attempt to belch up air in order to obtain relief. X-ray studies indicate that the only way a person can belch is by first swallowing air and then bringing back part of it. This leaves air accumulating in the stomach, which commonly causes flatulence with accompanying discomfort. Also called *aerophagy*.

**aerophagy.** See AEROPHAGIA.

**aerosol.** A misty spray delivered from pressurized containers.

**Aesculapius.** The mythological God of Healing.

*According to legend Aesculapius, son of Coronis and Apollo, was taken from his mother's womb as her body was conveyed to the funeral pyre—the first record of a cesarean operation. Another legend records that his mother was Ascinoe, who abandoned him at birth, and that he was suckled by a goat. Aesculapius married twice, and by his first wife had a daughter, Hygeia. His second wife was Lampetia, daughter of the Sun God. Hygeia became Goddess of Health and her name survives in such words as hygiene and hygienic. Having been artificially born and*

5

*reared, it was natural that Aesculapius should study medicine, and his instructor was the centaur Chiron who, although half horse and half man, was the most versatile of the celestial professors. Aesculapius's very success was his undoing. Pluto, God of the Underworld, complained to Zeus, God of the Heavens, that Aesculapius was so effective as a doctor that there were not enough deaths to keep up the population in Hades. Therefore, to restore the balance, Zeus slew Aesculapius with a thunderbolt. The Greeks believed the healing powers of Aesculapius to be so great that they erected temples in his honor. These were not merely temples of worship but sanatoria called Aesclepieia, which were staffed by priests who employed sunlight, fresh air, pure water, exercise and diet for the restoration of health. Neither did they hesitate to use drugs or perform operations, even though their medical procedure was strongly tinged with superstitious and religious practices. Only those considered to be moribund and women about to give birth were refused treatment. Later the Emperor Antoninus Pius provided a building at Epidaurus in which confinement cases might be lodged and tended, and it was, in effect, the first maternity hospital. The temples were also used for the study of medicine, and at the end of their course pupils were made to take the Oath of Hippocrates, the principles of which are still held dear by doctors. Eventually the temples became the seat of corruption and dishonesty. The sick brought with them an offering, such as a cockerel or a goat, which was placed on the altar in front of which the patient knelt and, with bowed head, recited his symptoms. Then, from behind a secret door, the priest removed the gift and replaced it with a pot of salve or balm. The priests also encouraged harmless snakes, stipulated to be sacred and therefore not to be destroyed, to inhabit the temples. When Christianity came to Rome the Christians took sticks, entered the temples, killed the snakes and beat the priests. The sticks and snakes are now incorporated into medical badges as a symbol, called the caduceus, of the determination of doctors to eradicate from medicine all forms of chicanery and charlatanism.*

**afebrile.** 1. Running no temperature. 2. Without a fever.

**affection.** 1. Feeling, love. 2. A morbid condition. 3. A disease.

**afferent.** 1. Leading towards the center. 2. Medically, the center is frequently the brain, so that nerves carrying impulses from the outside of the body towards the brain are called afferent nerves.

**affiliation.** In law, deciding who is the father of a child.

**affiliation order.** An order made by a magistrate that a sum of money for the child's maintenance be paid to the mother by the putative father, whether married to the woman or not.

**afflux.** The flowing of blood or some other fluid to any part of the body. Also called *affluxion*.

**African lethargy.** A form of sleeping sickness.

**African tick fever.** Also called *relapsing fever*. See FAMINE FEVER.

**afterbirth.** The popular name for the placenta, umbilical cord, and membranes. See also PLACENTA, UMBILICAL CORD.

**aftercare.** The care and nursing of people convalescing from illnesses.

**afterhearing.** The sensation of hearing sounds which have stopped.

**afterimage.** The persistent impression of seeing something after it has gone out of sight.

**afternystagmus.** Nystagmus is the coarse or fine movement of the eyeball. When this movement persists after the abrupt stopping of a rotation, it is called afternystagmus.

**afterpains.** The cramplike feeling in the pelvis suffered by some women after childbirth, and due to contraction of the womb.

**afterperception.** The persistence of a sensation long after the cause for it has ceased.

**aftersensation.** A sensation that persists after the original cause has stopped.

**aftersound.** The hearing of a sound after the original vibration has ceased.

**aftertaste.** A taste that persists long after the food has been swallowed.

**aftertreatment.** The treatment of a convalescent patient.

**agar-agar.** A gelatinous substance derived from seaweed. It is used in bulk-forming laxative medicines, sometimes combined with liquid paraffin, and in certain preparations for the treatment of obesity. It fills up the stomach with bulk without producing any nourishment.

**agenesia.** 1. Aplasia. 2. Sterility or sexual impotence. Also called *agenesis*.

**agglutination.** A clumping together of red blood cells or of bacteria, due to the presence of specific substances, the agglutinins and agglutinogens.

**agglutinin.** An antibody that causes clumping of blood cells and bacteria.

**agglutinogen.** Any substance which, acting as an antigen, stimulates the production of an agglutinin. These substances are found in bacteria and red blood cells. The agglutinin then clumps together the bacteria or red blood cells, rendering them inactive

and easier for the body to destroy. This process forms the basis of all the prophylactic inoculations against disease.

**agitographia.** Compulsion to write very fast, with the unconscious omission of words or whole sentences.

**agitolalia.** Excessive rapidity of speech in which words, syllables, and sounds are slurred, left out, or distorted.

**aglaucopsia.** Color blindness, especially to green color.

**aglutition.** Inability to swallow. Also called *dysphagia*.

**aglycaemia.** See AGLYCEMIA.

**aglycemia.** The absence of sugar in the blood. See HYPOGLYCEMIA.

**agnate.** In Scottish law, the name given to the responsible relative of an insane person, usually the closest relative on the paternal side.

**agnathia.** A congenital condition in which the lower jaw is either absent or defectively developed.

**agnosia.** Inability to recognize a sensory perception, due to disorders of the brain or nervous system.

**auditory agnosia.** Word deafness, or the inability to recognize the sounds of words.

**tactile agnosia.** Inability to recognize objects by touch.

**visual agnosia.** Inability to recognize objects by their shape or color.

**agonad.** A person without sex glands.

**agonal.** Related to agony, usually associated with the death agony.

**agoraphobia.** The neurotic fear of open spaces, resulting in the individual always remaining indoors.

**agrammatism.** A type of aphasia in which the patient can say various words but cannot put them together to make an intelligible sentence.

**agranulocyte.** One type of white blood cell which is devoid of granules.

**agranulocytosis.** A disease caused by the depression of the blood-forming mechanism of the body from the use of certain drugs or poisons. It is associated with ulceration and inflammation of the throat or the vagina and is a grave general disease, which may in some cases be fatal.

**agraphia.** Inability to write due to disease of part of the brain.

**agromania.** A morbid desire to be left alone or in solitude.

**agrypnia.** Insomnia.

**ague.** The old name for malaria, it really refers to the sweating and shaking attacks that come on with an attack of malaria.

**A.I.** Artificial insemination. A method of inducing pregnancy in which semen is introduced into the woman's womb by artificial means.

**A.I.D.** Artificial insemination by donor. A method of inducing pregnancy in which semen from a donor other than the husband is introduced into the womb by artificial means.

**A.I.H.** Artificial insemination by husband. A method of inducing pregnancy in which the husband's semen is introduced into the wife's womb by artificial means.

**air pollution.** Air pollution is a major international medical problem and is being studied by governmental health departments throughout the world. Some evidence suggests that cancer is caused by the chemicals released into the atmosphere by automobile exhaust, chemical factories, and the burning of coal. The chief poisons causing concern are carbon particles, or soot, benzpyrene chemicals, lead, and sulfur dioxide. The carbon particles are released principally by gasoline and diesel engines. The benzpyrene chemicals are found in tobacco smoke and have long been associated with cancer. Lead emerges from the combustion of leaded fuels in motor cars and is a notorious poison. Sulfur dioxide reaches the atmosphere mostly from coal fires, dissolves in the air moisture, and forms the sulfuric acid responsible for the erosion of the stone surfaces of city buildings. Governments throughout the world have tried various methods to deal with these pollution problems. Western nations all agree that automobile emissions must be controlled, and several nations, including the United States, have set strict emission standards which went into effect in 1975. Many nations have also limited cigarette advertising in an attempt to cut down tobacco consumption. In the United States, cigarettes may not be advertised on television. Although many countries have depended almost exclusively on coal fires to produce their electricity, new smoke filtration methods have considerably reduced pollutants. Several countries are also investigating the possibility of nuclear power plants to produce electricity. When properly engineered and regulated, nuclear power plants produce no pollution at all.

**airsickness.** A form of motion sickness allied to seasickness experienced by nervous individuals when flying.

**akinesia.** The marked absence of movements, caused by a disease of the nervous system.

**ala.** A winglike process.

**alalia.** The inability to speak.

**alar.** Pertaining to any winglike structure. The term usually refers to the shoulder blade, but it is loosely used to refer to the shoulder or armpit.

**alastrim.** A mild form of smallpox, found in South Africa.

**alba.** The white matter of the brain.

**albedo.** Whiteness.

**albicans.** Something white.

**albinism.** Congenital absence of the pigment normally present in skin, hair, and other parts of the body. An individual suffering from this condition is called an albino.

**albuginea.** A layer of white tissue surrounding an organ.

**albuginea oculi.** The sclerotic coat of the eye.

**albuginea ovarii.** The covering of the ovary.

**albuginea testis.** The covering of the testicle.

**albumin.** A protein substance present in egg white, milk, other animal tissues, and plant tissues. Albumin coagulates on heating, providing the method by which albumin is usually detected in the urine in order to diagnose disturbances of the kidney. A test tube is two-thirds filled with urine, and the top part of the tube is heated in a Bunsen flame. If albumin is present, it coagulates to form a white cloud at the top, which persists after the addition of a few drops of weak acetic acid. This may or may not indicate a disturbance in kidney function because, although albumin is present in the urine in some kidney diseases, it may be present in young people following exercise, and be only a spillover reaction.

**albuminuria.** The presence of albumin in the urine. See also ALBUMIN.

**alcaptonuria.** See ALKAPTONURIA.

**alcohol.** A derivative of an aliphatic hydrocarbon which contains an hydroxyl group (OH). There are many kinds of alcohols but most commonly known are ethyl alcohol and methyl alcohol. Methyl alcohol is cheap but unfit for human consumption. Taken internally, it may cause insanity, blindness, and even death. Ethyl alcohol is the spirit in normal alcoholic drinks. It creates an initial stimulation with mental excitement, followed by depression of the nervous system, which, in the early stages, slows up the body's reaction time, so that a motorist would be slow to take action or to realize impending danger. It is imperative that people taking sedatives and tranquilizers should know that the combination of these tablets and alcohol heightens the effect of each — sometimes to an alarming extent. Many drug overdose deaths are believed due to this combination. Having "one for the road" to keep out the cold actually has the opposite effect. Alcohol dilates the skin's blood vessels, and, though the individual may feel warmer, he is in fact losing body heat and is even more susceptible to cold.

**alcoholic.** 1. Pertaining to alcohol. 2. A person addicted to alcohol.

**alcoholic dementia.** The final stage of mental deterioration resulting from overdrinking and chronic alcoholism.

**alcoholic hallucinosis.** Hallucination resulting from overdrinking.

**alcoholic psychosis.** The complete and ultimate deterioration that may occur in the chronic alcoholic. In one type, Korsakow's psychosis, there is complete mental, moral, and social degeneration. See KORSAKOW'S PSYCHOSIS.

**alcoholism.** The state of suffering from the results of too large and too frequent intake of alcohol.

**acute alcoholism.** Drunkenness or the temporary disturbance caused by the excessive intake of alcohol.

**chronic alcoholism.** The condition resulting from the long-continued excessive intake of alcohol, characterized by severe disturbance of the digestive and nervous systems with cirrhosis of the liver.

**alcoholophilia.** A morbid craving for alcohol.

**alcoholuria.** The presence of alcohol in the urine. Alcoholuria resulting from drinking alcoholic beverages is the basis of tests for determining the ability of a driver to have proper control of a vehicle after drinking alcohol.

**alethia.** The inability to forget.

**aleucocytosis.** The absence or insufficient formation of white blood cells. An increase in the formation of white blood cells is called leucocytosis.

**aleukaemia.** See ALEUKEMIA.

**aleukemia.** A blood disease in which white cells are either deficient or absent. It may occur in the course of leukemia.

**alexia.** Word blindness. The inability to recognize written and printed words even though the individual has previously been able to read. It is due to a disturbance or disease of the brain.

**alga.** A low form of plant life found in water; the green slime that occurs on stagnant ponds.

**algesia.** Pain or increased sensitivity to pain.

**algesic.** Painful.

**algesiogenic.** Producing pain.

**algid.** 1. Chilly or cold. 2. A pernicious type of malaria in which the patient is severely shocked.

**algid pernicious fever.** A very severe malarial attack characterized by collapse, cold skin, and a tendency to fatal syncope.

**alginuresis.** Pain on passing urine. Also called *dysuria*.

**algophobia.** The fear of suffering or of witnessing pain.

**algospasm.** Any painful spasm.

**alienation.** 1. Estrangement. 2. A mental derangement.

**alienism.** An infrequently used term for the study of mental disorders, especially in their legal ramifications.

**alienist.** A psychiatrist who gives legal testimony.

**aliment.** Food or nourishment.

**alimentary.** Pertaining to the bowels or intestinal tract.

**alimentary tract.** All organs that make up the passage taken by food in its route from the mouth to the anus. Also called *alimentary canal, digestive tract.*

**alimentation.** The supplying of food.

**alimentology.** The science of nutrition.

**alinasal.** Pertaining to the wings of the nose at the opening of the nostrils.

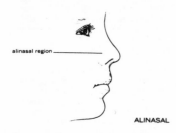

alinasal region _____

ALINASAL

**alkalaemia.** See ALKALEMIA.

**alkalemia.** Uncompensated alkalosis.

**alkali.** A chemical which is the complete opposite in its function to an acid.

**alkaline.** The presence of hydroxyl ions in an aqueous solution.

**alkalinity.** The presence of an excess of alkali.

**alkalinuria.** The presence of alkali in the urine.

**alkali reserve.** The total amount of available alkali in the body which can be used as a buffer against acids.

**alkaloid.** A class of organic nitrogenous chemicals which may be of plant or synthetic origin. They include such potent drugs as morphine, cocaine, hyoscyamine, and nicotine.

**alkalosis.** A disturbance of the body's acid-base equilibrium, characterized by sweating, vomiting, or diarrhea.

**alkaptonuria.** A defect of the body present at birth and characterized by the excretion in the urine of a substance called homogentisic acid. Also called *alcaptonuria.*

**allantoic.** Pertaining to the allantois.

**allantois.** A membrane growing out from the yolk sac in the early stage of the developing embryo and contributing to the formation of the placenta and umbilical cord.

**allelomorph.** One of two or more alternative hereditary units or genes or the characters they produce. As an example, the gene responsible for brown eyes is an allelomorph of the alternative gene for blue eyes. Also called *allele.*

**allergen.** Any substance which can produce a state of allergy.

**allergy.** There are probably no more abused words than this one. People say they are allergic to this and that when they really mean they are hypersensitive to such things. Properly defined, allergy is "the condition which results from the introduction into the body of certain substances, usually of a protein nature, which cause a disease complex called allergy." This may be manifested by such conditions as asthma, urtica or nettle rash, or certain skin diseases. The allergen responsible may be something in the air, such as pollen from plants, which produces hay fever; it may be something in the diet, such as eggs, fish, or other food products, which produce asthma; or it may be something in contact with the skin, producing an allergic dermatitis. This last mentioned type is frequently associated with an oversensitive nervous system.

**allobarbital.** One of the barbiturate drugs used as a hypnotic and sedative. Also called *allobarbitone.*

**allopath.** One who practices allopathy.

**allopathy.** A system of treating disease by administering drugs which produce phenomena different from those of the disease. This is the complete opposite of homeopathy, where treatment consists in using drugs in minute states of dilution to produce a like effect to the disease.

**allopsychic.** Relating to mental contact with the external world.

**allopsychosis.** A delusional state of extreme suspicion; a form of persecution complex.

**all or none laws.** A principle relating to nerve fibers and muscles in which they either react to a complete degree or do not act at all.

**allotopia.** Malposition of an organ. Also called *dystopia.*

**allotoxin.** Any substance developed within the body which has antitoxic properties.

**allotropism.** A condition or state where the same chemical substance has two differing appearances, for instance, phosphorus may occur as red phosphorus or yellow phosphorus.

**almoner.** Hospital social worker; one who helps hospital patients with family, financial, and social problems.

**alochia.** Absence of lochia, the vaginal discharge that takes place for some days following childbirth.

**aloes.** A purgative drug derived from aloe plants.

**alopecia.** Baldness. It may be congenital or acquired, localized or general. The acquired forms may be due to destruction of the hair follicles by scarring, to a chemical or bacterial poison, or of nervous origin.

*Alopecia is to be distinguished from the hairless patches on the heads of children in which the skin shows signs of inflammatory reaction. This latter condition is due to a fungous disease called ringworm of the scalp, and requires special medical treatment to kill off the attacking fungus.*

**alopecia areata.** A condition where the areas of baldness are round and often multiple and the skin is normal but the hairs on the edge of the patch may be shrunken at the base leaving a palisade of hairs like a row of exclamation marks. The bare patches may merge into total baldness. Sometimes the fingernails become atrophic and are also shed. Poor health and nerve trouble contribute to this condition, and in some people, recurrent attacks are almost a signal that the body is under a strain. Alopecia areata may occur at puberty, during pregnancy, and at the change of life, and often occurs in several members of the same family. Recovery is usual in three to four months without treatment.

**alopecia cicatrisata.** This occurs in young adults and the cause is unknown. The skin becomes wasted, and the hairs fall, leaving white depressed areas like "footprints in the snow." However, there are no broken hairs. Wasting of the nails occurs. Treatment to the scalp is useless, though the condition has been treated with gold injections. Also called *pseudo-pelade of Brocq.*

**alopecia totalis.** The complete dropping out of the hair. It may be due to nervous shock or emotion.

**atrophic alopecia.** The skin of the scalp wastes and the hair follicles disappear. The causes include scars, burns, scalds, and scarring from infected skin conditions such as pustular ringworm, chicken pox, smallpox, carbuncles, boils, syphilis, and leishamaniasis. Wasting and atrophic skin diseases such as lupus erythematosus and lichen conditions are also causes and so is the excessive use of x-rays and radioactivity. Treatment is of the activating cause, where possible. Also called *cicatrical alopecia.*

**folliculitis decalvans.** A condition in which bald patches occur with inflammation of the hair follicles surrounding the patch. Sulpha drugs by mouth and painting the scalp with tincture of iodine have been used as treatment.

Another variety of this same condition seems to be an extension of barber's rash from the beard area.

**secondary alopecia of the diffuse type.** This type of baldness may be produced by severe illnesses, especially influenza, pneumonia, and infectious fevers; by pregnancy; by severe electric shock, severe fright, or emotional shock; by some extensive skin diseases; and by syphilis. In infantilism the hair may refuse to grow, and baldness may follow ovarian disease. Myxedema may be followed by baldness, but the improvement is quite dramatic after taking thyroid tablets.

**senile or masculine type alopecia.** This begins about the age of 30 years, frequently runs in families, and is often associated with worry, overwork, and dietetic irregularities. Constriction of the scalp blood vessels by hats and caps may be a factor. Baldness starts at the forehead and tonsure areas, which gradually converge, leaving the shiny dome of the so-called "egg head." In advanced cases treatment is of no avail, but in the early stages much can be done to check its progress. Scurf and seborrheic dermatitis of the scalp require treatment, and hormone tablets help, though they may make men temporarily impotent. Improvement in the general health assists and so do a sedative and measures taken to relieve anxiety. Scalp massage makes the condition rapidly worse.

**tension alopecia.** This occurs at the sides of women's heads, due to the use of too-tight hair curlers, and in young children who pull out the hairs at the sides of the scalp. Infants also get bald patches on the back of the scalp from always lying on a pillow. The condition usually corrects itself without treatment.

*Hair is an extrusion from a hair cell like toothpaste from a tube and, like the nails, is a completely dead structure. For this reason it is painless to cut it, bleach it, or bend it into short-lived "permanent" waves; and nothing that is applied to it, left on for only a few seconds, and then rinsed off can have a beneficial effect—whether the shampoo contains lanolin, beer, egg yolk, or champagne. The term alopecia is derived from the Greek for fox mange, alopex, and comes from the time when Greek farmers added to their incomes by trapping foxes for their pelts. Sometimes, however, foxes contracted mange, which caused bare patches on the pelts, and over the years the bald patches on the human head have been likened to those on a mangy fox pelt— hence the term alopecia.*

**altitude sickness.** A condition resulting from lack of oxygen while flying at high altitudes or climbing high mountains without a supply of oxygen. The symptoms are headache, rapid breathing, general bodily distress, mental anxiety, lassitude, sleepiness, fatigue, depression, or wild excitement. Repeated flying at high altitudes without supplementary oxygen gives rise to the production of headache, mental and physical fatigue, increased appetite, irritability, nervousness, insomnia, poor mental concentration, lack of will power, and a total disregard for danger in the air.

**alum.** Potassium aluminum sulphate. One teaspoonful to a pint of water produces an astringent lotion often used to dry up and harden the skin of sweaty feet. Alum is also used as a vaginal douche in some special conditions, and is an ingredient of many proprietary antiperspirant lotions.

**alum precipitated toxoid.** Diphtheria vaccine.

**aluminosis.** A type of occupational chest disease caused by inhaling aluminium dust. Also called *pneumoconiosis*.

**alveolar abscess.** An abscess at the root of an infected tooth.

**alveolus.** A small cavity or cell. The term usually refers to a bony tooth socket or an air cell in the lung.

**alymphocytosis.** Gross deficiency or complete absence of lymphocytes in the blood.

**Alzheimer's disease.** Presenile sclerosis. See PRESENILE SCLEROSIS.

**A.M.A.** American Medical Association.

**amalgam.** A soft alloy of mercury and any other metal.

**dental amalgam.** A combination of metals used for filling teeth. It may contain silver, tin, copper, and mercury, or various combinations of these metals.

**amara.** Bitters.

**amaranth.** A red-brown powder used to color medicine, food, and cosmetics.

**amastia.** Absence of breasts.

**amaurosis.** Blindness, partial or total; particularly blindness without apparent damage of the eye.

**amaurotic idiocy.** A form of mental deterioration. See IDIOCY: AMAUROTIC IDIOCY.

**ambidextrous.** Able to use both hands with equal dexterity.

**ambilateral.** Pertaining to both sides.

**ambivalence.** The ability to hold opposing emotional states, such as love and hate, for the same object or action.

**amblyopia.** Dimness of vision or blindness that may be caused by toxins.

**amblyopia alcoholica.** Amblyopia due to the excessive consumption of alcohol.

**amblyopia ex anopsia.** The suppression of vision in a squinting eye.

**tobacco amblyopia.** Loss of vision due to excessive tobacco smoking. It is caused by nicotine poisoning, which prevents the body from absorbing and using vitamin B. It is now possible to correct this form of blindness with injections of vitamin $B_{12}$.

**ambosexual.** Pertaining to both male and female or exhibiting characters common to both, as axillary hair. Also called *ambisexual*.

**ambulant.** Able to walk about.

**ambulatory.** Pertaining to a disease or condition which can be dealt with while the patient is able to walk about and is not confined to his bed.

**ameba.** A microscopic unicellular animal, some species of which are parasitic in the body and cause disease.

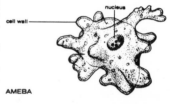

nucleus

cell wall

AMEBA

**amebiasis.** The state of having within the body the organism, *Entamoeba histolytica*, which causes amebic dysentery.

**amebic abscess.** An abscess found in the liver or lung, being a complication of amebic dysentery. Also called *tropical abscess*.

**amelioration.** The improvement in a patient's condition.

**amenorrhea.** The absence of the menstrual periods. This may be due to the onset of pregnancy or to some disturbance of the body, which suppresses the periods.

**amenorrhoea.** See AMENORRHEA.

**amentia.** 1. Feeble-mindedness. 2. Idiocy.

**amino acids.** Chemical compounds which represent the end products of protein digestion in the body and from which the body resynthesizes its protein. The amino acids considered essential for life are arginine, histidine, isoleucine, leucine, lysine, methionine, phenylalanine, threonine, tryptophane, and valine.

**aminosalicylic acid.** A derivative of aspirin. This drug is the familiar P.A.S. used for the treatment of tuber-

9

amnesia

culosis. Also called *para-aminosalicylic acid.*

**amnesia.** Inability to remember, especially past experiences.

**retrograde amnesia.** Inability to remember events prior to an accident in which the brain was damaged.

**amnion.** The innermost membrane, consisting of two layers, which surrounds the embryo in the womb and contains the fluid in which the embryo floats. Also called *amniotic membrane.* See CAUL; LIQUOR AMNII.

**amnionitis.** Inflammation of the amnion.

**amniorrhea.** Loss of the fluid, liquor amnii, surrounding the fetus within the womb shortly before birth.

**amniorrhoea.** See AMNIORRHEA.

**amoeba.** See AMEBA.

**amoebiasis.** See AMEBIASIS.

**amok.** A demented condition characterized by extraordinary behavior without self-control. The word is of Malayan origin describing the behavior of certain Malay tribesmen who, in a frenzy, would snatch a weapon and attack everybody within reach. Also called *amuck.*

**amorphous.** Not in a crystalline state and without form or structure, as in certain chemicals.

**amphetamine.** A drug which stimulates the activity of the nervous system.

**amphoric breath sounds.** These are sounds similar to those produced by blowing over the neck of a bottle, and which are heard through a stethoscope placed over a lung cavity. As the patient breathes, air is blown over the cavity, creating these hollow sounds.

**amphoteric.** In chemistry, a double-sided reaction in which certain chemicals act as both acids and bases, depending on environmental circumstances.

**amplitude.** The difference between the two extremes of a swinging pendulum.

**amplitude of accommodation.** The two extremes of the eyes' ability to focus.

**ampoule.** See AMPULE.

**ampule.** A miniature sealed glass bottle holding one dose of a sterile solution prepared for injection into the body.

**ampulla.** The bell-like mouth of a canal, such as in the tear duct of the eye and the milk duct of the breast.

**amputation.** Surgical removal of a limb or other part of the body.

**amputation neuroma.** A small, painful, and tender growth which sometimes develops at the cut end of nerve following amputation of a limb.

**amusia.** Inability to produce or understand musical sounds.

**amyasthenia.** Muscular weakness.

**amychophobia.** Fear of being scratched.

**amyelia.** Congenital maldevelopment of the spinal cord.

**amyelineuria.** Paralysis or other defective functioning of the spine.

**amyloid.** Starchlike.

**amyloid degeneration.** A waxy degeneration occurring in cases of long-standing disease, such as tuberculosis, in which the tissues of the body have deposits of starchlike substances which prevent the various organs such as the liver, kidneys, spleen, and intestine from carrying out their functions, and which contribute to the worsening of the patient's condition.

**amyloidosis.** The state of suffering with an amyloid disease. Also called *lardaceous degeneration, waxy degeneration.* See AMYLOID DEGENERATION.

**amylorrhea.** The presence of excessive quantities of starch in the stools.

**amylorrhoea.** See AMYLORRHEA.

**amylum.** Starch.

**amyocardia.** Weakness of the heart muscle.

**amyosthenia.** Muscular weakness.

**amyotonia congenita.** A disease of early childhood, usually congenital and sometimes familial, characterized by extreme flaccidity, smallness, and weakness of the muscles, which are not actually paralyzed. The disease is easily recognizable at birth and it has a tendency to improve slowly over the years. Also called *Oppenheim's disease.*

**amyotrophic.** Relating to diseases in which wasting of muscles is a feature.

**amyotrophic lateral sclerosis.** A chronic disease in which there is degeneration of the nerve tracts that supply certain muscle groups, resulting in a progressive atrophy of these muscles with concomitantly progressive weakness and virtual paralysis.

**amyotrophy.** Wasting of muscles, commonly the deltoid muscle, and accompanied by pain. Also called *amyotrophia.*

**Amytal.** A proprietary preparation of one of the barbiturate drugs.

**A.N.A.** American Nurses' Association.

**anabolism.** The building up of more complex nutrients and their conversion into protoplasm in the body. The breaking down of nutrients in the body is called catabolism.

**anachlorhydria.** The absence of hydrochloric acid in the gastric juice. Also called *achlorhydria.*

**anacousia.** See ANAKUSIS.

**anadipsia.** Intense thirst.

**anaemia.** See ANEMIA.

**anaerobe.** A bacillus or other microorganism capable of living and developing in the absence of air or oxygen.

**anaesthesia.** See ANESTHESIA.

**anaesthetic.** See ANESTHETIC.

**anaesthetist.** See ANESTHETIST.

**anakusis.** Total deafness. Also called *anacousia.*

**anal.** Referring to the anus, the lower opening of the digestive tract.

**analeptic.** 1. A restorative medicine or agent. 2. A drug which acts as a stimulant to the nervous system, as caffeine.

**analgesia.** Relief of or insensibility to pain, without loss of consciousness.

**analgesic.** A drug that relieves pain.

**analysis.** The determination of the composition of a substance by breaking it down into its component parts.

**anaphia.** Lack or loss of the sense of touch.

**anaphoresis.** 1. Too little or defective perspiration. 2. The movement of electropositive particles into tissues, induced by the presence of an electric field.

**anaphoretic.** A substance which prevents sweating.

**anaphrodisia.** Sexual impotence.

**anaphylaxis.** A special form of severe shock that sometimes follows the second injection into the body of a substance, usually a soluble protein, to which the individual was sensitized by an injection some 10 to 12 days previously. However, the reaction is not necessarily restricted to the tenth or twelfth day but may become manifest if the second dose of the sensitizing substance is received weeks or months after the initial dose. A bee sting is capable of causing anaphylactic shock in certain rare and highly sensitive people. The reaction occurs if such an individual is stung, and then, after 10 or 12 days have elapsed, receives a second sting. Whereas the first sting produced no reaction, the second sting causes a state of severe collapse with a swelling of the tissues, especially dangerous when the tissues in the throat swell and produce a choking effect. Emergency relief is given by the prompt injection of adrenaline. Subsequently, these rare and highly sensitive people have to be desensitized by progressively increasing injections of bee venom over a period of time. This type of shock may occur following many kinds of injection and is not known to doctors, who are always on the lookout for it when injecting second doses of such substances as sera. It is for this reason, in some cases, that a patient is not allowed to leave the doctor's presence until 15 or 20 minutes after an injection, for should such a reaction start, it can then be stopped by a prompt injection of adrenaline.

**anaplasia.** The reversion of some highly developed cells of organ or tissue in the body to a more primitive type, accompanied by excessive tendency to multiply, such as is seen in cancer growths.

**anaplastic.** Pertaining to anaplasia.

**anarrhexis.** The surgical operation of breaking a bone again in order to reset it into a better position.

**anarthria.** The loss of power to articulate remembered words as the result of a brain lesion. See also APHASIA.

**anarthrous.** Being without distinct joints.

**anaspadias.** See EPISPADIAS.

**anastomose.** To join up or provide a communication between two different hollow parts or hollow organs.

**anastomosis.** The joining of two arteries by a surgical operation is an arterial anastomosis.

**anatomy.** The study of the structure of the animal body.

**artistic anatomy.** The external form and shape of man and animals as a result of the underlying bony and muscular structure, as applied to painting and sculpture.

**comparative anatomy.** The study of the comparison of the anatomy of different animals.

**general anatomy.** Anatomy of the body tissues in general.

**morbid anatomy.** See PATHOLOGICAL ANATOMY, below.

**pathological anatomy.** Anatomy of diseased organs.

**regional anatomy.** Anatomy of a particular region, or related to certain parts of the body.

**special anatomy.** Anatomy of a particular organ.

**surgical anatomy.** Anatomy of various parts of the body which are of particular interest to the surgeon when planning an operation.

**topographical anatomy.** Anatomy of a part of the body in its relationship to other parts.

**ancylostomiasis.** A disease, usually of tropical and subtropical countries, in which certain worms are found in the intestinal tract of human beings. The presence of these worms can produce severe anemia, digestive upsets, and mental lethargy. Also called *ankylostomiasis, hookworm disease.*

**androgen.** A substance which produces the same effects as the male sex hormone.

**androsterone.** An androgenic steroid excreted in the urine of both men and women.

**anemia.** Literally translated, the term means without blood. Medically, it refers to a state of the blood in which there is a diminution of the number of red cells or the amount of hemoglobin. Broadly speaking, there are two main types of anemia. In one kind, iron deficiency anemia, the treatment is to administer iron in some form or another; the other type, pernicious anemia, responds to the injection of vitamin $B_{12}$. Neither treatment works for the other kind of anemia. It is quite useless to make a self-diagnosis of anemia and then hopefully take iron tablets obtained from the druggist. A proper diagnosis of anemia can only be made by placing a bead of blood under the microscope to see whether the cells are normal or altered in character and then by testing for the amount of hemoglobin present. Just to guess that anemia is present is a total waste of time and is frequently wrong. In any case, the anemia may be only the first sign of some other complaint; therefore the sooner anemia is correctly diagnosed the sooner the patient can receive the correct treatment for whatever is making him ill. The symptoms for practically all forms of anemia are the same: pallor, breathlessness, and a feeling of weakness. See also CASTLE'S FACTORS.

**anemophobia.** The morbid fear of wind and drafts.

**anesthesia.** Total or partial insensibility to pain or touch in a part. It may be due to disease or be produced by the application, injection, or inhalation of anesthetic agents.

**anesthesia dolorosa.** Severe pain in a part, which at the same time is insensible to touch; seen in certain diseases of the spinal cord.

**basal anesthesia.** Partial anesthesia produced by injecting a drug in order to reduce the amount of inhalation anesthetic necessary to produce complete anesthesia.

**block anesthesia.** See NERVE-BLOCK ANESTHESIA, below.

**caudal anesthesia.** Anesthesia produced by injecting the anesthetic into the caudal part of the spinal canal.

**dissociated anesthesia.** Anesthesia characterized by insensibility to pain and temperature, but sensibility to touch.

**field-block anesthesia.** Anesthesia produced by encircling the operative field with injections of a local anesthetic.

**general anesthesia.** The production of complete unconsciousness and absence of pain sensation.

**glove and stocking anesthesia.** Absence of pain sensation in the lower arms or lower legs.

**inhalation anesthesia.** Anesthesia induced by the inhalation of an anesthetic vapor.

**intravenous anesthesia.** Anesthesia induced by the injection of an anesthetic substance into a vein.

**local anesthesia.** Anesthesia which is confined to one part of the body.

**nerve-block anesthesia.** Anesthesia produced by injecting an anesthetic into or near the nerves serving the part to be operated upon.

**rectal anesthesia.** Anesthesia induced by introducing the anesthetic into the rectum.

**refrigeration anesthesia.** Anesthesia induced in a limb by packing it in ice chips for several hours.

**regional anesthesia.** See FIELD-BLOCK ANESTHESIA, above.

**spinal anesthesia.** Injection of anesthetic solutions into the spinal canal to freeze the whole area below the level of the injection.

*Patients are not now required to inhale the anesthetic in the first instance, which was for some people a terrifying ordeal, but are given an injection into a vein and asked to start counting. Few people get farther than ten before they are completely out—silently, painlessly, and with no distress. Before this occurs, however, children and nervous adults may be given a drug to render them sleepy and indifferent, and an injection of atropine to dry up the secretions in the mouth and lungs—a procedure known as premedication. Once the patient is unconscious the anesthetist may inject a derivative of curare (the South American Indian arrowhead poison) to relax the muscles, after which he can administer a much milder inhalation anesthetic to keep the patient unconscious. There are now so many anesthetics at the disposal of the anesthetist that he administers a veritable surgical cocktail, planned and designed to produce for the surgeon the conditions best suited to the type of operation, and for the patient total unconsciousness with a quick, calm, effortless recovery and no after-effects.*

**anesthetic.** 1. A substance which produces anesthesia. 2. Devoid of sensibility to touch or pain.

**anesthetist.** A doctor or other trained person who is an expert at administering anesthetics.

**anestrus.** 1. The period between two menstrual cycles in the human female. 2. The period during which the female is not "in heat" in mammals other than man.

**aneurin.** Vitamin $B_1$. A deficiency of aneurin in the diet is the cause of beriberi. Also called *thiamine.*

**aneurine.** See ANEURIN.

**aneurysm.** The dilation or ballooning of the wall of an artery or vein weakened by disease or injury.

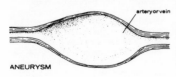

ANEURYSM

**angeitis.** See ANGIITIS.

**angel's wing.** The abnormal prominence of both shoulder blades. Also called *winged scapulae.*

**angiitis.** Inflammation of a blood or lymph vessel. Also called *angeitis, angitis.*

**angina.** Spasmodic pain associated with a sensation of choking or suffocation.

**angina pectoris.** Pain in the chest coming on after mild or severe exercise or excitement. It is due to local mechanical obstruction of the arteries that supply the heart with blood. The result of this poor blood supply is that the heart muscle goes into cramp, which causes the pain.

**angiocardiogram.** An x-ray of the heart and large blood vessels after the injection into the blood stream of radio-opaque substances to outline the shape of these organs.

**angiocarditis.** Inflammation of the heart and larger blood vessels attached to the heart.

**angioid.** Resembling a blood vessel.

**angioma.** A growth that has a tendency to form blood vessels; a tumor made up of either blood or lymph vessels.

**angionecrosis.** Death of a blood vessel or part of a blood vessel.

**angioneurectomy.** Surgical removal of blood vessels and nerves.

**angioneurotic edema.** A condition in which loose tissues of the body, notably the face and the scrotum in the male, swell up. It may be a manifestation of allergy or emotional disorder. Also called *giant urticaria.* See EDEMA: ANGIONEUROTIC EDEMA.

**angioneurotic oedema.** See ANGIONEUROTIC EDEMA.

**angioplasty.** Surgical repair of blood vessels.

**angiopoiesis.** Growth of new blood vessels.

**angiospasm.** A spasm in the blood vessels.

**angostura.** A bitter substance which is used as a stimulant and to reduce fever. It is derived from the bark of a tree which was originally found near Angostura in Venezuela.

**Angstrom unit.** A unit for measuring wavelengths of ultraviolet light, x-rays, and radium. The unit is equivalent to one hundred-millionth of a centimeter.

**anhidrosis.** Abnormal decrease or absence of sweat.

**anhydraemia.** See ANHYDREMIA.

**anhydremia.** The lessening or lowering of the fluid content of the blood.

**anhydrous.** Lacking in water, especially the water of crystallization.

**anhydrous glycerine.** Pure glycerine that contains no water.

**animal magnetism.** The name given by Mesmer to a power which enables one to induce hypnosis.

**aniridia.** A congenital defect of, or absence of, the iris of the eye.

**aniseed.** The seed of anise. It is used as a carminative in medicine to bring comfort to the stomach and aid in digestion. It is a frequent constituent of the gripe water marketed for babies.

**anisocytosis.** Unequal size of the red blood cells and an indication of the presence of a blood disease.

**ankle.** The joint between the lower leg and the foot.

**ankle clonus.** A greatly increased ankle jerk and a sign to the doctor of a disorder of the nervous system.

**ankle jerk.** The jerk of the foot produced by the calf muscles when the Achilles tendon at the back of the heel is tapped with a hammer.

**ankylocolpos.** Narrowing or partial closure of the vagina from adhesions.

**ankyloglossia.** Tongue-tie.

**ankylosed.** Fused together. This term is normally used when referring to joints in which the two surfaces are fused together by surgical operation. This results in a joint that is solid and is no longer usable.

**ankylosis.** The union of bones in a joint so that the joint becomes stiff. May be the result of chronic rheumatoid arthritis or a surgical operation.

**Ankylostoma.** The name of a genus of worms which can be found inhabiting the intestines of human beings. Also called *hookworm.*

**ankylostomiasis.** See ANCYLOSTOMIASIS.

**annular.** Shaped like a ring.

**anodinia.** Painless childbirth.

**anodmia.** Having no sense of smell. Also called *anosmia.*

**anodontia.** Being without teeth; edentulous.

**anodyne.** A pain-relieving drug.

**anoestrus.** See ANESTRUS.

**anomia.** Loss of ability to name objects or to recognize and recall names.

**anonychia.** Congenital absence of nails.

**Anopheles.** A genus of mosquito, certain species of which produce malaria.

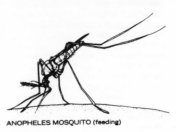

ANOPHELES MOSQUITO (feeding)

**anorectal abscess.** See ISCHIORECTAL ABSCESS.

**anorexia.** Lack of appetite.

**anorexia nervosa.** A condition which occurs in certain unhappy, neurotic, and young females, in which they become grossly wasted and yet have some curious ability to still continue to live and move about. The condition is characterized by an extreme aversion to all forms of food, extreme wasting, the cessation of the monthly periods, and loss of hair. These people can only be cured after prolonged psychoanalysis and the unraveling of the reason that makes them adopt this form of self-destruction. This complaint may follow emotional upsets.

**anosmia.** See ANODMIA.

**anospinal.** Pertaining to the spine and the anus.

**anovesical.** Pertaining to the anus and the urinary bladder.

**anovulation.** The cessation of egg cell production by the ovaries.

**anoxaemia.** See ANOXEMIA.

**anoxemia.** A deficiency of oxygen in the blood.

**anoxia.** Lack of oxygen.

**antacid.** A substance which neutralizes an acid.

**antagonism.** 1. Opposition. 2. Action by one agent such as a drug, in opposition to another.

**antagonist.** Something which acts in an opposite way and neutralizes something else. For example, a drug that neutralizes the effect of another drug is called an antagonist. The term is also applied to nerves and muscles which act in opposition to each other. For instance, the muscles which bend a limb at a joint are antagonists to those which straighten it, and vice versa.

**ante cibum.** Before a meal and indicated on a prescription as a. c.

**antecubital.** In front of the elbow joint.

**anteflexion.** Bending forwards.

**ante mortem.** Before death.

**antenatal.** Before birth.

**antepartum.** Before the delivery of a child.

**anteprandial.** Before the midday meal.

**anterior.** In front.

**antero-.** A prefix signifying in front, before, or in advance.

**anteroexternal.** Pertaining to the front of the outer side.

**anterograde.** Projecting or extending forwards.

**anteroinferior.** Relating to the area in front of and below.

**anterointerior.** Pertaining to the area situated in front and internally.

**anterointernal.** Situated in front and to the inner side.

**anterolateral.** Situated in front and towards one side.

**anteromedian.** Situated in front and towards the middle.

**anteroposterior.** From front to back.

**anterorotation.** A rotation forwards.

**anterosuperior.** Situated in front and above.

**anteversion.** The inclining forward of an organ.

**anteversion of the uterus.** A malposition of the uterus or womb, in which it is bent forward. See also RETROVERSION OF UTERUS.

**anthelmintic.** A drug which kills off worms in the intestinal tract.

**anthema.** A rash.

**anthophobia.** A morbid fear of flowers.

**anthracene.** A chemical derived from coal. It is used in the manufacture of certain dyes and purgatives.

**anthracosis.** A disease, common among coal miners, in which carbon particles, soot, or coal dust are deposited in the lungs.

**anthrax.** An acute, infectious disease of cattle and sheep transmissible to man, and caused by the anthrax bacillus. There are three clinical forms, each named according to the site of the lesion. If it occurs in the skin it is called malignant pustule; pulmonary anthrax when it attacks the lungs; and intestinal anthrax when it affects the intestines. It is an occupational disease of those working with animals or animal products. Also called *quarter evil, ragpicker's disease, tanner's disease, woolsorter's disease.*

**anthropoid.** Resembling man.

**anthropology.** The scientific study of man, including his origin, physical characteristics, and cultural development.

**anthropometry.** The measurement of the human body.

**antibacterial.** An agent acting against or destroying bacteria.

**antibiotic.** A substance derived from living microorganisms, especially fungi, which will destroy or inhibit the growth of germs in the body.

**antibody.** A substance found in the body fluids, which may be normally present or provoked into appearing by the injection of substances called antigens. This is the basis of protective inoculation, whereby a germ poison in small amounts is injected into the body to provoke the appearance of antibodies or immune bodies, which will provide immunity to a disease. See also IMMUNITY.

**anticardium.** The pit of the stomach.

**anticoagulant.** A substance which prevents the clotting of blood.

**antidote.** Something which neutralizes a poison.

**antigalactic.** An agent which dries up the supply of milk in a lactating breast.

**antigen.** A substance which, when injected into the body, is capable of provoking the manufacture of antibodies. See also IMMUNITY.

**antihistamine.** A substance that counteracts the liberation of histamine in the tissues. Histamine occurs naturally in the tissues and is a powerful dilator of blood vessels. Antihistamine drugs are swallowed as tablets or capsules to treat allergic diseases and applied to the skin as ointment to counteract itching and swelling from such things as wasp stings, bee stings, and mosquito bites.

**antimalarial.** Curing or preventing malaria.

**antimicrobic.** An agent acting against or destroying microbes or germs.

**antimony.** A bluish, crystalline metallic substance, whose action in the human body is similar to that of arsenic but is less poisonous. Antimony compounds can produce nausea, vomiting, and inflamation of the intestines and kidneys. In small doses antimony is occasionally used to cough medicines, and some preparations are used to treat diseases caused by protozoa.

**antimycotic.** An agent acting against or destroying fungi.

**antimydriatic.** A substance which, when applied to the eye, contracts the pupil.

**antipathy.** 1. An opposing characteristic or quality. 2. A feeling of revulsion or aversion.

**antiperistalsis.** Peristalsis taking place in the reverse direction. Also called *antistalsis.* See also PERISTALSIS.

**antiphlogistic.** An agent which counteracts fever or inflammation.

**antiphlogistine.** A proprietary preparation in the form of a poultice, which can soothe and relieve pain in muscles and joints. It is similar to the kaolin poultice, which has a basis of china

clay or kaolin and a mixture of many essential oils.

**antipruritic.** An agent that relieves itching.

**antipyretic.** An agent that reduces fever.

**antiscorbutic.** An agent that relieves or cures scurvy.

**antisepsis.** The prevention of infection.

**antiseptic.** Something which inhibits the growth of microorganisms, such as bacteria, without necessarily destroying them. See also GERMICIDE.

**antiserum.** A serum containing antibodies.

**antisocial.** Against the commonly held laws governing society.

**antispasmodic.** Something which relieves muscular spasm.

**antistalsis.** See ANTIPERISTALSIS.

**antisudoral.** An agent which lessens excessive sweating. Also called *antisudorific.*

**antitetanus.** An agent acting against or destroying the germ of tetanus or lockjaw.

**antitoxin.** A specific antibody, a substance found in the bloodstream, produced as a result of a germ toxin and capable of neutralizing that particular germ poison. See also ANTIBODY; IMMUNITY.

**antivenene.** A serum produced for the treatment of snake bite and an antidote to snake poison. Also called *antivenin.*

**antivenin.** See ANTIVENENE.

**antiviral.** Something which is effective in the treatment against a virus.

**antivivisection.** The opposition to laboratory experiments conducted on living animals to determine whether remedies are safe to be used on man.

**antral.** Relating to an antrum.

**antrum.** A cavity, particularly a cavity in a bone.

**anuresis.** Retention of urine in the bladder.

**anuria.** Absence of excretion of urine from the body due to a kidney disorder.

**anus.** The lower or terminal opening of the digestive tract—more specifically, the distal opening of the large intestine.

**anvil.** One of the three tiny bones in the ear which form part of the hearing apparatus. Also called *incus.*

**anxiety neurosis.** A form of nervous disorder in which generalized apprehension, fear, and agitation are the principal features. See also NEUROSIS.

**aorta.** The main artery from the heart. See also ARTERY.

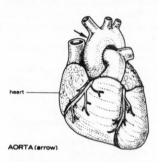

heart —

AORTA (arrow)

**aortic.** Pertaining to the aorta.

**aortic aneurysm.** A blood-filled sac communicating with the aorta and produced by disease of the arterial wall, weakening it and resulting in a thin-walled swelling having a tendency to burst with fatal results.

**aortic stenosis.** Narrowing of the aortic valve of the heart due to rheumatic heart disease. The heart enlarges in an attempt to force more blood through the narrowed valve but ultimately the heart fails.

**aortitis.** Inflammation of the aorta.

**apareunia.** The inability to have sexual intercourse.

**ape hand.** A deformity of the hand seen in progressive muscular atrophy and in amyotrophic lateral sclerosis.

**aperient.** A laxative or gentle purgative.

**aperitive.** Something which stimulates the appetite.

**A.Ph.A.** American Pharmaceutical Association.

**aphagia.** The inability to swallow.

**aphakia.** Congenital absence of the crystalline lens of the eye.

**aphalangia.** Congenital absence of one or more fingers or toes.

**aphasia.** Inability to use some or all words as symbols of ideas, or to comprehend the spoken or written language.

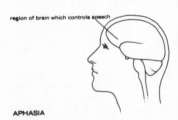

region of brain which controls speech

APHASIA

**aphonia.** Inability to speak due to a defect in the larynx.

**aphonogelia.** Inability to laugh out loud.

**aphrasia.** Inability to speak in continuous sentences or phrases. It is a nervous disorder.

**aphrodisia.** Sexual desire.

**aphrodisiac.** Any substance which increases sexual desire or power. These substances act by depressing inhibitory influences from the brain, as in alcohol, by stimulating the nerve centers in the spinal cord, as in strychnine, or by causing congestion of the sexual organs. Many are far too dangerous to use, such as cantharadin, which is a violent irritant if taken internally and which may cause kidney disease. Yohimbine, derived from the bark of an African tree and locally used, causes its effect within ten minutes by stimulation of the spinal cord nerve centers. Such drugs are used to cure sexual frigidity and impotence, though the vast majority of these cases, when not due to old age, are basically of a psychological nature.

**aphtha.** A small ulcer. These ulcers occur in the mouth, especially in children. Also called *stomatitis*.

**aphthous fever.** Known as foot-and-mouth disease in animals, this virus disease can be transmitted to man. The incubation period is from two to five days and commences with a slight headache, a slightly raised temperature, and dryness of the mouth. This is succeeded by a period of salivation, followed by the formation of vesicles upon the lips and tongue. Also called *aphtha epizootica, epidemic stomatitis.*

**apiotherapy.** The treatment of disease by bee stings. At one time used as a means of treating allergic disorders and rheumatism, it has now fallen into disuse. Bee venom is still used to desensitize patients hypersensitive to bee stings, but that is not strictly what is meant by apiotherapy.

**apiphobia.** A fear of bees.

**aplasia.** Congenital absence or maldevelopment of a tissue or organ.

**aplastic.** Structureless or without form.

**apnea.** Absence or the temporary stopping of breathing; may also mean asphyxia.

**apnoea.** See APNEA.

**apocrine.** A type of cell secretion in which the end of a gland cell is nipped off, leaving behind the nucleus and most of the cytoplasm, which then recovers and repeats the process. This occurs in sweat glands found in the armpit and around the pubis.

**apogee.** The highest point or climax in a disease.

**apomorphine.** A drug which causes vomiting.

**aponeurosis.** A fibrous membrane which encloses a muscle or gives attachment to a muscle.

**apoplexy.** A stroke due to a sudden hemorrhage into the brain. This may be the result of high blood pressure bursting a blood vessel in the brain. The patient becomes suddenly unconscious and falls to the ground, has a red face, breathes noisily, and is often paralyzed on one side of his body. See also COMA.

**appendectomy.** Surgical removal of the appendix. Also called *appendicectomy.*

**appendicitis.** Inflammation of the appendix. This may be acute or chronic.

**acute appendicitis.** In this type the patient suffers with pain of acute onset in the lower right-hand corner of the abdomen known as the right hypogastrium or right iliac fossa. Occasionally, however, the pain starts in the region of the navel before settling in the right iliac fossa. Vomiting often occurs after the onset of pain, and the patient has some degree of rising temperature, a rapid pulse, often a coated tongue, and tenderness to touch over the appendix area. The muscles over the appendix may go into protective spasm and supply the sign called abdominal rigidity. The importance of recognizing these symptoms as a possible case of acute appendicitis cannot be overemphasized because some mothers give purgatives to relieve abdominal pain. If this is done there is a grave risk of bursting the appendix and converting a straightforward case of appendicitis, requiring a relatively simple surgical operation to remove the inflamed appendix, into a case of acute peritonitis. This has a much graver significance, requiring drainage of the abdominal cavity.

**chronic appendicitis.** The picture here is somewhat different—the patient is constantly having low-grade attacts of abdominal pain and windy indigestion. This is usually due to either a blockage of the appendix by something entering from the bowel and becoming trapped, such as a small hard piece of feces, or to a stricture in the formation of the appendix, allowing feces to putrefy in a spot which has inadequate drainage. The only effective treatment is surgical removal of the appendix.

**left-sided appendicitis.** A condition so called because the symptoms resemble those of appendicitis but occur on the left side of the abdomen. It is, in fact, diverticulitis. However, there is a rare condition in which the appendix does actually lie on the left side of the abdomen.

**appendix.** Strictly, any appendage or adjunct, but medically the term usually refers to the appendix vermiformis, the blind tube that is about as thick as a pencil and from two to six inches long, which emerges from the cecum.

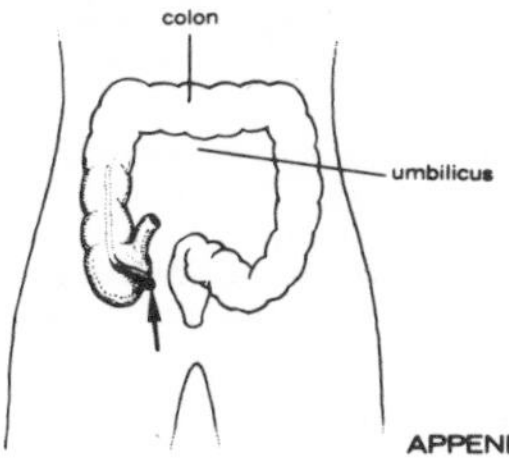

APPENDIX (arrow)

**A.P.T.** The abbreviation for alum precipitated toxoid, a diphtheria vaccine.
**apyretic.** Without fever.
**apyrexia.** The absence of fever.
**aquae.** Medicated waters used to flavor medicines. Aquae are produced by thoroughly shaking one of the essential oils, such as caraway or peppermint, in lukewarm water and then allowing the mixture to settle. The water is then decanted.
**aqueous.** Watery.
**aqueous humor.** The fluid in the front chamber of the eyeball.
**arachnids.** The class of animals which includes spiders, scorpions, and ticks. Also called *Arachnida.*
**arachnodactyly.** A congenital spider-like deformity of the fingers and toes—the digits being abnormally long and slender.
**arachnoid.** Weblike.
**arachnoid membrane.** The center membrane of the three that surround the brain and spinal cord.
**arctation.** A narrowing.
**arcuate.** Arc-shaped or bow-shaped.
**arcus.** Latin for a bow or an arch.
**arcus senilis.** The whitish circle that appears in old age around the edge of the colored part of the eye. It is due to the depositing of cholesterol.
**arc-welder's disease.** See SIDEROSIS.
**area.** Any delimited surface.
**areola.** **1.** A space between two tissues. **2.** The brownish ring around the breast nipple. **3.** That section of the iris surrounding the pupil of the eye.

*One of the signs of pregnancy is that the areola around the nipple becomes more deeply pigmented and obvious, but this change varies in women of different complexions, being more marked in brunettes than in blondes.*

**Argyll Robertson pupil.** A pupil of the eye which fails to contract when light falls upon it but will contract when the eye tries to focus on near objects. Sometimes the condition is found in people suffering with syphilis.
**ariboflavinosis.** A disease characterized by eruptions of the skin around the mouth, nose, and eyes and due to lack of riboflavin, one of the vitamin B complex, in the diet.
**arnica.** A flowering plant from which at one time an extract was obtained for use as a cardiac stimulant. An alcoholic extract called tincture of arnica was a popular remedy for bruises and sprains. Also called *leopard's bane.*
**aromatic.** The fragrant odor or taste which comes from certain essential oils, most of which are derived from plants.
**arrector pili.** The minute muscles surrounding the hair follicles, which, when stimulated, cause the hair to become erect. These muscles are responsible for "the hair standing on end" and "goose flesh." Also called *erector pili.*
**arrowroot.** A starchy preparation derived from certain plants. At one time it was popularly used as a remedy for diarrhea.
**arrythmia.** Absence of rhythm.
**cardiac arrythmia.** Irregular action of the heart, of which there are many types.
**sinus arrythmia.** The waxing and waning of the pulse rate, often synchronous with the breathing cycle. It is a normal manifestation.
**artefact.** See ARTIFACT.
**arteria.** A hollow tube or artery.
**arteriectomy.** Surgical removal of an artery or part of an artery.
**arteriocapillary.** Pertaining to arteries and capillaries.
**arteriolar.** Pertaining to arterioles.
**arteriole.** A very small artery.

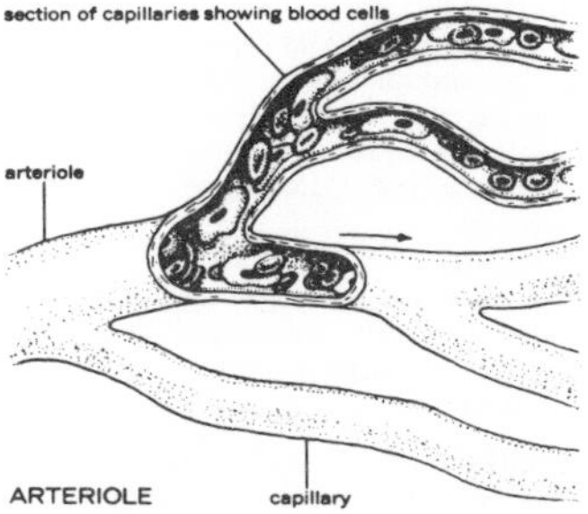

ARTERIOLE

**arterioplasty.** An operation for the cure of an aneurysm or the making of a new channel out of the walls of an aneurysm.
**arteriosclerosis.** Thickening of the lining of arteries causing loss of elasticity and resulting in diminished blood supply to the tissues and a rise in blood pressure. The cause is unknown.
**arteriospasm.** Spasm of an artery.
**arteriostenosis.** The narrowing of the bore of an artery.
**arteriovenous.** Referring to both arteries and veins.
**arteritis.** Inflammation of an artery.
**artery.** A blood vessel that carries blood away from the heart. It is composed of an outer coat, the tunica adventitia; a middle muscular coat, the tunica media; and an inner coat, the tunica intima. An artery is thicker than a vein, largely because of the artery's muscular middle coat, which responds to the heartbeat by converting a series of blood pulsations from the heart into a continuous flow. Contraction of the muscular coat narrows the bore of the artery, raises the blood pressure, and increases the work of the heart, while relaxation of the artery coat dilates the artery and causes a drop in blood pressure. When an artery is cut, this coat contracts, narrows

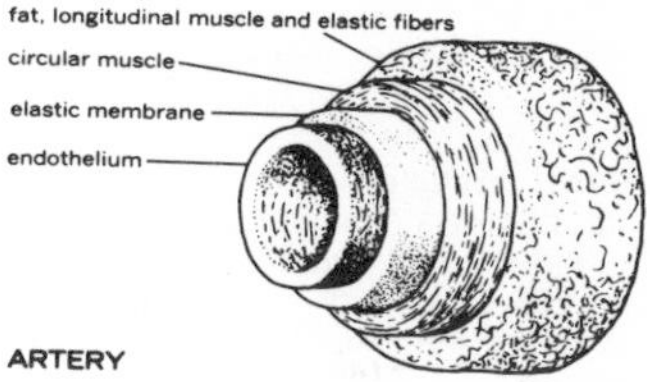

ARTERY

the opening, and assists in limiting bleeding. Although all arteries carry blood away from the heart, they do not all carry arterial blood, that is, blood which is bright red and full of oxygen. The pulmonary artery carries the dark-colored venous blood from the right side of the heart to the lungs. There the blood is reoxygenated, collected by the pulmonary veins, and returned to the left side of the heart. The term artery is derived from the Greek term for airway. This was due to the fact that the ancients found the arteries to be empty after death and concluded that they contained air in life.
**arteries of the chest.** The main artery of the body is the *aorta,* which immediately after it emerges from the heart branches into two small arteries—the *anterior coronary artery* and the *posterior coronary artery*—which supply the front and back of the heart muscle, respectively. The aorta then curves downwards to form the *arch of the aorta,* from which arise three arteries. The first of these is the *innominate artery* which divides into (1) the

*right subclavian artery,* which passes behind the collarbone to the armpit where it becomes the *axillary artery* and enters the arm as the *brachial artery,* and (2) the *right common carotid artery,* which passes up into the neck. The second branch from the arch of the aorta is the *left common carotid artery,* which also passes up into the neck. The third main artery to come off the aortic arch is the *left subclavian artery,* which follows the same course as the right subclavian artery but on the opposite side. From the subclavian arteries branch the *internal mammary arteries,* which pass to the inside of the breast; the *inferior thyroid arteries,* which supply the thyroid gland in the neck; and the *vertebral arteries,* which supply the spinal column. The *thoracic aorta* commences at the aortic arch and travels down the back wall of the chest until it passes through the diaphragm. It gives off the *posterior intercostal arteries,* which travel around the chest between the ribs to supply the intercostal muscles. **arteries of the neck and head.** Both the *right common carotid artery,* which arises from the subclavian artery, and the *left common carotid artery,* which arises from the arch of the aorta, divide in the neck into the external carotid artery and the internal carotid artery. The *external carotid artery* gives off various branches, including the *superior thyroid artery* to the thyroid gland; the *lingual artery* to the tongue; the *facial, maxillary,* and *transfacial arteries* to the face; the *occipital artery* to the back of the scalp; and the *posterior auricular artery* to behind the ear. The *internal carotid artery* passes up the neck, enters through an opening in the base of the skull, and then breaks up into various branches to supply the brain. Surgically, the most important of these branches within the brain is the *middle meningeal artery,* which passes either in a groove or in an actual bony canal at the side of the skull. This artery is sometimes ruptured in fractures of the side of the skull, causing a hemorrhage which can only be stopped surgically. **arteries of the arm.** The *axillary artery* is a continuation of the subclavian artery and passes behind the armpit to enter the arm, where it is called the *brachial artery.* This descends as far as the elbow joint, where it divides into the *radial artery,* which passes down the thumb side of the forearm, and the *ulnar artery,* which passes down the opposite side of the forearm. At the palm of the hand both arteries divide into two branches, which join up, resulting in two arched arteries which

cross the palm. These are known as the *superficial palmar arch* and the *deep palmar arch,* both of which give off smaller blood vessels to supply the hands and fingers.
**arteries of the abdomen.** The thoracic aorta enters the abdomen through an opening in the diaphragm, where it becomes the *abdominal aorta.* It then passes down the back wall of the abdomen giving off branches to the various organs until at the pelvis it divides into the two *common iliac arteries.* Each iliac artery then divides into an *internal iliac artery,* which passes backwards to supply the pelvis and buttocks, and an *external iliac artery,* which passes downwards via the groin to enter the leg.
**arteries of the leg.** The external iliac artery from the pelvis enters the leg and becomes the *femoral artery,* which continues downwards until at the level of the knee it divides into the *anterior tibial artery* and the *posterior tibial artery.* These continue downwards to the foot and each joins by loops to form two arterial plantar arches in the sole of the foot and in turn give off blood vessels to the toes.
**arthralgia.** A painful joint or pain in the joint.
**arthritic.** Relating to arthritis.
**arthritis.** Inflammation of a joint. See also OSTEOARTHRITIS; RHEUMATOID ARTHRITIS.
**arthrodesis.** A surgical operation which fixes a joint by sawing off the two surfaces of a joint and then placing the two parts together so that the bones fuse.
**arthrography.** The visualization of the inside of a joint by x-rays, usually performed by introducing into the joint a substance opaque to x-rays.
**arthropathy.** Disease of a joint or joints.
**arthroplasty.** 1. The repair of a joint. 2. The making of an artificial joint. 3. The reconstruction of a joint which has become fixed.
**arthrosclerosis.** Hardening of a joint or joints.
**arthrosis.** 1. A joint. 2. Any disease causing degeneration of a joint.
**arthrosynovitis.** Inflammation of the membrane lining a joint.
**articular.** Pertaining to a joint.
**articulate.** 1. Divided into joints. 2. Having distinct and clear speech.
**articulation.** 1. A joint. 2. A distinct or clear speech.
**artifact.** Anything that is not of natural occurrence in living tissue; artificial.
**artificial fever.** Fever deliberately induced by injecting various substances, the fever so produced having a benefi-

cial effect on the disease from which the patient is suffering.
**artificial respiration.** The induction of respiration by manual or artificial means.
**mouth-to-mouth and mouth-to-nose methods.** In these methods the position of the tongue is important. If the unconscious patient is on his back, his tongue falls backwards and will obstruct the air passages, but if his head is tilted fully backwards and his jaw pushed forwards and upwards towards the sky, then the tongue will be pushed out of the way and there will be no obstruction from it. Maintaining this grasp, the person giving aid should place his mouth in an airtight fit around the patient's mouth, blocking the nose by pressure of his cheek or by pinching the nostrils. Alternatively one can blow through the patient's nose, sealing off his mouth by closing his lips. Having taken a double deep breath, the attendant then forces his breath into the patient's lungs. This can be done once every six seconds for an adult, and the first few breaths should be given as rapidly as possible. If, however, it is found that air will not go into the lungs, then the patient will have to be turned on his side and his back thumped to dislodge any obstruction in his throat, and the mouth may have to be cleared with the finger. If after 10 or 12 successful inflations there is no apparent change in the patient's condition, such as improvement in his color, then the attendant should feel for the cardiac artery pulse by placing a finger below the angle of the jaw and just in front of the thick muscle bundle to be found there. If there is no pulse, then external cardiac massage may be started, provided that the person administering the massage has been carefully trained in this procedure. With infants and young children one must take very special care when blowing into the lungs. The attendant should place his mouth over the child's nose and mouth and blow gently with shallow puffs of air; he should do this rather more quickly than with adults, one every three seconds.
**external cardiac massage method.** While continuing mouth-to-mouth breathing, the giver of first aid should place the patient onto a hard surface. Then he should give the lower half of the breastbone six sharp, but not violent, pushes downwards, after each inflation of the lungs. If he can then feel the pulse return in the neck it means the heart has started beating again; the attendant can then continue with just the mouth-to-mouth breathing. It must be remembered that external cardiac massage is not without its dan-

gers. The pushes must be on the breastbone, not any lower down; they must be firm without being violent, and they must be related to the build and age of the patient. A too violent push might crack the ribs, particularly in old people, who have fragile bones. Should it be necessary to do external cardiac massage on an infant, one should apply only very gentle pressure on the lower part of the breastbone, as the internal organs are easily damaged.

**Silvester's method.** Follow these steps in administering this type of first aid. Clear the air passages of any obstruction that can be reached with the finger and lay the patient on his back, placing something under his shoulders to raise them, Allow the head to drop back. Kneel at the patient's head and grasp his arms at the wrists; then cross his arms and press them firmly over the lower chest—this forces air out of the lungs. Release the pressure and, with a sweeping movement upwards and outwards above his head, pull the arms backwards towards the ground —this movement should cause air to enter the lungs. Repeat these movements about 12 times a minute, taking two seconds for the chest pressure and three seconds for the arm movements. With the patient on his back there is a danger of his inhaling vomit, mucus, or blood, and this risk can be reduced by keeping his head extended, turned to one side, and a little lower than the trunk. If an assistant is available, he should press the lower jaw so that the chin juts out; this carries the tongue out of the way and prevents it from falling backwards and causing an obstruction.

*International experts are in favor of mouth-to-mouth or mouth-to-nose breathing as the methods for artificial respiration, with the Silvester method second and the Holger Nielsen method third. The Schaefer method seems to be definitely out. Some people are puzzled about mouth-to-mouth breathing and say, quite logically, "I can't see that it can do much good. All you are doing is breathing into the casualty carbon dioxide which you are trying to get rid of as a waste product from your own body. What the casualty really needs is oxygen." The explanation is simple and somewhat surprising. In approximate figures the air you breathe in contains 21 percent oxygen, while that you breathe out still contains 15 percent oxygen, plus about 4 percent carbon dioxide. If you take a very deep breath and then breathe it out, the figures are even better, the expired air containing as much as 18 percent oxygen, almost as much as fresh air and more than*

*enough to resuscitate a patient. The reason for the success of the mouth-to-mouth method is that it can be started immediately with little or no preparation wherever the patient is found, and, because of the forcible pressure used by the operator, air can be forced through any minor obstructions in the patient's air passages. In addition, it is not necessary to delay in order to try to drain water from the chest, as in drowning cases. Then there are other advantages: mouth-to-mouth respiration gives greater ventilation of the lungs and thus the blood is better oxygenated; you can see immediately if air is getting into the lungs and the casualty's chest can be watched for the first sign of natural breathing; it is much less tiring to perform than the other methods and takes no great physical strength—even a child can do it. There are just two snags. The casualty may also have facial injuries, which make the method impractical, or he may have some poison on the face and lips, which might make it dangerous to the person giving aid. Then the second choice will have to be the Silvester method. This also has the advantage in that you can watch the casualty's face and chest for the first signs of natural breathing. It should be remembered that artificial respiration must be continued until either the casualty starts to breathe or a doctor has pronounced further efforts useless.*

**artificial selection.** The selection for breeding of plants or animals which have particularly desirable and inheritable characteristics. Such a selection of chickens, for instance, might be made to provide a crossbreed of hen which would inherit the characteristic of profuse egg-laying as well as providing desirable table meat.

**arytaenoid.** See ARYTENOID.

**arytenoid.** Shaped like a pitcher. The term usually refers to the arytenoid cartilage at the back of the larynx.

**asbestos.** Magnesium silicate. It is used in the manufacture of fireproof materials.

**asbestosis.** A disease caused by the inhalation of asbestos dust, which results in fibrosis of the lungs and pleural adhesions.

**ascariasis.** The presence of worms within the body and the symptoms caused by them.

**ascaris.** An intestinal worm.

**ascending.** Taking an upward course.

**ascending colon.** The part of the colon which starts at the cecum and travels upwards towards the liver.

**ascites.** The presence of free fluid in the abdominal cavity due to disease.

**ascorbic acid.** Vitamin C, a substance present in fruit and green vegetables. Most animals manufacture vitamin C within their bodies, but the guinea pig, the monkey, and man cannot and have to obtain the vitamin from the diet. If the diet is deficient in this factor, scurvy develops.

**asecretory.** Having no secretion.

**asepsis.** The absence of infection by pathogenic organisms.

**aseptic.** Free from organisms capable of causing disease.

**asexual.** Without sex.

**aspect.** Appearance; a surface seen from any particular direction.

**aspergillosis.** A disease caused by the fungus of the genus *Aspergillus*.

**aspermia.** Failure of formation or emission of male cells or sperm in the seminal fluid.

**asphyxia.** Suffocation.

**asphyxia livida.** A form of asphyxia neonatorum. The baby's color is blue and the condition is caused by obstruction of the breathing mechanism.

**asphyxia neonatorum.** Asphyxia in newborn babies. It occurs in two forms. See ASPHYXIA LIVIDA; ASPHYXIA PALLIDA.

**asphyxia pallida.** This is a form of asphyxia neonatorum in which the baby is pale in color. The condition is due to shock and collapse.

**aspiration.** 1. The act of using an aspirator. 2. To draw or suck in.

**aspirator.** An apparatus for withdrawing fluids or gases from a cavity by suction.

**aspirin.** Originally a specific treatment for rheumatic fever, aspirin's pain-relieving qualities and relatively non-poisonous character resulted in its being used widely as a pain-relieving agent for all manner of slight disorders. It is now recognized that aspirin is not as safe as it was once thought to be. If one examines the lining of the stomach through a gastroscope, and some aspirin is passed down the tube onto the stomach lining, the normal gray appearance of the stomach wall immediately turns fiery red, demonstrating the amount of irritation that aspirin causes. There is little difference between soluble aspirin and ordinary aspirin in producing this effect. Research has also revealed that people who take aspirin in regular daily amounts frequently pass blood in their stools—further evidence of the irritation and inflammation that this drug causes. These findings suggest that aspirin should only be regularly used under doctor's orders for specific complaints and that some other tablet should be used for the relief of pain. Paracetamol (panadol) can be taken in the same dosage and has none of the disadvantages of aspirin but all the qualities of a safe, harmless, reliable, pain-relieving drug. An occasional dose of aspirin for a cold is harmless, but it should be crushed and taken on a full stomach. Also called *acetylsalicylic acid.*

**Assam fever.** A disease characterized by a continued, irregular fever, great wasting, anemia, blood disorders, and alterations in the cell structure of the liver and spleen. There are two types: the Indian, which affects older children and adults in India, Indo-China, and the Sudan; and the Mediterranean, which attacks infants `in countries bordering the Mediterranean Sea. Also called *dumdum, kalaazar, leishmaniasis.*

**assault.** In forensic medicine, an unlawful attack on a person.

**astereognosis.** Inability to recognize objects by touch.

**asthenia.** 1. Weakness. 2. Constitutional make-up characterized by tallness and slenderness of build.

**neurocirculatory asthenia.** See EFFORT SYNDROME.

**asthenic.** Characterized by asthenia.

**asthenopia.** Weakness of the eye muscles or of visual power.

**asthma.** A paroxysmal attack of severe shortness of breath with wheezing and a feeling of suffocation. See also BYSSINOSIS.

**bronchial asthma.** Asthma caused by a spasm of the smaller divisions of the air tubes or bronchi, with the pouring out of large quantities of sputum. It is usually due to hypersensitivity to an allergen combined with a psychological disturbance. Asthmatic people are supersensitive and frequently capable of a high degree of intellectual development. They have, in fact, the artistic type of temperament. One can explain the asthma syndrome by comparing the asthmatic patient to a loaded pistol with a hair trigger; the explosion of the pistol being the asthma attack. The triggering off may be caused by an emotional upset, an allergen to which the individual is highly sensitive, or to the onset of an infection. One can also use as an analogy a brick wall built of three types of bricks: nerve bricks, consisting of worry or emotion; allergen bricks, consisting of allergens of dust, food, or pollen; and germ bricks, consisting of infection such as a cold. When the wall reaches a certain height—and regardless of whether it is composed of one type of brick or all three types—the attack develops. The patient often protests that he has not been anxious or worried but has caught a cold; or he may say that he

has been worried by something at home or at work; or, again, for this particular attack he blames some food or dust. Therefore before treatment of bronchial asthma can be attempted, the patient must be reviewed in his entirety. His nervous make-up, his diet, the conditions of his home for dust, and his resistance to infections all have to be considered, and it is only after this complex picture has been broken down and assessed that the doctor can decide the treatment best calculated to relieve or cure.

**cardiac asthma.** An asthmatic attack which comes on suddenly, often in the middle of the night, due to spasm of the lungs from heart disease.

**uremic asthma.** Asthma caused by kidney disease.

**asthmatic.** Pertaining to asthma; a person suffering from asthma.

**astigmatism.** Poor sight caused by irregular curvature of the cornea of the eye.

**astringent.** A substance which tightens up the soft tissues of the body.

**asymmetry.** Unevenness or unlikeness; the absence of symmetry.

**asystole.** The failure of the heart to perform a complete systole.

**atavism.** The appearance in an individual of characteristics of a remote ancestor; reversion to an earlier type.

**atavistic.** Characterized by atavism.

**ataxia.** Muscular incoordination.

**atelectasis.** 1. Failure of the lungs to expand at birth. 2. The collapse of a lung due to disease.

**atheroma.** 1. Fatty degeneration of the lining of arteries. 2. A sebaceous cyst.

**athetosis.** A rhythmical and involuntary movement of muscles of the limbs, usually the fingers, due to a disease of the brain.

**athlete's foot.** An inflammatory reaction set up in the skin of the toes, which, having become spongy by perspiration, lose their resistance, and become contaminated with a fungus, *Tinea pedis.* It is probably true that the fungus does not attack normal skin but only that of very sweaty feet. Foot baths of potassium permanganate will effect a cure. These baths are prepared by adding to a basin of lukewarm water just enough crystals of potassium permanganate to color the water a rich red. The feet are placed in this for ten minutes night and morning for seven to ten days, after which the fungus is usually destroyed. The next stage in treatment consists of restoring the spongy skin to normal by exposing the feet to the air whenever possible. One method of doing this is to make up the bottom of the bed with the sheets folded in a similar way to the top of the bed, so that the feet are

exposed to the fresh air all night. This may not be very comfortable but it is effective in allowing the sweat to evaporate and so preventing the skin from becoming spongy again. Also, people who suffer with sweaty feet should, when possible, wear shoes rather like open Indian sandals, which allow the perspiration to evaporate during the day, instead of being encased in the shoe and sock, thus creating a wet atmosphere for the toes. The skin can then be hardened by bathing the feet in a strong brine solution, or in alum foot baths made up by dissolving one teaspoonful of powdered alum to each pint of water. These foot baths should be taken night and morning. After bathing, the skin should be dried carefully. Surgical spirit should be applied liberally to all crevices in and around the toes, and the foot should then be freely dusted with a dusting powder. Clean socks should be worn daily. Also called *ringworm of the foot.* See TINEA PEDIS.

**athrombia.** Defective blood clotting.

**atlas.** The first vertebra in the neck, on which the head rests.

**atmosphere.** 1. The air surrounding the earth. 2. A unit of pressure. The earth's atmosphere exerts a pressure equivalent to 14.7 pounds to the square inch.

**atomizer.** An apparatus producing a fine spray.

**atonicity.** Lack of tone. Also called *atony.*

**atopic.** 1. Out of position. 2. Relating to atopy.

**atopy.** Acquired or inherited hypersensitivity of the skin to a drug or external agent. The term commonly refers to allergic disorders.

**atresia.** The narrowing or closure of a body orifice, such as the anus or vagina, caused by failure of development or by disease. The term is also used to describe congenital absence of such an orifice.

**atrium.** One of the two upper chambers of the heart. Blood from the body enters the right atrium, is pumped into the right ventricle, and then into the lungs. The oxygenated blood from the lungs then passes into the left atrium, which pumps it into the left ventricle. The left ventricle in turn pumps the blood into the aorta. The term atrium is also applied to that part of the middle ear cavity below the head of the malleus, and to the front region of the nasal cavity. See also AURICLE; HEART.

**atropa.** A genus of plants belonging to the family *Solanaceae.* One of the best-known species of the genus is *Atropa belladonna,* or the deadly nightshade, whose purple-black berries contain belladonna, a source of atropine. See also ATROPINE; BELLADONNA.

**atrophy.** The wasting away of cells, organs, or muscles.

**atropine.** An alkaloid derived from hyoscyamine, the active principle of *Atropa belladonna*, or deadly nightshade. It paralyzes the sympathetic nervous system, dries up the secretions, and acts as an antispasmodic. It is used to dilate the pupil of the eye, lessen the gastric juice, dry up sweat, phlegm in the chest, or a running nose, and to stop colic. It has no effect when applied to the skin surface; therefore, belladonna plasters are completely useless.

**attenuate.** To make thin or to draw out; to weaken.

**attic.** A cavity in the ear above the eardrum.

**atypical.** Not conforming to type.

**audiogram.** A record of the ability to hear.

**audiometer.** An instrument used for measuring the ability to hear.

**auditory.** Pertaining to hearing or the organs of hearing.

**aura.** A sensation immediately preceding an epileptic fit. This may take the form of flashes of light before the eyes, an irritation of some part such as the thumb, or some other sensation, and it may enable the patient to get into a position of safety before the fit develops.

**aural.** Pertaining to the ear.

**aural vertigo.** An attack of giddiness precipitated by some disturbance of the labyrinth organ in the ear. See also MÉNIÈRE'S DISEASE.

**aureomycin.** An antibiotic drug.

**auricle.** 1. Literally a little ear but broadly a place into which something flows. Medically it commonly refers to the ear flap situated on the side of the head, a skin-covered piece of cartilage; also called *pinna*. 2. Quite erroneously, the term is sometimes applied to the upper chambers of the heart which are called the atria. The auricle is in fact an appendage of the atrium into which blood first flows from the blood vessels. It is also the point through which heart surgeons gain entry into the heart. See also ATRIUM; HEART.

**auricular.** 1. Relating to the ear. 2. Relating to the cardiac auricles.

**auricular extrasystole.** An extra heartbeat which arises in an auricle.

**auricular fibrillation.** A completely irregular beating of the heart due to impulses starting in the auricle.

**auriscope.** An instrument used for examining the eardrum.

**aurotherapy.** The use of gold in the treatment of disease.

**auscultation.** Listening for sounds within an organ or the body either with the ear or by using a stethoscope.

**autism.** A characteristic of schizophrenia. The individual is withdrawn within himself and more concerned with himself than with the realities of life.

**auto-antitoxin.** An antitoxin produced by the body itself to protect it from the toxin or poison of a disease.

**autoclave.** An apparatus used to sterilize objects by means of high-pressure steam.

**autodigestion.** Destruction of cells or tissues by their own secretions.

**autogenous.** Generated from within the body.

**autogenous vaccine.** A vaccine produced from bacteria harbored within the patient.

**autograft.** The taking of tissues from one part of the body to be used at another point in the same body.

**autohaemotherapy.** See AUTOHEMOTHERAPY.

**autohemotherapy.** The treatment of disease by taking some of the patient's own blood and injecting it into a muscle.

**autohypnosis.** A self-induced hypnotic state.

**auto-immunization.** Immunization produced by an attack of a disease.

**auto-infection.** An infection coming from within the body.

**autointoxication.** A disease process produced from poison manufactured within the body.

**autolysis.** The spontaneous destruction of tissues by the action of the tissues' own enzymes occurring in certain diseased conditions and after death. See AUTODIGESTION.

**automatism.** Actions performed without the individual's being aware of them. This automatic state sometimes follows an epileptic fit. See also EPILEPSY.

**autonomic nervous system.** This system comprises the parasympathetic and sympathetic nerves, which are responsible for those organs which function automatically and are not under the control of the will.

**autopsy.** Examination of the body after death; a post-mortem examination.

**autosuggestion.** Suggestions arising from within oneself.

*Autosuggestion assumed a new meaning about the period of the First World War when a Monsieur Couéelaborated in France a system of treatment in which the individual said out loud such optimistic phrases as "Every day and in every way I am getting better and better." This method was said to*

*produce a feeling of self-optimism which encouraged one to progress or recover.*

**autotherapy.** 1. The spontaneous cure of a disease. 2. The treatment of disease by using the patient's own body secretions as, for example, in autohemotherapy. At one time this treatment was much used for allergic disorders.

**avascular.** 1. Bloodless. 2. Without blood vessels.

**avitaminosis.** Disease due to lack of one or several vitamins.

**avulsion.** The tearing or wrenching away of a part of a structure of the body.

**axilla.** The armpit.

**axis.** An imaginary line drawn through the center of a body.

**axon.** A fiber which conducts impulses, projecting from, and an extension of, a nerve cell.

**azoospermia.** A deficiency of spermatozoa in the seminal fluid.

**azotaemia.** See AZOTEMIA.

**azotemia.** A condition of the blood, usually due to kidney disease.

**azygos.** A structure which has no counterpart; unpaired.

# B

**B.** The abbreviation for the genus *Bacillus*. See BACILLUS.

**Babinski's phenomenon or reflex.** An upward movement of the big toe when the sole of the foot is tickled. This is a normal reflex in infants but a sign of certain diseases of the central nervous system in adults. If no disease is present the toe goes in a downward direction.

**baby.** An infant; a child before it begins to walk. The birth weight of most normal infants is between 6 pounds and 8½ pounds with a broad average of 7¼ pounds. The newborn baby loses weight during the first two to five days but this is regained by the seventh to tenth day. The first stool passed by the baby is of a greeny-brown color and is called meconium, and although its appearance may frighten the mother it is quite normal. The average newborn baby is approximately 20 inches long and the circumference of the skull is 13½ inches. There is a deficiency in the skull bone on the top of the head where the brain is covered only by the scalp. It is called the anterior fontanelle, and automatically closes by the time the baby is 18 months old. If the fontanelle bulges unduly, other than during bouts of crying, it indicates an increase in intracranial pressure. A dehydrated baby has a sunken fontanelle.

**blue baby.** A baby with congenital heart disease causing blueness of the skin.

**newborn baby.** A baby during its first month of life. Should death occur during this period it is classified as a neonatal death.

**premature baby.** Any baby who weighs 5½ pounds or less at birth. These babies require special care if they are to survive, and the more the infant is below 5½ pounds the more precarious is its hold on life.

**Rhesus baby.** See RHESUS FACTOR.

**bacillaemia.** See BACILLEMIA.

**bacillary.** Related to or caused by bacilli.

**bacillemia.** The presence of bacilli in the blood.

**bacilli.** The plural of bacillus.

**bacilluria.** The presence of bacilli in the urine.

**bacillus.** A straight rod-shaped bacterium.

**bacitracin.** An antibiotic.

**backache.** Pain in the back and especially in the lower regions. The pain is sometimes acute, more often dull. See LUMBAGO.

**backbone.** The fairly rigid column formed by the vertebrae and extending posteriorly from the neck to the pelvis.

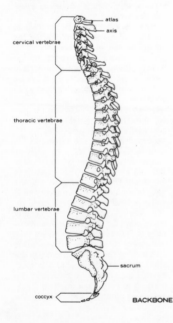

atlas
axis
cervical vertebrae
thoracic vertebrae
lumbar vertebrae
sacrum
coccyx
BACKBONE

**bacteraemia.** See BACTEREMIA.

**bacteremia.** The presence of bacteria in the blood.

**bacteria.** Unicellular plant microorganisms. They are classified according to their characteristics: *cocci* are round-shaped; *bacilli*, rod-shaped; *spirilla*, spiral-shaped; and *vibrios*, shaped like a comma. *Cocci* and *bacilli* may occur singly, grouped in pairs called *diplococci;* in a chainlike forma-

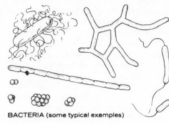

BACTERIA (some typical examples)

tion called *streptococci;* or in grapelike clusters called *staphylococci.* Bacteria are further divided into two main classes: *aerobes,* or aerobic bacteria, which need oxygen to survive; and *anaerobes,* or anaerobic bacteria, which flourish in the absence of oxygen. Some bacteria are static, while others can move, such as the *vibrios,* which can wriggle their tails like tadpoles. Bacteria are either *parasitic* and live on a live host, or *saprophytic* and live on a dead host. Only a very small percentage cause disease. These are called *pathogenic,* while the harmless ones are called *nonpathogenic.* Bacteria are further classified by whether they can be stained with Gram's stain. If they retain the stain they are *Gram positive,* and if they do not retain the stain they are *Gram negative.* Some, like those causing tuberculosis, are called *acid-fast* when even the use of acid fails to decolorize them. Those which cause fermentation are called *zymogenic;* those producing gas are *aerogenic;* and those producing pigment are *chromogenic.*

**bacterial.** Pertaining to or caused by bacteria.

**bactericidal.** Destructive of bacteria.

**bacteriology.** The study of bacteria, viruses and fungi, both pathogenic and nonpathogenic.

**bacteriolysis.** The destruction and dissolving of bacteria.

**bacteriophage.** A minute object with the ability to dissolve bacteria. Bacteriophages are so small that they can pass through filters which ordinary bacteria cannot. Some authorities con-

sider them to be living, while others think they are an enzyme.

**bacteriophobia.** A neurotic dread of bacteria.

**bacterium.** The singular of bacteria.

**bag of waters.** A membranous bag of water surrounding the baby in the womb. When labor commences, this bag in front of the baby's head acts as a dilator of the neck of the womb. Also called *amniotic sac.* See AMNION.

**bakers' itch.** A form of dermatitis caused by handling yeast and dough.

**bakers' leg.** Also called *genu valgum.* See KNOCK-KNEE.

**B.A.L.** Abbreviation for British Anti-Lewisite.

**balanitis.** Inflammation of the glans penis.

**balanus.** The bulbous tip of the penis; the glans of the penis.

**baldness.** See ALOPECIA; RINGWORM.

**Balkan frame.** A frame erected over a bed and from which hang slings to support fractured legs. Pulleys and weights are then attached in order to pull the fractured bones out straight.

**ball and socket joint.** A joint which is powerful and strong in structure because the head of one bone fits into a deep well or socket in another bone. The most powerful ball and socket joint in the body is the hip joint.

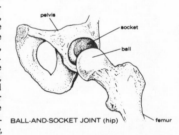

pelvis
socket
ball
BALL-AND-SOCKET JOINT (hip)
femur

**ballooning.** Distension of a body cavity by air or fluid.

**ballottement.** Maneuver in which pressure is placed on an organ and its rebound observed.

**balneotherapy.** Treatment of diseases by medicated baths; the standard treatment offered at various spas.

**balsam.** A mixture of oils and resins derived from certain plants.

**bandage.** A strip or piece of material, often gauze, for applying on a body structure. Bandages are used to protect an area against infection, to stop the flow of blood, to hold a splint in place, etc.

**Banti's syndrome.** Splenomegaly and anemia, together with cirrhosis of the liver and ascites.

**bandy leg.** Bowlegged.

**Barbados leg.** See ELEPHANTIASIS.

**barbed-wire disease.** A neurosis which occurs in prisoners of war due to the effects of total confinement.

**barbers' dermatitis.** A skin disease occurring in the hands of barbers.

**barbers' itch.** Also called *barbers' rash*. See SYCOSIS.

**barbiero fever.** A form of sleeping sickness caused by a Trypanosoma transmitted by the bite of insects. There are several forms of sleeping sickness (American, Gambian, Rhodesian) and all are characterized by irregular fever and enlarged glands. The patient slumps in bed and is roused only with difficulty.

**barbital.** The basic barbiturate, from which all the other barbiturate drugs arise; used as a sedative and for the treatment of insomnia.

**barbitone.** See BARBITAL.

**barbiturate.** One of several organic compounds used in medicine to induce sleep or sedation. Barbiturates are available only by prescription.

**Barcoo disease.** See VELDT SORE.

**barium enema.** A diagnostic procedure in which barium sulphate, a substance opaque to x-rays, is injected into the anus and allowed to flow around the large intestine, enabling the radiologist to see the intestine's outline on the x-ray screen.

**barium meal.** A flavored drink containing barium, a substance opaque to x-rays, which, when swallowed, outlines the intestines on the x-ray screen and enables the radiologist to diagnose whether the intestine is healthy or diseased; frequently used to detect gastric and duodenal ulcers.

**barognosis.** Ability to estimate weights.

**Bartholin's duct.** A duct opening into the floor of the mouth from a gland lying beneath the tongue. It is one of the glands that produces saliva.

**Bartholin's glands.** Glands situated in the walls of the vagina which produce and excrete the lubricating fluid that makes sexual intercourse possible.

**Bartholinitis.** Inflammation of Bartholin's glands.

**basal metabolic rate.** The minimum production of body heat after 12 hours of fasting and while lying completely at rest.

**basophil.** A pathological term descriptive of cells or tissues easily dyed with basic dyes.

**bathophobia.** The dread of looking down from high places.

**B.C.G.** Abbreviation for bacille Calmette-Guerin, a vaccine used to immunize against tuberculosis.

**Bedlam.** The abbreviated name of the Hospital of St. Mary of Bethlehem, an insane asylum established in London in 1547. During the 18th century Bedlam was one of the sights of London and visitors came from far and wide to watch the antics of the insane inmates. Some were kept in cages and exposed to view on payment of a fee. Occasionally some of these lunatics were allowed to go free, and they wandered the country begging. They wore a special badge and were known as "Tom O'Bedlams". There were no drugs, padded cells, or other methods of gentle restraint available and so when an inmate developed a maniacal attack he was ducked repeatedly in tanks of deep water until, exhausted and half-drowned, he was unable to be physically or mentally excited.

**bedsore.** Ulceration of the skin on the back of a patient who is allowed to remain for too long in one position. Pressure of the bed against the skin first squeezes out the blood supply and then, by friction, breaks down the tissues into an indolent ulcer. Apart from treatment to heal the ulcer, prevention consists in moving the patient regularly every two hours, massaging the back with surgical spirit and dusting with powder, and eliminating rucks and creases from the night clothes and lower sheet. Also called *decubitus ulcer, pressure sore.*

**bed-wetting.** Enuresis.

**belch.** The eructation of wind from the stomach, usually the result of aerophagy. Also called *eructation.*

**belladonna.** A drug obtained from the plant *Atropa belladonna,* popularly known as the deadly nightshade. An alcoholic tincture of belladonna is used in the treatment of spasms and colics, and to dry up secretions, such as those in the lungs. See also ATROPA; DEADLY NIGHTSHADE.

*Literally translated, belladonna means beautiful lady, and the ladies at the court of ancient Rome instilled the drug into their eyes to dilate the pupils. This, supposedly, gave them a soft and dreamy appearance presumed to be attractive to the opposite sex. The Borgias were familiar with belladonna and knew that the rabbit is immune to its poisonous effects, so when they desired to destroy an enemy secretly, they fed a rabbit on belladonna leaves until its muscles were saturated with the drug. The rabbit was then sent, alive and kicking, as a gift to the enemy, who, having killed and eaten it, was promptly overcome by belladonna poisoning.*

**Bell's palsy.** Facial paralysis.

**belly.** The abdomen.

**Benadryl.** One of the antihistaminic drugs.

**bends.** See CAISSON DISEASE.

**Benedict's test.** A test for sugar in the urine. Benedict's solution and a sample of urine are boiled in separate test tubes and then combined; if the urine contains sugar, the resulting solution is a bright orange.

**Benzedrine.** A proprietary preparation of amphetamine.

**benzpyrin.** A chemical which has come to popular notice since it was discovered that its derivatives, existing in car exhaust gases and tobacco tar, have the ability to cause cancer. See also AIR POLLUTION.

**beriberi.** A disease caused by the total lack of vitamin $B_1$ in the diet. It produces a form of peripheral neuritis, increasing dropsy of the body, profound weakness, paralysis, mental disturbance, heart failure, and death.

**beta rays.** One of the rays given off by radioactive substances.

**bezoar.** Any concretion formed in the gastrointestinal tract.

*The term is derived from the Persian for "poison". Bezoar stones were used extensively in the Middle Ages and earlier as a medical remedy. They were either worn as a charm to ward off disease or were put in a cup of wine in the belief that they would neutralize any poison put into the wine by an enemy. Their efficacy as a remedy was in direct proportion to their fantastic cost, for the charlatans who sold them claimed they were difficult to obtain. They explained that deer in the rutting season frequently stamped on the ground, and this caused snakes to emerge from among the rocks. The deer then swallowed the snakes, which caused such pain that the deer dashed into the lakes, where they stood neck-high in water and cried piteously. The crying resulted in a stone forming in the tear ducts and this stone was alleged to be a bezoar. The truth is that the bezoar stone was a gallstone obtained from horse slaughterhouses and was neither of any value nor of any cost.*

**bi-.** A prefix meaning two or twice.

**biceps.** Having two heads. The term is applied to various muscles, notably the biceps muscles in the arm and thigh.

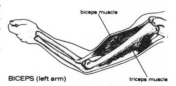

BICEPS (left arm)

**bicuspid.** Having two cusps. See VALVE.

**b.i.d.** To be taken twice daily, from the Latin *bis in die.*

**bifid.** Divided into two; forked.

**bifocal.** Having a double focus. Bifocal spectacles are those in which each lens has two portions, one for distance vision and one for close vision.

**bifurcation.** Division into two branches.

**bile.** The greenish-yellow secretion from the liver, which is stored in the gall bladder and at intervals is passed into the duodenum, to assist in the digestion of fats.

**bilharzia.** A parasitic worm which enters the body and causes bilharziasis.

**bilharziasis.** A disease which causes bloody urine. Also called *Bill Harris disease, schistosomiasis.*

**biliary.** Pertaining to the bile or gall bladder.

**bilious.** Pertaining to the bile or to bilious attacks, so called because of the presence of bile in the vomit.

**biliousness.** Bilious. See also CYCLIC VOMITING.

**bilirubin.** One of the bile pigments.

**bilirubinaemia.** See BILIRUBINEMIA.

**bilirubinemia.** The presence of bilirubin in the blood.

**bilirubinuria.** The presence of bilirubin in the urine.

**bilobed.** Having two lobes.

**bilocular.** Having two compartments.

**bimanual.** Involving the use of both hands.

**binocular.** Pertaining to both eyes, as in binocular vision; the vision produced by two eyes.

**binovular.** Arising from two eggs. The term most commonly refers to binovular twins, where each baby arises from a separate egg. See also TWINS.

**biochemistry.** The chemistry of the living body.

**biology.** The study of plant and animal life.

**biopsy.** The removal of a piece of living tissue from the body and its examination in various ways, such as under a microscope, to determine its structure and the presence or absence of disease.

**bipara.** A woman who has had two separate pregnancies and been delivered of one or more children from each pregnancy.

**biparietal.** Pertaining to both parietal bones, which form part of the sides of the skull.

**biparous.** Giving birth to twins.

**bipartite.** Composed of two parts.

**biped.** Having two feet.

**biperforate.** Having two openings.

**birth.** The act of being born. See also LABOR.

**cross birth.** A birth in which the baby lies transversely across the womb with no part presenting at the opening of the womb.

**multiple birth.** The occurrence of two or more babies at the same birth.

**posthumous birth.** Birth of a baby after its father has died.

**premature birth.** Birth of a baby before the 40th week and after the 28th week of pregnancy. Prior to the 28th week, termination of pregnancy is called an abortion or miscarriage.

**stillbirth.** The birth of a dead baby.

**birth control.** Contraception, regulation, or prevention of pregnancy. *Occlusive methods.* The male may wear a rubber sheath or the female may use an occlusive rubber cap over the neck of the womb, either with or without sperm-killing pessaries, to prevent the male sperm from fertilizing the female egg. *Oral method.* In this method, the woman takes hormone pills in order to prevent an egg cell from maturing in the ovary. The whole subject is unsettled from many points of view. Some doctors are not certain that it is harmless, and controversy still rages as to whether it can produce phlebitis or be conducive to the later formation of cancer. There are also objections to the method on religious and social grounds. *The "safe" period.* This is defined as the two or three days before the onset of the menstrual period during which the female is unlikely to conceive. In order to arrive at what is the "safe" period, it is necessary to do extensive calculations and these can only be done if the woman knows with precision when her periods are likely to start. If she is at all irregular the calculation is impossible.

**birthmark.** A birth anomaly in which there is a profusion of small blood vessels at some point in the skin. The majority of birth marks disappear by the age of 18 months and the remainder seldom require treatment before the age of five years. The superstition that they are caused by the mother being frightened during pregnancy is, of course, totally untrue. See also NEVUS.

**birth palsy.** A form of paralysis caused by damage to the baby during birth.

**birth rate.** The proportion of live births per thousand of the population.

**birth trauma.** Any injury occurring to a baby during the act of birth. In psychiatry it refers to mental trauma alleged to occur during birth and which may subsequently be the starting point of a neurosis. Although this may seem a little far-fetched, experimental work, in which groups of babies were subjected to various sounds while they slept, revealed that those who were most relaxed in sleep were those subjected to a sound simulating the pumping of the mother's heart and circulation, to which, presumably, the baby had been attuned while within the

womb. Some psychiatrists also claim that there is less neurosis in breast-fed babies than in those brought up on the bottle, and deprived of the natural instinct to suckle at the breast. The whole question is open to conjecture, and it is probable that the nervous temperament that dries up the mother's milk also provides the nervous background in which the child is reared, and that it is this environment that leads to neurosis, not the lack of the act of suckling.

**bisexual.** Having the characteristics of both sexes; hermaphroditic; ambosexual. Some animals are bisexual, as for example the earthworm, in which alternate segments are male and female and thus can fertilize each other.

**bisexuality.** 1. Hermaphrodism. 2. Sexual attraction to individuals of both sexes.

**bismuth.** A white crystalline metal with a reddish tint. The insoluble salts of bismuth are commonly used in stomach mixtures to act as an inert protective covering to the irritable or ulcerated lining of the stomach or duodenum. As an injection, bismuth salts are used in the treatment of syphilis.

**bistoury.** A long, slender, straight or curved surgical knife.

**bitemporal.** Relating to both temporal bones.

**bituminosis.** A form of pneumoconiosis caused by inhaling coal dust. Also called *anthracosis.*

**biurate.** A salt of uric acid.

**black death.** See PLAGUE.

**black eye.** A contusion of the tissues around the eyeball caused by a blow, and often treated by lumps of raw meat, which have not the slightest effect on the condition. Cold water compresses applied soon after the blow or soon after the discoloration appears will limit the bruising. The condition is due to a small quantity of blood emerging from broken blood vessels under the skin and spreading down and around the eye, making the injury look much worse than it really is. Gradually the blood undergoes chemical changes, and, as the hemoglobin becomes oxidized, the color changes from dark blue-black ranging through green and yellow until it finally disappears.

**blackhead.** A comedo. See also ACNE.

**blackout.** Momentary unconsciousness with failure of vision, due to diminished circulation of the blood in the brain and eye.

**black sickness.** Kala-azar.

**black spit.** The sputum of coal miners, containing particles of coal.

**black vomit.** A condition due to bleeding occurring in the stomach or intestines. Being partly digested, the blood changes from red to black and is then vomited. See also VOMIT: COFFEE-GROUND VOMIT.

**black-water fever.** A form of malaria characterized by marked prostration, rigors, restlessness, vomiting, black urine, and collapse. It is a serious disease in malarial countries and has been precipitated by the administration of quinine to a malarial patient. The red blood cells are destroyed and the altered hemoglobin is excreted in the urine, giving the characteristic black urine or black water. Also called *malarial hemoglobinuria.*

**bladder.** The reservoir of the urine secreted by the kidneys. It lies at the pit of the abdomen in front. Normally when 8 to 10 ounces of urine have accumulated the distension of the bladder wall sets up a sensation that calls for emptying. In cases of obstruction to the outlet, the bladder is capable of enormous distension, holding several pints, 50 ounces being not at all uncommon. This degree of distension causes agonizing pain.

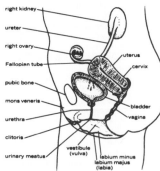

BLADDER (female)

**bland.** Soothing.

**blastoderm.** The germinal membrane of an egg, which forms the growing embryo.

**blastoma.** A tumor originating in immature or embryonic cells.

**blastomycosis.** A general term for diseases produced by yeastlike fungi.

**bleaching powder.** Chlorinated lime, a powerful antiseptic, disinfectant, and deodorizer. It releases chlorine, which reacts with moisture to produce a mixture of hypochlorous and hypochloric acids; the former decomposing and liberating nascent or newly liberated oxygen. The free chlorine has an affinity for the hydrogen in the protein that is contained in bacteria. This re-

placement and the effect of the hydrochloric acid and nascent oxygen kill the bacteria.

**bleb.** A vesicle or blister.

**bleeder.** A person who suffers with hemophilia, a condition in which the blood lacks the ability to clot. See HEMOPHILIA.

**bleeding.** See HEMORRHAGE.

**bleeding sickness.** Hemophilia.

**bleeding time.** The time taken by a needle prick to stop bleeding, normally four to five minutes.

**blennorrhagia.** Any profuse mucous discharge from anywhere in the body, particularly the profuse purulent gonorrheal discharge from the penis or the vagina. Also called *blennorrhea.*

**blennorrhoea.** See BLENNORRHAGIA.

**blepharism.** Rapid winking of the eye; a spasm of the eyelids.

**blepharitis.** Inflammation of the free margins of the eyelids. In a run-down child it may be due to unhealthy and poor living conditions, and is sometimes associated with seborrhea of the scalp, which produces dandruff. The dandruff then infects the eyelids.

**blepharon.** The eyelid.

**blind, blindness.** Absence of vision. See also AMAUROSIS.

**blind spot.** A spot on the retina, insensitive to light and located where the optic nerve enters the eye to form the retina. Also called *optic disc, optic papilla.*

**blister.** A bleb, vesicle, or fluid-filled swelling arising within and on the skin.

**blood.** The fluid that circulates through the heart, arteries, and veins, carrying nutriment and oxygen to the body tissues. Blood is composed of a clear yellow fluid, the plasma, containing the erythrocytes (red blood cells), the leukocytes (white blood cells), and the thrombocytes (blood platelets). The erythrocytes contain hemoglobin, a red oxygen-carrying chemical. The leukocytes have various functions. They assist in the repair of injured tissues of blood and are part of the body's defense against infection. When germs enter the body, the leukocytes rush to the scene, then engulf and destroy the germs. The thrombocytes assist in the coagulation of the blood. Blood is formed in the marrow of the long bones, and, varying with the size of the individual, the body contains six to twelve pints. An adult can lose two pints of blood without ill effect, larger losses producing severe surgical shock and collapse. One cubic millimeter of blood contains between four and five million erythrocytes (each of which has a diameter of seven-thousandths of a millimeter), four to eleven thousand leukocytes, and up to five hun-

dred thousand thrombocytes. Blood circulates under the pressure of the heart pump equivalent in the healthy adult to 120 millimeters of mercury. A drop of blood takes from nine to sixteen seconds to travel from the arm to the tongue and from four to eight seconds to travel from the arm to the lung. See also PRESSURE: BLOOD PRESSURE.

**blood groups.** Four types of blood are differentiated according to (1) the presence or absence of A and B agglutinogens found in the red blood cells, and (2) the presence or absence of anti-A and anti-B agglutinins in the plasma. The plasma of one individual may have an agglutinin that will agglutinate or clump and destroy the red cells of another. Therefore in carrying out a transfusion it is imperative to know whether the blood of both individuals involved is compatible. Individuals are placed into one of the following groups: A, B, AB, and O, which indicate the agglutinogens present in their respective blood cells. Blood type is an inherited trait and can be explained by the existence of a series of three alternative genes, every individual having any two (a pair) and making possible six types of genotypes. Group A individuals are either pure or hybrid and can give blood safely to A and AB individuals. Group B are either pure or hybrid and can give blood to B and AB individuals. Group O can give blood to any group but can receive from only Group O and are called universal donors. Group AB cannot be given to the other groups but can receive blood from any group and are called universal recipients. In addition, blood is classified into a number of other types including Rhesus positive and Rhesus negative, and M and N. See also RHESUS FACTOR.

**bloodless.** Anemic.

**bloodletting.** The removal of blood by opening a vein.

**blood pressure.** The pressure of blood on the walls of the arteries. See also PRESSURE: BLOOD PRESSURE.

**blue baby.** A baby with a congenital heart disease in which the blood is not being properly oxygenated, resulting in cyanosis—blueness of the skin. Occasionally a baby may suffer with "blue turns" as a result of inadequate expansion of the lungs after birth. See also RHESUS.

**blue pill.** A pill containing mercury; not much in use today.

**blue sclerotics.** An intense blue coloration of the sclerotic membranes or the whites of the eyes, occurring in osteogenesis imperfecta.

**blue-yellow blindness.** A rare form of color blindness in which the individual is unable to recognize the difference between blue and yellow.

**B.M.A.** The initials of the British Medical Association.

**B.M.R.** Abbreviation for basal metabolic rate.

**Bockhart's impetigo.** See IMPETIGO FOLLICULARIS.

**boil.** An abscess occurring in the depths of a hair follicle and resulting in a collection of pus underneath the skin. In the past the standard treatment was to apply hot boracic fomentations, a practice now largely discontinued because they sodden the skin, lower its resistance, and provoke the appearance of further boils. The treatment today is to leave it alone, administer an antibiotic drug, and if pus collects but does not discharge of its own accord, to let it out by a small incision. A boil should not be squeezed, for this only tends to spread the infection.

**bolus.** A rounded mass of large size.

**bone.** A hard tissue forming the skeleton. Bone is composed of a dense form of connective tissue containing ossein and osseomucoid impregnated with mineral salts, especially calcium phosphate. Dense, smooth bone is described as compact, while that with a spongelike structure is called cancellous. Bones are of four shapes: long, such as those in the limbs; short, such as in the wrist; flat, as in the skull; and irregular, as in the spine. The long bones contain marrow, a substance which manufactures the blood cells. Each bone is enveloped by a thin membrane, the periosteum, containing many blood vessels and nerves, which assists in the growth of the bone and in the repair of fractures. There are 208 bones in the body—30 in the head, 54 in the trunk, 64 in the upper limbs and 60 in the lower limbs—but only the principal ones are listed below.

**bones of the skull.** These are arranged in two groups, those of the cranium and those of the face. The cranium consists of the *occipital* bone at the back; two *parietal* bones, which form most of the sides; the *frontal* bone, which forms the front and forehead; the *temporal* bones, which form the areas of the temple and are pierced in the center for the organ of hearing; and the *sphenoid* and *ethmoid* bones, which form the base of the skull. The bones of the face consist of the *maxilla*, which forms a large part of the face and supports the upper teeth; the *mandible*, which supports the lower teeth; and the *zygomatic* bones.

**bones of the spinal column.** These bones are called vertebrae. They number 33 and comprise 7 *cervical* bones in the neck, 12 *thoracic* or *dorsal* bones in the region of the chest, and to which the ribs are attached, 5 *lumbar* bones in the small of the back, 5 *sacral* bones, which are fused together to form the *sacrum* (rump bone), and 4 *coccygeal* bones, which are also fused together to form the *coccyx* (tailbone).

**bones of the chest.** There are 12 pairs of ribs, which extend from the thoracic vertebrae to the front of the body. They are numbered as first, second, and so on, commencing from above. The upper seven pairs are the *true ribs* and are attached at their front ends to the *sternum* (breastbone). The lower five pairs are the *false ribs*, the upper three pairs being attached by cartilage to the ribs immediately above them. The last two pairs are unattached and are called the *floating ribs*.

**bones of the upper limb.** The *clavicle* (collarbone) extends from the sternum to the *scapula* (shoulder blade); the bone of the upper arm is the *humerus*, while those on the forearm are the *radius* on the thumb side with the *ulna* on the opposite side. These two bones end at the *carpus* (wrist), which consists of eight bones arranged in two rows of four. Those of the first row, from the thumb side, are the *scaphoid*, *lunate*, *triquetal*, and *pisiform*. The second row consists of the *trapezium*, *trapezoid*, *capitate*, and *hamate*. Attached to the carpus are the five long *metacarpal* bones, one going to each finger, and to these are connected the *phalanges*, each finger having three, while the thumb has two.

**bones of the pelvis.** The true pelvis cohsists of two halves formed by the *innominate* bones, above which rise the two *ilium* (wing or hip) bones. The back of the pelvis consists of the *sacrum*, formed by the fusion of the five sacral vertebrae; the front, the *pubis*, is formed by the fusion of the two *innominate* bones. The *ischial tuberosity* is the rear portion of the innominate bone, and can be felt as a hard bony knob in the center of the buttock.

**bones of the lower limb.** In the upper part of the leg is the *femur* (thigh bone), the top of which fits into the pelvis, while the lower end forms part of the knee joint, in front of which is the *patella* (knee cap). Below the knee come the *tibia* (shinbone) and the *fibula* (calf-bone). These join with the *tarsus*, which is composed of seven short bones, namely, the *talus* (ankle bone), the *calcaneum* (heel bone), the *navicular* bone, three *cuneiform* bones, and the *cuboid* bone. These connect with the five *metatarsal* bones (the metatarsus), which in turn connect with the *phalanges* (toe bones).

**borborygmi.** Intestinal rumblings due to the movement of gas or fluid in the bowels. They may be a manifestation of a nervous disorder and can occur in threatened conditions of intestinal obstruction.

**Bornholm disease.** An epidemic disease rather like influenza accompanied by muscle pains, and named after a Danish island in the Baltic. Also called *Devil's grip, pleurodynia.*

**botulism.** A very severe and sometimes fatal form of food poisoning of abrupt onset and violent symptoms. It is caused by food (often canned food) which has become contaminated by the poisons produced by the germ *Clostridium botulinum.*

**bougie.** A long, slender surgical instrument used for dilating a tube or canal in the body. It derives its name from a town in Algeria that was famous for making wax candles that were used as bougies and imported into Europe as such.

**boutonneuse fever.** A rickettsial disease transmitted to man by a dog tick and occurring on the shores of the Mediterranean. It has all the characteristics of typhoid fever.

**bowel.** The intestine.

**bowleg.** Outward curvature of the legs and separation of the knees. Also called *genu varum.*

**B.P.** The abbreviation for British Pharmacopoeia.

**B.P.C.** The abbreviation for British Pharmaceutical Codex.

**brachial.** Pertaining to the arm.

**brachialgia.** Pain arising in the arm.

**brachiocephalic.** Pertaining to the arm and the head.

**brachiocrural.** Pertaining to the arm and the leg.

**brachiocubital.** Pertaining to the arm and the forearm.

**brachiofacial.** Pertaining to the arm and the face.

**brachium.** The arm, especially the arm above the elbow.

**brachydactyly.** Abnormal shortness of the fingers.

**bradycardia.** Abnormal slowing of the heartbeat and pulse.

**bradyuria.** Passing urine extremely slowly.

**brain.** The central organ of the nervous system, contained within the cranium. The brain is divided into three main parts—the cerebrum, the cerebellum, and the medulla oblongata. The largest part is the *cerebrum*, which controls the movements of the limbs, facial expression, sight, hearing, speech, and other functions. It is also the center of intelligence and responsible for the memory and emotions. Below the cerebrum is the *cerebellum*, which is responsible for the balance and the co-ordination of the limbs. The third, and smallest, portion is the *medulla oblongata*, containing the vital nerve centers controlling breathing and the heartbeat. The brain is protected by three membranes, the *meninges*. The principal and outermost of these is the *dura mater*, and the middle membrane is the *arachnoid mater*. These two membranes are practically in contact, but between them is a small quantity of liquid, the cerebrospinal fluid. The innermost membrane, the *pia mater*, is very delicate and closely applied to the brain. Cavities within the brain, the *ventricles*, contain a clear, colorless liquid, the *cerebrospinal fluid*, which also surrounds the spinal cord. This fluid is derived from the blood and undergoes changes in the presence of disease. The average weight of the adult brain is about 48 ounces in the male and 44 ounces in the female, though intelligence is not related to size. The average brain is said to contain some 15,000,000,000 cells.

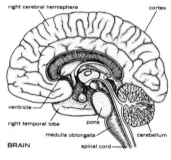

BRAIN

right cerebral hemisphere — cortex
ventricle
right temporal lobe — pons
medulla oblongata — cerebellum
spinal cord

**brain fever.** A disease in which the cardinal symptoms are severe headache, high temperature, and vomiting. An important feature of the disease is that it apparently only occurs during the winter and spring. Modern antibiotic treatment has cut short this disease process and largely abolished the serious complications that used to occur. Also called *cerebrospinal meningitis, cerebrospinal fever.*

**branchial.** A word derived from the Greek for gills. In the early stage of the developing human embryo the appearance of the fetus is not unlike that of a tadpole with marks which would grow into gills. From these areas in the human fetus different parts and organs of the body develop. If a remnant of the original gill formation found in the neck becomes a cyst, it is called a branchial cyst to denote its origin.

**Brazilian spotted fever.** A type of typhus fever.

**breakbone fever.** See ADEN FEVER.

**breast.** 1. The front of the chest. 2. The mammary gland, the milk-producing gland of the female, which is composed of 15 to 20 lobes, each lobe having a minute milk duct coverging towards the nipple. The nipple is sometimes

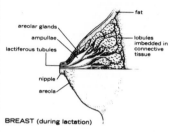

fat
areolar glands
ampullae
lactiferous tubules — lobules imbedded in connective tissue
nipple
areola

BREAST (during lactation)

found to be enlarged in a newborn baby, and milky fluid called "witch's milk" has even been found issuing from the baby's nipples. This precocious development is caused by the presence of female sex hormone supplied by the mother. The condition subsides quite quickly without treatment.

**breastbone.** See STERNUM.

**breathing.** The normal rate of breathing is 16 breaths per minute. This rate increases with exercise or certain chest disorders and decreases in comatose conditions or when the patient is under the influence of certain drugs. See also ARTIFICIAL RESPIRATION; RESPIRATION.

**breech.** The buttocks.

**bricklayer's itch.** A form of dermatitis caused by irritation from mortar and cement.

**Bright's disease.** Acute or chronic nephritis. The disease is named after Dr. Richard Bright (1789-1858), who first differentiated between the dropsy due to heart disease and that due to kidney disease. There is now a much more complete classification of acute and chronic nephritis, and the term is falling into disuse.

**brilliant green.** An antiseptic dyestuff.

**British Anti-Lewisite.** An antidote to heavy metal poisoning, such as mercury. Chemically the antidote is 2:3-dimercaptopropanol. It was invented during the Second World War as an antidote to arsenical war gases. Also called *B.A.L., dimercaprol.*

**British Pharmaceutical Codex.** A book issued voluntarily by the Pharmaceutical Society of Great Britain as a service to drug manufacturers, pharmacists, and doctors. The book stipu-

lates the standards of purity for drugs and includes articles on their dosage and usage.

**British Pharmacopoeia.** A book issued by the General Medical Council under the authority of an Act of Parliament, and containing the standards of purity for the manufacture of drugs in Great Britain.

**Brodie's abscess.** A chronic abscess of bone occurring in osteomyelitis, usually situated in the head of the tibia of young adults.

**Brodmann's areas.** Areas of the surface of the brain which were originally differentiated by their cellular structure. The term is now more commonly used to differentiate the function of that part of the brain. Thus Brodmann's area No. 4, the posterior part of the precentral gyrus, is the motor area of the brain from which messages are sent to various muscle groups. Areas 41 and 17 are concerned with the senses of hearing and vision.

**bromhidrosis.** Foul-smelling sweat.

**bromidrosiphobia.** Fear of body odor.

**bronchadenitis.** Inflammation of the lymph glands in the chest.

**bronchi.** The two main branches of the trachea; the plural of bronchus.

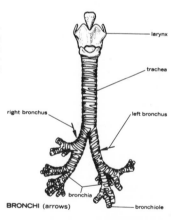

BRONCHI (arrows)

larynx
trachea
right bronchus — left bronchus
bronchia
bronchiole

**bronchiectasis.** A condition that sometimes follows diseases such as whooping cough, in which there is dilation of the bronchi or bronchioles—the air pipes in the lungs. This dilation sometimes progresses to the point of forming a cavity and results in a pooling of the secretions in the chest. The secretions become infected, causing a severe paroxysmal cough, the production of large amounts of foul-smelling sputum, and eventually lead to clubbing of the finger ends, blood spitting, and a general deterioration in health. Sometimes, however, the condition is confined to one lobe of a lung and in these cases the lobe can be removed, resulting in complete recovery of the patient.

**bronchiole.** A minute end branch of a bronchus.

**bronchiolitis.** Inflammation of the bronchioles.

**bronchiospasm.** Spasm of a bronchus or bronchi. Also called *bronchiospasmus*.

**bronchitic.** A person suffering with bronchitis.

**bronchitis.** Bronchitis is an inflammation of the bronchial tubes. Unquestionably it is bound up with air pollution and cigarette smoking, though other contributory factors are sinus disease and upper respiratory infections which migrate down on to the chest.

*Bronchitis patients need clean air; therefore they should avoid smoky and fume-laden atmospheres, should not smoke cigarettes, and should guard against catching influenza by having an injection of influenza vaccine in October or November, well before winter sets in. The chronic bronchitic must also wear warm clothing during bad weather. During fog or smog chest sufferers simply must stay indoors and close all the windows. Fumeless appliances should be used for heating. If fog invades the home, the patient must consider wearing a mask, which is quite easy to make. From a 5-yard roll of gauze make a pad the size of the face with 12 or 16 layers of gauze, stitch round the edges and sew tapes to the corners. Then damp the pad with water and wear it over the nose and mouth to act as a filter.*

**bronchodilator.** A drug which dilates the bronchial tubes.

**bronchomycosis.** A form of bronchitis caused by a fungus. Also called *bronchomoniliasis*.

**bronchopathy.** Any disease of the bronchi.

**bronchopneumonia.** Inflammation of the lungs commencing in the bronchi, sometimes patchy and localized. In lobar pneumonia, a whole lobe of a lung is affected.

**bronchopulmonary.** Pertaining to both bronchi and lungs.

**bronchoscope.** An instrument which is passed down the main airway to examine the lungs and air passages.

**bronchoscopy.** Inspection of the interior of the bronchus with a bronchoscope.

**bronchotracheal.** Relating to both bronchi and trachea.

**bronchus.** One of the main branches of the trachea, the main airway of the chest.

**bronzed diabetes.** See HEMOCHROMATOSIS.

**brow.** The forehead.

**Brucella.** A genus of bacteria in man and domestic animals. See ABORTUS FEVER.

**brucellosis.** A generalized infection caused by one of the species of the genus *Brucella*.

**bruise.** A superficial injury to the skin or soft tissues in which the minute blood vessels are broken, causing slight bleeding into the tissues, and producing the characteristic blue staining. During the ensuing ten days the blood becomes absorbed, and the skin color changes from blue to green to yellow until the color fades away completely. The only useful first-aid treatment is an ice pack or cold compress—raw steak and other gimmicks, such as tincture of arnica, have no effect. Spontaneous bruising, a bruising without any history of a blow, is seen in some people suffering from certain blood diseases, such as leukemia.

**bruit.** An abnormal sound heard during auscultation with a stethoscope.

**bubo.** An inflamed and swollen lymph gland, particularly the glands in the groin. It is a marked feature of bubonic plague, in which the buboes enlarge and discharge a mixture of pus and blood.

**bubonic plague.** See BUBO; PLAGUE.

**bucca.** The mouth or cheek.

**buccal.** Pertaining to the mouth or cheek.

**Buerger's disease.** A disease of unknown cause, characterized by acute inflammation with thrombosis, affecting both arteries and veins, principally in the lower leg. Seen chiefly in young or middle-aged men, it affects almost exclusively heavy tobacco smokers. Also called *thromboangiitis obliterans*.

**bulla.** A blister; a bulging structure.

**bullous fever.** A febrile illness accompanying pemphigus.

**bunion.** A swelling over the inner side of the big toe due to wearing for many years shoes that are too narrow and pointed. As a sequel, the big toe is forced towards the outer side of the foot. This, plus the friction from the narrow shoe, sets up irritation and swelling over the big toe joint and its bursa, initiating a vicious circle of friction, swelling, and inflammation. The only cure is surgical removal of some of the bone and the wearing of shoes that will allow the big toe to lie in a straight line. Nearly all bunions occur in the feet of women.

**burns.** Injuries caused by any form of dry heat, an electric current, or strong corrosive chemical whether acid or alkali. Given below are brief details of first-aid treatment for various types of large burn. *Acid burns.* Neutralize the acid by flooding the burn with a solution of bicarbonate of soda made up by dissolving one or two teaspoonfuls of bicarbonate of soda in a pint of clean water. Apply a clean dressing and transfer the patient to a hospital. *Alkali burns.* Corrosive alkalis—quicklime or caustic soda, for example—should be washed off the skin with large quantities of clean water. A dry dressing should be applied, and the patient should be taken to a hospital. *Dry heat burns.* Cover with clean dry dressing and take patient to a hospital.

*Electrical burns.* Cover with clean dry dressing and transfer patient to a hospital. Electrical burns may, however, be overshadowed by the need for artificial respiration, after the patient has been removed from contact with the electric current. See ARTIFICIAL RESPIRATION. *Scalds.* Small scalds merely need covering with a sterile dressing, while larger ones, not amounting to emergency treatment, need antibiotic treatment under medical supervision.

*Small burns.* Clean gently, apply a mild antiseptic, a dry dressing, and a bandage to hold it in place. If blisters form after a burn they should be left severely alone and not pricked, even with a sterile needle. These blisters protect the burnt tissue beneath, keep out infection, and will absorb in time. Some people have a firm conviction that they get relief from a thick paste of bicarbonate of soda and water, and since it is a harmless first-aid treatment it may be worth trying. Putting butter on small burns or holding them against a warm object to obtain relief are popular fallacies and valueless as treatment.

*The great danger in burns is that they can produce profound surgical shock. The question of whether surgical shock will arise in any given case depends on how much of the surface area of the body is involved. In an adult, if 30 percent of the body surface is burned surgical shock will occur. It may be far less than that figure in the case of a small child or baby. As a guide, the head is 10 percent of the body surface, the front of the trunk 18 percent, the back of the trunk 18 percent, each leg 18 percent, and each arm 9 percent. Therefore a burn involving the front of the trunk and both legs equals 54 percent of the body area—well over the 30 percent danger level.*

**bursa.** A small sac or bag containing fluid interposed between a bone and the skin surface. There are many bursae, nature placing them over bony prominences to prevent the bone rubbing through the skin.

*Many inflammatory conditions of bursae have names associated with the occupation of the patient. Housemaid's knee is a swelling of the preputellar bursa over the knee cap, attributed (in the days when there were maids!) to constant pressure on the knee cap when kneeling and scrubbing floors. Student's elbow is inflammation and swelling of olecranon bursa over the point of the elbow. Students claim it is due to supporting the head on the hands with the elbows resting on the hard surface of a desk while studying their textbooks. Their professors, however, claim it is due to the students going to sleep in that position!*

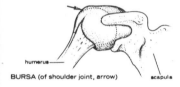

BURSA (of shoulder joint, arrow)

humerus

scapula

**bursectomy.** The surgical removal of a bursa.

**bursitis.** Inflammation of a bursa.

**byssinosis.** A lung disease caused by inhaling cotton dust over a long period. Three stages of the disease are recognized. In the first stage there is an irritating cough with tightness of the chest and breathlessness, usually occurring on a Monday, after which the individual remains well for the rest of the week, hence the name "Monday fever." The second stage is characterized by the above symptoms continuing all through the week. In the third stage the condition causes tightness of the chest and severe shortness of breath, due to chronic bronchitis and emphysema of such severity that the individual is permanently disabled. Also called *strippers' asthma, grinders' asthma, cotton card room asthma.*

*Other allied and somewhat similar disorders due to inhaling cotton dust cause a condition characterized by loss of appetite, headache, vomiting, abdominal pain, and sometimes rigors, which usually last for about a week.*

# C

**cachectic.** Characterized by cachexia.
**cachet.** A flat capsule in which disagreeable-tasting drugs are enclosed so that they can be swallowed without unpleasantness. The cachet is soluble and dissolves in the stomach.
**cachexia.** The extreme state of wasting found in people suffering from serious diseases such as cancer.
**cachinnation.** Hysterical laughter.
**cacidrosis.** Excessive and offensive sweating.
**cadaver.** Corpse.
**cadaveric.** Relating to a corpse.
**cadaverous.** Resembling a corpse.
**caduceus.** The wand of Mercury; the symbol of the medical profession. See AESCULAPIUS.
**caecal.** See CECAL.
**caecostomy.** See CECOSTOMY.
**caecum.** See CECUM.
**caesarean section.** See CESAREAN SECTION.
**caffeine.** A chemical which has a stimulating effect on the nervous system.
**caisson disease.** A condition which occurs in people working under high atmospheric pressure, such as divers and tunnel workers. It is caused by a too rapid return to normal pressure. When subjected to high pressure the body tissues absorb not only oxygen but nitrogen, and if decompression takes place too rapidly bubbles of nitrogen appear in the tissues, especially in the brain tissue, and cause severe damage. Excruciating pain in the muscles is the first sign of trouble. Decompression must therefore be gradual so that nitrogen can come out of the tissues and be absorbed by the blood slowly and in small quantities. Also called *the bends.*
**calamine.** Zinc carbonate. It is used to make soothing lotions, ointments, and dusting powders.
**calcaneal.** Relating to the calcaneus.
**calcaneus.** The heel bone or os calcis. Also called *calcaneum.*
**calcarea.** Quicklime or calcium oxide.
**calcareous.** Containing calcium or lime.
**calcariuria.** The presence of calcium salts in the urine.
**calciferol.** Vitamine $D_2$, created by the action of ultraviolet light on ergosterol. Vitamin $D_3$ occurs naturally in fish-liver oils, milk, and animal fats, usually in company with vitamin A, and is produced in the skin by the action of sunlight or ultraviolet light on 7-dehydrocholesterol. Vitamin D,

which covers both $D_2$ and $D_3$, acts by raising the phosphorus and calcium present in the blood, aids their absorption from the gut, and assists the bones to use these chemicals. Deficiency of vitamin D produces rickets and osteomalacia, and overdosage produces lethargy, causes withdrawal of calcium from the bones, and creates stones in the kidneys.
**calcification.** The hardening up of tissues by deposits of chalk or lime.
**calcination.** The roasting of a substance to drive off water.
**calcinosis.** A state characterized by the abnormal deposition of calcium salts in the tissues.
**calcipenia.** The absence or deficiency of calcium salts in the body.
**calcium.** The basic element of lime, it is very abundant in nature, and in the pure state is a brilliant, silver-white metal, having a strong affinity for oxygen. It is an essential ingredient of the bones and although calcium is added to bread flour, the human being's intake is largely derived from milk and milk products.
**calculous.** A stonelike state.
**calculus.** A stone found in the gall bladder, salivary glands, bile ducts, or urinary system. Its chemical composition depends on where it is found.
**calf.** The fleshy part of the leg at the back of the shin bone.
**caliber.** The inner diameter of a tube.
**calipers.** Steel bars fitted to the heel of a boot and extended up the leg to act as a support in cases where the leg muscles are paralyzed or have to be rested.
**callosity.** A thickened portion of the skin.
**callous.** A hard, indurated area.
**callus.** The new bone that is deposited around a fracture site, and which unites the ends of a broken bone.
**caloric.** Relating to calorie or to heat.
**calorie.** A heat unit; the amount of heat required to raise the temperature of one gram of water one degree Centigrade. The unit used in calculating the nourishment value of a diet.
**calorific.** Heat-producing.
**calvaria, calvarium.** The skull.
**calvities.** Baldness. See ALOPECIA; RINGWORM.
**calx.** 1. The heel. 2. Calcium oxide.
**calyx.** One of the funnel-shaped structures surrounding the pyramids in the kidneys.
**camp fever.** See TYPHUS FEVER.
**camphor.** A substance originally derived from the camphor plant but now produced synthetically from turpentine. It has been used as a carminative, antispasmodic, and diaphoretic, but has fallen into disuse. Camphorated

oil, so extensively used as a liniment for rubbing into chests, sore muscles, and painful joints, is one percent of camphor in cottonseed oil.

**canal.** A channel or passage.

**canalicular.** Relating to a small channel or passage.

**canaliculus.** A small channel or groove.

**canalization.** The making of channels or grooves.

**cancellate.** A web or latticework type of structure. Also called *cancellated, cancellous.*

**cancellus.** The spongy, latticelike texture of bone.

**cancer.** A term loosely used to describe any form of malignant growth. Every organ in the body is composed of cells, and the cells of each organ have specialized functions and distinctive shapes recognizable under the microscope. A cancerous change takes place when, for as yet no explicable reason, some cells of an organ suddenly take on violently rapid multiplications in a different form. Since cancer cells have no function, they cannot carry out any useful work, and, in time, they replace all the functioning cells of the organ. Cancer spreads through the body either by direct spread and invasion or by entry into the blood and lymph streams, being distributed round the body as emboli. Some cancers are amenable to treatment with deep x-rays and radium, and some to drugs and hormones. The prospect in the future is that cancer may be controlled by the injection of some chemical as yet unknown, which will prevent normal cells from taking on this malignant power of rapid multiplication.

**cancerocidal.** Destroying cancer cells.

**cancerogenic.** Capable of causing cancer.

**cancerophobia.** The dread of having cancer.

**cancerous.** Of the nature of cancer.

**cancrum oris.** A rare form of gangrene. See NOMA.

**canker.** An ulceration, chiefly of the mouth and lips.

**canker sore.** Small ulcerations of the lining of the mouth. Many have no known cause, though some may be due to food allergy. The number of treatments advised for the condition is legion and is an indication that nobody really knows the exact cause. These small ulcers can be touched with either pure carbolic acid or a solution of chromic acid, which induces them to heal. Also called *aphthous ulcer.*

**cannabis.** The plant from which marihuana is obtained. Also called *Indian hemp.* See MARIHUANA.

**cannula.** A surgical instrument, usually a tube which surrounds a trocar,

that is thrust into a cyst. The trocar is then pulled out and the cannula left in position so that fluid can drain out of the cyst. Also called *canula.*

**cantharides.** A chemical derived from Spanish flies. It acts as a blistering agent when applied externally and as a violent purgative when taken internally. It has the reputation of stimulating the sex organs, but if used for this purpose it produces the most violent ill effects, especially in the kidneys. Also called *cantharidin.*

**canthus.** The angle at the junction of the two eyelids.

**canula.** See CANNULA.

**caoutchouc.** Gum elastic or India rubber.

**capillary.** Minute blood vessels communicating between the arteries and the veins; a minute lymph vessel; pertaining to capillaries.

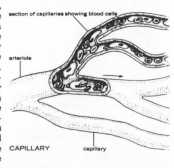

section of capillaries showing blood cells

arteriole

CAPILLARY       capillary

**capillary attraction.** The phenomenon that allows fluid to rise in a very small diameter tube because the adhesive force between the liquid and the side walls of the tube exceeds the gravitational force per unit of weight of the liquid.

**capitate.** In the shape of a head.

**capitation fee.** In England, the fee paid to a family doctor in the National Health Service for each patient on his list.

**capitatum.** One of the small bones in the hand.

**capitellum.** 1. The bulb of a hair. 2. A small rounded knob on a bone. 3. The rounded eminence at the lower end of the humerus.

**capsicum.** The pepper plant. Extract of pepper is applied to the skin as a counterirritant and is an ingredient of the colored wool sold as soothing pads for painful joints.

**capsular.** Relating to a capsule.

**capsule.** 1. A sheath enclosing a structure. 2. A soluble gelatine shell for enclosing drugs.

**capsulectomy.** The surgical removal of a capsule.

**capsulitis.** The inflammation of a capsule.

**caput.** 1. The head. 2. The chief part of an organ.

**caput medusae.** A condition named after Medusa, described in mythology as having a head of snakes, and very descriptive of the appearance of large dilated veins which occur on the abdominal wall, especially surrounding the navel, in cases of portal obstruction due to cirrhosis of the liver. The veins provide an alternative channel for blood from the abdominal organs to get back to the liver and the heart.

**caput succedaneum.** An edematous swelling found on the baby's skull as a result of pressure during the process of birth. Most of it disappears within 24 hours and all of it usually within the first week after birth.

**caraway.** A plant which supplies an essential oil; used as a carminative.

**carbhaemoglobin.** See CARBHEMOGLOBIN.

**carbhemoglobin.** See CARBOXYHEMOGLOBIN.

**carbohydrates.** The starches and sugars that occur in the diet.

**carbolic acid.** A powerful disinfectant derived from coal tar. Also called *carbolic, phenol.*

**carbon.** A nonmetallic element, which in its purest form is found as a diamond; a constituent of graphite, coal, and all plant and animal tissues.

**carbon dioxide.** A gas excreted from the lungs as a waste product. See also ARTIFICIAL RESPIRATION.

**carbon dioxide snow.** Solid carbon dioxide produced by the rapid expansion of liquid carbon dioxide. Because of its extremely low temperature it is used in medicine as a cauterizing agent or as a freezing agent to remove small blemishes or growths on the skin. When carbon dioxide snow is applied for one or two minutes, the part freezes solid and its blood supply is cut off; this in turn produces a form of aseptic gangrene and, after preliminary blister formation, the growth drops off. The advantage of the method is that it only affects the very superficial layers of the skin, which then grow again, leaving little or no scar.

**carbonic acid.** An unstable chemical produced by dissolving carbon dioxide in water.

**carbonize.** To char.

**carbon monoxide.** A very poisonous, colorless, and odorless gas arising from the incomplete combustion of coal and other products. It is present in domestic coal gas, and people who have unsuccessfully attempted suicide by inhaling carbon monoxide state that long before consciousness is lost the entire system of muscles of the body is paralyzed, thus preventing the victims, after a change of mind, from moving away from the danger of the gas. Carbon monoxide is also a constituent of sewer gases and of afterdamp (the poisonous gas found in coal mines following explosions). The gas has been found after explosions of shells or bombs in confined spaces. The skin of those who have died from carbon monoxide poisoning displays a curiously attractive pink coloration.

**carboxyhaemoglobin.** See CARBOXY-HEMOGLOBIN.

**carboxyhemoglobin.** A chemical produced by the combination of carbon monoxide and hemoglobin. Carbon monoxide has 30 times the affinity for hemoglobin as oxygen, thus when carbon monoxide is breathed it rapidly abolishes the ability of the hemoglobin to carry oxygen and as a result, in many cases, the body dies from oxygen starvation.

**carbromal.** A mild sedative and hypnotic.

**carbuncle.** An infection under the full thickness of the skin, caused by the pus-forming germ staphylococcus. It produces a large infected area from which the pus escapes by making numerous openings for itself through the skin, producing a sievelike appearance. A carbuncle is tremendously debilitating, very painful, and very much more serious than a boil, which is an infection of a hair follicle by the same organism.

**carcinogen.** A cancer-forming agent.

**carcinogenesis.** The development of cancer.

**carcinogenic.** Of or pertaining to the production of cancer.

**carcinoid.** A benign tumor arising either from cells of the appendix or other intestinal tissue. Microscopically it resembles cancer, but does not give rise to any symptoms.

**carcinoma.** See CANCER.

**carcinomatophobia.** A dread of cancer.

**carcinomatosis.** The general spread of cancer throughout the body.

**carcinomatous.** Cancerlike.

**cardia.** 1. The heart. 2. The region of the stomach which opens into the esophagus.

**cardiac.** Relating to the heart.

**cardiac asthma.** A type of asthma associated with heart disease. See ASTHMA.

**cardiac cycle.** The succession of beats of the chambers of the heart.

**cardiac decompensation.** Heart failure.

**cardiac failure.** The inability of the heart to maintain the circulation.

**cardiac hypertrophy.** An enlargement of the heart to compensate for a defect in circulation.

**cardialgia.** See HEARTBURN.

**cardiazol.** A heart stimulant.

**cardiogram.** A record of the heartbeat taken through the chest wall.

**cardiograph.** An instrument for recording the heartbeat graphically.

**cardiography.** Examination with a cardiograph.

**cardiologist.** A heart specialist.

**cardiology.** The science of the study of the heart.

**cardiomegaly.** Enlargement of the heart.

**cardioneurosis.** A nervous disorder characterized by palpitations. See VAGAL ATTACK.

**cardiopathy.** Any heart disease.

**cardiopericarditis.** Inflammation of the heart and pericardium.

**cardiophobia.** The fear of heart disease.

**cardiopulmonary.** Pertaining to the heart and the lungs.

**cardiorenal.** Pertaining to the heart and the kidneys.

**cardiosclerosis.** Hardening of the heart muscle due to the deposition of fibrous tissue.

**cardiospasm.** Spasm of the cardiac sphincter, a valve of the stomach, preventing the proper passage of food from the esophagus to the stomach.

**cardiosphygmograph.** An instrument for recording the apex beat, radial pulse, and venous pulse.

**cardiotomy.** Surgical incision into the heart or the cardia of the stomach.

**cardiovalvulitis.** Inflammation of the heart valves.

**cardiovascular.** Relating to the heart and blood vessels.

**carditis.** Inflammation of the heart.

**cardophyllin.** A respiratory stimulant.

**caries.** Destruction by inflammation of bone or teeth.

*Interest in dental caries has increased since it was proved beyond doubt that those who live in areas where the water supply contains one part per million of fluoride suffer with far less dental decay than those who live in areas where fluoride is not naturally present. This subject has been fully investigated in 18 countries, and the collective results of the research have been incorporated in a report by the World Health Organization. It is suggested that the domestic water supply in areas where there is a deficiency of fluoride should now be treated with fluoride to bring it up to the level of one part per million. In the experimental trials where this has been done in several countries, especially in the United States, the number of fillings performed on children's teeth dropped by as much as 78 percent. Attempts to treat teeth by painting them with a fluoride solution, by the*

*use of chewing gum impregnated with fluoride, and by brushing them with toothpaste containing fluoride do not compare with the results obtained by introducing fluoride into the water supply. That this is a harmless and safe procedure is self-evident when one considers that in areas where fluoride is a natural constituent of the water many generations have lived and drunk it without coming to any harm. The consensus of opinion of the experts is that to have the greatest effect fluoride should be introduced into the tooth structure while the teeth are developing during the first eight years of a child's life.*

**carminative.** A drug employed to have a soothing effect on the stomach.

**carnivorous.** Flesh eating.

**carnophobia.** The dislike of eating meat.

**carotene.** A yellow pigment found in carrots, leafy vegetables, milk, egg yolk, and animal fat; a precursor of vitamin A, into which it is converted in the human body.

**carotid.** The principal artery on each side of the neck, which carries blood from the heart to the brain and the tissues of the head and neck.

**carotid sinus.** The area where the carotid artery divides into the internal and external carotid arteries and which is richly provided with nerves.

**carotid sinus reflex.** If the carotid sinus is squeezed or pressed it can inhibit or stop the action of the heart. It is the basis of garrotting as opposed to strangulation, for by pressing on these areas on either side of the neck the victim can be made to drop unconscious.

**carotid sinus syndrome.** Attacks of giddiness, fainting, and sometimes convulsions, associated with a fall in blood pressure and slowing of the pulse; caused by excessive irritability of the carotid sinus. The attacks may occur without warning, follow an emotional upset, or be caused by pressure over the carotid sinus.

**carpal.** Relating to the carpus.

**carpometacarpal.** Pertaining to the carpus and the metacarpus.

**carpopedal spasm.** Spasmodic movements of the hands and feet due to lack of calcium from a disease of the blood.

**carpophalangeal.** Pertaining to the carpus and the phalanges of the finger bones.

**carpus.** The eight small bones of the wrist.

**carrier.** Someone who harbors within his body a germ which is capable of infecting other people although the carrier is apparently immune.

*Carriers are dangerous people who unwittingly start or spread epidemics, and one such epidemic was produced by a man working in a water well. Being too lazy to climb to the surface, he urinated at the bottom of the well. Unknowingly he was a carrier of typhoid fever and as a result of his action an epidemic of the disease occurred in the area.*

**car sickness.** A form of motion sickness.

**cartilage.** The gristle or specialized connective tissue found in association with bony tissue.

**cartilaginous.** Of the nature of cartilage.

**caruncle.** A small, fleshy, red mass or nodule.

**lacrimal caruncle.** The small, pink pad normally seen at the inner corner of the eye.

**urethral caruncle.** A small, fleshy mass seen attached to the back wall of the opening of the female urethra and the cause of pain and bleeding. It is not malignant.

**cascara.** A purgative made from the bark of a North American shrub.

**caseation.** A form of tissue death seen in cases of tuberculosis and syphilis in which the dead tissue has a cheeselike appearance.

**casein.** The protein of milk.

**caseous.** See CASEATION.

**caseous abscess.** An abscess containing cheeselike material, usually tuberculous. Also called *cheesy abscess.*

**cassia.** A plant which yields senna, used as a purgative.

**cast. 1.** A mass of body tissue or exudate that has taken the shape of the lining of a cavity. Casts are classified according to the cavity from which they originated, such as bronchial casts from the lungs, intestinal casts from the intestines, renal casts from the kidney. The most important are the renal casts, which are classified according to their constitution as blood, epithelial, fatty, fibrinous, granular, hyaline, mucous, and so on, and each has a significance in the investigation of kidney disease. The next most important are the intestinal casts, which are shed in some forms of colitis. **2.** The term also refers to a mold made of plastic or plaster of paris.

**Castle's factors.** So named after Dr. Castle, an American physician whose research uncovered the cause of pernicious anemia. Castle described an intrinsic factor, contained in the gastric juice, which, when combined with an extrinsic factor, contained in certain foods, provides the antianemic factor normally stored in the liver. As a result of this work it was found that administering liver extract or dried, powdered hog's stomach produced the factors necessary to cure pernicious

anemia. It is now known that injections of vitamin $B_{12}$ provide the antianemic factor so that liver extract and hog's stomach are seldom used.

**castor oil.** A vegetable oil used as a purgative and as inert bland oil drops to soothe the eyes. The advantage that castor oil has over other purgatives is that it acts from the very top of the intestinal tract as a thorough clearing agent to the entire intestinal system. It is used in midwifery for clearing out the bowels prior to labor, but its disadvantage in this respect is that, having emptied the entire bowel, it produces constipation for several days. However, for this reason it is also used to treat some kinds of diarrhea.

**castration.** Removal of the sex glands either in the male or female.

**casualty.** A person injured by an accident.

**catabolism.** Destructive metabolism, the breakdown of the constituents of the diet into simpler substances with an attendant release of energy—the basic process by which an organism supplies itself with the energy needed for all body functions. The building up of substances in the body is called anabolism.

**catabolite.** One of the breakdown products produced in the metabolism of the body.

**catalepsy.** A trancelike state associated with hysteria and schizophrenia; a stage of self-hypnotic sleep. In localized catalepsy a single muscle or group of muscles is affected, and the patient will keep, say, an arm raised for an indefinite period without apparent fatigue. See also CATATONIA.

**cataleptic.** Relating to catalepsy; a person with catalepsy.

**cataleptiform.** Resembling catalepsy. Also called *cataleptoid.*

**catalysis.** A chemical reaction between two chemicals resulting in the addition of a small quantity of a third chemical, the third chemical being called a catalyst.

**catalyst.** A substance effecting catalysis.

**catamenia.** The menstrual period in women; the menses.

**cataphora.** A state of coma punctuated by brief lucid intervals.

**cataphoresis.** The diffusion of electrically charged drugs through the skin or mucous membrane.

**cataphoretic.** Relating to cataphoresis.

**cataphoria.** The condition in which the visual axis of each eye tends to incline below the horizontal plane.

**cataplasm.** A poultice.

**cataract.** The milky opacity of the lens of the eye or of its capsule, which oc-

curs either in old people as evidence of age or in others from disease. It is one of the commonest causes of poor vision or blindness in elderly people, and it was at one time thought that a cataract could not be removed surgically until it was so-called "ripe." This was proved untrue, and today surgeons like to remove a cataract before vision has diminished beyond recovery. To leave a cataract to the last possible moment results in the patient having poor vision even after it has been removed, whereas early removal and the wearing of adequate spectacles preserves the eyesight.

**cataract extraction.** The surgical removal of a cataract.

**catarrh.** Mild inflammation of a mucous membrane. Medically speaking, this refers to any mucous membrane in the body, but popularly refers to nasal or bronchial catarrh.

**bronchial catarrh.** Bronchial catarrh may be caused or maintained by nasal catarrh dropping down the air passages into the lungs. Unquestionably the most potent factor in the production of bronchial catarrh is the inhalation of tobacco smoke, although infection and allergy also play a part. See also NASAL CATARRH, below.

**nasal catarrh.** Before treatment can effectively cure this condition, investigations have to be made to ensure there is no nasal obstruction caused by enlarged adenoids or by a bent and twisted nasal septum. X-rays need to be taken of the nasal sinuses, because if one is blocked and infected its constant contribution of sepsis to the nose maintains the catarrhal state. It also has to be established whether hay fever, allergic rhinitis, or any allergy is present, because until the allergic factor has been dealt with the catarrh cannot be cured. If allergy, infection, and nasal obstruction can be excluded then tremendous improvement can be obtained by using an alkaline nasal douche or sniff prepared by adding one teaspoonful of bicarbonate of soda and one teaspoonful of ordinary salt to a pint of water. The solution, which is used three times a day over a period of many weeks or months, can produce dramatic results. It is sufficiently harmless to be used even in children. The common use of very powerful oily nasal drops to shrink the swollen lining of the nose is to be deprecated, because after the initial shrinkage the drops encourage a much worse swelling of the lining and paralyze the cilia in the nose. These cilia are minute hairlike roots, which protrude from the cells of the membrane lining the nose into the nasal cavity. They move in an orderly direction, removing particles of dust and debris, playing a useful and important part in maintaining a healthy nose. Therefore it is not in the interest of the patient to paralyze them with powerful nasal drops. The use of oily nasal drops is further deprecated because there is a risk that the oil may get into the lungs and set up oil pneumonia. Nasal drops should therefore be in a watery base. See also AIR POLLUTION; BRONCHITIS.

**catarrhal.** Pertaining to catarrh.

**catarrhal fever.** An old-fashioned term for the common cold.

**catatonia.** A symptom of mental illness, usually schizophrenia, in which limbs are retained in a posture for long periods. For instance, if the patient's arm is placed above his head he will keep it there for a period which in a normal person would be impossible owing to fatigue and pain. Also called *catatony.*

**catatonic.** Pertaining to catatonia.

**catechu.** A powerful astringent derived from a plant, used in medicines in conjunction with prepared chalk as a treatment for diarrhea.

**catgut.** A substance made from the intestines of sheep and other animals. It is used for stitching up inside the body or as a ligature around blood vessels. In time catgut is absorbed by the body.

**catharsis.** 1. Purgation; effecting an evacuation of the bowels by a cathartic medicine. 2. In psychoanalysis it refers to the elimination of worry or anxiety by bringing it from the subconscious mind to the conscious mind where it can be faced and dealt with more logically.

**catheter.** A hollow tube made of rubber or gum elastic used for passing into a body canal or opening to effect drainage. The commonest type is that introduced through the urethra for draining the bladder of urine in cases of urinary obstruction.

**catheterization.** The passing of a catheter.

**cathode.** The negative electrode in an x-ray tube, from which x-rays emerge.

**cat-scratch fever.** An illness characterized by enlarged glands, skin rash, and general systemic disturbances, occurring 7 to 14 days after a person receives a cat scratch. No infecting agent has been identified, but a virus is suspect.

**cauda.** A tail or termination.

**cauda equina.** The group of nerve roots which resemble a horse's tail and is found in the lower part of the spinal column.

**caudal.** Relating to a cauda.

**caudate.** Having or resembling a tail.

**caul.** Part of the amnion that sometimes covers the baby's head at birth. These membranes are considered by superstitious seamen to be a source of great luck, and an effective protection against drowning.

**causalgia.** The burning pain sometimes present in injuries of the sensory nerves, particularly those nerves supplying sensation to the skin of the palms of the hands and soles of the feet, and sometimes associated with changes in the tissues of the hands and feet. It has also been loosely used to explain the symptoms that arise in the so-called "phantom limb."

**caustic.** A chemical which burns away tissues.

**cauterize.** To burn with a cautery or caustic chemical.

**cautery.** An instrument for destroying tissue by burning, usually operated by electricity which heats a platinum loop to a dull red.

**cava.** 1. Any body cavity. 2. Either of the large veins which open into the right atrium of the heart: the superior vena cava drains blood from the head and neck towards the heart, and the inferior vena cava brings blood from the trunk and limbs towards the heart. These veins are the largest in the body.

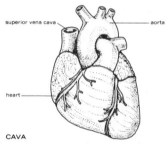

superior vena cava — aorta

heart —

CAVA

**cavernoma.** A tumor composed of large vessels, usually blood vessels. Also called *cavernous angioma.*

**cavernous.** Containing hollow spaces.

**cavernous sinus syndrome.** Paralysis of the muscles supplied by the third, fourth, and sixth cranial nerves. The paralysis is due to thrombosis of the cavernous sinus (a widened blood vessel at the base of the brain).

**cavitation.** The formation of cavities.

**cavity.** 1. Any hole or hollow space. 2. In dentistry, a hole in a tooth made by caries.

**abdominal cavity.** The space between the diaphragm and the pelvis containing the abdominal organs.

**amniotic cavity.** The fluid-filled cavity within which the unborn baby lies.

**cerebral cavities.** The spaces within the brain filled with cerebrospinal fluid. Also called *ventricles.*

**cranial cavity.** The total space within the skull holding the brain and its membranes.

**glenoid cavity.** The hollow in the scapula into which the humerus bone fits.

**nasal cavity.** The space in the head behind the nostrils.

**oral cavity.** The space in the mouth.

**pelvic cavity.** A cavity within the pelvis.

**pericardial cavity.** A cavity between the heart and the membranous sac surrounding it.

**peritoneal cavity.** The potential space between the membrane enveloping certain abdominal organs and that lining the inside of the abdominal cavity.

**pleural cavity.** The potential space between the membrane enveloping the lungs and that lining the inside of the chest.

**serous cavity.** Any cavity lined by serous membrane, such as the peritoneal and pleural cavities.

**thoracic cavity.** The space containing the heart and lungs.

**tympanic cavity.** The cavity of the middle ear located behind the eardrum containing three vibrating ear bones, which transmit sounds to the internal ear. It communicates with the postnasal space by means of the Eustachian tube. Also called *cavum tympani, tympanum.*

**cecal.** Relating to the cecum.

**cecostomy.** An operation to establish a communication between the surface of the abdomen and the cecum so that the intestinal contents will emerge through the abdominal outlet, not through the anus.

**cecum.** The blind pouch which lies in the right lower region of the abdomen (the right inguinal area or right iliac fossa). The ascending colon commences at the top of the cecum and at its lower end is the insertion of the small intestine, the appendix being attached close to this. In man, the cecum, which is about three inches long and of the same diameter, is of no importance, but in herbivorous animals, which depend on a large intake of vegetable material, the cecum is very large and is associated with the digestion of cellulose.

**celiac.** Relating to the abdomen.

**celiac disease.** A disease of childhood in which the child is born with a defect in its digestive processes which prevents absorption of fat and calcium from the diet. The child produces bulky greyish stools containing an abnormal amount of fat, has a general wasting of the body, a pot belly, porous bones, and retardation of growth. In the past celiac disease was treated with curious diets of apple or banana pulp, but dramatic results are now achieved by injections of crude liver extract and large doses of vitamin B, together with a gluten-free diet. Also called *Gee's disease, Heuber-Herter's disease, intestinal infantilism.* See also SPRUE: NON-TROPICAL SPRUE.

**celiotomy.** See VENTROTOMY.

**cell.** The ultimate unit of animal and plant structure.

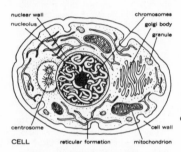

CELL

**cellular.** Composed of cells.

**cellulitis.** Widespread inflammation, especially of tissues that lie beneath the level of the skin.

**cellulose.** The substance that forms the cell walls in plants.

**centesis.** The act of puncturing or perforating.

**centigrade.** A description applied to anything divided into a hundred parts, but usually to the centigrade scale of temperature. The centigrade thermometer is divided into 100 degrees with zero as the freezing point of ice and 100 as the boiling point of water. It is also known as Celsius's thermometer after the Swedish astronomer who introduced it in the early 1700s. See also THERMOMETER: CENTIGRADE THERMOMETER.

**centipetal.** Traveling towards the center; the opposite of centrifugal.

**cephalad.** Towards the head.

**cephalalgia.** Pain in the head; headache.

**cephalhaematoma.** See CEPHALHEMATOMA.

**cephalhematoma.** A collection of blood found beneath the scalp, usually the scalp of a newborn baby, due to pressure during birth.

**cephalic.** Pertaining to the head.

**cephalohydrocele.** A collection of cerebrospinal fluid situated beneath the scalp, which can only arise in cases of fracture of the skull with a wound leading to the spaces of the brain occupied by cerebrospinal fluid.

**cera.** Beeswax.

**ceraceous.** Waxy; like wax.

**cerebellar.** Relating to the cerebellum.

**cerebellum.** The back portion of the brain. It controls muscular coordination and equilibrium. Also called *little brain.* See also BRAIN.

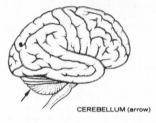

CEREBELLUM (arrow)

**cerebral hemorrhage.** Cerebral hemorrhage is caused by a blood vessel bursting in the brain. The absence of any suggestion of accident gives a clue, because a stroke may occur while the patient, usually an elderly or middle-aged person, is in bed or sitting in a chair. His face is red, breathing noisy, and he may be paralyzed down one side of his body. Treat by placing in propped-up sitting position, remove dentures, and seek medical aid. Also called *stroke.*

**cerebral thrombosis.** A clot in a blood vessel in the brain. Also called *stroke.*

**cerebration.** Mental activity.

**cerebrospinal.** Pertaining to the brain and spinal cord.

**cerebrospinal fluid.** The clear colorless liquid occupying the space between the arachnoid and pia mater membranes of the brain. The fluid, manufactured by the choroid plexuses inside the brain ventricles, serves as a buffer for the central nervous system, and as a means for the exchange of food to the nervous system. Its normal constitution varies in the presence of certain brain diseases and is of the utmost diagnostic significance when removed by lumbar puncture. It would be almost impossible to make a correct diagnosis of brain disease or injury without performing lumbar puncture, which determines not only the pressure of the fluid but also the presence of germs and other chemical variations.

**cerebrospinal fever.** See BRAIN FEVER.

**cerebrum.** The front and main part of the brain. See also BRAIN.

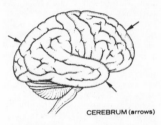

CEREBRUM (arrows)

**cerumen.** The wax secreted in the ear. See EAR WAX.

**cervical.** Pertaining to the neck, to the neck of the womb, or to a necklike structure.

**cervicitis.** Inflammation of the cervix uteri.

**cervico-axillary.** Pertaining to the neck and armpit.

**cervicobrachial.** Pertaining to the neck and the arm.

**cervicodorsal.** Pertaining to the neck and the back.

**cervicofacial.** Pertaining to the neck and the face.

**cervicohumeral.** Pertaining to the neck and the upper arm.

**cervico-occipital.** Pertaining to the neck and the back of the head.

**cervicoplasty.** Plastic surgery of the neck.

**cervicoscapular.** Pertaining to the neck and the shoulder blade.

**cervicothoracic.** Pertaining to the neck and the thorax.

**cervicovaginal.** Pertaining to the neck of the womb and the vagina.

**cervix.** The neck.

**cervix uteri.** The neck of the womb. It is frequently referred to as the cervix without qualification.

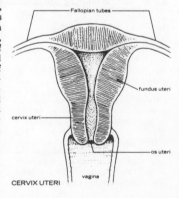

CERVIX UTERI

**cervix vesicae.** The neck of the urinary bladder.

**cesarean section.** The operation by which a baby is removed from the mother's abdomen instead of being born naturally.

*The operation derives its name from the allegation that Julius Caesar was the first known human being delivered by this method. The story is untrue, but originated from the Caesarean law that on the death of a pregnant woman the baby must be removed from the womb before her body was buried. Legend also attributes Aesculapius to be the first god to be born in this manner.*

**Cestoda.** A class of flatworms to which tapeworms belong.

**cetrimide.** A detergent and antiseptic chemical.

**Ceylon sickness.** Beriberi, a disease due to a deficiency of vitamin B in the diet.

**Chagas' disease.** A grave disease, usually affecting children, found in Brazil and caused by a protozoan parasite transmitted to man by the bite of certain types of bugs. Also called *South American trypanosomiasis.*

**chalazion.** A cyst of the meibomian glands in the eyelid. See MEIBOMIAN CYST.

**chalicosis.** See SILICOSIS.

**chancre.** The primary ulcer produced by an attack of syphilis.

**chancroid.** A soft venereal sore that appears in a similar situation to a syphilitic chancre but is not syphilitic in origin.

**chancroidal.** Relating to chancroid.

**chancrous.** Chancrelike.

**change of life.** Also called *climacteric.* See MENOPAUSE.

**chapped hands.** The cracking or roughening of the skin produced by cold and moisture. Some people are more prone to this condition than others, and in these either the skin is deficient in grease or the hands are constantly in contact with degreasing agents, such as washing detergents, soda, petroleum products, oven cleaners, washing-up liquids, paraffin, cement, lime, and garden fertilizers. Drying the hands carefully after washing, the wearing of protective gloves, the use of barrier creams, and the replacement of the lost grease in the skin by rubbing in olive oil every night all help to keep this condition at bay. Exposure and rough work may produce painful cracks at the ends of the fingers in some people, especially in the winter months. When the cracks have appeared they can be filled with cobbler's wax, durofix, or collodian. The skin must be protected while the cracks are trying to heal. A first-class general hand lotion to be

used after washing the hands is the following: powdered tragacanth 44 grains, tincture of tolu 72 minims, glycerine 5 fluid ounces, water to 20 fluid ounces. A small quantity should be well rubbed into the skin of the hands several times a day.

**Charcot joint disease.** A disease of joints, commonly the knee joint, resulting in internal disorganization of the joint accompanied by swelling and an almost complete absence of pain. It is a manifestation of syphilis.

**Charcot's triad.** A triad of symptoms occurring in disseminated sclerosis consisting of intention tremor, nystagmus, and hesitant type of speech. When present, Charcot's triad is diagnostic of disseminated sclerosis, but rarely is the triad seen except in the later stages.

**chart.** A record on which are put all the relevant details about the patient: temperature, respiration, pulse, and the number of times that the bowels have been open.

**cheek. 1.** The side of the face. **2.** Any rounded prominence, such as the buttock.

**cheesy abscess.** See CASEOUS ABSCESS.

**cheilitis.** Inflammation of the lip.

**cheilosis.** A condition in which ulcers and fissures appear at the angles of the mouth, and due to a deficiency of vitamin B. Both Bemax and Marmite are rich in vitamin B and their addition to the daily diet will effect a cure. Alternatively the patient has to take tablets of vitamin B complex.

**cheiropompholyx.** A skin disease affecting the hands and feet, most commonly the hands, in which masses of minute irritating blisters appear, associated with an intense burning sensation. It can be caused by the fungus that produces athlete's foot. If this is not the cause, then it is due to a highly strung, emotional nervous system and an outside irritating factor to the skin. Calamine lotion is a soothing first-aid measure, but many layers must be put on and not washed off. The patient will also need sedatives to calm the irritable nerves in the skin.

**cheirospasm.** See CHIROSPASM.

**cheloid.** An exaggerated amount of scar tissue, the scar becoming heaped up, hard, and unsightly. See also KELOID.

**chemotherapy.** Treatment of disease with chemicals—that is, medication. When the term was first introduced it applied only to infectious diseases but is now used for all illnesses.

**cheromania.** A mental disorder characterized by excessive cheerfulness.

**cherophobia.** The fear of rejoicing or pleasure.

**chest.** See THORAX.

**Cheyne-Stokes asthma.** See ASTHMA: CARDIAC ASTHMA.

**chiasma.** A crossing. Also called *chiasm.*

**optic chiasma.** The junction of the nerves to the eyes, the optic nerves, where the nerve fibers from the nasal half of each retina cross and join the optic nerve of the opposite side. Thus in disease of one half of the brain there may be blindness affecting half of the retina of not only the eye on the same side but also on the opposite side.

**chiasma syndrome.** Impaired vision, headache, giddiness, and limitation of the visual fields due to a lesion in the optic chiasma.

**chickenpox.** Chickenpox is a contagious infection, principally of children, usually mild in course and characterized by a papular rash and slight elevation of temperature. The incubation period is from 10 to 14 days, but may be as long as 23 days. The rash is composed of spots, each spot being a small pink papule that later develops a blister on top. The spots first appear on the trunk, soon spreading to the face, scalp, and the upper part of the limbs. Occasionally they invade the mucous membranes, painful spots being formed inside the mouth, on the back of the throat, and even in the eye. Frequently the rash appears as crops of a few spots over a period of several days, but it may cover the whole back and front of the trunk. Treatment in most cases consists of liberally dabbing the rash with calamine lotion every four hours (avoiding the eyes and mouth) to build up a crust to protect the spots from infection, thus lessening the risk of scarring. The rash should not be washed, and children must be prevented from picking the scabs off the spots or this may result in permanent scarring. The course of the disease is from one to three weeks, the child being free from infection when the scabs dry and fall off. Also called *varicella.*

*Caused by a virus, the disease is universally prevalent and highly infectious but in most cases is not very severe. There are also two rare forms: one in which the skin becomes gangrenous and which may be fatal to severely debilitated children, and the even rarer hemorrhagic form, in which the blisters fill with blood. However, many doctors with 30 or 40 years of experience have never seen these rare forms and only know about them from medical textbooks. Chickenpox is usually spread by droplet spray from coughing and sneezing but can be communicated by a patient's clothing, which may remain infectious for a considerable period, or by the dried scabs of the spots, which probably become powdered, wafted into the air, and inhaled. The disease can also be carried by a healthy intermediary. The rash is very much like that of smallpox, except in distribution. The smallpox rash always comes out primarily on face, hands, and feet, whereas the rash of chickenpox first appears on the trunk. Chickenpox is mainly a disease of childhood, and is uncommon after the age of ten years, but adults, even of advanced years, may contract it and infants are not completely immune. One attack usually affords complete protection, second attacks being extremely rare. Convalescents from diseases such as measles and scarlet fever are especially liable to contract chickenpox. There is a strong association between the disease and herpes zoster or shingles. The elderly person in contact with chickenpox may develop shingles and, conversely, a case of shingles may provide the virus which gives a child chickenpox. Therefore it is important when children have chickenpox to keep elderly relatives away from the house until the child is cured. Shingles can be a very severe disease and extremely painful for elderly people to endure.*

**chigger.** A sand flea of tropical countries, which causes chigger disease, a condition in which the female chigger burrows into the skin of the feet and legs to lay its eggs, causing irritation and, if not treated, ulceration. Also called *chigoe.*

**chilblain.** A red, swollen, irritating area usually localized to those parts of the body at the ends of the circulation, such as the heels, the back of the calves, and the flap of the ear. Chilblains are in effect areas of paralyzed or sluggish circulation—hence their congested appearance. Since chilblains are caused or aggravated by cold and damp, every effort should be made to avoid or remove these two possible causes. Suitable clothing should be worn to keep the circulation warm and active, standing on cold surfaces such as tiled or concrete floors should be avoided, and so should sedentary occupations. Tight garters, tight elastic in the legs of children's knickers, overtight shoes or stockings, and any constriction that tends to slow the circulation should be removed, and every effort should be made to stimulate the circulation by vigorous exercise. Numerous remedies have been advocated, from thyroid tablets, calcium tablets, and large doses of vitamin $D_2$, down to tablets of nicotinamide, which dilate the peripheral circulation. No one treatment works in all cases. In mild cases of early chilblain formation a lot can be done by rubbing the chilblains with lotion if ulceration has not

started. An old-fashioned treatment that works in some cases of early chilblains is to place the hands or feet into a bowl of lukewarm water and then add boiling water until the water in the bowl is as hot as the patient can tolerate. This dilates the circulation and may help to stop or reverse the stagnation in the chilblain. Also called *pernio.*

**childbed fever.** A severe form of blood poisoning, caused by a streptococcal germ, occurring in women following childbirth, and promptly cured by antibiotics. It was at one time called milk fever because it occurred two or three days after delivery and about the time that the breasts became engorged with milk. In the past the disease killed tens of thousands of mothers, and it was not until 1847-49, when Dr. Semmelweis of Vienna made his observations, that its true nature was recognized. Semmelweis was appointed to the Lying-in Hospital in Vienna, which was divided into two halves; in one half the mothers were delivered by nurses and midwives, and in the other half by medical students. Semmelweis noticed that the death rate in mothers delivered by the students was much greater than in those delivered by the midwives and he came to the conclusion that the students, who were also attending the post-mortem room to study the causes of death among corpses, were transmitting something of an unknown nature to the labor wards. Semmelweis therefore installed, outside the post-mortem room, a bath of bleaching powder solution in which the students had to rinse their hands before leaving, and from then on the death rate from childbed fever became equal in both halves of the hospital. His observations were received with scorn by the medical profession at the time. Also called *puerperal fever.*

**chill.** A feeling of cold and the shivering that occurs with a fever. There is no medical word which is more popularly used and with less scientific reason. Almost the first thing that most patients blame for whatever is wrong with them is "catching a chill." It all harks back to the Middle Ages when there was no scientific explanation for disease and no knowledge of their infective origin from bacteria and viruses; thus the cold feeling experienced with the arrival of a raised temperature not only became a symptom, it also became the pathological explanation. It is true that being subjected to chilling conditions, such as standing in a cold draft, may temporarily lower the resistance of the body, so that germs, already present in the body,

find an opportunity to attack and cause illness. In most cases this popular expression really means that the person has contracted a cold in the head.

**chiropodist.** One who treats corns, bunions, and nail disorders of the hands and feet.

**chiropractic.** A system of treatment based on the conception that all disease is due to defects in the central nervous system, which it is alleged can be cured by spinal manipulation.

**chiropractor.** A practitioner of chiropractic.

**chirospasm.** Writer's cramp. See NEUROSIS: OCCUPATIONAL NEUROSIS.

**chirurgia.** Surgery.

**chirurgical.** Surgical.

**chitin.** The principal substance forming the exoskeletons of invertebrates.

**chloasma.** A condition in which pigment is deposited in the skin in patches of various shapes and sizes and of any color from yellow, brown, to black; often associated with some disorder of the endocrine glands.

**chloasma uterinum.** Pigmented areas occurring on the forehead, temples, cheeks, nipples, and abdomen, which may become more marked during pregnancy or the menstrual periods. It may also occur with tumors or disorders of the ovaries. Also called *chloasma gravidarum.*

**chloral.** A liquid sedative drug. It does not keep indefinitely and in time degenerates into a poisonous substance. It should, therefore, only be used over a period of two or three weeks after it has been dispensed, after which it should be thrown away.

**chloramphenicol.** An antibiotic. Its trade name is Chloromycetin.

**chlorbutol.** A sedative and pain reliever, formerly much used to relieve nausea and vomiting.

**chlorination.** A saturation with chlorine. The process is used in public baths to sterilize the water and in some instances to sterilize drinking water.

**chlorodyne.** A pain-relieving drug containing chloroform, ether, alcohol, and morphia with small quantities of dilute hydrocyanic acid. At one time this drug was popular for the relief of stomach disorders. It should not be given to children except under medical supervision.

**chloroform.** A general anesthetic. Its very much favored these days because of the poisonous effect it can have on the heart muscle.

**chloroma.** A condition mainly affecting children and young people, characterized by a blood disorder and the appearance of greenish tumors in some bones.

**Chloromycetin.** A brand of chloramphenicol, an antibiotic.

**chlorophyll.** The green pigment used by plants in the process of photosynthesis to manufacture carbohydrates.

**chlorosis.** A disease characterized by iron-deficiency anemia and a greenish-yellow tint to the skin. At one time commonly met with in young women, it is now relatively rare.

**chlorotic.** Relating to chlorosis.

**chloroxylenol.** A powerful and nonirritant bactericide. Dettol belongs to this class of disinfectant.

**choked disc.** See PAPILLEDEMA.

**cholaemia.** See CHOLEMIA.

**cholagogue.** A drug that promotes the flow of bile.

**cholangiectasis.** Dilation of the bile ducts.

**cholangioma.** A tumor arising from the cells of the bile ducts.

**cholangitis.** Inflammation of a bile duct.

**cholecyst.** See GALL BLADDER.

**cholecystectomy.** Surgical removal of the gall bladder.

**cholecystitis.** Inflammation of the gall bladder.

**cholecystogram.** An x-ray film of the gall bladder.

**cholecystography.** The x-ray visualization of the gall bladder by administering drugs which are stored in the gall bladder and opaque to x-rays.

**cholecystolithiasis.** The presence of stones in the gall bladder.

**cholecystopathy.** The presence of any disease in the gall bladder.

**cholecystostomy.** The operation of bringing the gall bladder to the surface of the abdomen so that bile is discharged through the abdominal opening, performed to permit drainage of the gall bladder.

**cholecystotomy.** Surgical incision into the gall bladder.

**choledochectomy.** Surgical incision into the common bile duct.

**choledochitis.** Inflammation of the common bile duct.

**choledocholith.** A stone in the common bile duct.

**choleic.** Relating to the bile.

**cholelithiasis.** The presence of stones in the gall bladder.

**cholelithotomy.** Surgical incision into the gall bladder to remove gallstones.

**cholelithotrity.** The crushing of a gallstone.

**cholemia.** The presence of bile in the blood. It leads to jaundice.

**cholera.** An acute infectious disease caused by the bacterium Vibrio cholerae, and characterized by violent vomiting, profuse diarrhea with the passage of watery stools, severe dehydration, painful muscle cramps, inability to speak, suppression of urine, and collapse. Cholera is nearly always present in Far Eastern countries and travelers to such countries should obtain inoculations against the disease.

**choleraic.** Pertaining to cholera.

**choleric.** A particular type of temperament, the possessor being subject to wild attacks of rage and irritability. In ancient times it was thought such people possessed or made too much bile. Hence the term choleric from the Greek khole, meaning bile.

**cholerine.** An Asiatic form of cholera of sudden onset, mild course, and rapid recovery.

**cholesteatoma.** 1. A tumor occurring in the ear as a result of chronic middle ear disease and constant purulent discharges. 2. A rare form of brain tumor, arising from remnants of embryonic cells and which can also occur in the spinal cord. Also called pearly tumor.

**cholesterol.** A chemical constituent of all animal fats and oils, and of bile and gallstones. Its presence in the blood in excessive quantities, due to the large intake of dairy products such as butter, milk, and cheese, has been blamed for some cases of coronary thrombosis. For this reason some patients are put on noncholesterol diets, replacing animals fats by vegetable fats such as corn oil and sunflower seed oil. Not all doctors, however, accept that cholesterol in the blood damages the lining of arteries enough to cause coronary thrombosis.

**chololith.** A gallstone.

**cholorrhea.** Excessive secretion of bile.

**cholorrhoea.** See CHOLORRHEA.

**choluria.** The presence of bile pigments in the urine.

**chondral.** Cartilaginous.

**chondralgia.** Pain arising in a cartilage.

**chondritis.** Inflammation of a, cartilage.

**chondroma.** A tumor arising in cartilage.

**chondromalacia.** A softening of the cartilages.

**chondro-osteodystrophy.** A condition of childhood characterized by interference with the growing ends of bone, resulting in disturbances of height and growth. It resembles achondroplasia. Also called Morquio's disease, Brailsford-Morquio's disease.

**chondropathy.** Any disease involving cartilage.

**chondrosis.** Pertaining to the formation of cartilage; a tumor composed of cartilage.

**chorda.** 1. Any cord, tendon, or nerve filament. 2. The notochord, that part of the embryo around which the vertebral column forms.

**chordae tendinae.** Fibrous bands which tether the atrioventricular valves.

**chorda tympani.** A branch of the facial nerve.

**chordee.** An intensely painful and violent erection of the penis, the result of irritating inflammatory processes near that organ.

**chorditis.** Inflammation of the vocal chords.

**chorea.** Chorea is a disease of the nervous system affecting girls more frequently than boys and characterized by spontaneous, uncontrollable movements, irregular both in time and extent, by muscular weakness, and by a variable degree of emotional disturbance. It is thought to be due to a diffuse inflammatory reaction occurring in the brain and its membranes. The patient becomes nervous and more impressionable, is increasingly unable to concentrate, becomes clumsy in his movements, and lets objects fall from his grasp. Anemia, apathy, languor, and irregularity of appetite are commonly present. There are slight involuntary movements of the face and fingers, often confined at first to one side of the body. Gradually the movements become more marked and spread to the limbs and trunk. The face is constantly grimacing, the hands and arms scarcely cease from turning about, and walking is irregular and clumsy. The child can no longer keep still, and even the breathing movements become irregular and spasmodic. At this stage the chorea is fully developed. There is a close association between this disease and rheumatic fever, in both of which the heart and its valves can be damaged. Also called Sydenham's chorea, rheumatic chorea, St. Vitus's dance. See also HUNTINGTON'S CHOREA.

Some 500 years ago there developed in Europe a form of semireligious hysterical compulsion to dance madly about until utter physical and emotional exhaustion set in. It was believed this dancing mania originated in the town of Tarantula in Italy, from which the tarantula spider also obtained its name. Because of this association of names it was believed that the dance was caused by the bite of the spider, which, of course, does not cause serious poisoning. The music composed for these dancing manias was called the tarantati, which survives today as the tarantella. St. Vitus was adopted as the patron saint of these sufferers, who implored him to stop the wild paroxysms of dancing and mania.

**choreiform.** Resembling chorea.

**chorioadenoma.** A growth developing in the afterbirth tissues. See also CHO-RIONEPITHELIOMA.

**chorioiritis.** Inflammation of the iris and choroid membrane of the eye.

**choriomeningitis.** Nonpurulent meningitis.

**lymphocytic choriomeningitis.** A virus disease of wild mice and possibly dogs which can on occasion be transmitted to man, causing a rare form of meningitis in the absence of any general cause of infection. It is characterized by the rapid onset of symptoms of meningeal irritation and a short, benign course with recovery.

**chorion.** The outermost membrane of the fetal bag, within which the unborn baby lives.

**chorionepithelioma.** A malignant tumor arising from the cells of the chorionic villi (threadlike projection from the chorion), left in the womb after childbirth or abortion.

**chorionic.** Relating to the chorion.

**chorioretinitis.** Inflammation of the choroid and the retina.

**choroid.** The middle membrane of the three which form the eyeball.

**choroiditis.** Inflammation of the choroid membrane of the eye.

**choroid plexus.** A fringelike growth which projects into the cavities of the brain and creates the cerebrospinal fluid.

**Christian-Schüller syndrome.** See SCHÜLLER'S DISEASE.

**chromatosis.** An abnormal pigmentation of the skin.

**chromidrosis.** The production of colored sweat.

**chromosome.** One of the minute bodies within the nucleus of a cell. They carry the characteristics (genes) of the individual. Certain chromosomes determine the sex of the individual. In

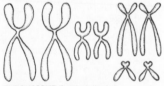

CHROMOSOME (four typical pairs)

man the nucleus of each cell contains 46 chromosomes, two of which are sex chromosomes (described as either X or Y chromosomes) while the remaining 44 are called autosomes. If a fertilized egg contains two X chromosomes it will develop into a female, but should it contain an XY combination it will develop into a male.

**chromosome test.** A test performed to determine the true sex should this be in doubt, as in hermaphrodism, or to discover whether certain congenital defects are liable to be passed on to future offspring. It is a painless procedure in which a few cells are scraped from the inside of the cheek for microscopical examination.

**chronic abscess.** An abscess of slow development with little local inflammatory reaction, usually tuberculous.

**chyle.** The fluid found in the intestinal lymph vessels during absorption. The fluid is white in color owing to its rich content of fat.

**chylocele.** The presence of fatty lymph under the membrane covering the testicle, seen as a result of rupture of lymphatics in elephantiasis.

**chylopericardium.** Chyle in the pericardial cavity.

**chyloperitoneum.** Chyle in the peritoneal cavity of the abdomen.

**chylopoiesis.** The production of chyle.

**chylorrhea.** The excessive production of chyle.

**chylorrhoea.** See CHLORRHEA.

**chylothorax.** An accumulation of chyle in the pleural cavity due to rupture of the thoracic duct.

**chylous.** Pertaining to chyle.

**chyluria.** The presence of chyle in the urine.

**chyme.** Food that has been digested by the stomach but not yet passed into the intestine for intestinal digestion.

**cicatrix.** A scar.

**cicatrization.** The process of healing by scar formation.

**cicatrize.** To heal by scar formation.

**cilia.** 1. The eyelashes. 2. The hairlike projections protruding from the cells of the lining of the upper respiratory tract and which move in a rhythmical pattern to pass on, in a sweeping action, dust, germs, and mucus.

**ciliary body.** A structure within the eyeball which connects the front edge of the choroid membrane to the rim of the iris. It contains the ciliary muscle which alters the shape of the lens and allows the eye to vary its focus between near and far objects.

**ciliary muscle.** The muscle that adjusts the shape of the eye lens enabling the eye to focus between near and far objects.

**cilium.** The singular of cilia.

**cillosis.** Twitching of the eyelid.

**cinchona.** A type of tree whose bark yields quinine.

*One legend records that when Spain was colonizing South America, the wife of a Spanish governor suffered from a disease in which she sweated violently for several days, to a point of exhaustion, and then the symptom re-*

*curred. Eventually her Inca maid begged the governor to allow her uncle to try to cure her mistress. When the maid's uncle arrived he placed some bark in a pot, poured boiling water over it, and then pounded it with a pestle. The liquid was then drunk by the patient, who within a few days was better and within ten days was cured. A Jesuit priest, impressed by this cure, ordered vast quantities of quinine bark to be shipped to Europe. There it was distributed amongst the Jesuit monasteries where it was used to treat malaria and was called the "Jesuit Bark."*

**cinnabar.** 1. Red mercuric sulphide. 2. Vermilion.

**cinnamon.** The dried bark of a tree, used as a spice and as a carminative. It had a vogue some years ago as a certain cure for a feverish cold.

**circinate.** Ring-shaped.

**circle of Willis.** See WILLIS'S CIRCLE.

**circulation.** The passing of blood through the heart and blood vessels of the body.

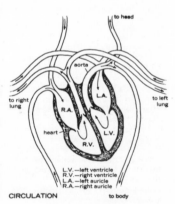

L.V.—left ventricle
R.V.—right ventricle
L.A.—left auricle
R.A.—right auricle

CIRCULATION

**fetal circulation.** The circulation of blood in the unborn baby through the umbilical cord and the placenta.

**portal circulation.** The vessels which carry blood between the intestines and the liver.

**pulmonary circulation.** The circulation of blood in the lungs.

**systemic circulation.** The circulation of blood in the body, with the exception of the pulmonary circulation.

**circumcision.** The removal of the foreskin, or prepuce, at the end of the penis. Originating as a religious rite of the Jews, the operation is now performed on many non-Jewish children to prevent infection.

**circumscribed.** Clearly defined or limited.

**circumtonsillar abscess.** See PERITONSILLAR ABSCESS.

**cirrhosis.** A disease of the liver characterized by destruction, irregular regeneration, and fibrosis of the liver substance. It ultimately leads to portal obstruction and ascites.

**cirrhotic.** Relating to cirrhosis.

**citrate.** Any salt of citric acid. Citrates taken internally neutralize the acid of the urine and make it alkaline. This brings great comfort to the patient suffering from inflammation of the bladder.

**citric acid.** An acid which gives the characteristic taste to lemons and limes.

**claudication.** Lameness or limping.

**intermittent claudication.** Intermittent limping due to the impairment of the arterial circulation in the legs. The poor supply of blood and oxygen to the muscles causes them to go into a cramplike spasm when they are used.

**claustrophobia.** The fear of being in closed spaces.

**clavicle.** The collarbone.

**clavicular.** Relating to the collarbone.

**clavus.** A corn; a horny growth on the skin.

**clawfoot.** See TALIPES.

**clawhand.** A deformity resulting from paralysis and wasting of some of the small muscles of the hand. Also called *main-en-griffe.*

**cleft palate.** Cleft palate and harelip are due to congenital failure of the two halves of the face to unite in the midline, and a baby may be born with one or both conditions. If the defects are severe they may prevent proper feeding, the food regurgitating down the nose instead of being swallowed. Harelip is usually repaired before the baby is three months old or is 10 pounds in weight, whichever happens first; cleft palate is repaired before the child has started to speak, that is, between a year and eighteen months old.

**cleidarthritis.** Inflammation of the sternoclavicular joint.

**cleidocostal.** Pertaining to both the collarbone and ribs.

**cleidocranial.** Pertaining to both the collarbone and skull.

**cleidotomy.** A surgical operation in which both collarbones are divided in the unborn baby in order to narrow the shoulders and permit the baby to be born; used in cases where the width of the baby is causing an obstructed labor.

**climacteric.** Also called *change of life.* See MENOPAUSE.

**clinic.** An institution for the treatment of patients.

**clinical.** 1. Relating to a clinic. 2. Relating to the signs of disease as observed by the doctor.

**clinician.** A doctor who examines and treats patients at the bedside.

**clitoris.** A small structure situated between the smaller lips of the vaginal opening and the remnant of what would become the penis in the male. Friction of the clitoris during sexual intercourse produces sexual orgasm in the female.

**cloaca.** 1. The common canal in the developing embryo into which open the intestines, the reproductive organs, and the urinary ducts. 2. A sinus originating in a diseased bone and opening on to the surface.

**clonic.** Relating to clonus.

**clonus.** The rapid and involuntary contraction and relaxation of opposing muscles, such as flexors and extensors.

**clostridium.** A genus *Clostridium,* of spore-bearing bacteria which grow in the absence of oxygen. Members of this genus of bacteria produce gas gangrene of wounds and tetanus.

**clot.** A semisolid mass, as coagulated blood or lymph.

**clotting.** The forming of a coagulated substance over the ends of broken blood vessel walls. This insures the stoppage of blood flow.

**cloudy swelling.** A degeneration and swelling of the tissues arising during the course of an inflammatory illness.

**clubbing.** A club-shaped deformity of the tips of the fingers or toes seen in long-standing heart and lung disorders.

**clubfoot.** See TALIPES.

**clubhand.** A congenital deformity of the wrist.

**clumping.** Agglutination; sticking together.

**coagulant.** An agent which promotes clotting.

**coagulation.** Clotting.

**coal gas poisoning.** Poisoning by the gas commonly used for heating and cooking. Open all windows and doors to let out the gas, remove the casualty to the fresh air, and administer artificial respiration until a doctor arrives. When sending for an ambulance the message should include an instruction to bring oxygen resuscitation apparatus.

**coarctation.** A narrowing of the caliber of a vessel or canal.

**coarctation of the aorta.** A congenital narrowing of the aorta so that blood pressure is raised on the side nearest the heart. The obstruction may occur between the points where the two arm arteries arise, causing blood pressure in the right arm to be higher than that in the left. The essential diagnostic feature of the condition is that the blood pressure in the upper part of the body is higher than that in the legs.

**coccal.** Relating to cocci.

**cocci.** The plural of coccus.

**coccidioidomycosis.** A disease of the lungs caused by a fungus of the genus *Coccidioides,* and somewhat resembling tuberculosis. Also called *San Joaquin Valley fever, desert fever.*

**coccus.** A round-shaped bacterium.

**coccygeal.** Relating to the coccyx.

**coccygectomy.** Surgical excision of the coccyx.

**coccygodynia.** Pain arising in the coccyx. The pain is worse on sitting and may originate from a heavy fall on to the buttocks or a kick, and it occasionally follows difficult childbirth, when the coccyx can be fractured.

**coccyx.** The bone situated at the end of the spine and between the buttocks. It is the remnant of the tailbone.

**cochlea.** The small structure shaped like a snail shell which is the fundamental organ of hearing.

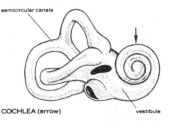

COCHLEA (arrow)

**codeine.** A drug derived from morphine, codeine has some pain-relieving qualities but is used largely to suppress a cough, and because of its constipating effect for allaying the irritable intestine in colitis.

**coeliac.** See CELIAC.

**coffee-ground vomit.** Aptly describes vomit from a patient who has had bleeding into the stomach, the blood having remained there long enough to be altered by the digestive juices. See also BLACK VOMIT.

**cogwheel breathing.** A form of jerky respiration usually seen in a neurotic person. See also RESPIRATION.

**cohabitation.** Literally the living together of a man and a woman, but in legal circles the term indicates that a couple is living together as man and wife without legal sanctions.

**cohere.** To stick together.

**coherent.** To be consistent, precise, clear, and logical in speech.

**coitus.** Sexual intercourse.

**coitus interruptus.** The attempt to achieve contraception by the male withdrawing prior to his reaching a sexual peak or orgasm. It is an unreliable method because during the period of sexual excitement prior to male orgasm the prostrate gland liberates a clear fluid which acts both as a lubricant and a nutrient medium in which the male cells can survive on their journey through the womb and into a Fallopian tube. It is possible for a male cell or sperm to escape in this fluid and fertilize the female cell or egg prior to the male's main ejaculation. This fact is the basis of many court cases in which the male denies paternity, because he is certain that although he had penetration he did not have an ejaculation.

**colchicine.** An alkaloid derived from colchicum, and the standard remedy for acute gout. A solution of colchicine is used in horticulture to promote root formation in plant cuttings.

**colchicum.** A drug obtained from the meadow saffron and used in the treatment of gout.

**cold.** The popular name for coryza or catarrh of the upper respiratory tract. It is caused by a virus. It has been stated, not without a core of truth, that without treatment a cold lasts two weeks and with treatment it lasts 14 days. Proprietary cold "cures" are largely useless, and so are antibiotics, vitamin C, quinine, cinnamon, and the like. Medical treatment consists of lessening the symptoms with belladonna to dry up the secretions, ephedrine nasal drops to shrink the membranes, and aspirin to reduce the fever.

**cold abscess.** See CHRONIC ABSCESS.

**cold sore.** A form of herpes. Believed to be due to a virus which inhabits the skin, these so-called cold sores occur as blisters around. the mouth and ultimately become crusted ulcers. Frequent applications of surgical spirit, followed by an antibiotic cream, help to heal them. The antibiotic may have to be applied to the nostrils at the same time, as frequently the germ also inhibits the nose. Success in the prevention of cold sores has been obtained by repeatedly vaccinating the individual against smallpox once a week for several weeks. No real explanation has been found as to why this treatment is successful, but in many cases it does work. Also called *herpes labialis.*

**colectomy.** Surgical removal of a part or the whole of the colon.

**coli.** Relating to the colon.

**Bacterium coli.** The microorganism which normally inhabits the large intestine. In this situation it is harmless

but if it migrates to other regions it sets up violent inflammation. For instance, if it invades the urinary tract it sets up cystitis.

**colic.** Relating to the colon; a griping pain in the abdomen.

**biliary colic.** The violent pain produced in the gall bladder by gallstones.

**lead colic.** Colic due to lead poisoning.

**renal colic.** Colic due to the presence of stones in the kidney or ureter.

**colitis.** Inflammation of the colon.

**mucous colitis.** In this condition the patient passes many stools a day, often accompanied by pain. The stools contain large shreds of mucus, sometimes even tubular shreds representing complete casts of the inside of the colon. This type often occurs in emotional, nervous people.

**ulcerative colitis.** Colitis characterized by ulceration and inflammation of the lining of the intestine. The patient passes numerous stools each day, mostly containing blood in obvious form, pus, and mucus. It is a serious disease leading to generalized loss of weight and severe anemia.

**collagen.** A constituent of the fibrous tissue in the body.

**collagen diseases.** A group of disorders which have in common a general disturbance of the connective tissues in the body. Included in this group are: rheumatic fever, rheumatoid arthritis, polyarteritis nodosa, disseminated lupus erythematosus, generalized scleroderma, and dermatomyositis. All these conditions show in different degree changes in the body's connective tissue including degeneration of collagen, excessive deposition of collagen, increase in altered ground substance to the tissues, proliferation of connective tissue with or without degenerative change, and inflammatory cell infiltration. All collagen diseases have much in common and there are many which cannot be designated but form a transitional picture between the various disorders listed. In some cases the disease is considered to be due to an allergic reaction to a germ poison. Temporal arteritis probably belongs to this group.

**collapse.** 1. Emotional or surgical shock. 2. The retraction of an organ.

**collar-stud abscess.** An abscess erupting on the surface but connected by a sinus with a deeper infection.

**Colles' fracture.** A fracture of the wrist in which the deformity of the bones gives the wrist and hand an appearance closely resembling a dinner fork. If the deformity is in the reverse direction it is called a Smith's fracture.

**collodion.** A flexible cellulose plastic varnish, often used to seal small cuts.

**colloid.** A homogeneous gelatinlike substance consisting of large molecules or groups of small molecules dispersed in another medium. An example is a solid dispersed in a liquid as in protoplasm. Colloids are not true solutions, hence cannot pass through semipermeable cell membranes.

**collunarium.** A nasal douche.

**collutorium.** A mouthwash or gargle. Also called *collutory.*

**collyrium.** An eye lotion.

**coloboma.** The congenital defect of any portion of the eye, especially a fissure.

**colocynth.** A drug derived from a plant and used as a purgative.

**colon.** That part of the large intestine extending from the cecum to the rectum. It is about five feet long and consists of the ascending colon, transverse colon, descending colon, iliac colon, and sigmoid colon, in that order.

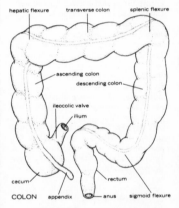

hepatic flexure    transverse colon    splenic flexure

ascending colon

descending colon

ileocolic valve

ilium

cecum

rectum

COLON    appendix    anus    sigmoid flexure

**color blindness.** The inability to recognize various colors. It is of importance when the individual is unable to distinguish between red and green, especially in these days of traffic lights. This type of color defect is called "color defective unsafe." There are many minor kinds of color defect which are of no practical importance.

**color index.** The term used to describe the amount of hemoglobin in the red blood cells.

**colostomy.** The surgical manufacture of an artificial anus by bringing the colon out onto the abdominal wall.

**colostrum.** A thin, white fluid; the first milk expressed from the mother's breasts during the two or three days after giving birth and before normal lactation begins.

**colour blindness.** See COLOR BLINDNESS.

**colour index.** See COLOR INDEX.

**colpitis.** Inflammation of the vagina.

**colpocele.** A hernia protruding into the vagina.

**colpocystocele.** Protrusion of the urinary bladder into the vagina.

**colphysterectomy.** Surgical removal of the womb via the vagina.

**colpoperineorrhaphy.** Repair of the vagina and perineal opening of the vagina.

**colpoplasty.** Surgical repair to the vagina.

**colpoptosis.** Prolapse of the vaginal walls.

**colporrhaphy.** A surgical operation for narrowing the vagina.

**colposcope.** An instrument for examining the vagina.

**coma.** A state of absolute unconsciousness. Partial unconsciousness is called stupor. If the casualty responds to a shouted question, providing he is not deaf, he is in stupor; if there is no response he may be in coma, fainting, hysterical, or dead. If the eyelids are retracted and flutter or resist being opened the casualty is in stupor. If the pupils contract when a torch is shined into the eyes and dilate when the light is turned off, the casualty is in stupor; in coma, the pupils are unresponsive to light, and if the coma is very deep they may be widely dilated as well as unresponsive. *First aid for the unconscious.* Remove any dentures and ensure there is no obstruction to the breathing. Slightly raise the shoulders and keep the head turned to one side in case the patient should vomit. If the breathing is noisy and sounds as though water is bubbling in the chest, place him half on his front and half on his side. Cover him with a blanket but do not warm with a hot-water bottle. Do not give anything to drink or he may choke, and do not leave him unattended but send for a doctor.

**diabetic coma.** The carbohydrate and fat in our food have to be broken down by digestion into a form in which the body can use them, and since they work together one cannot be digested without the other being present. In diabetes the pancreas fails to produce insulin, which controls carbohydrate metabolism, and so carbohydrate builds up to high levels in the blood in the form of glucose. At the same time fat is not properly broken down and leaves in the blood hydrobutyric acid, which, with other chemicals, acts as an anesthetic on the brain and produces diabetic coma. When diagnosed, diabetes is treated either by diet alone or by diet and injections of insulin, or by tablets. In diabetic coma the casualty is quiet and appears to be asleep,

and his breath may smell of acetone. He is in urgent need of insulin and should be removed to a hospital as quickly as possible. See also DIABETES.

**insulin coma.** If the diabetic does not eat he is therefore getting too much insulin, the effect of which is to completely empty his bloodstream of sugar, causing what is called insulin coma. This type of coma varies in intensity from mild confusion to complete coma. The patient sweats, his breath does not smell of acetone and for a time he may be excitable. Treatment consists of feeding him sugar and water before consciousness is lost, and if given in time recovery will be dramatic and rapid. Most of these patients carry a card stating that they are diabetic and they usually carry some lump sugar, often found in the waistcoat pocket of a man. A further indication of a diabetic are the pin-prick marks on the forearms or tops of the thighs caused by insulin injections. However, a doctor should be sent for or the patient removed to hospital. Also called *hypoglycemic attack, insulin reaction.* See also DIABETES.

**comatose.** In a state of coma.

**combined degeneration of the cord.** A form of paralysis of the arms or legs, usually the legs, occurring in pernicious anemia and curable by injections of vitamin $B_{12}$.

**comedo.** A plug of dried secretion in a sebaceous gland of the skin. Also called BLACKHEAD. See also ACNE.

**comminuted.** Broken into more than two pieces.

**comminution.** The process of breaking into little pieces.

**commissure.** A band of fibers joining corresponding opposite parts.

**communicable.** Capable of being transmitted.

**compatible, compatibility.** Usually refers to two drugs that can be mixed together safely without one canceling out or enhancing the effect of the other. To know which drugs are chemically compatible is of enormous importance when prescribing medicine, for the mixing of two drugs may start a chemical activity that will precipitate a powerful drug reaction at the bottom of the bottle so that the last dose contains a dangerous concentration.

**compensatory.** Effecting a condition of compensation.

**complement.** A complex substance found in the blood plasma, which, with the assistance of an antibody, destroys germs and other foreign substances.

**complemental, complementary.** Supplying a deficiency.

**complemental colors.** Any two colors of the spectrum which combine to produce white light.

**complemental space.** The lowest part of the chest cavity, which only becomes filled with the lungs on deep inspiration.

**complex.** A group of symptoms and signs which form a disease syndrome; a group of ideas or fears transferred from the conscious mind to the subconscious mind and which influence the behavior and personality of the individual.

**anxiety complex.** A form of neurosis characterized by fear and apprehension at the outcome of any situation; a morbid attitude to personal health and a constant feeling of impending disaster.

**electra complex.** A similar condition to the Oedipus complex, but in this case the attraction is between a daughter and her father.

**father complex.** See ELECTRA COMPLEX, above.

**inferiority complex.** An emotional conviction of inadequacy, real or imaginary, associated with depression and neurosis.

**mother complex.** Oedipus complex.

**Oedipus complex.** Sexual obsession by a son for his mother accompanied by resentment and aggression towards the father. Also called *mother complex.*

**superiority complex.** Exaggerated aggressiveness. This may be a manifestation of the onset of mania or a compensation attitude adopted to overcome a sense of inferiority due to failure to succeed, lack of education, or to physical shortcomings such as lack of height.

**component.** An ingredient of a mixture.

**compos mentis.** Of sound mind; sane.

**compound.** To mix, as in manufacturing a medicine or ointment.

**comprehension.** The ability to understand.

**compress.** A soft pad, usually of cloth, used as a means of applying pressure, moisture, cold, heat, or medication.

**compressed-air sickness.** Caisson disease.

**compression syndrome.** The liberation into the bloodstream, by severe crush injuries, of chemicals which affect the kidneys and produce profound symptoms of surgical shock. Also called *crush syndrome.*

**concave.** With a surface hollowed out.

**concavity.** A depression.

**concavo-concave.** Hollowed out on both sides.

**concavo-convex.** One side hollowed out and the other side rounded.

concentration. 1. The proportion of a substance dissolved in a liquid; the act of increasing the proportion of a substance in a liquid. 2. The ability to fix the attention.

concentration test. A kidney function test.

concentric. Circles having a common center.

conception. 1. An idea. 2. Fertilization of the ovum or egg by the sperm.

concha. The Latin for shell and descriptive of the appearance of the external ear. Any structure resembling a shell.

concomitant. Going with, accompanying.

concretion. A stone or calculus.

concubitus. Sexual intercourse.

concussion. Following a blow on the skull, the brain may be so rocked about that concussion results. It may last a few minutes or days, and the first sign of recovery is often an attack of vomiting. On becoming conscious the casualty may suffer from loss of memory and be unable to recall either the blow or how he arrived in his present position. Following recovery he may suffer with postconcussional headaches, which may persist for many months; in severe cases there may follow a change of personality—a happy man becoming quiet and moody. However, if the only brain damage is concussion and a general shaking-up, the patient gradually recovers. If there has been more severe damage, such as bleeding into the skull or brain laceration, blood collects and presses on the brain, producing cerebral compression. Concussion may pass into compression without the casualty regaining consciousness, and sometimes he may come around from concussion and then slip into coma from the late onset of compression. The concussion case is quiet and appears to be just deeply asleep, but when compression sets in the whole picture changes. The patient becomes deeply unconscious, red-faced, breathes noisily, and has a slow, bounding pulse. The pupils of his eyes may be unequal or widely dilated and not react to light. If, however, the bleeding has been only slight and stops spontaneously the casualty may show none of these signs, and since some people are born with unequal pupils this sign can sometimes be misleading. In either case the patient should be kept at rest in a propped-up sitting position, dentures should be removed, and medical aid should be summoned.

conditioned reflex. A reflex action artificially induced. For example: if every time a dog is given food a bell is rung simultaneously, the dog comes to associate the sound of the bell with food, and since the dog normally salivates in anticipation of food eventually it will salivate at the sound of the bell alone. This is a conditioned reflex.

condom. A thin sheath, often of rubber, worn over the penis during coitus for the purpose of preventing conception and transmission of infection.

Condy's fluid. A solution of permanganate of potash used as a disinfectant, and named after a nineteenth-century English physician.

condylar. Relating to a condyle.

condyle. A rounded knob of bone, usually part of a joint.

condylectomy. Surgical removal of a condyle.

condyloid. Pertaining to a condyle.

condyloma. A wartlike growth or tumor which usually arises near the anus or around the genitals.

condyloma acuminatum. Pointed wartlike growths of nonsyphilitic origin occurring on the genital organs. Also called *verruca acuminata*.

condyloma latum. A moist wartlike outgrowth seen in syphilis where two skin surfaces come into contact.

confabulation. A mental disorder in which the patient describes fictitious events he believes he has experienced. They are not hallucinations but are advanced by the patient to fill gaps in his memory. Confabulation is one of the main signs of Korsakow's syndrome, an end manifestation of chronic alcoholism.

confinement. The act of going into labor; childbirth.

confusion. A disturbance of the mind in which the patient is unable to think clearly and is disorientated.

congenital. Present at birth.

congenital syphilis. Syphilis present at birth. It is transmitted to the unborn child by an infected mother, and produces in the baby bony deformities such as saddlenose, frontal bossing (enlargement of the front of the skull), bulldog jaw, Hutchinson's teeth, saber-shaped tibial bones as well as skin eruptions, wasting of tissues, and other abnormalities.

*In the Middle Ages syphilis was popularly called the pox. One manifestation of syphilis is alopecia, and this was one reason why wigs became popular among courtiers. Syphilis was often treated by rubbing in mercury ointment.*

congested. An excess of blood in a part; a state of congestion.

congestion. Too much blood concentrated in one part.

conium. Hemlock.

conjugal. Relating to husbands and wives.

conjugate. To couple together.

conjunctiva. The mucous membrane covering the front of the eyeball.

conjunctival. Pertaining to the conjunctiva.

conjunctival reflex. The rapid closing of the eyelids when the eyeball is touched.

conjunctivitis. The inflammation of the conjunctiva. The white of the eye becomes red, congested, and sore, with a feeling of grittiness under the eyelids. Occasionally, when inflammation is severe, there is a complaint that ordinary daylight is too strong to endure. The redness is a part of the inflammatory process and is due to the dilated blood vessels that cross the white of the eye.

connective tissue. A tissue, present in every organ, which binds together and supports the various parts of the organ and is composed of an intercellular substance with either white or yellow elastic fibers arranged in bundles or weblike patterns.

consanguineous, consanguinity. Related or descended from the same ancestor.

consciousness. To be aware of one's existence and able to appreciate what is going on in one's surroundings.

conservation. Restricting or preserving without loss.

consistence, consistency. The degree of density or hardness.

consolidating. The process of healing of wounds or fractures.

consolidation. 1. The state of becoming solid. 2. In lobar pneumonia the lobe of the lung which has become inflamed and collapsed is referred to as being consolidated.

constant. Fixed, without change.

constipation. The inability to open the bowels. Just missing one daily bowel movement is not constipation. Some people have their bowels open only twice a week and for them this is quite normal; others have a bowel action night and morning every day and this, too, is normal for them. Therefore, if the individual who normally has the bowels open night and morning does not pass a motion for five days this would be constipation, whereas it is not constipation for the individual who lives happily and healthily with a bowel movement twice a week.

constitution. 1. The total make-up of a person's body. 2. An individual's ability to resist disease.

consumption. At one time a popular name for pulmonary tuberculosis.

consumptive. A person suffering from tuberculosis of the lungs.

**contact.** To be in touch or touching. An individual who has been exposed to an infectious or contagious disease.

**contact lens.** A lens applied to the surface of the eyeball.

**contagion.** Transmission of disease by direct transference from one person to another or through an intermediary.

**contagious.** A disease capable of being transmitted by contact.

**contiguous.** Close by or in actual contact.

**continence.** Self-restraining; the ability of the bowel or urinary bladder to retain their contents.

**continued fever.** A fever in which the temperature does not vary more than one or two degrees in 24 hours.

**contraception.** The prevention of pregnancy. See also BIRTH CONTROL.

**contraceptive.** An agent which prevents pregnancy.

**contracted pelvis.** A pelvis smaller than normal.

**contractile.** The property of being able to contract.

**contraction.** Becoming smaller; or the drawing together to make two parts nearer.

**contracture.** Permanent or spasmodic shortening of a muscle, tendon, or skin, or the deformity of a joint due to these causes.

**contraindication.** Evidence that a specific form of treatment is inadvisable or dangerous.

**contralateral.** Pertaining to the opposite side.

**contrast media.** Substances which, being denser than body tissues, are injected into cavities, organs, or vessels to outline their structure on an x-ray photograph. For instance, barium meals and enemas are given to outline the inside of the gastrointestinal tract, and other substances, such as iodized oil, are injected into the bloodstream to outline the kidneys, gall bladder, and other organs.

**contrecoup.** A French term for a condition in which a blow on one side of the skull can cause damage to the brain on the opposite side by transmit-. ted force.

**contuse.** To bruise.

**contusion.** A bruise; damage to the body in which the skin is not broken.

**convalescence.** The period of recovery after an illness.

**convalescent.** Somebody recovering from an illness.

**convergence.** Meeting or bringing to a central point, as in the coordinated movement of both eyes on fixation upon a near object.

**convergent.** Pertaining to convergence.

**conversion.** 1. In midwifery, the alteration of the position of the unborn baby in order to make it easier to deliver. 2. In psychiatry, a mental defense mechanism whereby unconscious emotional conflict is transformed into physical disability, the affected part always being symbolic of the nature of the conflict. For example, an unhappily married woman longing for a baby that her husband refuses to allow may complain of symptoms relating to the vagina, which, on examination, proves to be quite healthy and normal—the patient having concentrated her attention on the very part connected with her emotional upset. When the cause of her unhappiness is removed the symptoms disappear, without any medical treatment for the part.

**convex.** An outward curve on the surface.

**convexoconvex.** Curved outwards on both surfaces.

**convoluted.** Coiled or heaped up in coils.

**convolution.** A folding of an organ upon itself; usually refers to the appearance of the surfaces of the brain.

**convulsant.** A drug which causes spasms.

**convulsion.** A violent contraction of muscles due to a disturbance of the brain.

**convulsions in children.** Excessive heat on the brain can produce a convulsion or unconsciousness, or both, and illnesses and high body temperatures which produce only a shivering attack in an adult may cause a convulsion in a child. A child with a high temperature may suddenly become unconscious and have a convulsion—a trembling and shaking of the body muscles. It looks frightening, but the child nearly always comes out of it. Such a convulsion is due to the high temperature affecting the brain. First-aid treatment is to lower the temperature either by encouraging sweating or by tepid sponging with lukewarm water, and in some cases, by immersing the child in a warm bath. Prevention and cure of infantile convulsions consists of treatment for the illness creating the high temperature. See also HEAT EXHAUSTION; HEAT STROKE.

**convulsive.** Of the nature of a convulsion.

**coordination.** The rhythmical and harmonious action as of muscles.

**coprolalia.** An obsessive compulsion to use filthy words.

**coprolith.** A hard mass of feces in the bowel.

**coprophagy.** The eating of feces. Also called *skatophagy*.

**coprophilia.** The state of mind of being attracted to feces.

**coprophobia.** Abnormal repugnance to feces.

**coprostasis.** Constipation.

**copulation.** Sexual intercourse.

**coraco-acromial.** Related to the coracoid and acromion processes of the scapula.

**coracoid.** A bony process of the scapula.

**Coramine.** A proprietary drug used as a respiratory stimulant.

**cord.** Any stringlike body.

**corium.** The true skin.

**corn.** A small painful overgrowth of the horny layer of the skin of the toes with a central core, pressure on which causes pain. Those affected by sweat are called soft corns.

*Corns are caused by pressure from tight or ill-fitting shoes though undoubtedly some people have an inherited predisposition to them. They can be treated by soaking in hot water, paring down with a corn knife, and gradually digging the core out under strict antiseptic precautions. Salicylic collodion applied for several nights followed by a soaking in hot water is also often successful in removing them. The application of strong caustics is not advisable and since self-treatment seldom works, a chiropodist should be consulted.*

**cornea.** The clear, transparent part at the front and center of the eyeball.

**corneal.** Relating to the cornea.

**cornification.** The process of becoming hard as in a corn.

**corona.** A Latin word used to describe any structure in the body which resembles a crown.

**coronary arteries.** The two arteries encircling the upper part of the heart in the form of a crown.

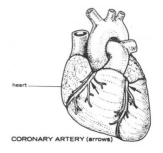

heart

CORONARY ARTERY (arrows)

**coronary occlusion.** Blockage of a coronary artery.

**coronary thrombosis.** A blood clot obstructing the coronary artery. The coronary arteries are end arteries, which means they are not connected to other arteries and that the area of heart muscle they supply has no alternative source of blood; therefore if an artery is blocked the part it supplies is deprived of blood and dies from lack of oxygen. Coronary thrombosis patients must therefore spend long periods in bed after an attack to enable the damaged area of muscle to scar up, fibrose, and replace the lost tissue. See also CHOLESTEROL; HEART ATTACK.

**coroner.** An official who holds inquiries into the unnatural cause of death of people for whom a doctor will not issue a death certificate.

**corpora.** The plural of corpus.

**corpulence, corpulency.** Obesity or fatness.

**corpulent.** Obese.

**cor pulmonale.** Huge enlargement of the heart seen in severe obstructive chest diseases.

**corpus.** A body; the main part of any organ.

**corpuscle.** 1. Any small round body. 2. The minute end organ of a sensory nerve. 3. A blood cell.

**corpuscular.** Relating to a corpuscle.

**corpus luteum.** A yellow mass formed in the space left in an ovary after an egg cell has been discharged from the ovary.

**correctant, corrective.** A substance that improves the taste, smell, or color of a drug.

**correlation.** A relationship between two or more objects or attributes.

**corrode.** To wear away.

**corrosion.** The process of corroding.

**corrosive.** Something which eats away or corrodes.

**cortex.** That layer of an organ which lies immediately under its covering membrane.

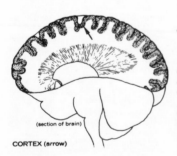

(section of brain)

CORTEX (arrow)

**cortical.** Relating to the cortex.

**cortisone.** A hormone secreted by the suprarenal gland and now synthesized in the laboratory. Its main action is anti-inflammatory, though its masking effect is not without danger since "silent" widespread infections can occur in those taking the drug. When first discovered, cortisone was hailed as a major advance in the treatment of rheumatoid arthritis, but it was found that improvement was short-lived and almost equal results could be obtained with aspirin. In fact it was suggested that aspirin stimulated the production of cortisone from the suprarenal glands. The forms of cortisone now manufactured have fewer side effects and are used to treat severe asthma, severe bronchitis, inflamed joints such as tennis elbow, and for lessening the violent inflammatory reactions of some virus diseases for which antibiotic drugs are useless, especially where there is an inflammation of central nervous system.

**coryza.** A cold in the head. See COLD.

**costal.** Relating to the ribs.

**costive.** Constipative, constipated.

**costoclavicular.** Relating to the ribs and the clavicle.

**costovertebral.** Relating to the ribs and vertebrae.

**cough.** The sudden violent expulsion of air from the lungs, which also removes phlegm and sputum.

**dry cough.** A cough without expectoration.

**moist cough or productive cough.** A cough accompanied by sputum.

**reflex cough.** Cough produced by irritation of a remote organ, such as syringing the ear, irritation of the stomach and indigestion, or disease of the vagina or neck of the womb.

**unproductive cough.** See DRY COUGH.

**whooping cough.** Also called *pertussis*. See WHOOPING COUGH, main entry.

**winter cough.** In the early stages of chronic bronchitis a cough only occurs during the winter. As the condition becomes more severe the cough occurs summer and winter.

**counterirritation.** The application of an agent to the surface of the body in order to have an effect on a deep-seated organ.

**cowpox.** See VACCINIA.

**coxa.** The hip joint.

**coxalgia.** Pain from disease of the hip joint.

**coxa plana.** See PERTHES' DISEASE.

**cramp.** A violent spasm of muscles which may be precipitated by cold, as when swimming, or which may occur in those unaccustomed to taking violent exercise. It may also occur during the course of severe general diseases when the existence of the disease overshadows the symptom of cramp. Night cramps, when not due to general disease, occur in some people merely by stretching the feet down the bed, causing the calf muscles to go into spasm. A warm bed plus resting the feet against a pillow pushed down to the bottom of the bed, and a quinine tablet before retiring, will usually cure this type of cramp.

**cranium.** The skull.

**creeping sickness.** Ergot poisoning. See ERGOTISM.

**cremaster muscle.** A muscle situated in the scrotum which, when it contracts, draws up the testicle.

**cremation.** The burning of dead bodies.

**crepitant.** Crackling.

**crepitation, crepitus.** The grating sound produced when the broken ends of a bone are moved against one another; the sound produced when the dry inflamed surfaces of the pleura touch each other during breathing in cases of pleurisy; and when tissues containing air are pressed. The sound is similar to that created by walking over a gravel path.

**cresol.** A mixture of coal tar derivatives. It can be a colorless, brownish, or pinkish fluid with a carboliclike odor, and is used chiefly as a surgical disinfectant, usually in the form of saponated cresol solution containing 50 percent cresol.

**creta.** Chalk.

**creta praeparata.** Prepared chalk as used in medicines.

**cretin.** One suffering with cretinism.

**cretinism.** A disease found in newborn babies and due to a deficiency of the thyroid gland. The child is stunted in growth with failure of mental and sexual development; the features are coarse and broad; the tongue is swollen and there are other symptoms of myxedema. The condition can be cured by doses of dried thyroid gland. Cretinism occurs in the same areas in which goiter in adults is endemic, but goiter in adults does not necessarily lead to mental deterioration, whereas the cretin is almost an idiot. It is thought that cretinism and myxedema are associated with a lack of iodine in the food in the areas in which these conditions occur, and in many countries, iodine is added to table salt. Also called *congenital myxedema*. See also GOITER; MYXEDEMA.

**cribriform.** Perforated like a collander or sieve.

**cribriform plate.** A bone in the skull perforated with numerous holes through which nerve filaments pass.

**cricoid.** One of the ring-shaped cartilages in the larynx.

**crinis.** Hair.

**crisis.** The turning point in a disease.

**critical.** Relating to a crisis.

**Crohn's disease.** See ILEITIS; REGIONAL ILEITIS.

**croup.** A condition met with in children, characterized by a harsh, brassy cough and a crowing noise accompanied by difficult respiration; occasionally the coughing sounds somewhat like the barking of a dog. It is due to a paralysis of the vocal cords brought about by inflammation that may be caused by nothing more serious than a cold in the throat. It is occasionally the result of laryngeal diphtheria, and in these cases the diphtheria membrane can be seen lining the throat, the neck glands are swollen, and the child is gravely ill. The "cold in the throat" variety rapidly responds to inhalations of steam medicated with half a teaspoonful of friars balsam or eau de Cologne. The child should place its mouth above the jug and breathe the steam in and out. This treatment, which can be repeated every one or two hours, usually effects relief within 24 hours. In preparing inhalations only hot, not boiling, water should be used, and an adult should hold the jug firmly so that it cannot be spilt and scald the child.

**crown.** The top part of a tooth. See also CORONA.

**crowning.** The appearance of a baby's head at the opening of the birth canal during labor.

**crucial.** 1. Resembling a cross. 2. Decisive or critical.

**cruciform.** Shaped like a cross.

**crude.** In its natural state; unrefined.

**crura.** The plural of crus.

**cruraeus.** See CRUREUS.

**crural.** Pertaining to the thigh or leg.

**crureus.** A muscle in the thigh.

**crus.** The leg or a limblike structure.

**crush syndrome.** See COMPRESSION SYNDROME.

**crust.** Dry exudate.

**cryosurgery.** The destruction of tissue by the use of extreme cold, as in certain cancerous lesions of the skin, and in Parkinson's disease where certain areas of the thalamus are destroyed, to relieve the patient's tremors.

**crypt.** A small cavity.

**cryptorchism.** Failure of the testicles to descend from the abdomen into the scrotum.

**crystal violet.** A bright purple-violet dye which has a special action in destroying fungus infections and Gram-positive bacteria. At one time much used by skin specialists, but now largely discontinued owing to the frightful mess it makes on clothing and bed clothes.

**C.S.F.** The abbreviation for cerebrospinal fluid.

**cubital.** Relating to the elbow.

**cubitus.** The elbow.

**cubitus valgus.** A deformity of the elbow in which the forearm when extended deviates outwards in relation to the upper arm.

**cubitus varus.** A deformity of the elbow in which the forearm deviates inwards in relation to the upper arm.

**Culex.** A genus, *Culex,* of malaria-carrying mosquitoes.

**culture.** The growth of microorganisms in suitable media.

**cumulative.** A heaping up or an increasing. Used to describe the action of a drug which is administered faster than the body can get rid of it so that its effect is exaggerated.

**curare.** The arrow poison of the South American Indians. It is used during surgical operations to paralyze and relax muscles, thus allowing the anesthetist to use far less anesthetic to render the patient unconscious, while at the same time giving the complete relaxation of the patient's muscles the surgeon must have to operate.

**curettage.** Scraping with a curette.

**curette.** A spoon-shaped instrument for scraping away tissue.

**curie.** The unit of measurement of radioactive substances representing the emanation equal to the radioactive emanation of a source in which 3.7 multiplied by $10^{10}$ atoms decay each second; named after Marie and Pierre Curie, the discoverers of radium.

**Cushing's syndrome.** A condition due to a disturbance of the pituitary gland and characterized by obesity of face and trunk, with muscular weakness, high blood pressure, diabetes, scanty or absent menstrual periods, and other defects.

**cusp.** 1. A pointed part of the top of a tooth. 2. A triangular segment of a heart valve.

**cuspid, cuspidate.** Having a sharp point. The cuspid, or canine, teeth are the four teeth having conical crowns.

**cutaneous.** Pertaining to the skin.

**cuticle.** 1. The thin layer of skin covering the base of a nail. 2. The epidermis.

**cutis.** The true skin or derma.

**cyanopia.** Vision in which all objects appear blue in color.

**cyanosed.** Affected with cyanosis.

**cyanosis.** A dusky-bluish tinge of mucous membranes or skin due to an excess of hemoglobin in the capillaries and indicating congestion of the part. Sometimes the blue color may be due to methemoglobin, which occurs in the blood due to the action of certain drugs, notably the sulphanilamide group, on hemoglobin. Generally, cyanosis of face and body is an indication of heart or lung disease. On the other hand, cyanosis of the fingers may be

due to some local cause, as in acrocyanosis.

**cyanotic.** Pertaining to cyanosis.

**cycle.** A succession of events or symptoms which recur.

**cyclic.** Pertaining to or recurring in cycles.

**cyclitis.** Inflammation of the ciliary body in the eye.

**cyclobarbitone.** A short-acting barbiturate drug.

**cycloplegia.** Paralysis of the ciliary muscles of the eye, resulting in loss of the ability to change focus.

**cyclothymia.** An emotional condition in which the individual has violent swings in mood, being alternately wildly excited and completely depressed.

**cyclotron.** A machine for smashing the atom.

**cyesis.** Pregnancy.

**cyst.** 1. A membranous bag or sac containing fluid. 2. A bladder.

**cystadenoma.** A growth containing an adenoma and cysts.

**cystalgia.** Any pain arising in a urinary bladder.

**cystectomy.** Surgical removal of a cyst, of the cystic duct, of part of the gall bladder, or of part of the urinary bladder.

**cystic.** Pertaining to a cyst, the gall bladder, or the urinary bladder.

**cysticercosis.** A tropical disease caused by infestation with cysticerci, a type of worm. It is characterized by muscular pain, general muscular weakness, utter fatigue, loss of weight, and nervous excitability. In the very worst cases, where the infestation is widespread and the brain has been invaded, general paralysis, epileptic fits, and convulsions occur.

**cysticercus.** A type of tapeworm.

**cystitis.** Inflammation of the urinary bladder.

**cystocele.** The protrusion of the urinary bladder into the vagina. One of the forms of prolapse seen in women following a series of pregnancies and childbirths.

**cystocolostomy.** An operation in which the gall bladder is joined to the colon and a permanent communication is made between them.

**cystoenterocele.** A rupture or hernia which contains portions of the bladder and the intestine.

**cystolithectomy.** Surgical removal of a stone from either the gall bladder or the urinary bladder.

**cystolithiasis.** The formation of a stone in the bladder.

**cystomerocele.** A hernia of the urinary bladder through the femoral ring into the groin.

**cystoparalysis.** Paralysis of the urinary bladder.

**cystopexia.** A surgical operation which fixes the urinary bladder to the abdominal wall.

**cystoplasty.** Surgical repair of the bladder.

**cystoptosis.** Prolapse of the lining of the bladder into the urethra.

**cystorectostomy.** Joining the urinary bladder to the rectum and making an opening so that the urine passes into the rectum.

**cystorrhagia.** Bleeding from the urinary bladder.

**cystoscope.** A long tubular metal instrument with a light in its tip used for examining the urinary tract and the inside of the bladder. There is also an operating cystoscope through which the surgeon can not only see into the bladder but also can pass in instruments to carry out certain maneuvers, such as crushing stones.

**cystoscopy.** Examination by means of a cystoscope.

**cystospasm.** Spasm or cramp of the urinary bladder.

**cystospermitis.** Inflammation of the seminal vesicles.

**cystostomy.** The formation of an opening into the bladder by sewing it to a hole made in the skin so that the urine passes through this aperture and not through the normal channels.

**cystotomy.** Surgical incision into the urinary bladder.

**cytoblast.** The nucleus of a cell.

**cytology.** The study of the formation and function of cells.

**cytoplasm.** The portion of the protoplasm within a cell that lies outside the nucleus.

# D

**Da Costa's syndrome.** See EFFORT SYN-DROME.

**dacryoadenitis.** Inflammation of a tear gland.

**dacryocele.** Protrusion of a tear sac. Also called *dacryocystocele*.

**dacryocyst.** The lacrimal sac.

**dacryocystalgia.** Pain arising in the lacrimal sac.

**dacryocystitis.** Inflammation of a lacrimal sac.

**dacryocystocele.** Protrusion of a tear sac. Also called *dacryocele*.

**dacryocystotomy.** Surgical puncture of a lacrimal sac.

**dacryolith.** A chalky stone in the tear ducts.

**dacryorrhea.** Excessive flow of tears.

**dacryorrhoea.** See DACRYORRHEA.

**dactyl.** A finger or toe.

**dactylar, dactylic.** Pertaining to a finger or a toe.

**dactylate.** Resembling a finger.

**dactylitis.** Inflammation of a finger or a toe, but usually inflammation of the bone.

**dactyloid.** Resembling a finger.

**dactylomegaly.** Having abnormally large fingers or toes.

**dactylospasm.** Spasm of a finger or toe.

**D.A.H.** The abbreviation for disordered action of the heart. See EFFORT SYN-DROME.

**Dakin's solution.** A solution used to irrigate wounds, consisting of a mixture of bicarbonate of soda, chlorinated lime, and water, with boric acid added as the last ingredient.

**dandruff.** Scurf. See PITYRIASIS. PITYRIASIS CAPITIS.

**dandy fever.** Also called *dengue fever*. See ADEN FEVER.

**Darier's disease.** See KERATOSIS. KERATO-SIS FOLLICULARIS.

**dartos.** The smooth muscle beneath the skin of the scrotum responsible for tightening up the scrotum as, for instance, in cold weather.

**D.D.T.** The abbreviation for dichlorodiphenyltrichloroethane, a synthetic insecticide first used during the Second World War to disinfest prisoners and refugees infested with body lice, which are carriers of typhus fever. It was also used in attempts to kill off malarial mosquitoes, but it was discovered that in time local insect populations became immune to D.D.T., and other chemicals had to be employed. D.D.T. is a frequent ingredient of flypapers. When the fly alights on them it collects on its feet a small quantity of D.D.T., which is then absorbed into its body, and after a short interval the fly dies. D.D.T. is also included in some forms of paint used for walls and wallpaper as a permanent insecticide.

**dead hand.** A condition marked by disturbances of the circulation in the fingers in various diseases, but found especially in workmen handling such vibrating tools as rotary cutters and road drills.

**deadly nightshade.** The popular name for the plant *Atropa belladonna*, the purple-black berries of which contain a poisonous alkaloid, belladonna. These berries are particularly attractive to children because of their sweet taste, but having eaten them a child becomes wildly excited and confused, with widely dilated pupils and a peculiar action of the arms, which can only be described as attempting to pick imaginary butterflies out of the air. The child should immediately be seen

by a doctor, who may send him to hospital for the stomach to be washed out and belladonna antidotes administered. See also ATROPA; BELLADONNA.

**deaf-mute.** A person who is unable to hear or speak, especially one in whom the inability to speak is due to congenital deafness or deafness occurring shortly after birth.

**deafness.** The loss of ability to hear. This term includes various degrees of loss of hearing.

**debility.** Weakness.

**débridement.** Surgical cleaning of a wound in which all damaged, infected, and dead tissue is cut away.

**decalcification.** The removal or loss of calcium salts from bone.

**decalcified.** Freed from calcium salts.

**decant.** To pour off liquid from a mixture, leaving behind the solid sediment.

**decapsulation.** Surgical stripping of the capsule of an organ, especially the capsule of a kidney that has stopped functioning, in an effort to get it to secrete urine.

**decibel.** A tenth of a bel, the unit for measuring the volume of sound. A decibel is the least intensity of sound at which any given note can be heard.

**decidua.** The mucous membrane lining the womb into which the fertilized egg embeds itself in order to develop as a baby. It is also known as the endometrium, and is responsible for the female monthly periods. See MENSES.

**decidua basalis.** The portion of the membrane covering the womb that is directly under the implanted fertilized egg.

**decidual.** Relating to the decidua.

**deciduous.** Something which is not permanent but cast off at maturity. A child's first teeth are referred to as the deciduous teeth or milk teeth.

**decipara.** A woman who has borne ten children.

**decline.** A wasting away of the body, or the period of abatement in a disease. At one time "going into a decline" was a favorite expression for describing somebody dying from pulmonary tuberculosis.

**decoction.** A term used in pharmacy to describe a preparation obtained by boiling a vegetable substance in water. Strictly speaking, jam is a decoction.

**decoloration.** Removal of all color.

**decompensation.** Failure of compensation; usually refers to failure of the heart and the circulation.

**decomposition.** Putrefaction.

**decompression.** The removal of pressure. Usually refers to a surgical operation performed to relieve pressure on the brain either by making burr holes in the skull or by raising a depressed fracture of the skull. It also refers to the slow process of bringing back to ordinary atmospheric pressure divers and caisson workers who have been working under highly pressurized conditions. See also CAISSON DISEASE; DECOMPRESSION SICKNESS.

**decompression sickness. 1.** Caisson disease. **2.** A disease that may occur in aviators climbing too fast into a rarefied atmosphere; the sickness can usually be aborted by descending to a lower altitude.

**decontamination.** Removing the clothes and cleaning the skin of individuals who have been exposed to such chemicals as mustard gas.

**decortication.** See DECAPSULATION.

**decrepit.** Infirm or worn out.

**decrepitude.** Senile debility.

**decrudescence.** A decline in the severity of a disease.

**decubital.** Relating to decubitus.

**decubitis.** The horizontal position of the patient in bed.

**decussation.** A crossing over from one side to the other, such as the crossing over of nerve fibers in the brain or spinal cord.

**deep x-ray.** The use of x-rays to treat disease within the body.

**defaecation.** See DEFECATION.

**defecation.** The act of opening the bowels.

**defect.** The absence of any part or organ; failure of a normal function; any lack or failure.

**deferent.** Carrying away.

**deferentitis.** Inflammation of the vas deferens, the excretory duct of the testicle.

**deferred.** Delayed or put back.

**deferred surgical shock.** Shock that comes on only after an interval following an accident. Also called *delayed surgical shock.*

**defervescence.** The cooling down of a feverish body to a more normal temperature.

**deficiency disease.** An illness caused by the absence of certain necessary food elements in the diet, such as vitamins, minerals, or some other needed dietary constituent.

**deflection.** A turning aside. In psychiatry, an unconscious diversion of ideas from conscious attention.

**deforming.** Disfiguring.

**deformity.** Malformation or distortion.

**degeneration. 1.** A change from a higher to a lower form. **2.** It may also refer to a deterioration of the mentality, personality, or character of an individual.

**deglutition.** The act of swallowing.

**degradation.** Degeneration.

**degustation.** The act of tasting.

**dehiscence. 1.** A bursting open, particularly of a wound. **2.** A defect in a bony canal or cavity.

**dehumanization.** The degeneration of some of those qualities which differentiate a human being from an animal.

**dehydration.** The removal of water.

**dehypnotize.** To arouse from a hypnotic sleep.

**déjà vu.** A French term literally meaning "already seen." Medically it refers to a state in which experiences seem to have happened before—the feeling that one has already been in a place or seen a person before, whereas in fact one has not. It is thought to be due to forgotten or repressed daydreams' about a different but similar situation on another occasion, and it is the basis of some of the contentions used by certain people who assert that their spirit has visited a place without their having been there in the flesh—in fact, it is a trick of the memory.

**dejecta.** Something thrown out, as for instance the feces.

**dejection.** Normally refers to depression.

**Déjerine-Roussy syndrome.** See THALAMIC SYNDROME.

**deleterious.** Harmful, dangerous.

**Delhi boil.** An ulcer caused by the germ of leishmaniasis. See DELHI SORE.

**Delhi sore.** A skin disease caused by infection by the germ of leishmaniasis transmitted by a species of fly. It is characterized by ulcers, which become secondarily infected with other germs. The secondary germs have to be destroyed by penicillin before attempting to cure the leishmaniasis. Kala-azar is also a member of this group of diseases, which are covered by the general term leishmaniasis. These ulcers have different names in various parts of the world, such as *Aleppo boil, tropical sore, Biskra button, Baghdad boil, Kandahar sore, Delhi boil, Tashkend ulcer, Ashkabad sore, Pendeh sore, Bouton d'Orient.*

**delinquency.** Antisocial behavior, especially in young people.

**deliriant.** Causing delirium.

**delirious.** Relating to delirium.

**delirium.** A confusional state consisting of hallucinations, delusions, restlessness, and disorientation.

**delirium tremens.** A type of mania associated with chronic alcoholism and which may be followed by Korsakow's syndrome. See also SYNDROME: KORSAKOW'S SYNDROME.

**deliver.** To remove, or to assist the act of birth.

**delivery.** The act of giving birth.

**deltoid.** A muscle in the shoulder, which raises the arm sideways away from the body.

**delusion.** A false impression that occurs in mental disorders, and a common feature of the last stages of untreated syphilis of the brain. The individual attaches to himself fantastic qualities of grandeur and wealth.

**delusional.** Characterized by delusions.

**demented.** Insane or of unsound mind.

**dementia.** Insanity.

**alcoholic dementia.** A prolonged form of dementia occurring in the late stages of chronic alcoholism.

**apoplectic dementia.** A form due to a stroke causing softening of the brain tissue.

**dementia agitata.** A form characterized by great excitement and hallucinations, seen in schizophrenia.

**dementia paralytica.** A form seen in the late stages of syphilis of the central nervous system.

**dementia praecox.** See SCHIZOPHRENIA.

**epileptic dementia.** Mental deterioration seen in some forms of severe epilepsy.

**senile dementia.** Mental deterioration in old age.

**traumatic dementia.** A form due to brain injury.

**demineralization.** The abnormal loss of mineral salts from the body.

**demonomania.** A form of madness in which the individual is convinced that he is possessed of a devil.

**demonophobia.** A fear of demons.

**demulcent.** Something having a soothing action.

**demyelinated, demyelination.** Relating to nerve fibers which have lost their myelin sheaths; the pathological condition found in such a disease as disseminated sclerosis.

**denature. 1.** To remove the original properties of a substance or to smooth out its rough texture. **2.** To render a substance unfit for human consumption.

**dendric, dendriform, dendrite, dendritic, dendron.** All refer to a nerve cell having a branching or tree-shaped process emerging from it.

**dengue.** An acute infectious disease caused by a virus transmitted by mosquitoes. See ADEN FEVER.

**dental.** Pertaining to the teeth.

**dentate.** Notched or toothed.

**dentation.** Any projection in the shape of a tooth.

**denticulate.** Having tooth-shaped projections.

**dentifrice.** A substance for cleaning teeth.

*Toothpastes and powders consist essentially of chalk or china clay mixed with glycerine to which are added many alleged tooth-saving ingredients. The mouth cannot be freed from germs even for a few minutes, and the amount of antiseptic needed to lower the bacterial count for just a few seconds would make toothpaste too unpalatable to use. Moreover, it is not in the mouth long enough for it to have any effect on bacteria, so it really does not matter which toothpaste you use. Brush the teeth night and morning, especially before going to bed, with a moderately stiff brush using an up and down movement to remove food particles from crevices. Toffee and sticky candies are far worse for children's teeth than boiled candies which dissolve and wash away. Eating apples daily is a good treatment for teeth and gums.*

**dentine.** That part of a tooth beneath the enamel surrounding the pulp or core.

**dentition.** The development and cutting of the teeth.

**dentoid.** Resembling a tooth.

**denture.** A set of artificial teeth, or the entire set of natural teeth.

**denudation.** Making something bare or naked.

**deodorant.** An agent for correcting offensive odors.

**deodorize.** To take away the smell.

**deossification.** The absorption of bone.

**deoxygenate.** To deprive of oxygen.

**deoxygenation.** Deprivation of oxygen.

**depersonalization.** A mental disorder in which the individual feels he has no personal existence.

**depigmentation.** The loss of color or pigment.

**depilate.** To remove hair. This can be done by electrolysis, in which an electric needle introduced into the hair follicle kills the hair root, causing the hair to fall out and not regrow. It is also done by applying x-rays to the scalp, which causes the entire head of hair to drop out and enables a scalp condition to be treated. Later, the hair regrows, unless, of course, the dose of x-rays has been excessive, in which case the loss is permanent. And, of course, there are the ointments, creams, and lotions sold to remove superfluous hair from the face and legs.

**depilation.** Removal or loss of hair.

**depilatory.** An agent capable of removing hair.

**depletion.** Removal of accumulated solids or fluids.

**deposit.** A sediment.

**depraved.** Perverted.

**depressant.** A drug which lowers the function of some organ.

**depressed.** 1. Melancholic. 2. Occupying a space lower than normal, as in depressed fracture of the skull where the bone is driven in and rests on the brain.

**depression.** 1. A hole or a hollow. 2. A lowering of the functional activity of an organ; refers principally to an emotional derangement involving feelings of dejection and withdrawal.

**agitated depression.** Melancholia associated with great restlessness.

**reactive depression.** Melancholia induced by some external factor, such as the loss of a dear one, being jilted, and the like.

**derangement.** A disorder, particularly a mental disorder.

**Dercum's disease.** See ADIPOSIS DOLOROSA.

**derma.** The true skin or cutis vera. See SKIN.

**dermabrasion.** The removal of extensive scars or marks on the skin by means of high speed abrasive brushes.

**dermal.** Pertaining to skin.

**dermanaplasty.** Skin grafting.

**dermatitis.** Inflammation of the skin. Despite popular frequent use, the term dermatitis is not a complete diagnosis in itself. There are so many causes of dermatitis that unless the term is qualified by an adjective descriptive of the type present neither the prognosis nor the treatment is obvious. In the main, dermatitis is due to irritation of a susceptible skin by external irritants. Too much sunlight can produce it, and so can petroleum and turpentine products, soda, detergents, soap, and other chemicals which degrease the skin. Other external irritants which can produce dermatitis are flour, sugar, plants, cement, fertilizers, industrial chemicals, and various insects and mites. It can also be caused by various allergies, by the high dosage or prolonged administration of drugs, and it may be the result of nervous irritability. Treatment, therefore, depends on the diagnosis, and the diagnosis consists of identifying the operative cause.

**dermatologist.** A specialist in diseases of the skin.

**dermatology.** The study and treatment of skin diseases.

**dermatolysis.** A congenital laxity of the skin that produces folds; small growths of the skin (fibromas) accompanied by lax sagging skin. Also called *cutis pendula, fibroma pendulum, chalazodermia.*

**dermatome.** 1. An instrument for cutting skin to produce a skin graft. 2. The side of an embryonic somite, the cutis plate. 3. An area of skin supplied by a single spinal nerve.

**dermatomycosis.** Any skin disease caused by a fungus, such as athlete's foot.

**dermatomyositis.** A degenerative rather than an inflammatory change in skin and muscles, causing muscular weakness and pain. The condition may be very extensive or slight. The skin reaction may be quite severe, with edema and reddening, or redness may be completely absent.

**dermatoneurosis.** A skin disease secondary to anxiety and nervous irritability.

**dermatophobia.** The fear of contracting a skin disease.

**dermatoplasty.** Plastic surgery; or the replacement of skin by skin grafts.

**dermatosis.** A general term covering any disease of the skin.

**dermis.** The true skin or corium. See SKIN.

**dermographia, dermographism, dermography.** A harmless congenital phenomenon in which the slightest touch on the skin by a firm object leaves for a few minutes a red mark. In a person with this condition, it is possible with the edge of the fingernail to write one's initials across his back, the initials appearing as raised, bright red streaks which take some minutes to disappear. The condition is not harmful or dangerous and there is no known cure.

**dermoid.** Resembling skin.

**dermoid cyst.** During development, the embryo is a flat plate that curves on itself to form a tube. Occasionally some cells become buried out of their proper position and later develop into a cyst, which may contain tissues from all parts of the body, such as hair, teeth, cartilage, and bone.

**desensitization.** 1. The reduction of sensitivity to an agent. For example, in hay fever due to hypersensitivity to pollens, it is possible, by giving small repeated and increasing doses of pollen extract, to gradually desensitize the body to the effect of pollens, thus curing the hay fever for at least one year. 2. In psychiatry, the removal of a mental complex.

**desert sore.** An ulcer that appears on the face, hands, and lower extremities in tropical climates. Also called *barcoo rot.* See also VELDT SORE.

**desiccant.** A drying agent.

**desiccate.** To render dry.

**desiccation.** The process of drying.

**desmoid.** Resembling a ligament, tendon, or fibroid.

**desmoid tumor.** A hard slow-growing fibroma, occurring in small numbers or even singly, on the bodies of either sex; fibroma which arises from either fascia or tendon. It is commonly seen in the sheath of the muscle of the abdominal wall and occurs mostly in women who have borne many children.

**desoxycorticosterone.** One of the hormones derived from the suprarenal gland; it is concerned with electrolytes and water metabolism. It is used in the treatment of Addison's disease. Also called *D.O.C.A.*

**desquamation.** Shedding or peeling of the skin. In arsenic poisoning the entire top surface of the skin can be shed, so that when the clothes are removed a cloud of skin scales drops to the ground. Desquamation of a fine type also appears following scarlet fever.

**deterioration.** Becoming worse.

**detoxication.** The removal of poisonous properties.

**detritus.** Any disintegrated waste product or substance.

**detrusion.** Ejection.

**detrusor.** 1. Serving to expel something. 2. The detrusor muscle of the urinary bladder, which aids in expelling urine.

**Dettol.** A proprietary disinfectant, whose active ingredient is chloroxylenol, in popular use for both its effectiveness and its painlessness on application; much used by doctors and midwives.

**detubation.** The removal of a tube.

**detumescence.** The subsidence of a swelling.

**deviation.** To turn aside from a regular or standard course.

**axis deviation.** A term used in electrocardiography to indicate that the electrical axis has shifted due to the position of the heart. It is referred to as right or left axis deviation or shift, depending on whether the axis is less than 0 degrees or greater than 90 degrees.

**conjugate deviation.** Persistent turning of the head and eyes to one side; a sign of brain disease.

**primary deviation.** A deviation in which a squinting eye deviates when the normal eye is fixed on an object.

**secondary deviation.** A deviation in which the healthy eye deviates when the squinting eye is fixed on an object.

**devil's grip.** Epidemic pleurodynia. Also called *Bornholm disease*. See PLEURODYNIA.

**devisceration.** Removal of the viscera.

**devitalization.** Loss of vitality.

**devolution.** Degeneration.

**dexter.** Right; to the right side.

**dextrocardia.** A congenital condition in which the heart is displaced to the right side of the chest, as opposed to the normal position somewhat to the left side of the chest.

**dextrose.** Dextroglucose.

**dextrorsuria.** The presence of dextrose in the urine.

**dextroversion.** Turning to the right.

**dhobie itch.** See TINEA: TINEA CRURIS.

**diabetes.** A term derived from a Greek word meaning "to pass through." Medically it applies to the passing from the kidney to the urine of sugar from the blood, and used without qua-

lification it refers to diabetes mellitus. However, the presence of sugar in the urine does not necessarily mean that the patient is suffering from diabetes mellitus.

**diabetes insipidus.** A disease caused by a lesion of the pituitary gland and characterized by severe thirst and frequent passage of weak unconcentrated urine.

**diabetes mellitus.** A condition, popularly known as sugar diabetes, caused by failure of the pancreas to produce the insulin the body needs to digest glucose, which then appears in heavy concentration in the blood and spills over via the kidneys into the urine. The symptoms are severe thirst, loss of weight, some nervous irritability, lack of energy, and an increased desire to pass urine. The condition is usually controlled by diet and insulin injections. See also COMA: DIABETIC COMA, INSULIN COMA.

**diabetic.** One who has diabetes; pertaining to diabetes.

**diabetophobia.** Fear of diabetes.

**diagnosis.** The determining of the nature and type of a disease; the decision so reached.

**clinical diagnosis.** A diagnosis made from recognition of the symptoms alone.

**differential diagnosis.** Distinguishing between similar diseases by comparing their symptoms and signs.

**laboratory diagnosis.** A diagnosis arrived at after performing various tests on tissues, excretions, or blood.

**microscopical diagnosis.** A diagnosis made after examining diseased tissues under a microscope.

**pathological diagnosis.** Diagnosis based on the structural lesions present.

**physical diagnosis.** The diagnosis made after inspection including palpation, percussion, or auscultation.

**dialysis.** Separating substances in solution by filtration through semipermeable membranes.

**diameter.** The length of any straight line passing through the center of a circle, body, or figure and connecting opposite points on its circumference, as the pelvic diameter.

**diamorphine.** Heroin, a drug of addiction, and a potent cough suppressor; very infrequently used owing to its ability to create addiction. Chemically it is diacetyl morphine. Its pain-relieving qualities are some four times stronger than morphine and it is principally used in patients dying of inoperable cancer, where the problem of addiction does not arise. Unlike morphine, it does not cause vomiting or severe constipation and controls pain without clouding the intellect. In can-

cer cases it produces a euphoria, which greatly mitigates the suffering.

**diaper rash.** Reddening of the skin in babies caused by constant irritation by wet diapers. Frequently it is due to a germ which breaks down the urea contained in urine into various substances; ammonia is one of these and it is this which attacks the skin. Prevention consists in either neutralizing the urine by administering sodium citrate by mouth or preventing the germs from developing by impregnating the diaper with antiseptic. After the diaper has been washed and rinsed it should be steeped in a mixture of Roccal antiseptic and water, wrung out, and allowed to dry. The skin can be treated by a bland cream or ointment, such as zinc and castor oil cream, which should be applied each time the diapers are changed, and for some part of each day the baby should be without a diaper so as to allow the free passage of air to the skin. Also called *diaper erythema*.

**diaphanous.** Thin, transparent.

**diaphoresis.** Sweating.

**diaphoretic.** A drug that causes sweating.

**diaphragm.** 1. The large musculotendinous sheet separating the chest cavity from the abdominal cavity. 2. Also used to name other separating structures.

**diaphragmatic.** Pertaining to a diaphragm.

**diaphragmatic pleurisy.** Inflammation of the pleural membrane covering the diaphragm and which causes severe pain even with shallow breathing.

**diaphragmatocele.** Rupture of an organ through the diaphragm.

**diaphysis.** The shaft of a long bone.

**diaphysitis.** Inflammation of the shaft of a long bone.

**diarrhea.** The passage of frequent loose stools.

**diarrhoea.** See DIARRHEA.

**diastalsis.** A form of peristalsis in which a wave of inhibition precedes a wave of contraction. See also PERISTALSIS.

**diastase.** An enzyme found in the saliva and intestinal juices, which converts starch first into maltose, and then into dextrose.

**diastase test.** Estimation of the quantity of diastase in the urine; used as a test of the functioning of the pancreas during acute infections of this gland.

**diastasis.** 1. A separation of parts normally joined together, such as separation of the epiphysis from the bone shaft without a true fracture being present; an incomplete dislocation. 2. The gap between the inner edges of the recti abdominis muscles on either side of the midline of the abdomen.

**diastole.** The resting phase of the heart during which the chambers fill with blood prior to systole.

**diastolic.** Pertaining to the diastole of the heart.

**diathermy.** Heat treatment by means of high-frequency currents.

**diathesis.** The constitutional liability of an individual to contract a particular disease.

**dichotomy.** A division in two parts.

**Dick test.** The test for immunity to scarlet fever. A tiny quantity of the germ poison is injected into the layers of the skin, and if it produces a pink-red area maximal in 24 hours the patient is susceptible to scarlet fever.

**dicoumarol.** See DICUMAROL.

**dicrotic.** Pertaining to dicrotism.

**dicrotism.** A condition in which there are two pulse beats to every heartbeat.

**dicumarol.** A substance used to prevent clotting of the blood. It is found in sweet clover and hay and can be prepared synthetically.

**didelphic.** Having a double womb.

**didymitis.** Inflammation of the testicle.

**dienestrol.** A synthetic female ovarian hormone.

**dienoestrol.** See DIENESTROL.

**dietetics.** The science of nutrition.

**dietitian, dietist.** A specialist who constructs diets.

**Dietl's crisis.** A phenomenon occurring when a kidney becomes misplaced and kinks the ureter—the tube carrying the urine from the kidney to the urinary bladder. There is a dramatic onset of severe pain in the loin, but if the patient lies down the kidney falls back into place, the ureter becomes unkinked, the pain stops, and there is a sudden passage of urine.

**differential.** Relating to a difference.

**differential blood count.** The counting under a microscope of the relative numbers of the different types of white blood cells in a sample of blood.

**differential diagnosis.** A diagnosis arrived at by comparing and excluding the symptoms of different diseases.

**differentiation.** 1. The act of distinguishing between. 2. The process of embryonic cells developing into diversified tissues as the embryo develops.

**diffraction.** The bending of light when it passes from one medium to another. For example, a stick partially placed in water, although known to be straight, appears bent where it enters the water.

**diffuse.** Scattered, generalized.

**diffusion.** A spreading or scattering.

**digest.** To convert food into substances capable of being absorbed by the body.

**digestant.** A substance promoting digestion.

**digestion.** The chemical changes that take place in food prior to absorption from the intestine to be used as fuel by the body.

**digestive.** Pertaining to the digestion.

**digestive tract.** See ALIMENTARY CANAL.

**digit.** A finger or toe.

**digital.** Pertaining to the fingers or toes.

**digitalin.** A pure drug derived from the foxglove and used in treatment of heart disease.

**digitalis.·** An extract from foxglove used in treating heart disease.

**digitate.** Having the appearance of fingerlike branches.

**dil.** The abbreviation for dilute.

**dilatation.** Expansion, especially of a cavity.

**dilate.** To enlarge or expand.

**dilator.** An object used to dilate or expand an organ.

**dilution.** Weakening the strength of a solution.

**diminution.** A reduction.

**dimorphism.** The state of having two forms.

**dimorphous.** Pertaining to dimorphism.

**dimple.** A small depression.

**diodine.** A radio-opaque substance used to outline the urinary tract to determine the presence of abnormalities.

**diopter.** The unit of measurement of the focus of a lens.

**dioptre.** See DIOPTER.

**dioptric.** Pertaining to diopters or dioptrics.

**dioptrics.** The branch of optics dealing with refraction.

**diphasic.** Having two phases.

**diphenan.** A drug used against threadworms.

**diphtheria.** An acute infectious disease accompanied by fever, heart weakness, prostration, anemia, and a swelling of the larynx and pharynx. Patchy membranes are commonly found on the lining of the throat.

*Preventive inoculation is a complete protection against diphtheria, which is becoming a rare disease. The incubation period is 3-4 days after which malaise and a sore throat develop in an insidious manner with the child not apparently very ill. A pearly-grey membrane forms in the throat, and attempts to detach it will cause bleeding. The disease may spread to or be confined to the larynx or nose (in the latter case there is a bloodstained discharge from one or both nostrils), and it may also attack wounds or other parts of the body. Treatment consists of early injections of antitoxin.*

**diphtheric, diphtheritic.** Pertaining to diphtheria.

**diphtheroids.** Germs similar in appearance to diphtheria germs, but which are in fact harmless. See also PSEUDODIPHTHERIA.

**Diphyllobothrium latum.** A tapeworm. It is one of the largest tapeworms and can attain a length of 20 to 30 feet.

**diplegia.** Paralysis of two comparable parts, such as two legs or two arms.

**cerebral diplegia.** The disease affecting persons who are popularly called spastics. The child has a spastic paralysis of the limbs, usually the legs, often associated with convulsions and varying degrees of mental deficiency. Also called *spastic diplegia, Little's disease.*

**diplobacillus.** A bacillus or germ which is found in pairs.

**diplobacterium.** Two bacteria adhering to each other to form a pair.

**diplococci.** Bacteria of the genus *Streptococceae,* which stay paired together.

**diploe.** The layer of bone of spongelike appearance between the inner and outer tables of the skull.

**diploic.** Pertaining to the diploe.

**diploic veins.** The veins between the tables of the skull.

**diplophonia.** The simultaneous utterance of two sounds from the larynx due to the paralysis of one of the vocal cords.

**diplopia.** Double vision.

**dipsomania.** Periodic bouts of compulsive drinking of alcohol.

**dipsophobia.** Fear of alcohol.

**disarticulation.** Surgical amputation of a limb by cutting through a joint.

**disc.** A circular flat plate or organ.

**discharge.** Emission from the body of a liquid which may be composed of pus, blood, mucus, or some other secretion.

**discrete.** Made up of separated parts; lesions which do not become blended.

**disinfect.** To destroy harmful germs.

**disinfectant.** An agent which disinfects.

**disinfection.** The destruction of dangerous germs and their poison.

**disinfestation.** Rendering free from insect or animal parasites; delousing.

**disjoint.** To remove a limb through a joint.

**disk.** See DISC.

**dislocation.** The tearing apart of two bones at a joint; or one bone's displacement at a joint.

**disordered action of the heart.** See EFFORT SYNDROME.

**disorganization.** Destruction of organic tissue. The act of deranging.

**disorientation.** Loss of normal relationship to one's surroundings, with the failure to comprehend time, place, and people. It occurs in some forms of brain disease and in some psychiatric and toxic states.

**dispar.** Unequal.

**displacement.** Removal from the normal position. In psychiatry, an unconscious device whereby anxiety arising out of a repressed feeling of guilt is discharged through a symbolic act or ritual, thus preventing the original and intolerable situation or experience from entering the conscious mind.

**disposition.** Susceptibility to disease.

**dissect.** To separate.

**dissecting aneurysm.** A condition in which blood enters between the lining and the middle coat of an artery to form a blood-filled sac.

**disseminated.** Scattered, disposed over a large area.

**disseminated sclerosis.** A chronic disease in which the nerve sheaths in the brain degenerate and disappear. This results in the exposed nerve fibers dying so that muscles and other parts lose their nerve supply. The cause is unknown.

*In the early stages symptoms are fleeting and may appear first in one area of the body and then in another. An early sign is weakness in the legs which comes and goes with intervening apparent recovery. Other symptoms include tremor of the hands on voluntary movement, numbness and tingling in the extremities, areas of sensory loss, loss of vibration sense, double vision, squint, nystagmus, loss of vision, emotional upsets such as euphoria, and disturbances of micturition. After a period, usually of many years, there is spastic paraplegia (spasm of the muscles of both arms or both legs) and the patient becomes increasingly helpless. In some cases the disease passes into a quiet or temporary recovery phase which may last from 5 to 15 years, making it extremely difficult to assess the usefulness of treatment.*

**dissolution.** The breaking up of a body into component parts; liquefaction; impending death.

**distal.** Remote; at the farthest place from the center.

**distension.** The state of being blown out or enlarged.

**distillation.** A chemical process by which liquids are heated to a gaseous state and then cooled to re-form into a fluid.

**dithranol.** The active ingredient of chrysarobin, which, in ointment form, is used to treat psoriasis.

**diuresis.** The increased flow of urine.

**diuretic.** A drug which promotes the secretion of urine.

**diuria.** Frequency of passing urine during daytime.

**divergence.** The going away from a common point; separation.

**divergent.** Going out in different directions from a common point.

**diver's paresis.** A form of paralysis occurring in caisson disease. See CAISSON DISEASE.

**diverticula.** The plural of diverticulum.

**diverticular.** Pertaining to a diverticulum.

**diverticulitis.** Inflammation of diverticula or a diverticulum. Diverticulitis is a disease of middle age, and because the symptoms are similar to appendicitis it has been called "left-sided appendicitis." The pain, however, is in the left side of the abdomen, not on the right as in appendicitis. In cases where there are many diverticula it may be necessary to remove part of the bowel to obtain permanent relief.

**diverticulosis.** A condition in which there are many diverticula.

**diverticulum.** A small blind pouch which appears in the wall of a hollow organ. It occurs most commonly in the colon and is in fact a hernia of the bowel lining through the muscular coat. Waste products become lodged in this pouch where they stagnate and putrefy, setting up the inflammatory condition called diverticulitis.

**dizziness.** Giddiness.

**Döderlein's bacillus.** This bacillus normally inhabits the vagina of the healthy virgin, appearing there during the first weeks of life. The bacillus is sugar-fermenting which results in the healthy vaginal secretion being acid and antiseptic from the presence of lactic acid. If this harmonious process is disturbed, either by infection entering the vagina or by a disturbance of general health which reduces glycogen production, then a low-grade vaginitis is induced which leads to a whitish vaginal discharge. This condition is called leukorrhea, popularly known as "the whites."

**dolor.** Latin for pain.

**dolorific.** Producing pain.

**dolorosus.** Painful.

**domatophobia.** Fear of being inside a house.

**dominant.** Overbearing or prevailing.

**donor.** One who gives living tissue for transfer to another person, particularly one who gives blood.

**dope.** Slang for any drug or medicine.

**doraphobia.** Fear of touching skins or fur.

**dormancy.** Being dormant.

**dormant.** Quiet or inactive.

**doromania.** A morbid desire to make gifts to people.

**dorsal.** Pertaining to the posterior, or back, of an organ.

**dorsalis.** Relating to the back.

**dorsiflexion.** Bending in a backward direction.

**dorsispinal.** Relating to the back of the spine.

**dorsoanterior.** Relating to both back and front.

**dorsocephalad.** Towards the back of the head.

**dorsolateral.** Pertaining to the back and the side of the body.

**dorsolumbar.** Pertaining to the back and lumbar region.

**dorsoposterior.** Pertaining to the back surface and the posterior part of a body.

**dorsoventrad.** In a direction from back to front.

**dorsum.** The back part of any organ or the back itself.

**dose.** The exact portion of a medicine, whether drug or radiation, that is to be given at any one time or in a given period of time.

**dosimetry.** The determination of medicinal doses or doses of x-rays.

**double quartan fever.** A form of malaria with a three-day cycle.

**douche.** A stream of water or watery solution directed into a cavity of the body.

**Dover's powder.** A powder containing 10 percent opium and ipecacuanha, sometimes used as a pain reliever but commonly used combined with aspirin to induce a heavy night sweat to sweat out a cold. Named after Dr. Thomas Dover, the 17th-century English physician who rescued Alexander Selkirk, the original of Robinson Crusoe, from the island of Juan Fernandez.

**draft.** 1. A single liquid portion of medicine. 2. A current of air in an enclosed space, as in a room.

**dragée.** A sugar-coated pill.

**drain.** 1. To draw off. 2. A tube or other appliance used in surgery to drain an operation site.

**draught.** See DRAFT.

**dreams.** A series of vivid images experienced during sleep.

**dream state.** The sleepy period following an epileptic fit.

*Sleep is the total withdrawal of the conscious, leaving the unconscious mind full play, which often results in dreams, during which are released urges, ambitions, and wishes, often in symbolic form. Children's dreams are uncomplicated, simple in type, and usually gratify a wish, for a toy perhaps, denied them during the day. In adults, dreams undergo varying amounts of distortion and the wish is disguised in symbolic form. According to Freud, no instinct has been so repressed as sex and he holds that it is the sexual element in the unconscious which is constantly striving for expres-*

*sion in dreams. The most vivid part of the dream is not always the most significant, for even the unconscious tries to conceal the true meaning. Freud maintained that many dream symbols are fixed and recurrent. For instance: The king and queen in the dream are the parents; a prince or princess represents the dreamer; boxes, rooms, bottles, or hollow spaces are the female sex organs; long objects, sharp and penetrating weapons are the male organ; complicated mechanisms, machinery, and landscapes represent both male and female sex organs; movements such as ascent, descent, floating, flying, and jumping represent the sexual act. These generalizations are only partly true, and to interpret dreams the psychiatrist needs to have detailed knowledge of the patient.*

**dresser.** A medical student who dresses wounds.

**dressing.** A covering applied to a wound to protect it from further injury and to aid in the healing process.

**drip.** The administration of medicaments, blood, plasma, and the like by slowly introducing them either into a vein or the subcutaneous tissues.

**drivel, driveling.** Salivation.

**droplet.** A minute drop.

**dropped organs.** See VISCEROPTOSIS.

**dropsical.** Pertaining to dropsy.

**dropsy.** The abnormal accumulation of fluid in the tissues. See EDEMA.

**drug.** Any substance used as a medicine for the purpose of treatment or prevention of disease, for diagnosis, or for relieving pain.

**drug coma.** Coma produced by an overdose of drugs. The victim lies quiet, relaxed, and cannot be roused; if deeply under the effects of morphine or other narcotic, his pupils are contracted to pinpoints. Often a container of sleeping tablets or the like is found nearby and it is imperative that this should not be touched, for it may be necessary to identify the drug. There is really no first-aid treatment for this sort of case apart from sending for an ambulance.

**drug fever.** Fever resulting from the administration of drugs to which the patient is particularly sensitive.

**drum.** The tympanic membrane or eardrum.

**duct.** A tube or channel, particularly one carrying excretions or secretions.

**ductile.** Capable of being drawn out, as into a wire.

**ductless glands.** The endocrine glands. See ENDOCRINE.

**ductule.** A small duct.

**ductus.** A duct.

**ductus arteriosus.** A tube in the unborn baby carrying blood from the pulmonary artery into the aorta, thus by-passing the lungs. After birth this tube should become a fibrous cord and be no longer capable of carrying blood, but if it remains open (patent ductus arteriosus) it may result in serious heart disease. The condition can be cured completely by surgery.

**Duke's disease.** A disease resembling scarlet fever and measles. Also called *fourth disease.*

**dull.** Not resonant.

**dullness.** Lack of resonance found on percussion over an area of pneumonia, collapsed lung, or pleural effusion.

**dumb.** Unable to speak.

**dum-dum.** See KALA-AZAR.

**dumping syndrome.** Abdominal pain, palpitations, and cold sweats experienced following removal of a part or the whole of the stomach. Any attempt to eat a normal-sized meal causes distension of the stump of the stomach and the duodenum. Some cases are relieved by insulin.

**duodenal.** Pertaining to the duodenum. See also ULCER: DUODENAL ULCER.

**duodenectomy.** Surgical excision of part or all of the duodenum.

**duodenitis.** Inflammation of the duodenum.

**duodeno-.** A prefix indicating a relationship with the duodenum.

**duodeno-enterostomy.** An operation in which a connection is made between the duodenum and another part of the small intestine.

**duodenojejunostomy.** An operation in which the duodenum is joined to the jejunum, the second part of the small intestine.

**duodenostomy.** Formation of an artificial opening through the abdominal wall into the duodenum.

**duodenotomy.** Surgical incision into the duodenum.

**duodenum.** The first part of the small intestine extending from the valve of the stomach to the jejunum. It is similar in shape to a horseshoe and is about 11 inches long.

**Dupuytren's contraction.** Contraction of the tissues of the palm in which the fingers become bent into the palm and remain fixed in that position. Workmen using tools such as screwdrivers, which by pressure irritate the palm, may in time develop this condition, though often the little finger of both hands are the only fingers affected. There seems to be an hereditary factor in this complaint as often it is found in more than one member of a family. The only cure for this deformity is a surgical operation.

**dural.** Relating to the dura mater.

**dura mater.** The outermost of the three membranes covering the brain and spinal cord. Also called *dura.*

**dwarf.** An individual of stunted growth.

**dwarfism.** The state of being a dwarf, See also ACHONDROPLASIA.

**dynamograph.** An instrument for recording muscular strength.

**dynamometer.** An instrument for measuring muscular strength.

**dyne.** The unit of force. It is the amount of force necessary to move a mass weighing one gram and to increase its velocity by one centimeter per second.

**dysacousia.** Discomfort derived from hearing normal sounds. A state of hypersensitivity of the hearing mechanism. Also called *dysacusis.*

**dysarthria.** Inability to speak clearly due to a disorder of the nervous system.

**dysarthrosis.** A deformed joint.

**dysbasia.** Difficulty in walking.

**dyschezia.** Constipation; difficulty in emptying the rectum.

**dyschondroplasia.** A disease of unknown cause which attacks the long bones of the skeleton and the bones of the hand. It is characterized by the normal growth of cartilage which only very slowly turns into bone. Also called *skeletal enchondromatosis.*

**dyscrasia.** Any abnormal condition, particularly of the blood.

**dysenteric.** Pertaining to dysentery.

**dysentery.** A group of diseases characterized by inflammation of the colon, resulting in pain, spasm of the rectum, intense diarrhea, with frequent passage of small amounts of mucus and blood with symptoms of generalized poisoning of the body. The two main types are amebic dysentery and bacillary dysentery. See also SONNE DYSENTERY.

**dysfunction.** Bad performance; impaired function of some part of the body.

**dysgerminoma.** A firm, elastic, solid tumor of the ovary or testicle. It is a slow-growing form of cancer which does not produce cancerous deposits in distant regions.

**dysgraphia.** Inability to write due to a disease of the nervous system.

**dyshidrosis.** Any disturbance in sweating. Also called *dysidrosis.*

**dyskinesia.** The inability to perform certain muscular movements.

**dyslalia.** Inability or impairment of articulation of speech due to disease of the nervous system.

**dyslogia.** Inability to express ideas in speech.

**dysmenorrhea.** Excessively painful menstruation. There are two main types, in both of which there is often a pronounced emotional factor which aggravates the condition.

**primary or spasmodic dysmenorrhea.** The pain occurs with the flow of blood, is usual in teenagers, and investigation fails to reveal any abnormality in the pelvic organs. It is relieved by childbirth. Treatment consists of simple analgesics; if these fail the neck of the womb can be stretched, for it is thought the pain is due to cramp of the womb muscles. In very severe cases it may be necessary to cut the nerves to the womb (presacral neurectomy).

**secondary or congestive dysmenorrhea.** Pain starts before the menstrual flow and is due to congestion and tension in the tissues. Occasionally it is caused by disease of the pelvic organs, such as salpingitis and retroverted uterus. When not due to disease, treatment consists of exercise, hot baths, purgatives, and simple analgesics. Sometimes the administration of a hormone for the week prior to the period is of value.

**dysmenorrhoea.** See DYSMENORRHEA.

**dysostosis.** Congenital malformation of bone.

**dyspareunia.** Difficult or painful sexual intercourse in the female. Difficult coitus may be due to spasm of the vagina from fear or emotional factors, poorly developed vagina, rigid hymen, tumors, or severe ankylosing hip disease. In the absence of disease or malformations, psychological factors are usually responsible, fear being the commonest cause. The fault may also lie with the male partner due to ineffective erections or excessive size of the penis. Painful coitus can result from almost any gynecological disease or abnormality. Inflammation, painful scars, and tender swellings in the pelvis, such as a dropped ovary, are among the more common causes. Alleged pain at intercourse due to nervous spasm is a frequent complaint in women who fear pregnancy or pain, or dislike the sexual act.

**dyspepsia.** Indigestion.

**dyspeptic.** One who suffers with indigestion.

**dysphagia.** Difficulty in swallowing.

**dysphasia.** Impairment of speech due to a disease of the nervous system.

**dysphoria.** An uneasy feeling.

**dysphrasia.** Impaired speech or understanding of the spoken word occurring in mentally retarded patients.

**dysplasia.** Abnormal development or growth.

**dyspnea.** Shortness of breath usually caused by heart, lung, or kidney disease.

**dyspneic.** Short of breath.

**dyspnoea.** See DYSPNEA.

**dyspnoeic.** See DYSPNEIC.

**dystocia.** Difficult childbirth.

**dystonia.** Any disorder of tone or lack of tone in the muscular tissues.

**dystrophic.** Pertaining to dystrophy.

**dystrophy.** A state of defective nutrition, abnormal development, or degeneration. The term is usually qualified by an adjective indicating the organ or site of degeneration.

**progressive muscular dystrophy.** A disease of childhood or early adolescence, in which the muscles become weak and degenerate. There are several forms of this disorder, and in the pseudohypertrophic type, instead of the muscles actually wasting, they appear to be of normal size or even larger than normal. Also called *dystrophia*.

**dysuria.** Difficulty or pain in passing urine.

# E

**ear.** The organ of hearing. The external ear consists of the pinna or ear flap and the external auditory meatus, the tube from the outer ear to the eardrum. The middle ear is the cavity between the eardrum and the bony wall of the inner ear; it contains three small bones—the incus, the malleus, and the stapes. These small bones,

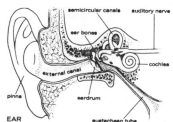

EAR

which articulate with one another, are attached to the eardrum, or the tympanic membrane, and transmit its vibrations to the inner ear. The inner ear, or labyrinth, consists of the vestibule (a cavity containing a fluid), into the front of which open the cochlea, or spiral canal, containing the essential organ of hearing (the organ of Corti), and the semicircular canals responsible for the sense of balance. Extreme motion upsetting the movements within the semicircular canals causes severe vertigo and the sensations of motion sickness, as seasickness and airsickness.

**eardrum.** The tympanic membrane. It vibrates with sound waves and aids in producing the sense of hearing.

**ear wax.** A waxy substance secreted by glands in the ear passage; nature's provision for trapping germs, dust, and small insects to protect the eardrum. This wax can collect and become very hard, either irritating the eardrum or blocking the ear passage, causing temporary deafness. Providing the eardrum is not perforated, the wax can be removed by filling the ear with a bland oil, such as olive oil, three or four times a day until the wax is softened, when, as a rule, it will discharge as an oily waxy substance. In some cases, however, it can only be removed with syringing by a doctor, and it is imperative that unqualified people do not attempt to remove it either by syringing, or poking down the ear opening with a knitting needle, for the drum may become damaged and the hearing permanently ruined. Also called *cerumen*.

**eburnation.** An increase in the density of bone or cartilage seen in joints affected with osteoarthritis.

**ecbolic.** A substance which causes the womb to contract.

**eccentric.** 1. Peculiar in behavior. 2. Situated away from the center.

**ecchondroma.** A tumor of cartilage; a chondroma.

**ecchymosis.** The presence of blood underneath the skin causing a small hematoma, a tumor containing blood. It later shows all the color changes seen in bruising.

**eccrine.** Any gland which delivers its secretion to the surface of the body, such as the sweat glands in the skin. Also called *exocrine*.

**E.C.G.** The abbreviation for electrocardiogram.

**echinococcus.** A tapeworm which forms cysts in the brain, liver, and lungs.

**echolalia.** Meaningless repetition of words spoken by others; a symptom in some cases of schizophrenia.

**eclampsia.** A toxemia of pregnancy in which the blood pressure rises and the urine contains large amounts of albumin. If not treated in time, the condition may produce severe epileptic-type fits.

**ecology.** The study of the relations between living organisms and their environment.

**Economo's disease.** Encephalitis lethargica or sleeping sickness, first described by Von Economo, an Austrian nerve specialist.

**ectasia.** Distension or dilation.

**ecthyma.** A form of skin disease usually found on the lower limbs, characterized by large superficial pustules, which develop into ulcers covered with thick crusts. It is probably caused by the germ that produces impetigo. Also called *ulcerative impetigo.*

**ectoderm.** The outer of the three primary germ layers of the embryo from which develops, among other things, the skin. See also EMBRYO.

**ectogenous.** Capable of growth outside the body; usually refers to parasites or microorganisms.

**ectoparasite.** A parasite that lives on the surface of its host.

**ectopia.** The abnormal position of an organ.

**ectopic.** In an abnormal position.

**ectopic pregnancy.** A pregnancy occurring either in the abdomen or in the Fallopian tube instead of in the womb. See also PREGNANCY.

**ectoplasm.** The outer area of the protoplasm of a cell.

**ectromelia.** Congenital absence of the whole or a part of a limb or limbs.

**ectropic.** Everted.

**ectropion.** Eversion of a part, especially of an eyelid.

**eczema.** A skin disorder, the cause of which may be unknown, characterized by inflammation, itching, secondary infection, and a rash which may appear as vesicles, papules, or pustules, with scaling, thickening, and discharges. When, however, the cause is known, the term eczema is usually abandoned in favor of the term dermatitis coupled with an adjective indicating its origin. For example, eczema due to an external irritant is called contact dermatitis. Nerves, diet, and heredity may all be causative factors.

**eczematoid.** Resembling eczema.

**eczematous.** Pertaining to eczema.

**edema.** The abnormal accumulation of fluid in the tissues.

**angioneurotic edema.** A condition marked by acute, transitory, localized swellings, often about the face or loose tissues between the legs; resembling urticaria but affecting somewhat larger areas. Some cases appear to be hereditary; others may be due to a food allergy, or are a manifestation of a neurosis. Also called *giant urticaria, giant edema, Quincke's disease.*

**cardiac edema.** Edema occurring in heart failure, due to raised pressure in the veins, most marked in the lowest parts of the body, such as the lower limbs and lower part of the back, where gravity allows fluid to collect.

**cerebral edema.** Edema of the brain, due to toxic or nutritional causes. It is usually associated with delirium, convulsions, or coma.

**collateral edema.** The edema found in the region of an inflamed part.

**heat edema.** Edema in which swelling of the hands and feet occurs in hot weather, due to increased blood volume and dilatation of the capillaries.

**hereditary edema.** Chronic edema of the legs, often appearing in families, usually at or after adolescence and without obvious or known cause. Also called *Milroy-Meige-Nonne's disease.*

**hunger edema.** See NUTRITIONAL EDEMA, below.

**inflammatory edema.** See COLLATERAL EDEMA, above.

**lymph edema.** Edema due to obstruction of lymph vessels, such as is seen in elephantiasis.

**malignant edema.** Edema occurring in infections with gas-forming bacilli

**nutritional edema.** Edema occurring in nutritional states, due to low concentration of protein in the blood plasma.

**pitting edema.** Edema of such severity that pressure on the surface by the fingers leaves behind small depressions or pits.

**pulmonary edema.** Edema in which there is an effusion of fluid into the lungs, usually due to heart failure.

**renal edema.** The edema present in kidney disease.

**edentate, edentulous.** Without teeth.

**E.E.G.** The abbreviation for electroencephalogram.

**effect.** The end result or consequence.

**effeminate.** Unmanly, or pertaining to a female.

**efferent.** Carrying away or going away from, such as a nerve carrying impulses away from the central nervous system or blood vessels carrying blood away from a part.

**effervescence.** The bubbling condition which occurs when gas escapes from a liquid.

**effleurage.** The stroking movements given in massage.

**efflorescence.** An eruption or rash.

**effluvium.** 1. A shedding, as of the hair. 2. A bad smell.

**effort syndrome.** A psychoneurotic condition characterized by shortness of breath, palpitations, and pain in the chest. Also called *neurocirculatory asthenia, Da Costa's syndrome, disordered action of the heart (D.A.H.).*

**effusion.** The presence in a body cavity of a fluid, which may be a clear serous liquid, pus, or blood.

**purulent effusion.** A liquid composed of pus.

**ego.** The self or that part of the personality in conscious contact with reality.

**egocentric.** Self-centered or selfish.

**egophony.** The curious noise, sometimes described as like the bleat of a goat, that is heard through a stetho-

scope applied over a layer of pleural effusion in the chest. The patient is asked to say "99" so that the doctor may hear the sound coming through the chest wall. When egophony is present, instead of a clear "99," the sound has a nasal quality, as though the patient has a cold in the head.

**eighth nerve.** The nerve for hearing and for position and movement of the head. Also called *eighth cranial nerve.*

**ejaculate.** 1. To throw out suddenly. 2. Usually refers to the male sexual orgasm in which the seminal fluid is discharged.

**ejaculation.** The emission of seminal fluid.

**electrocardiogram.** The graphic record of the minute electrical waves produced by contraction of the heart muscle; reveals to the heart specialist the type and nature of the disorder present. Often abbreviated to E.C.G. See also LEAD, ELECTROCARDIOGRAPHIC.

**electrocardiograph.** The instrument used to produce an electrocardiogram.

**electrocardiography.** The study and recording of electrocardiograms.

**electrocautery.** An instrument with a platinum wire tip which can be heated to a dull red by electricity and which is used to burn tissues and small growths or to coagulate small blood vessels. Some surgeons use it instead of a knife to cut through certain tissues.

**electrocoagulation.** Coagulation of tissues by an electric current.

**electroencephalogram.** A graphic record of the electrical waves produced by various parts of the brain; used to aid in the diagnosis of diseases and disorders of the brain. These graphic records show characteristic waves in such disorders as epilepsy and brain tumors. Often abbreviated to E.E.G.

**electroencephalography.** The study and recording of brain waves.

**electrolysis.** The destruction of tissue by an electric current. This method is used to destroy superfluous hair, by passing an electric current into the hair root. See also DEPILATE.

**electronarcosis.** A state of deep sleep produced by means of electrical currents.

**electrophoresis.** The movement of particles charged with electricity through the medium in which they are dispersed, when placed under the influence of an applied electric current.

**electropneumograph.** An instrument used to study breathing.

**electropuncture.** The application of electric current via a needle.

**electroshock.** A treatment used for certain mental illnesses in which shock is produced by applying an electric current to the brain. See also SHOCK THERAPY.

**electuary.** A medicinal preparation containing honey.

**element.** Any ultimate part of which something is composed. In chemistry, a substance that cannot be decomposed into simpler substances by ordinary chemical means and consisting of atoms of one type only.

**elephantiasis.** A disease characterized by gross enlargement or swelling of the lower limbs and external genitals. The commonest form is a tropical disease due to filaria entering the lymph channels and causing obstruction. Other varieties occur as birth malformations and in leprosy. Also called *Barbados leg.*

**elimination.** 1. Getting rid of or casting out. 2. Usually refers to the expulsion of waste products from the body.

**elixir.** A medicinal preparation containing honey or syrup.

**elm.** A tree of the genus *Ulmus.*

**slippery elm.** A species of elm from which the powdered, dried, inner bark has in the past been used for a variety of purposes, including the relief of catarrh and diarrhea, on which it had no effect. It has also been used as a corrective for the menses, it being firmly believed by the users that it would start menstruation and possibly produce an abortion. It has no possible value in this connection.

**emaciation.** Wasting.

**embalm.** The preservation of a corpse by injecting into the main leg artery a mixture of carbolic, glycerine, and formaldehyde, to replace the blood and prevent putrefaction.

**embedding.** 1. A term used mainly to refer to the fixation of a pathological specimen in paraffin wax to support the tissue structure while it is cut into thin sections for microscopical examination. 2. The implanting of the fertilized egg into the wall of the womb.

**embolectomy.** Surgical removal of an embolus.

**embolic.** Relating to an embolus.

**embolic abscess.** An abscess starting at the final resting place of a septic embolus such as a blood clot.

**embolism.** The obstruction of a blood vessel, usually an artery, by an embolus.

**embolalia.** The inclusion of meaningless words into speech.

**embolus.** A piece of foreign matter circulating in the bloodstream. It may be a blood clot, an air bubble, cancer cells, fat, vegetation from a heart valve, clumps of bacteria, or a foreign body, such as a needle or bullet, which gains entrance to the circulation and is carried by the bloodstream until it lodges in and obstructs a blood vessel.

**embryo.** The early stages of the development of the fertilized egg in the womb. The embryo consists of three layers: the ectoderm, or outer layer, from which develop the skin, hair, eyes, nails, and nervous system; the mesoderm, or middle layer, from which develop the circulatory, muscular, and skeletal systems; and the entoderm, or inner layer, from which develop the digestive apparatus, liver, lungs, bladder, and thyroid gland.

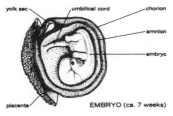

EMBRYO (ca. 7 weeks)

**embryology.** The science of the developing embryo.

**emesis.** Vomiting.

**emetic.** Something which causes vomiting.

**emetine.** A drug derived from ipecacuanha; used in the treatment of amebic dysentery.

**emissary veins.** The veins which pierce the bones of the skull and form a connecting circulation between the veins on the skull surface and the dural sinuses within. These veins also provide a means by which infection can be transmitted from outside the skull to the brain, and a particularly important one is at the root of the nose. Therefore if an infection, such as a boil, occurs on the cheeks there is a special risk that bacteria may travel via this vein into the skull and cause catastrophic damage. For this reason the front of the cheeks is regarded as a danger area, and infections in this region are always given very special attention. Despite the patient's protests, he is usually put to bed and kept quiet and still until the infection has been mastered.

**emission.** 1. An ejaculation. 2. The radiation of light and heat.

**nocturnal emission.** Ejaculation of semen during sleep. Also called *wet dream.*

**emmenagogue.** A drug used for promoting menstrual flow. Also called *menagogue.*

**emmenia.** The monthly periods.

**emmetropia.** Normal vision.

**emmetropic.** Relating to emmetropia.

**emollient.** A soothing or a softening preparation.

**emotion.** A feeling or sentiment, but may also refer to a violent feeling, usually of an agitated nature, involving mental and physical reactions such as changes in heart action and disturbances of circulation, including blushing, palpitations, rapid pulse, fast breathing, sweating, dry mouth, or pallor.

**emphysema.** The abnormal presence of air or gas in tissues. It can be detected by the creaking sensation felt when the part is pressed with the fingers.

**pulmonary emphysema.** A condition in which the normal air spaces in the lungs are enlarged, causing the lungs to become more bulky. It usually accompanies chronic bronchitis and causes shortness of breath and discomfort to the lungs and heart. In the advanced state it is recognized by the barrel shape of the chest and a very poor degree of chest expansion, which may be as little as half an inch. Also called *pneumonectasia, pneumonectasis.*

**subcutaneous emphysema.** Air or gas beneath the skin due to injury or infection by a gas-forming organism.

**surgical emphysema.** The distension of the subcutaneous tissues after a surgical operation by air coming from a wound communicating with the lungs.

**emphysematous.** Pertaining to emphysema.

**empiric, empirical.** 1. Based on observation and experience and not necessarily on scientific reasoning. For example, it may refer to the knowledge that a drug is effective without knowing precisely the reason for its effectiveness. 2. Also describes a charlatan who practices medicine without scientific training.

**emplastrum.** A plaster.

**empyema.** The presence of pus in the chest, usually a purulent pleurisy.

**emulsion.** A suspension of oil in water, often by means of gum arabic, which effects a very fine division of the oil.

**enamel.** The outer covering of the teeth.

**encapsuled, encapsulated.** Enclosed.

**enceinte.** Pregnant.

**encephalic.** Pertaining to the brain.

**encephalitis.** Inflammation of the brain.

**encephalitis lethargica.** Sleeping sickness.

**encephalography.** X-ray investigations of the brain after replacing some of the cerebrospinal fluid by injections of air.

**encephaloid.** Resembling brain tissue.

**encephaloma.** A brain growth.

**encephalomalacia.** Softening of the brain resulting from cutting off of the blood supply by embolism or thrombosis.

**encephalomeningitis.** Inflammation of the brain and its coverings.

**encephalomyelitis.** Inflammation of both brain and spinal cord.

**encephalon.** The brain.

**encephalopathy.** A growth composed of cartilage growing in tissue where cartilage is not ordinarily found, such as the interior of a bone.

**enchondrosis.** A cartilaginous tumor.

**encysted.** Enclosed in a cyst.

**endarteritis.** Inflammation of the inner layer of the wall of an artery. This can produce so much thickening that obstruction results.

**end artery.** An artery which ends finally without communication with the small branches of any other artery.

**endemic.** Pertaining to any disease constantly present in a particular area, as opposed to epidemic, which implies a sudden explosive outburst of a disease.

**endemiology.** The science of endemic diseases.

**endocardial.** Pertaining to the endocardium.

**endocarditis.** Inflammation of the endocardium, especially that part which covers the heart valves; frequently due to rheumatic fever or to a bacterial infection.

**endocardium.** The lining membrane of the heart.

**endocervical.** Pertaining to the inner part of the neck of the womb.

**endocervicitis.** Inflammation of the membrane lining the neck of the womb.

**endochondral.** From within a cartilage.

**endocolitis.** Inflammation of the lining of the colon.

**endocolpitis.** Inflammation of the lining of the vagina.

**endocranial.** Contained within the cranium.

**endocranium.** The inner surface of the skull.

**endocrine.** Pertaining to the endocrine glands and their secretions.

**endocrine glands.** Ductless glands that secrete hormones into the blood and that have a particular effect on other organs. They are also known as ductless glands and include the following. The adrenal (sometimes called the suprarenal) is situated above the kidney. The cortex (outer layer) of the gland produces many steroids with cortisonelike activity that affects car-bohydrate metabolism, increases protein breakdown, produces an antiinflammatory reaction, acts on the kidney in controlling the elimination of salt and water, and affects the sex glands. The medulla (inner part) of the gland produces epinephrine and norepinephrine, which raise the blood pressure, stimulate metabolism, and mobilize glycogen as glucose. The pancreas, situated within the abdomen, produces insulin and glucagon, which controls carbohydrate metabolism, and produces digestive enzymes (an exocrine function). The parathyroid gland, situated in the neck, controls calcium in the body. The pineal gland, situated in the brain, produces melatonin. This gland calcifies with age and serves as a useful radiologic landmark. The pituitary gland, situated in the brain, has three parts; between them they liberate a large number of hormones including a growth hormone, a thyroid-controlling hormone, an adrenocorticotrophic hormone, gonadotrophin, a milk-stimulating hormone (prolactin), an oxytocic hormone, which contracts the womb, a vasopressor hormone, which raises blood pressure, and an antidiuretic hormone, which reduces the output of urine. From the thymus, situated in the chest, no specific hormone has been isolated, though there does appear to be a connection between this gland and myasthenia gravis. The thyroid gland, situated in the neck, produces thyroxine, which controls growth and development. This gland influences other glands and has been described as the master gland.

Glands of Internal Secretion:
Pi — Pineal body
H — Hypophysis (pituitary)
Td — Thyroid & parathyroids
Ts — Thymus
A — Adrenals
Pa — Pancreas
D — Duodenum
O — Ovaries (F)
Pr — Prostate (M)
T — Testes (M)
(The stomach and liver also perform grandular functions)

ENDOCRINE GLANDS

**endocrinology.** The study of the endocrine glands.

**endocrinopathy.** Any condition caused by a disorder of the endocrine glands.

**endocystitis.** Inflammation of the lining of the urinary bladder.

**endoderm.** See ENTODERM.

**endoenteritis.** Inflammation of the lining of the intestine.

**endogastritis.** Inflammation of the lining of the stomach.

**endogenous.** Produced from within the body.

**endointoxication.** Poisoning of the body by a poison produced within itself.

**endolymph.** A fluid contained in the labyrinth of the ear.

**endometrial.** Pertaining to the endometrium, the lining of the womb.

**endometrioma.** A tumor arising in the lining of the womb. Occasionally, tissue similar to that lining the womb occurs in the ovary, the Fallopian tube, or other unusual situations where it undergoes the same monthly change as the womb lining, bleeds during menstruation, and may form a blood cyst or tumor.

**endometriosis.** The general term applied to the presence in the body of endometriomas.

**endometritis.** The inflammatory state of the lining of the womb.

**endometrium.** The membrane lining the womb into which the fertilized egg is embedded in order to develop. It is also responsible for menstruation. See MENSES.

**endoneuritis.** Inflammation of the connective tissue which forms a framework for the support of individual fibers in a nerve.

**end organ.** The final termination of a nerve fiber in muscle, skin, or other structure.

**endoscope.** An instrument for examining the interior of a hollow organ. It is equipped with an electric bulb and a series of lenses which provide a well-lit visual examination.

**endoscopic.** Relating to endoscopy.

**endoscopy.** Examination with an endoscope.

**endothelial.** Pertaining to the endothelium.

**endothelioma.** A tumor or growth derived from cells forming the endothelium.

**endothelium.** The single-celled membrane lining the inside of the heart, blood, and lymph vessels, the wall of capillaries, the lymph spaces, and serous cavities.

**endothermy.** Surgical diathermy.

**endothrix.** The group name for fungi which cause such skin disorders as tinea capitis.

**endotoxin.** A poison contained within a germ and only liberated when the germ disintegrates. It is not the usual poison which the germ manufactures and excretes into the blood to produce disease.

**end plate.** The expanded end of a nerve fiber supplying a muscle.

**enema.** Liquid introduced into the rectum to wash out the rectum, to cure constipation, to treat the lining of the bowel with a medical lotion, and to introduce food products or drugs which will be absorbed through the lining of the lower bowel.

**engorgement.** Congestion; the damming back of blood in a tissue or organ and indicative of obstruction to the normal flow of blood in the part.

**enophthalmos.** Receding of the eyeball into the orbital cavity; sunken eye.

**ensiform.** Shaped like a sword; usually refers to the ensiform cartilage at the end of the breastbone.

**E.N.T.** The abbreviation for ear, nose, and throat.

**entamoeba.** A group of protozoa which cause such diseases as amebic dysentery.

**enteral.** Within the intestine.

**enterectomy.** Surgical removal of part of the intestine.

**enteric.** Pertaining to the intestine.

**enteric fever.** See TYPHOID FEVER.

**enteritis.** Inflammation of the intestine.

**enterococcus.** A streptococcal germ found in the intestinal tract; and which may cause such inflammatory conditions as appendicitis.

**enterocolitis.** Inflammation of both small intestine and colon.

**enterocolostomy.** A surgical operation to join together the small and large intestines. It usually implies that a portion of diseased intestine has been removed and the cut ends of the colon and small intestine have been joined together.

**entero-enterostomy.** A surgical operation to join together two loops of the intestine. This usually means that an intermediate portion of diseased intestine has been removed.

**enterogastritis.** See GASTROENTERITIS.

**enterogenous.** Originating in or pertaining to the intestine.

**enterolith.** A stonelike body formed within the intestine.

**enterologist.** A specialist in intestinal disorders.

**enterology.** The study of the intestinal tract, including its diseases.

**enterolysis.** Surgical removal of intestinal adhesions.

**enteromegaly.** Enlargement of the intestines.

**enteropexy.** Surgical fixation of part of the intestine to the abdominal wall to secure it from dropping.

**enteroplasty.** Surgical repair of the intestine.

**enteroplegia.** Paralysis of the intestines that sometimes follows surgery

within the abdomen, not necessarily on the intestines themselves. It is a form of surgical shock of the intestines.

**enteroptosis.** Sagging of the intestines from their normal position down to the bottom of the abdomen.

**enterospasm.** Intestinal spasm or colic.

**enterostenosis.** A narrowing or stricture of the intestinal tube.

**enterostomy.** A surgical operation by which a piece of intestine is brought through the abdominal wall to the surface and then opened so that the contents of the intestinal tract emerge through this abdominal opening instead of through the anus.

**entoderm.** The innermost of the three germinal layers of the embryo, from which develop the lining of the digestive tract, pancreas, liver, middle ear, respiratory tract, thyroid, parathyroid, and thymus glands, and other parts. Also called *endoderm.*

**entopic.** Situated in the usual place; as opposed to ectopic, which means out of position.

**entropion.** Inversion of the eyelid in which the eyelashes rub against the eyeball.

**enucleation.** Surgical removal of the eyeball from its socket; or the shelling out of a tumor or organ from its capsule.

**enuresis.** Incontinence of urine; or the spontaneous emptying of the bladder. **nocturnal enuresis.** Bed-wetting.

**environment.** The external conditions which surround, act upon, and have effect on an organism or its parts.

**enzyme.** A chemical substance produced by tissue cells, which has a specific effect in promoting a chemical change.

**eosin.** A rose-colored dye used in the pathological laboratory to dye tissue specimens. It is also used as a dye in some kinds of lipstick, and was originally used to discover leaks in sewers because it is easily recognized by normal eyesight.

**eosinophil.** A white blood cell having a great affinity for eosin. Its normal percentage is much increased when the body has been invaded by parasites, and in some allergic diseases.

**eosinophilia.** The condition of having an increased number of eosinophils in the blood.

**Epanutin.** A drug used in the treatment of epilepsy.

**ependyma.** The membrane lining the cavities of the brain and the central canal of the spinal cord.

**ephedrine.** A drug used as follows: to relieve asthma; to reduce shortness of breath in chronic bronchitis and em-

physema; to cut short migraine headaches; to treat bed-wetting in children; for certain muscle disorders; as a spray in the treatment of hay fever; and in the treatment of narcolepsy—a disorder in which the patient has an irresistible urge to sleep for short periods. Ephedrine was originally discovered to be present in a plant found in China, but is now synthesized, making it much cheaper to buy.

**ephemeral.** Transient.

**epicanthus.** A half-moon-shaped skin fold covering the inner angle of the eye.

**epicondyle.** A bony prominence situated on the femoral and humeral condyles.

**epicritic.** Pertaining to certain skin nerve fibers which enable one to appreciate very fine distinctions of temperature and touch.

**epidemic.** The unusual and sudden prevalence of a disease in a given area or locality.

**epidemic catarrhal fever.** Influenza.

**epidemic parotitis.** See MUMPS.

**epidemiology.** The study of epidemics and their occurrence throughout the world.

**epidermalization.** The conversion of tissue into skin.

**epidermatoplasty.** Skin grafting.

**epidermis.** The outer layer of the skin.

**epidermophytosis.** A fungus disease of the skin. Also called *foot rot.* See also ATHLETE'S FOOT.

**epididymis.** A small structure lying behind and above each testicle and part of the seminal tract.

**epididymitis.** Inflammation of the epididymis.

**epididymo-orchitis.** Inflammation of the epididymis and testes.

**epidural.** Situated upon or over the dura mater, one of the brain coverings. **epidural injection.** A spinal anesthetic injected into the epidural space at the lowest part of the spine. **epidural space.** The space, potential or real, external to the dura mater. **epidural abscess.** An abscess pressing on the coverings of the brain or spinal cord.

**epigastric.** Referring to the epigastrium.

**epigastrium.** The upper-middle region of the abdomen just below the chest plate.

**epiglottic.** Pertaining to the epiglottis.

**epiglottis.** The valve in the throat below and behind the tongue, which cuts off the air passages during swallowing to prevent food and liquid from entering the lungs.

**epignathous.** A tumor arising from the palate, filling the mouth and protruding from it.

**epilate.** To remove hair by destroying the roots.

**epilation.** Removal of hair by destroying the roots.

**epilatory.** Removing hair permanently; a chemical which destroys hair.

**epilepsy.** A convulsive condition of the nervous system, due to a disturbance of the brain's electrical activity, which results in a characteristic fit. During a fit, the subject suddenly cries out and falls to the ground. He often suffers an injury because he is unconscious in the upright position and falls during this period. At first the body is stiff and in a complete muscular spasm, but after a time this passes and the muscles of the body begin to jerk—the patient throws himself about and may need gentle restraint to avoid further injury. The jerking gradually passes, and later a very sleepy person regains consciousness and looks surprised. During the attack he may have passed urine or feces. The danger during the jerking stage is that the tongue may be bitten through; the first-aid treatment is to get between the patient's teeth something on which he can bite without damaging the tongue—a piece of wood wrapped in a handkerchief or a roll of bandage will do. If the tongue is bleeding freely the patient should be turned face downwards or half on his front and half on his side so that blood can run out of the mouth and not down the throat. As soon as the attack has passed and the mouth can be safely opened, the tongue can be examined to see if any treatment is needed. The patient will, however, require medical aid and a doctor should be sent for or the patient removed to hospital. In minor fits of epilepsy, consciousness is not lost but there is a split-second pause in whatever the patient is doing and he seems a bit vacant. This form of the disease is more of a nuisance than a danger; some people have as many as thirty or forty attacks a day.

*It is alleged that following an epileptic fit some individuals suffer from a period of automatic action in which there is complete loss of memory, and it has been advanced in murder trials that the accused man was in such a state at the time of the crime and therefore not responsible for his actions. Susceptibility to epilepsy can be verified by having the brain's electrical activity measured by an electroencephalograph, which shows characteristic records in an epileptic type of person.*

*Many epileptics are of normal intelligence, or even above average, while a percentage of them are subnormal. Treatment is by various antispasmodic and sedative drugs which have to be* taken regularly for at least three years after the last attack followed by a further period of twelve months, during which the patient is slowly and gradually weaned off his tablets, before it is safe to say he is cured. Epileptics are not allowed to drive motor vehicles and, for obvious reasons, certain jobs such as employment involving moving machinery or working at great heights are closed to them.

**grand mal.** In this, the major form of epilepsy, the patient usually calls out and then falls to the ground unconscious. At first the whole body goes stiff and rigid (tonic spasm) which passes off fairly quickly after which all the muscles of the body start to twitch (clonic spasm). This persists for two or three minutes and then stops, after which the patient slowly becomes conscious and is at first dazed and sleepy. See also COMA.

**Jacksonian epilepsy.** In this type, first described by the English neurologist, Hughlings Jackson, the patient may not lose consciousness but has a twitching of the muscles. The fits are due to something irritating the surface of the brain, and the irritant can often be removed by operation resulting in an outright cure.

**myoclonic epilepsy.** This very rare form of epilepsy appears in children, usually between the ages of 5 and 15 years, while in adults it commences between the ages of 25 and 40 years. The characteristic symptom is sudden muscle contractions which may vary in intensity from simple twitching to violent movements of the limb. The condition may remain stationary for years, having little tendency to shorten life, or it may end fatally within a few months of onset, with progressive mental deterioration and ultimately coma. Recovery may take place spontaneously but the condition is very prone to recur.

**petit mal.** In this condition the patient does not lose consciousness but for a moment has an arrest of all muscular activity. For instance, he may be drinking soup and for a split second he may hold the spoon poised between plate and mouth, after which he finishes the movement. There may be as many as 30 or 40 attacks per day and at one time there was no treatment for this type of epilepsy but there are now drugs which do mitigate the number of fits. Also called *minor epilepsy.*

**epileptic.** Pertaining to epilepsy; a person affected with epilepsy.

**epileptic psychoses.** A series of mental disturbances, among which are automatism, confusion, depression, dream states, and actual mania, which either follow or replace an epileptic fit.

**epileptiform.** Resembling an epileptic attack.

**epimenorrhagia.** Excessive loss at the monthly periods.

**epimenorrhea.** Having more than one menstrual period in a month.

**epimenorrhoea.** See EPIMENORRHEA.

**epinephrectomy.** Surgical removal of a suprarenal gland.

**epinephrine.** Adrenaline, the internal secretion of the suprarenal glands. Epinephrine is also produced synthetically. See ADRENALINE.

**epinephritis.** Inflammation of a suprarenal gland.

**epinephros.** Another name for a suprarenal gland.

**epiphora.** An excessive outpouring of tears. This may be due to blockage of the duct which carries the tears away from the eye into the nose or to excessive manufacture of tears by the lacrimal gland.

**epiphyseal.** Referring to an epiphysis.

**epiphysis.** 1. The pineal body. 2. Each end of the shaft of a long bone.

**epiphysitis.** Inflammation of an epiphysis. See also PERTHES' DISEASE.

**epiploic.** Relating to the omentum.

**episclera.** The connective tissue between the conjunctiva of the eyeball and the coat underneath.

**episcleritis.** Inflammation of the episclera.

**episiotomy.** Surgical incision of the back part of the vaginal opening to allow the baby's head to come through at childbirth in order to avoid extensive tearing. After birth the incision is stitched up.

**epispadias.** A congenital deformity of the penis in which the urethra opens on the top surface of the penis instead of at the tip. If the urethra opens on the undersurface of the penis the condition is known as hypospadias. Also called *anaspadias.*

**epistaxis.** Nosebleeding, nasal hemorrhage. In the majority of cases nosebleeding is due to a small ulcer on the fore part of the nasal septum and is frequently associated with nosepicking—the septum is the dividing wall between the nostrils and is generously supplied with blood vessels. The first-aid treatment is simple enough: the patient should be made to sit up, bend slightly forward, and breathe through the mouth while the person giving first aid pinches the nostrils together for five or ten minutes—this usually stops the bleeding and clots up the ulcer. If this treatment fails, then a doctor may have to pack the nose with ribbon gauze soaked in adrenalin, which contracts the blood vessels and stops the bleeding by pressure. Very severe bleeding, fortunately rare, has to be treated by an electric cautery. The old-fashioned belief that a nosebleed was "good for you" is a survival of the days when practically the only treatment was bloodletting. Nosebleeding does you neither good nor much harm, since the quantity of blood lost is so small, and by far the biggest factor in any nosebleed is the panic it engenders either in the patient or among the relatives. Also called *rhinorrhagia*.

**episternum.** The upper part of the breastbone. Also called *manubrium*.

**epithelial.** Pertaining to or composed of skinlike cells; often refers to the whole skin.

**epithelioma.** A form of skin cancer.

**epithelium.** The layer of cells which covers the surfaces and lines the internal cavities of the body; it is also a general term for the various types of surface membrane, such as the skin itself, the lining of blood vessels (endothelium) and that lining body cavities (mesothelium). Other names are given to various kinds of epithelia, either because of their function or the microscopical structure that distinguishes them, such as *pigmented epithelium*, in which cells contain granules of pigment, and *ciliated epithelium*, where the cells have a protruding, whiplike moving filament, as in the nasal passages and cheeks.

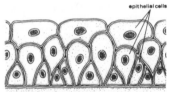

epithelial cells

EPITHELIUM (from the lining of the bladder)

**epithelization.** The growth or regrowth of epithelium over a raw surface or wound; the process of repair.

**Epsom salts.** Chemically known as magnesium sulphate, Epsom salts has various uses. Taken by mouth as a purgative, it can be used in two ways: a teaspoonful dissolved in about a quarter tumbler of water draws fluid out of the body and produces a watery stool; this is also used as a method of dehydration in certain diseases. The second method, in which a teaspoonful is dissolved in a half pint or more of water, also acts as a purgative but only because the Epsom salts prevents water from being absorbed by the body, and the half pint that is swallowed goes through the gut unabsorbed,

washing as it goes, and producing a watery stool. This is the better way of using Epsom salts as a purgative because it is merely a mechanical washing out of the bowel, whereas if the salts are taken in a small quantity of water, although opening the bowels, it makes one feel low in spirits. Injected into the blood, a solution of Epsom salts provokes dehydration of the brain and is used in certain nervous disorders. Epsom salts is also incorporated with glycerine to form a paste known as magnesium sulphate paste, which, because of its drawing action, is used on boils to bring them to a head, or on dirty wounds to draw out body fluid to wash the wound clean. A saturated solution of magnesium sulphate, made by dissolving as much Epsom salts as possible in water, makes a hypertonic lotion for use as a soothing application for such conditions as sunburn.

**equilibrium.** An even balance, or a state in which no change can take place.

**Erb's disease.** A condition in which there is wasting and paralysis of muscles. The condition of the muscles is masked by their becoming apparently bigger than normal.

**Erb's palsy.** A paralysis of the upper arm due to nerve damage during the course of birth.

**erection.** Specifically refers to the alteration to the penis in which it becomes blown up with blood, erect, and stiff.

**eremophobia.** Fear of being lonely; fear of desolate places.

**erepsin.** A proteolytic enzyme found in the intestinal juice.

**ergometrine.** A drug derived from ergot.

**ergophobia.** A morbid fear of work.

**ergot.** A drug derived from *Claviceps purpurea*, a fungus found on growing rye. Ergot or one of its derivatives is used in midwifery to contract the womb, to prevent bleeding after delivery, and as an ingredient of tablets used for the relief of migraine headaches. If taken in excessive amounts, ergot constricts the tiny blood vessels in the extremities of the fingers and toes, causing numbness, tingling, severe pain, and gangrene. It was first discovered in the fifteenth century on the plains of Italy among growers of rye, who inevitably ate a lot of their crop, and as a result absorbed so much of the fungus that they sustained ergot poisoning, which in those days was called St. Anthony's fire. Curiously enough, St. Anthony's fire still appears sporadically in patients who, instead of taking migraine tablets only for the first two days in order to cut

short an attack, go on taking them without reason for long periods.

*Erysipelas, often erroneously called St. Anthony's fire, was in the past an overwhelming infection of the skin and soft tissues, and the patient usually died from toxemia while those that recovered were not crippled. On the other hand, ergotism was a terribly crippling complaint that resulted in hordes of crippled vagrants roaming Europe until the Hospital Brothers of St. Anthony were inaugurated in 1093 by Gaston de Dauphiné in thanksgiving for his son's recovery from the disease.*

**ergotism.** Ergot poisoning. See ERGOT.

**erosion.** An ulceration. Commonly refers to erosion of the cervix, an ulcer on the neck of the womb, which sometimes follows childbirth. It causes a white, occasionally blood-stained, vaginal discharge which continues until the ulcer has been cauterized. The discharge is popularly known as "the whites." See also. LEUKORRHOEA.

**erotic.** Pertaining to the sexual passions; moved or roused by sexual desire; a lustful or amorous person.

**eroticism, erotism.** Pertaining to the erotic state.

**erotomania.** Morbid or abnormally strong sexual desire.

**erotopath.** A sexual pervert.

**erotophobia.** A neurotic fear of sex.

**eructation.** Belching. See also AEROPHAGIA.

**eruption.** A bursting forth; the tooth erupting through a gum.

**eruptive fever.** Any fever with a skin rash.

**erysipelas.** An acute, contagious inflammation of the skin due to infection with a streptococcal germ and characterized by a fever, headache, and spreading red oval patches on the skin. It is controlled and cured within two or three days by antibiotic drugs. In the prepenicillin era erysipelas was an extremely serious disease in persons over sixty and tantamount to a death sentence. Often erroneously called St. Anthony's fire. See also ERGOT.

**erysipeloid.** An inflammatory skin disease resembling erysipelas. It does not disturb the patient's general health, and is due to a germ which causes erysipelas in pigs. The disease is to be found usually in butchers, fishmongers, and cooks who handle infected meat or fish.

**erythema.** A diffuse redness of the skin caused by congestion of the skin blood vessels.

**biological erythema.** Erythema produced by mammals, insects, plants, and bacteria.

**erythema ab igne.** Erythema produced by artificial heat and seen in stokers and ladies who "toast" their legs in front of the fire.

**erythema annulare centrifugum.** A chronic form of erythema consisting of large rings with smooth pink, red, or brown coloration.

**erythema bullosum.** Erythema accompanied by bullae or vesicles.

**erythema chronica migrans.** A form of erythema with large rings, often following an insect bite.

**erythema circinatum.** Ringed lesions having a pale center and red margins. If two or more of the rings fuse together it is called *erythema figuratum.*

**erythema granuloma annulare.** Small papules arranged in rings, usually on the arms or legs. The condition disappears spontaneously. It is commonly seen in New Zealand.

**erythema infectiosum.** A form of erythema occurring in children during the summer and characterized by a rash, sore throat, lassitude, but no temperature. It may occur as an epidemic. Also called *fifth disease.*

**erythema iris.** A variety of erythema that has varicolored rings resembling an archery target.

**erythema marginatum.** See TOXIC ERYTHEMA, below.

**erythema multiforme.** A toxic erythema of unknown cause; characterized by red patches of various shapes, sizes, and pattern accompanied by vesicles and crust formation. It can vary from a mild and recurrent skin condition to a grave illness accompanied by pneumonia. The severe form is called *erythema multiforme exudativum.* See also STEVENS-JOHNSON SYNDROME.

**erythema nodosum.** A toxic erythema causing nodular swellings, usually on the shins. It is considered to be an allergic reaction to a drug or germ poison. In children, a large number of cases are due to tuberculosis.

**erythema papulatum.** Erythema accompanied by dome-shaped papules.

**erythema pernio.** Chilblains.

**erythema solare.** Erythema produced by ultraviolet light, such as sunburn.

**erythema traumaticum.** Erythema produced by mechanical irritation of the skin.

**erythema vesiculosum.** Erythema accompanied by vesicles.

**toxic erythema.** Erythema caused by the toxins of disease such as in scarlet fever, German measles, rheumatic fever, and drug eruptions. One of the distinctive erythemas under this heading is erythema marginatum, which occurs as red rings or patterns in rheumatic fever, rheumatic endocarditis, and chorea. Certain foods,

such as strawberries, plums, and rhubarb, can cause toxic erythema and so also can drugs such as arsenic, lead, mercury, sulphonamide, and quinine.

**x-ray erythema.** Radiodermatitis produced by x-rays.

**erythematous.** Pertaining to erythema.

**erythraemia.** See ERYTHREMIA.

**erythrasma.** A fungus disease of the skin characterized by reddish or brownish scaly patches, usually occurring on the upper part of the inner thigh, the armpits, the folds beneath the breasts, and in other moist regions.

**erythredema.** See PINK DISEASE.

**erythremia.** See POLYCYTHEMIA.

**erythrism.** The condition of being red-haired.

**erythritol tetranitrate.** A drug used in the treatment of angina pectoris.

**erythroblast.** An immature cell with a nucleus from which an erythrocyte or red blood cell develops. At maturity the nucleus is absent.

**erythrocyanosis.** A skin condition due to a disorder of the local circulatory system, found especially in young girls and young women, characterized by a bluish-red discoloration, especially in the feet and legs but more marked over the calves, and accompanied by a burning or itching sensation, sometimes with swelling of the affected areas.

**erythrocyte.** A mature red blood cell.

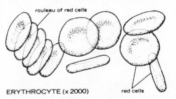

ERYTHROCYTE (x 2000)

rouleau of red cells

red cells

**erythrocytosis.** An abnormal increase in the number of red blood cells in the blood.

**erythroderma.** Any skin disease characterized by an abnormal redness of the skin together with infiltration in which the whole thickness of the skin is involved. Also called *erythrodermia, generalized exfoliative dermatitis.*

**erythroderma desquamativum.** Erythroderma occurring in infants, characterized by redness of the skin and a scaling eruption. Also called *Leiner's disease.*

**erythroderma exfoliativa.** Pityriasis rubra, a skin disorder having a rash similar to scarlet fever; The disorder lasts from six to eight weeks with free desquamation of the skin surface.

**erythroderma ichthyosiforme congenitum.** A congenital form of erythroderma characterized by generalized redness, especially over the front of the neck and flexor surfaces of the large joints, and associated with thickening of the skin on the soles of the feet, with deformities of the nails, and seborrhea of the scalp.

**erythroderma maculosa perstans.** A variety of psoriasis in which the areas involved are about a half-inch in diameter and without marked scaling.

**erythroedema.** See ERYTHREDEMA.

**erythromelalgia.** A skin disorder characterized by congestion and reddening of the skin of the hands or feet and accompanied by severe neuralgic pains. Also called *Weir-Mitchell's disease.*

**erythrophobia.** Blushing, when a neurotic manifestation.

**erythroplakia.** The early changes seen in a mucous membrane which can ultimately develop squamous carcinoma (cancer).

**esophageal.** Pertaining to the esophagus.

**esophagectasis.** Dilatation of the esophagus.

**esophagectomy.** Surgical removal of part or the whole of the esophagus.

**esophagismus.** Spasm of the esophagus.

**esophagitis.** Inflammation of the esophagus.

**esophagocele.** A blind tube leading out from the wall of the esophagus.

**esophagoduodenostomy.** A surgical operation in which a great part of the esophagus is removed and the cut end joined to the duodenum.

**esophago-enterostomy.** A surgical operation in which part of the esophagus is removed and the cut end joined to any portion of the small intestine.

**esophagogastrostomy.** A surgical operation in which part of the esophagus is removed and the cut end joined to the stomach.

**esophagojejunostomy.** A surgical operation in which part of the esophagus is removed and the cut end joined to the jejunum.

**esophagomycosis.** Any fungus disease of the esophagus.

**esophagoplasty.** Surgical repair of the esophagus.

**esophagoscope.** An instrument used to examine the lining of the esophagus.

**esophagospasm, esophagismus.** Spasm of the esophagus.

**esophagostenosis.** A constriction of the esophagus.

**esophagostomy.** A surgical operation to make an artificial opening into the esophagus.

**esophagotomy.** Surgical incision into the esophagus.

**esophagus.** The gullet. Composed of an outer layer of muscular tissue and an inner one of mucous membrane, it is about nine inches long and reaches from the pharynx, passing downwards on the back wall of the chest and through the diaphragm, to the stomach.

**esophoria.** Tendency to squint inwards.

**esophoric.** Relating to esophoria.

**esotropia.** A convergent squint.

**essential fever.** Any fever of unknown cause.

**estivo-autumnal fever.** See MALARIA.

**estradiol.** A female sex hormone.

**estrin.** A female sex hormone.

**estrogen.** Any substance which has the property of the female hormone to produce estrus. Estrogens may arise in the ovaries, adrenal glands, and placenta, and be present in the urine. They can be produced synthetically.

**estrone.** A female sex hormone.

**estrum, estrus.** 1. The sequence of changes which occur in the ovary and womb and correspond with the menstrual cycle. 2. The period when sexual desire is highest in the lower animals; the mating period of animals, especially of the female; also called *being in heat, rut.*

**ethmoid.** A bone at the base of the skull.

**ethmoidal.** Relating to the ethmoid bone.

**ethmoidectomy.** Surgical removal of the ethmoid sinus cells.

**ethmoiditis.** Inflammation of the ethmoid bone or the ethmoid sinuses.

**ethmoid sinuses.** Air-containing cavities in the ethmoid bone situated at the back of the nose.

**ethnic.** Pertaining to racial characteristics.

**etiology.** The study of the causes of diseases.

**eugenics.** The science of improving the hereditary characteristics of the human race.

**negative eugenics.** Measures which aim to decrease the incidence of hereditary defects.

**positive eugenics.** Measures under social control which aim to increase the families having desirable and superior traits.

**eunuch.** A castrated male.

**eunuchoidism.** A condition found in the male in which most of the male characteristics are poorly developed, accompanied by obesity of the female type.

**euphoria.** A sense of well-being.

**euphoric.** Relating to euphoria.

**eustachian tube.** See TUBE: EUSTACHIAN TUBE.

**euthanasia.** The painless induction of death in people suffering from incurable disease, the invitation coming from the patient himself. Also called *mercy killing.*

**evacuant.** Emptying an organ; a purgative which empties the bowels.

**evacuation.** The act of emptying the bowels.

**evanescent.** Tending to disappear quickly.

**eventration.** The protrusion of the contents of the abdomen through the abdominal wall so that they are only covered by the skin. This very large hernia may contain most of the intestine and some of the abdominal organs.

**eversion.** To turn outwards, as for instance eversion of the eyelid.

**evolution.** A process of development going on in all living species through the millions of years that life has been on the earth; this involves change which in general makes for more complex differentiation of body parts.

**evulsion.** The forcible tearing away of a part. Commonly refers to a piece of bone being torn off by violent strain by a muscle or ligament, or knocked off by a blow.

**exacerbation.** An increase in the severity of a disease.

**exaltation.** A mental state characterized by self-satisfaction, ecstatic joy, abnormal cheerfulness, optimism, or delusions of grandeur.

**exanthem, exanthema.** An erruption of the skin or a rash, but commonly refers to an infectious fever, such as measles, accompanied by a rash.

**exanthrope.** Any external origin for a disease.

**excipient.** An inert substance combined with a drug to make a tablet easier to manufacture.

**excise.** To remove some part or organ by surgical operation.

**excision.** The cutting off of part of an organ or tissue.

**excitability.** Irritability; the readiness of response to a stimulus.

**excite.** To cause an increase in activity; to stimulate.

**excitement.** The state of increased activity of an organ.

**excoriation.** Abrasion of the skin.

**excrement.** Feces.

**excreta.** The waste products of the body such as urine and feces.

**excrete.** To expel waste products from the body.

**excretion.** Waste products of the body; the act of excreting.

**exenteration.** 1. Removal of the thoracic or abdominal organs. 2. Protru-

sion of the abdominal organs through a surgical incision. 3. Removal of the contents of an organ, such as the eye.

**exfoliation.** Shedding the layers of the skin.

**exfoliative.** Causing exfoliation.

**exhalant.** Breathing out; exhaling.

**exhaustion.** 1. Loss of strength, or fatigue. 2. The emptying of a vessel of air, thus causing a vacuum.

**exhibit.** To administer a drug or medicine.

**exhibitionism.** A sexual perversion in which pleasure is obtained by exposing the genital organs to one of the opposite sex.

**exhibitionist.** A person addicted to exhibitionism. The word is also popularly used to describe somebody who shows off.

**exhumation.** Digging up a dead body after burial.

**exocrine.** Pertaining to a gland which delivers its secretion through a duct to a specific area of the body.

**exophoria.** Tendency to squint outwards.

**exophthalmic.** Relating to exophthalmos.

**exophthalmos.** Abnormal prominence or protrusion of the eyeballs. This may be a familial characteristic, when it is of no significance, or be associated with overactivity of the thyroid gland, when the patient suffers from nervousness, rapid pulse, and loss of weight—the condition known as hyperthyroidism or Graves' disease. Surgical removal of part of the thyroid gland, situated in the front of the neck, cures the hyperthyroidism but not always the prominent eyeballs, which may persist. Protrusion of a single eyeball may be an indication of a tumor or abscess behind the eye. See also GOITER.

**exostosis.** A bony outgrowth.

**exoteric.** Developed outside the body.

**exotoxin.** A poison freely excreted by a germ.

**exotropia.** A divergent squint.

**expectorant.** A cough mixture which promotes the spitting up of mucus from the lungs.

**expectorate.** To spit up from the lungs.

**expectoration.** Spitting.

**expiration.** 1. The act of breathing out. 2. Death.

**expire.** 1. To breathe out. 2. To die.

**exploration.** A diagnostic surgical operation, during which the surgeon can examine some part inside the body.

**expression.** The act of pressing out; expulsion.

**expulsion.** The act of driving out.

**expulsive.** Relating to the act of expelling.

**exsanguinate.** To render a surgical field of operation bloodless, usually by binding elastic bandages round the limb beginning from below and moving upwards.

**exsiccant.** A drying agent.

**exsiccate.** To drive out moisture.

**extirpate.** To completely remove or eradicate.

**extirpation.** The total removal of a part.

**extra-.** A prefix meaning beyond, outside, or additional.

**extra-articular.** Outside a joint.

**extradural.** Outside the dura mater, one of the membranes covering the brain.

**extragenital.** Outside the genital organs.

**extrasystole.** A premature heartbeat. When these occur repeatedly, the patient complains of a thumping and bumping of the heart, commonly called palpitations.

**extra-uterine.** Outside the womb.

**extra-uterine pregnancy.** A pregnancy in which the fetus develops outside the womb. It may occur in the Fallopian tube, the ovary, or the abdominal cavity. See also PREGNANCY.

**extravasate.** The escape of fluid into the surrounding tissues.

**extreme unction.** A sacrament of the Roman Catholic Church administered to those in danger of death. The term "anointing of the sick" is now generally preferred to "extreme unction."

**extremity.** A limb or the distal portion of any organ.

**extrinsic.** Originating from outside a part.

**extroversion. 1.** The state of being inside out. **2.** A mental attitude in which a person's interests are directed to persons other than himself.

**extrovert.** One whose interests tend to extroversion.

**extrude.** To thrust out; to expel.

**extrusion.** A thrusting out or expulsion.

**exuberant.** Prolific or copious.

**exudate.** During inflammation, material that has passed through the wall of vessels into adjacent tissues or spaces.

**exudation.** During inflammation, the passage of various constituents of the blood through the walls of blood vessels into adjacent tissues or spaces.

**eye.** The organ of sight. It consists of a tough, dense membrane forming a globe, the front translucent portion of which is called the *cornea.* The front of the globe is covered by mucous membrane, which also lines the lids, called *conjunctiva,* and when this becomes inflamed the eye becomes red and irritable the condition is called conjunctivitis. Inside the eye is the *crystalline lens,* which can have its shape altered by muscles in order to focus clearly. When the lens becomes opaque it is called a cataract. In middle life the lens becomes stiff and inelastic and thus cannot be focused so well on near objects. The condition is called presbyopia and can be recognized by the need to wear reading spectacles. The chambers of the eye both in front of and behind the lens are filled with a substance called the *aqueous humor.* At the back of the eye the *optic nerve* enters from the brain and expands to form a visual sensitive plate, the *retina,* which has a small blind spot where the nerve enters it. The retina can be examined by an instrument called an ophthalmoscope. This blind spot is important to doctors because it is the one spot where veins and arteries can be examined under working conditions and because this area shows the early signs of pressure within the skull.

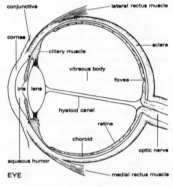

EYE

**eyecup.** A cup-shaped device that fits over the eye and is used for cleansing or applying medication to the exposed portion of the eyeball.

**eye drops.** Drugs used for the treatment of eye diseases; administered by pulling down the lower eyelid and dropping the liquid into the conjunctival sac. It cannot be too strongly emphasized that eye drops should never be kept long after the disease for which they were ordered has recovered, for most deteriorate after a week or so and some, such as penicillin eye drops, after seven days.

**eyelash.** One of many hairs growing on the edge of the eyelids.

**eyelid.** Either of two folds, upper and lower, that are moveable and protect the front surface of the eyeball.

**eyestrain.** Irritation and weariness of the eye resulting from excessive use or uncorrected visual defects. In the ordinary course of events these symptoms disappear after a night's sleep.

**eye teeth.** The upper canine teeth. See TOOTH: CANINE TOOTH.

# F

**facet.** A small surface, usually on a bone.

**facial.** Pertaining to the face.

**facies. 1.** A specific surface of the body. **2.** The appearance of the face, which can be quite revealing in the diagnosis of disease.

**factitious.** Artificial; unnatural.

**facultative.** Applied to bacteria capable of living both in the presence and in the absence of oxygen.

**faecal.** See FECAL.

**faeces.** See FECES.

**faeculent.** See FECULENT.

**Fahrenheit.** A temperature scale devised by the German physicist Gabriel Daniel Fahrenheit (1686-1736), in which the freezing point of water is marked as 32° and boiling point as 212°.

**faint.** To lose consciousness.

**fainting.** This is due to a sudden lowering of the blood pressure causing anemia of the brain. It may follow a fright, be caused by an overheated room, or occur on getting up from bed after a debilitating illness. The patient becomes deathly white, complains of feeling ill, and collapses.

**fainting sickness, falling sickness.** Obsolete terms for epilepsy.

**falling sickness.** Epilepsy.

**Fallopian tube.** See TUBE: FALLOPIAN TUBE.

**Fallot's tetralogy.** A form of congenital heart disease. See TETRALOGY OF FALLOT.

**familial.** A characteristic affecting several members of a family, or a disease to which a family is prone.

**faradism.** The application of induced currents; used in physiotherapy.

**farcy.** See GLANDERS.

**farinaceous.** Made from flour.

**far-sighted.** See HYPERMETROPIA.

**fascia.** Layers of fibroelastic tissue under the skin (superficial fascia) and between muscles, forming the sheaths of muscles or covering other deep structures, such as nerves and blood vessels (deep fascia).

**fascial.** Pertaining to fascia.

**fascicle.** A small bundle of muscle or nerve fibers.

**fascicular.** Bundle-shaped.

**fascitis.** Inflammation of a fascia.

**fastigium.** The summit.

**fat.** A soft or solid glycerol ester of the higher fatty acids occurring in plant and animal tissues. Fats serve as soft pads between organs, round out the bodily contours, and furnish a reserve supply of energy.

**fauces.** The back of the throat.

**faucial.** Pertaining to the fauces.

**favus.** A contagious fungus disease of the skin, usually affecting the scalp; characterized by round, yellow cup-shaped crusts, and a peculiar mousy odor.

**febrifuge.** An agent that brings down the temperature.

**febrile.** The state of running a temperature.

**fecal.** Relating to feces.

**fecal abscess.** An abscess containing feces and indicating a connection with the inside of the intestines.

**feces.** The waste products discharged from the anus.

**feculent.** Containing feces.

**fecundate.** To fertilize.

**felo de se.** Suicide.

**felon.** A whitlow.

**femoral.** Pertaining to the femur or femur region.

**femur.** The thigh bone, the longest bone in the body.

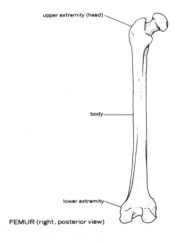

upper extremity (head)

body

lower extremity

FEMUR (right, posterior view)

**fenestra.** Latin for window or opening.

**fenestration.** A surgical operation involving a new opening in the internal ear, performed to relieve deafness.

**fermentation.** The decomposition of substances such as carbohydrate un-der the influence of ferments or enzymes. It is the process on which brewing of beer is based, during which starchy substances are broken down to yield alcohol.

**ferric.** Pertaining to or containing iron.

**fertilization.** Fecundation; fusion of a male and female sex cell.

**fester.** To suppurate.

**festination.** A type of walking seen in such nervous diseases as paralysis agitans, when the patient trots along in little bursts, getting faster and faster until he has to stop and then start off again; otherwise he would fall over.

**fetal.** Pertaining to a fetus or embryo.

**fetish.** Any object to which has been ascribed supernatural powers by the ignorant and superstitious.

**fetus.** The unborn baby after the second month of pregnancy.

**fever.** Pyrexia. A rise in the normal temperature of the body, which is about 98.6° F. though in children and old people it may normally be as high as 99° F. without being a sign of illness. In the past, the term fever referred specifically to scarlet fever, which was then much more serious and was dreaded by the general public. Nowadays, because of modern methods of treatment, it is a comparatively trivial disease. See also TEMPERATURE.

**fibrillation.** Twitching of muscle fibers. The condition is seen in diseases such as progressive muscular atrophy, syringomyelia, and uremia.

**auricular fibrillation.** A disorder of the heart producing a grossly irregular beat. Also called *atrial fibrillation.*

**fibrin.** A substance deposited when blood coagulates, and which then contracts to form a clot.

**fibrinogen.** The precursor of fibrin. In the presence of calcium and thromboplastin, the thrombin in the blood converts fibrinogen into fibrin during the process of blood coagulation.

**fibroadenoma.** A harmless growth composed of glandular and fibrous tissue, especially referring to fibroadenoma found in the breasts of young women.

**fibrocystic.** A fibrous degeneration which produces cysts.

**fibrocystic disease of bone.** A condition in which there is excessive loss of calcium and phosphorus in the urine and resorption of bone, which is replaced by fibrous and to a small extent by osteoid tissue, leading to the formation of cysts and tumorlike masses in the affected bones. Also called *osteitis fibrosa cystica generalisata, von Recklinhausen's disease.*

**fibrocystic disease of the pancreas.** A disease of infants and young children, characterized by cyst formation in the pancreas, the passage of undi-gested fat in the stools, and chronic chest trouble.

**fibroid.** A noncancerous benign growth that occurs in the womb. It can occur inside the cavity, inside the wall, and on the outer surface. Fibroids grow very slowly and cause trouble either by their size or by creating an irritation of the womb. Those occurring inside the womb can cause heavy menstrual periods, prevent pregnancy, or cause early miscarriages. Those occurring in the wall of the womb can cause heavy menstrual periods, and those occurring on the outside of the womb can grow large and may obstruct labor. Some fibroids hang by a stalk which may become twisted. This cuts off their blood supply and they degenerate, causing pain and other symptoms. They often require an operation for their removal.

**fibroidectomy.** Surgical removal of a fibroid.

**fibroma.** A benign harmless growth composed of fibrous tissue and frequently seen as hard, pink growths in the skin.

**fibromatosis.** The production of many fibromas such as occurs in neurofibromatosis.

**fibrosis.** The abnormal increase of fibrous tissue in an organ.

**fibrositis.** Inflammation of fibrous tissue, such as ligaments, tendons, muscle sheaths, and fasciae. Also called *muscular rheumatism.*

**fibrotic.** Relating to fibrosis.

**fibula.** The slender outer and smaller of the two bones of the lower leg. It is a nonweight-bearing bone. Also called *strap bone.*

**fifth disease.** A mild infectious disease of childhood, characterized by a rash which commences over the cheeks and forehead, forming rose-red patches with raised edges, the color of which fades in the center. It is a cross between measles and scarlet fever.

**filaria.** A type of threadworm.

**filarial.** Pertaining to filaria.

**filariasis.** Any disease in which filaria gain entrance to the lymphatic ducts causing inflammation, fibrosis, and blocking, which results in gross swelling of the area and the production of elephantiasis.

**filiform.** Threadlike.

**filix mas.** Male fern, a drug used to destroy intestinal worms.

**finger-agnosia.** Inability to recognize the individual fingers due to disease in the cerebral hemisphere of the brain.

**Finsen light.** Light from which the heat rays have been absorbed by filters, leaving only violet and ultraviolet rays; called after the Danish physician who advocated sun-ray treatment. In the past, Finsen light concentrated on small areas by means of lenses and was used for treating tuberculous skin diseases.

**first aid.** Emergency treatment while waiting for medical aid.

**first intention.** The healing of a wound by immediate union. This implies that the wound is clean and not likely to become infected.

**fissure.** A groove or cleft.

**anal fissure.** A very painful crack in the lining of the anus. It is initially caused by passing an excessively large stool, which overstretches the anus. Sometimes a fissure is associated with an anal polyp or skin tag.

**fistula.** An abnormal communication or channel between hollow organs, or between an organ and the skin surface.

**fit.** A convulsion or sudden paroxysm. See also EPILEPSY.

**fixation abscess.** An abscess caused by injection of an irritant beneath the skin.

**flaccid.** Soft, relaxed, or flabby; usually refers to the state of tone in a muscle.

**flagellation. 1.** Massage by strokes or blows. **2.** Flogging practiced by some religious orders, whose members whip themselves in expiation of their sins.

**flagellum.** A whiplike appendage, the organ of locomotion of spermatozoa and certain bacteria.

**flail joint.** An abnormally mobile joint.

**flatfoot.** A lowering of the bony arch of the foot. When complete in a mobile foot it is painless and causes no disability—in fact, most ballet dancers are completely flat-footed. Pain arises when the foot is only partially flat and this induces strain on the foot ligaments.

**flatulence.** See ERUCTATION.

**flatulent.** Characterized by flatulence.

**flatus.** Gas or air in the gastrointestinal tract.

**flexibility.** The property of being able to be bent without breaking.

**flexion.** The process of bending.

**flexor.** A muscle that causes bending of a limb or part.

**flexure.** A bent or curved structure within the body.

**hepatic flexure.** The curve of the colon on the righthand side of the body near the liver.

**sigmoid flexure.** The part of the colon between the descending colon and the rectum.

**splenic flexure.** The bend in the colon on the left side of the body in the region of the spleen.

**floating kidney.** Nephroptosis.

**flooding.** Excessive bleeding from the womb, usually occurring in and around the change of life.

**flora.** The normal bacterial content of a part, such as the intestine.

**florid.** Bright pink or red, usually the result of congestion.

**fluid dram.** A pharmaceutical measure for liquids which equals one-eighth ounce or 3.55 cubic centimeters.

**fluid ounce.** A pharmaceutical measure which equals 8 fluid drams.

**fluke.** A group of worms of the class *Trematoda.*

**fluorescein.** A chemical with a powerful dye property instilled into the eye to detect the edges of a corneal ulcer, which glow an orange-red under the dye's influence.

**fluoride.** A chemical which, if present in the local water supply, is almost a guarantee of sound teeth. See also CARIES.

**fluoroscope.** An apparatus used for examining internal organs by means of x-rays.

**fluoroscopy.** Examination by means of a fluorescent screen.

**flush.** Redness of the face.

**flutter.** Usually refers to auricular or atrial flutter, a gross irregularity of the heartbeat in which the atrium of the heart, instead of beating 70 to 80 beats a minute, may be beating as fast as 350 beats a minute.

**focus. 1.** The principal seat of disease. **2.** The meeting point of rays of light made convergent by a convex lens.

**foetal.** See FETAL.

**foetus.** See FETUS.

**folic acid.** A vitamin substance used in the treatment of anemia.

**follicle.** A small secretory cavity or tubular gland in the skin.

**follicular.** Pertaining to a follicle.

**follicular tonsilitis.** Inflammation of the crypts, or follicles, of the tonsils.

**folliculitis.** Inflammation of a follicle.

**fomentation.** The application of moist heat to relieve pain by causing a dilatation of the skin vessels. At one time a very popular treatment for all manner of ailments such as boils but now largely discontinued in favor of drugs. See also POULTICE.

*A fomentation is prepared by taking a piece of lint of the size required, rolling it up in a piece of material, such as a handkerchief, and then pouring boiling water over it. After squeezing out excess water, the lint is then ready to apply.*

**fomes.** Any item, such as bedding or clothing, capable of transmitting infectious germs.

**fomites.** The plural of fomes.

**fontanel, fontanelle.** The area of a baby's skull where the bones have not yet grown together and the brain in this area is only covered by its membranes and the scalp. The region bulges in conditions causing pressure within the skull and is depressed in conditions where the baby is dehydrated. Normally this fontanel closes by 18 to 22 months of age. There are six possible fontanels in a baby's skull.

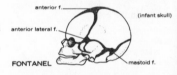

anterior f.
(infant skull)
anterior lateral f.
FONTANEL
mastoid f.

**food poisoning.** An acute disease characterized by an explosive onset with vomiting, diarrhea, and colic. In the past it was erroneously called ptomaine poisoning because it was believed that food proteins decomposed into poisonous substances called ptomaines. It is now known that the cause is either due to a definite germ or to its poison. Germs can be killed by cooking or heating, but many of their toxins cannot and so cause poisoning. The causative germ may be a staphylococcus, or one of the Salmonella group, which are similar to the germs of paratyphoid. Botulism, another form of food poisoning, is caused by a germ poison contaminating tinned meat, ham, sausages, fish, or vegetables. Food poisoning occurs as a result of the food having become infected with germs due to a lack of hygiene in its preparation, storage, or deep freezing. Contamination by flies, the refreezing of frozen food after it has been thawed

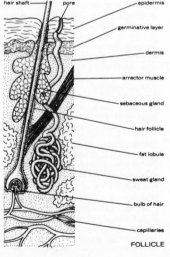

hair shaft
pore
epidermis
germinative layer
dermis
arrector muscle
sebaceous gland
hair follicle
fat lobule
sweat gland
bulb of hair
capillaries
FOLLICLE

out, and partial cooking of sausages, and duck eggs can all cause food poisoning.

**foot and mouth disease.** A virus disease of cattle and very rarely found in man; when it does occur it mainly causes ulceration of the mouth. Also called *aphthous fever.*

**foot drop.** A dropping of the foot due to paralysis of certain leg muscles.

**foot rot.** Epidermophytosis.

**foramen.** A term much used in anatomy to describe the natural openings, usually in bones, through which special organs pass, as for instance the *foramen magnum* situated at the back of the skull, through which the spinal cord passes into the brain.

**forceps.** Any two-bladed instrument used for grasping, extracting, or compressing.

**dental forceps.** Forceps used to extract teeth.

**midwifery forceps.** Forceps used to extract a baby from the birth canal.

**forensic medicine.** The study of medical facts as they relate to legal problems.

**foreskin.** The prepuce, the retractible skin covering the end of the penis. See also CIRCUMCISION.

**forme fruste.** An atypical form of a disease.

**formication.** A sensation as though ants were crawling across the skin.

**formula.** 1. The constituents of a medicine. 2. The chemical composition of a compound.

**formulary.** A collection of formulas for making up medicines.

**fornix.** Any vaultlike structure, it commonly refers to the vault of the vagina.

**fortification figures.** Rings of colored light and altered images seen by the patient during a migraine headache attack.

**fossa.** A depression. In anatomy the term is applied to various hollows in the body.

**foundling.** An abandoned infant.

**fourchet, fourchette.** A fold of mucous membrane at the back of the vulva.

**fovea.** A small pit or depression.

**fovea centralis retinae.** The area on the retina which records the most distinct vision.

**Fowler's position.** See POSITION: FOWLER'S POSITION

**foxglove.** A flowering plant from which is derived digitalis, a drug used to treat heart disease. Digitalis slows the heart rate but increases the force and strength of the beat.

**fracture.** The breaking of a part, especially a bone.

**Bennett's fracture.** Fracture of the first metacarpal bone of the thumb. Also called *boxer's fracture.*

**boxer's fracture.** See BENNETT'S FRACTURE, above.

**closed fracture.** A fracture which does not produce a wound in the skin through which infection can pass.

**Colles' fracture.** Fracture of the lower end of the radius giving the characteristic upward deformity said to resemble the back of a dinner fork.

**comminuted fracture.** A fracture in which the bone is broken into many fragments.

**complicated fracture.** Fracture complicated by other injuries, the jagged end of the bone being driven into nearby arteries, nerves, or organs. It always requires surgery.

**compound fracture.** See OPEN FRACTURE, below.

**depressed fracture.** Fracture of a flat bone like that of the skull, in which a fragment is depressed below the surface and may press on the brain.

**Dupuytren's fracture.** Fracture in which the anklebone is forced backwards between the tibia and fibula.

**fatigue fracture.** A fracture at the lower end of the fibula seen in athletes, or of a metatarsal. Also called *march fracture, stress fracture.*

**greenstick fracture.** Fracture in which the bone is partly cracked and partly bent, as happens with a green stick. It occurs in the pliable bones of children.

**impacted fracture.** Fracture in which one fragment of bone is firmly driven into the other. The commonest is the neck of the femur, and is frequently met with in old ladies who have fallen on to their sides.

**Monteggia fracture.** Fracture of the ulna and dislocation of the head of the radius at the elbow joint.

**open fracture.** Fracture in which a wound occurs in the skin over the site of the fracture. The wound may not be caused by the broken bones pushing through the skin but by the blow that produced the fracture. This is a serious complication because germs can gain entrance to the blood clot around the fracture and set up infection. It always requires surgical toilet of the wound.

**Pott's fracture.** External rotation fracture of the tibia and fibula at the ankle joint.

**simple fracture.** See CLOSED FRACTURE.

**Smith's fracture.** Fracture similar to a Colles' fracture, but the deformity is downwards instead of upwards. Also called *reverse Colles' fracture.*

**stress fracture.** See FATIGUE FRACTURE.

**Wagstaffe's fracture.** An adduction fracture of the ankle involving the internal malleolus.

*Principal signs and symptoms of fractures.* (1) Pain at or near the seat of the fracture. (2) Tenderness or discomfort on gentle pressure over the affected area of bone. (3) Swelling about the fracture site. Such swelling frequently masks other signs of a fracture and care must be taken not to treat the condition as a less serious injury. (4) Loss of power because the injured part cannot be moved normally. (5) Deformity of the limb, which may assume an unnatural position. The contracting muscles may cause the broken bone ends to override each other, producing shortening of the limb. (6) Irregularity of the bone, which may be actually felt, if the fracture is near the skin. (7) Crepitus, or bone-grating, may be heard or felt as the bone ends touch. (8) Unnatural movement at the seat of the fracture. If such movement occurs where there is no joint, obviously the bone is broken. Any or all of these signs and symptoms may or may not be present and may vary in degree. Comparison with the uninjured side will assist in diagnosis. The casualty may be aware of his condition enough to be able to point to the site of the fractured bone.

*First-aid treatment of fractures.* Treat the fracture on the spot. Do not move the casualty until the injured part has been immobilized, unless life is in immediate danger from some other cause. If, however, final immobilization cannot be completed on the spot, temporary fixation should be carried out before moving the casualty to a more suitable and safer surrounding. Bleeding and severe wounds must be treated before the fractures, with due regard to the requirements of both types of injury.

Steady and support the injured parts at once so that movements of the broken bones are impossible. This prevents any increase in the bleeding which always occurs at the fracture site, and also prevents the broken bones from damaging blood vessels, nerves, and muscle, or from piercing the skin.

Immobilize the fracture. The application of bandages using the casualty's own body as a means of support will be adequate for ordinary purposes, but splints also will be required if long or difficult transport is necessary to reach medical aid. Splints will also be needed when the casualty's body cannot be used as a "natural splint," such as tying a broken leg to the uninjured leg, but obviously if both legs are fractured this cannot be done. If in doubt always treat as though a fracture is present and remember that more than one bone may be broken. Never tie a bandage over the fracture site, for this may alter its position and make it more serious. Bandages must be applied sufficiently firmly to prevent harmful movements but not so tightly as to stop the circulation of blood. In the case of a fractured limb, delayed swelling may occur, causing the bandages to become too tight and cutting off the circulation. Should this occur, and it will be obvious from the swelling and congestion of the limb below the level of the bandages, then the bandages must be loosened and reapplied to allow the circulation to return. Padding must always be placed between the ankles and knees if these are tied together. When the casualty is lying down and it is necessary to pass a bandage round the body or limbs, double the bandage over the end of a splint or stick and pass it under the body's natural hollows, such as the neck, the loins, the knees, and the regions above the heels. Avoid jarring the patient while working the bandages into their correct positions. Splints should always be long enough to immobilize the joint above and the joint below the fracture site and be sufficiently firm, wide, and well padded. The padding is necessary to make the splint fit accurately to the limb; it can be applied over the clothing. Any stiff object can be used as a splint: a splint may be improvised from a walking stick, an umbrella, broom, a brush handle, a piece of wood, stout cardboard, or even rolls of firmly folded paper. In fracture of the upper arm and collarbone it is frequently only necessary to apply a wide arm sling to support the limb.

**fraenum.** See FRENUM.

**fraenum linguae.** See FRENUM LINGUAE.

**fragilitas.** Fragility.

**fragilitas ossium.** See OSTEOGENESIS IMPERFECTA.

**fragmentation.** A separation into small parts.

**frambesia.** See YAWS.

**freckle.** A small pigmented spot in the skin occuring commonly on the face and the backs of the hands caused by exposure to the sun in some people but sometimes of congenital origin and an inherited factor. Also called *lentigo*.

**fremitus.** A vibration that can be felt by the hands.

**friction fremitus.** The rubbing sensation sometimes felt by the doctor in dry pleurisy when two inflamed dry surfaces of the pleural membrane rub together during the act of breathing.

**vocal fremitus.** The vibration which the doctor feels when he places his hand on the patient's chest and asks him to say "ninety-nine."

**frenum.** A fold of skin or mucous membrane limiting movements of an organ.

**frenum linguae.** A fold of skin fixing the tongue to the floor of the mouth and limiting the tongue's movements. Also called *frenulum linguae*. See also TONGUE.

**frenzy.** Violent excitement.

**frequency.** The number of times that something happens. Commonly refers to an increase in the number of times a patient needs to pass urine. If this occurs during the day it is called *diurnal frequency*, and if at night, *nocturnal frequency*. This commonly occurs either in an old man with an enlarged prostate gland or in some forms of inflammation of the genitourinary tract.

**Freudian.** Relating to doctrines expounded by Sigmund Freud, an Austrian doctor who propounded that emotional upsets and disorders in the adult can be traced back to subconscious sexual impressions acquired in childhood and thereafter repressed, and can be cured by bringing these suppressed emotions and subconscious sexual desires to the conscious· mind by psychoanalysis.

**friable.** Easily crumbled.

**friar's balsam.** Compound Benzoin Tincture (*B.P.*); it is frequently used with great effect as a steam inhalation for the relief of laryngitis and chest troubles. See also CROUP.

**Friderichsen-Waterhouse syndrome.** Acute adrenal insufficiency caused by bleeding into the suprarenal gland during meningococcal meningitis; more common in infants than in adults.

**frigidity.** A revulsion against sexual intercourse or the inability to respond to sexual stimuli. See also IMPOTENCE.

**Fröhlich's syndrome.** Failure of sexual development associated with obesity and dwarfism. Also called *adiposogenital dystrophy*.

**Froin's syndrome.** See LOCULATION SYNDROME.

**frontal.** Pertaining to the front of an organ or the body, or to the forehead.

**frostbite.** A form of gangrene of the extremities set up by severe cold stagnating and stopping the blood circulating to a part and characterized by redness, swelling, and pain. It cannot be too strongly emphasized that rubbing the affected part with snow or some other friction method simply causes more damage. The proper treatment for frostbite is to leave the part untouched and bring the casualty into a sheltered place, such as a hut or house, where the frostbitten part is allowed to thaw out slowly and gradually while being treated as a wound which may well become infected.

**fugitive.** Fleeting or transient.

**fugue.** An abnormal mental state in which the individual carries out rational behavior for which he has a complete loss of memory. For instance, a man might leave home, travel by train to the other end of the country, and then be found wandering, unable to explain how he got there, yet he has carried out the procedure of buying a ticket, entering a train, perhaps even taking a meal on the train and getting off the train.

**fulguration.** The destruction of tissue, usually growths, by means of an electric current.

**fulminant.** Sudden and severe.

**fumigation.** Sterilization by exposure to the fumes of a disinfectant.

**functional.** 1. Relating to the special action of an organ. 2. In a wider connotation it refers to a disorder not due to disease of an organ but to an alteration in its nervous control which sets up symptoms like those of a disease while the organ itself is completely normal. For example, functional dyspepsia, which gives all the symptoms of a gastric ulcer, may, in fact, be due to chronic anxiety upsetting the nervous control to the stomach.

**fundal.** Pertaining to a fundus.

**fundus.** The base, or that part of a hollow organ farthest from its mouth.

**fundus uteri.** The top end of the womb; its position is used to calculate the duration of a pregnancy.

**fungal.** Relating to a fungus.

**fungi.** The plural of fungus.

**fungicide.** An agent which destroys a fungus.

**fungoid.** Resembling a fungus.

**fungus.** One of a lower group of plants characterized by absence of flowers, leaves, and chlorophyll and including molds some of which are pathogens.

**funny bone.** A popular name for a part of the elbow. When it is struck in a certain position the ulnar nerve is concussed and produces a slightly painful tingling sensation from the elbow to the hand.

**fur.** A morbid coating of the tongue which may be associated with a disordered stomach, mouth breathing, or heavy tobacco smoking.

**furfur.** An alternative name for dandruff or scurf.

**furred.** See FUR.

**furuncle.** A small boil.

**furuncular.** Pertaining to a furuncle.

**furunculosis.** A condition characterized by the presence of numerous boils.

**fusion.** 1. The process of melting. 2. The process of uniting. 3. The coming together of the vision from two eyes, called binocular fusion.

# G-H

**gag.** 1. An instrument for holding the mouth open. 2. To retch or try to vomit.

**gait.** An individual's manner of walking.

**galactagogue.** A substance that promotes the secretion of milk.

**galactin.** The hormone that stimulates the production of milk. Also called *prolactin.*

**galactorrhea.** Excessive production of milk.

**galactorrhoea.** See GALACTORRHEA.

**galactostasis.** The stagnation of milk in the breast.

**galenicals.** Medicines containing organic substances as contrasted with chemical ingredients; named after the great ancient Greek physician, Galen. See also HUMOR.

**gall.** The bile.

**gall bladder.** A pear-shaped organ about four inches in length situated on the under surface of the liver, in the right upper corner of the abdomen, and which acts as a storage depot for the bile manufactured in the liver.

**gallop rhythm.** The rhythm, resembling that of a galloping horse, heard when the heart makes three sounds instead of two. When the third sound is heard over the apex of the heart during diastole, it denotes that the right ventricle is under strain during failure of the left ventricle. A third sound heard during the systolic phase of the heartbeat is of no significance.

**gallstone.** A stone found in the gall bladder or bile ducts.

**galvanism.** Electricity generated by chemical action.

**galvanocautery.** An instrument with a platinum-loop tip which is heated to a dull red by a galvanic current and used to cut or destroy tissues.

**galvanometer.** An instrument for measuring the magnitude of electric currents.

**gamete.** The name given to the male or female reproductive cell, whether it occurs in animals, man, or plants. In human beings the female ovum and the male sperm are the gametes. In plants, the male gamete is part of the pollen grain, while the female ovum is contained in the ovule.

**gametogenesis.** The production and development of gametes. Also called *gametogeny.*

**gamgee tissue.** A form of surgical dressing, consisting of cotton wool between two layers of gauze and used either as padding or as a means of soaking up discharges.

**gamma.** A unit of weight equivalent to a microgram, one-millionth part of a gram.

**gamma rays.** Rays emitted by radioactive substances and of shorter wavelength than x-rays.

**ganglial, gangliar.** Relating to a ganglion.

**gangliectomy.** Surgical excision of a ganglion.

**ganglion.** 1. A subsidiary nerve center in the brain or other part of the nervous system. 2. A localized fluid-filled swelling found mainly on the wrist, the back of the hand, and the back of the foot and due to a tiny rupture of a tendon sheath.

**ganglionectomy.** Excision of a ganglion.

**gangrene.** Mortification or death of tissue due to failure of the arterial blood supply from disease or injury; the putrefactive changes in dead tissues.

**diabetic gangrene.** A type of gangrene due to thickening or coating of the blood vessels, cutting off the blood supply and usually affecting the extremities.

**dry gangrene.** Local death of a part that becomes mummified.

**gas gangrene.** Gangrene due to infection of a wound with a gas-producing germ.

**moist gangrene.** Local death of a part that becomes infected.

**senile gangrene.** A type occurring in old age and due to arteriosclerosis. It usually affects the extremities.

**Ganser's syndrome.** A disturbance involving amnesia, hallucinations, and disturbances of consciousness; thought to be of emotional origin.

**gargoylism.** An inherited condition characterized by mental deficiency, defective vision, a very large head, a prominent abdomen, and short arms and legs, and so called because the facial features resemble those of a gargoyle.

**gargarism.** A gargle.

**gargle.** Any liquid preparation for rinsing the mouth and throat.

**garrot.** A tourniquet.

**garrotting.** The popular interpretation of this word as strangulation is not quite correct. On each side of the neck there is a carotid artery which supplies the brain with blood. If both carotid arteries are compressed, the blood supply to the brain is cut off and causes unconsciousness. This, strictly speaking, is garrotting and not strangulation, which implies compression of the windpipe.

**gastralgia.** Pain in the stomach.

**gastrectomy.** Surgical removal of part of the stomach.

**gastric.** Pertaining to the stomach.

**gastric crises.** Paroxysms of abdominal pain with vomiting which occur in tabes dorsalis.

**gastric influenza.** A form of gastroenteritis caused by the influenza virus.

**gastric juice.** The secretion from stomach glands; a digestive juice.

**gastric ulcer.** An ulcer in the lining of the stomach.

**gastritis.** Inflammation of the stomach lining.

**gastrocnemius.** A muscle in the calf of the leg.

**gastrocolic.** Relating to both stomach and colon.

**gastrocolic reflex.** The nerve stimulus given to the lower colon when food is taken into the stomach; one of the symptomatic urges which indicates that the bowel needs to be emptied.

**gastroduodenal.** Relating to both stomach and duodenum.

**gastroduodenitis.** Inflammation of both the stomach and the duodenum.

**gastroenteric.** Relating to both stomach and intestine.

**gastroenteritis.** A disease characterized by inflammation of the lining of the stomach and small intestine, causing abdominal pain, nausea, and sometimes vomiting and diarrhea. It can be caused by food contaminated with germs or chemical poisons which irritate the gut, and frequently occurs as localized epidemics for which no cause can be found.

**gastroenterology.** The branch of medicine relating to diseases of the stomach and intestines.

**gastroenteroptosis.** Downward displacement of the stomach and intestines.

**gastroenterostomy.** A surgical operation in which the small intestine is joined to the wall of the stomach, to by-pass the duodenum.

**gastroesophagal.** Pertaining to both the stomach and the esophagus.

**gastrointestinal.** Relating to both stomach and intestines.

**gastrojejunal.** Relating to both the stomach and the jejunum (a part of the small intestine).

**gastrojejunostomy.** A surgical operation to join the jejunum to the stomach so that food passes directly from the stomach into the jejunum.

**gastrology.** The study of the diseases of the stomach.

**gastromalacia.** Abnormal softness or softening of the wall of the stomach.

**gastronephritis.** Inflammation of both stomach and kidneys.

**gastro-oesophageal.** See GASTROESOPHA-GEAL.

**gastroparalysis.** Paralysis of the stomach.

**gastropathy.** Any disease or disorder of the stomach.

**gastropexy.** An operation in which the stomach is stitched to the abdominal wall to cure displacement.

**gastrophrenic.** Pertaining to both the stomach and the diaphragm.

**gastroplegia.** Paralysis of the stomach.

**gastroptosis.** A sagging downwards of the stomach.

**gastrorrhagia.** Hemorrhage into the stomach.

**gastrorrhaphy.** Suture of the stomach.

**gastrorrhexis.** Rupture of the stomach.

**gastroscope.** An instrument for visual examination of the inside of the stomach.

**gastroscopy.** Examination of the inside of the stomach by means of a gastroscope.

**gastrostenosis.** Stricture of the stomach.

**gastrostomy.** An operation in which an opening made in the stomach is sewn to an opening in the abdominal skin. The patient can then be fed through this opening instead of swallowing food.

**gastrotomy.** An incision into the stomach.

**gathering.** An abscess.

**gatophobia.** Fear of cats.

**gauze.** A thin open-meshed material used as a surgical dressing. Its loose texture soaks up blood and exudates and creates a greater surface area which rapidly increases the blood-clotting time and helps to stop minor bleeding. In the days before asepsis or surgical gauze it was a common practice to lay a cobweb over a bleeding wound. This acted in a similar manner to gauze but was by no means surgically sterile.

**Gee's disease.** See CELIAC DISEASE.

**gene.** A hereditary unit, of which there are many arranged linearly in a chromosome, and having the ability to transmit a particular characteristic from one generation to the next. Examples are eye color, skin pigmentation, and blood types. See also CHROMOSOME.

**genetic.** Pertaining to genes, or development.

**genetics.** The science of heredity, the processes by which the overall system and specific characteristics of the body are inherited.

**genital.** Relating to the genitalia.

**genitalia, genitals.** The sex organs.

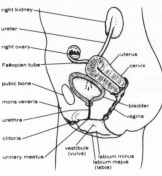

GENITALIA, GENITALS (female)

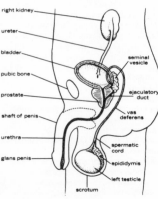

GENITALIA, GENITALS (male)

**genitourinary.** Relating to the genitals and the urinary organs.

**gentian.** A bitter tonic plant extract which stimulates the appetite and provides the astringent flavor of many Continental aperitifs.

**genuflex.** To bend the knee.

**genupectoral.** The position of the patient when he rests on his knees and chest.

**genu valgum.** Knock-knee.

**genu varum.** Bowleg.

**geriatic.** Relating to old age.

**geriatrics.** The science which studies the diseases of old age.

**germ.** 1. A microbe. 2. A spore, a seed, or any embryo in its early stage.

**German measles.** A mild contagious disease characterized by a rash and general enlargement of the glands in the body. The usual incubation period is 17 to 18 days. Sometimes the en-larged tender glands in the neck appear before the rash, which is paler than that of measles (rubeola), quickly spreads across the body and, usually, just as quickly fades away. There is very little general disturbance. The temperature may not be raised more than one or two degrees, and often is not raised at all. The importance of the disease lies in the fact that 25 percent of the women contracting it in the first two or three months of pregnancy will bear infants with cataracts, heart malformations, deaf-mutism, and other defects. A woman coming in contact with a case of German measles in the early weeks of pregnancy and not previously having had the disease herself, can be given temporary protection by an injection of gamma globulin. By far the best prophylactic, however, is to ensure that all girls contract German measles during childhood, for one attack apparently gives protection for life. It has been suggested quite seriously that when the disease appears in a district all the little girls should get together at tea parties with the infected child so that they all get it and so remove the risk to their own babies should they eventually become mothers. Also called *rubella*.

**germicidal.** Destructive to germs.

**germicide.** An agent which destroys germs.

**gerontology.** Geriatrics.

**gestation.** See PREGNANCY.

**Gibraltar fever.** See ABORTUS FEVER.

**giddiness.** A sensation of rolling or unsteadiness which may be due to anxiety, anemia, or general debility. It should not be confused with vertigo, a much more definite and severe disorder due to disease of the ears, eyes, brain, stomach, or blood.

**gigantism.** A condition of abnormal size and of height usually in excess of 79 inches caused by overproduction of the growth hormone secreted by the front part of the pituitary gland in the brain.

**acromegalic gigantism.** Gigantism in which the characteristics of acromegaly are superimposed on those of gigantism.

**eunuchoid gigantism.** Gigantism in which there is sexual inefficiency, impotence, and sterility.

**normal gigantism.** Gigantism in which all the body functions are normal.

**gingiva.** The gum.

**gingival.** Relating to the gum.

**gingivitis.** Inflammation of the gums.

**girdle.** A band around the body.

**girdle pains.** Sensations of pain and constriction around the abdomen which occur in certain diseases of the spinal cord.

**glabrous.** Smooth and hairless.

**gland.** A group of cells or an organ which manufactures and discharges a substance into the bloodstream, or into a cavity, each substance performing its own special function.

**glanders.** A highly contagious disease of horses, mules, and donkeys. Caused by a germ, it is communicable to dogs, goats, sheep, and man, but not to cattle. It is characterized by fever, inflammation of lining membranes, especially of the nose, enlargement of the lymph glands, and the formation of nodules which have a tendency to collect to form deep ulcers. In man the disease usually runs an acute feverish course and terminates fatally. Also called *farcy, equinia.*

**glandular.** Pertaining to a gland.

**glandular fever.** An acute infectious disease characterized by fever, glandular enlargement, and the appearance in the blood of somewhat abnormal white cells. See also MONONUCLEOSIS.

**glans.** The bulbous tip of the penis.

**Glauber's salt.** Sodium sulphate. It has a similar action to Epsom salts. See also EPSOM SALTS.

**glaucoma.** A disease of the eye characterized by raised internal pressure of the eyeball, making it hard and stonelike when felt. It produces severe pain in the eye, vomiting, and, if not relieved, blindness.

**gleet.** Chronic inflammation of the urethra, the tube carrying the urine from the bladder to the outside.

**glenoid.** Having a shallow socket.

**glenoid cavity.** The shallow depression on the scapula which with the head of the humerus forms the shoulder joint.

**glia.** The tissue that composes part of the central nervous system. Also called *neuroglia.*

**glioma.** A tumor of the central nervous system.

**globe.** The eyeball.

**globulin.** A general name for a group of proteins different from albumins.

**immune globulin.** A sterile solution of antibodies taken from an individual who has recovered from measles and used as an injection treatment for measles in those who need an urgent passive immunity.

**serum globulin.** The globulin contained in blood serum.

**globus.** A ball or globe.

**globus hystericus.** The neurotic sensation of having a permanent lump in the throat.

**glomerule, glomerulus.** A coil of minute blood vessels in the kidney in contact with a cup-shaped uriniferous tubule, which collects the waste products passed into it from the glomerule. A normal kidney contains about one million glomerules. This kidney apparatus produces from the blood a protein-free liquid which is converted into urine by the reabsorption of water and certain salts by the renal tubules emerging from the cup.

**glomerulonephritis.** A type of nephritis in which there is inflammation of the glomeruli of the kidney.

**glomus.** The primitive glomerule present in the developing embryonic kidney.

**glomus cell.** A cell at the junction of the minute arteries and veins in the skin of the fingers and toes.

**glomus choroideum.** An enlargement of the choroid plexus of the lateral ventricle of the brain.

**glomus tumour.** An extremely tender, small, purple-colored tumor, composed of minute blood vessels and nerves, occurring mostly under a fingernail or toenail.

**glossa.** The tongue.

**glossal.** Relating to the tongue.

**glossectomy.** Excision of the tongue.

**glossitis.** Inflammation of the tongue.

**glossopharyngeal.** Relating to the tongue and the pharynx.

**glossy skin.** A painful condition of the skin, usually affecting the fingers, characterized by a shiny stretched appearance of the skin.

**glottic.** Relating to the glottis.

**glottis.** The vocal apparatus of the larynx.

**glucaemia.** See GLYCEMIA.

**glucose.** A naturally occurring sugar.

**glucosuria.** The presence of glucose in the urine. It may indicate the presence of diabetes or just that the kidney, due to a peculiar characteristic, is spilling out glucose in the urine. It is then not evidence of disease. See also DIABETES.

**gluteal.** Relating to the buttocks.

**glutei.** The large muscles which form the buttocks.

**gluteofemoral.** Relating to the buttocks and the thigh.

**gluteoinguinal.** Relating to the buttocks and the groin.

**gluteus.** One of the large muscles in the buttock.

**glycaemia.** Glycemia.

**glycemia.** A condition in which sugar is found in the blood.

**glycogen.** A chemical which the body forms from glucose and then stores in the liver as a fuel which it can quickly convert back to glucose and release when the body requires it for muscular exertion.

**glycosuria.** The excretion of glucose in the urine. See GLUCOSURIA.

**goat fever.** See ABORTUS FEVER.

**godemiche.** An artificial penis used, largely by women, to simulate the action of the penis in various sexual acts. Also called *dildo.*

**goiter.** An enlargement of the thyroid gland in the front of the neck. A goiter may irritate the thyroid gland to overactivity or have no effect on it except by reason of its size and pressure symptoms. If it irritates the thyroid it produces Graves' disease, or hyperthyroidism, characterized by prominent staring eyeballs, a rapid pulse, loss of weight, and sometimes heart disorders. The treatment is removal or destruction of part of the thyroid gland to lessen its function. The large swelling sometimes seen in the front of the neck of otherwise healthy people has various names, and one used in Great Britain is Derbyshire neck, because of its prevalence in that county.

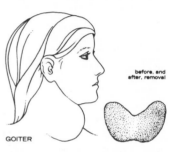

before, and after, removal

GOITER

**goitre.** See GOITER.

**gonad.** One of the sexual glands, a testicle or an ovary.

**gonadal.** Relating to a gonad.

**gonadotrophins.** Substances which stimulate the sex glands. A sex hormone.

**gonadotropic.** Stimulating the function of the sex organs.

**gonococcal.** Relating to the gonococcus.

**gonococcus.** The germ that causes gonorrhea.

**gonorrhea.** A venereal disease characterized by a profuse discharge of pus from the urethra. Treated early, gonorrhea can be completely cured, but untreated it can lead to prolonged and severe ill health.

**gonorrheal.** Relating to gonorrhea.

**gonorrhoea.** See GONORRHEA.

**gonorrhoeal.** See GONORRHEAL.

**goose flesh.** Skin marked by the prominent appearance of the hair follicles which stand up as the result of a stimulus to a minute muscle called the arrectores pilorum. Spasm of this muscle is usually a sequel to cold, but sometimes to fright. Also called *horripilation.*

**gout.** A constitutional hereditary condition mainly affecting males, in which biurate chemicals are deposited in and around joints, leading to acute inflammation, the big toe joint being most commonly affected. Relief of the acute attack can be obtained by taking tablets of butazolidin or colchicum. The prophylactic treatment consists of dietary restrictions and the use of drugs, such as probenecid, which alter the concentration of uric acid in the blood and increase its excretion in the urine.

**G.P.I.** The abbreviation for general paralysis of the insane. It is due to disease of the brain. Also called *dementia paralytica.*

**gr.** The abbreviation for grain. There are 437½ grains to one avoirdupois ounce and 480 to one troy ounce.

**graft.** Skin, muscle, bone, nerve, or other tissue taken from a living organism and employed to replace a defect in a corresponding structure.

**Gram's stain.** A mixture of iodine in potassium iodide used for staining bacteria. Those bacteria which hold the stain are called Gram positive and those that do not Gram negative. The method is named after the Danish bacteriologist who introduced it.

**grand mal.** The major fits of epilepsy.

**granulation.** The tiny red granules visible in the base of an ulcer; or, the process of formation of granulation tissue in or around the site of inflammation, and the method by which the body repairs an ulcer or wound devoid of skin.

**granuloma.** A tumor formed of granulation tissue. One form of granuloma is the so-called "proud flesh" that develops in a surface ulcer.

**granulomatous.** Characterized by granulation tissue.

**gravel.** The sandlike substance which is passed down the urinary tract and which, if congealed, would form a stone in either the kidney or the bladder.

**Graves' disease.** See GOITER.

**gravid.** Pregnant.

**gravida.** A pregnant woman.

**gravitation abscess.** A collection of pus that has dropped by gravity from an infected area higher in the body.

**green sickness.** Chlorosis, the severe iron-deficiency anemia of young girls, accompanied by a greenish-white appearance of the face; now rarely seen in civilized countries.

**Gregory's powder.** A mixture of rhubarb and magnesium carbonates flavored with ginger; used as a purgative.

**grinder's asthma.** Also called *grinder's rot.* See SILICOSIS.

**grip, grippe.** See INFLUENZA.

**gripe.** A severe pain or spasm of the bowels.

**gristle.** Cartilage.

**groin.** The depression between the abdomen and the thigh.

**growth.** 1. Progressive development in a living organism both in size and differentiation and by which the organism ultimately reaches its complete physical development. 2. An abnormal tissue development, as a tumor.

**Guillian-Barré syndrome.** A form of polyneuritis in which paralysis and altered sensations occur at the distal parts of the limbs.

**gullet.** The esophagus.

**gum.** The fleshy tissue which covers the necks of the teeth and the parts of the jaws in which the teeth are set. Also called *gingiva.*

**gumma.** A localized lesion of a consistency resembling India rubber, with a tendency to necrosis and caseation. It is one of the features of syphilis.

**gummatous.** Of the nature of gumma or affected with gumma.

**gustation.** The sense of taste.

**gustatory.** Relating to the sense of taste.

**gut.** The intestine.

**gutta.** A drop.

**gymnophobia.** Fear of naked bodies.

**gynaecologic, gynaecological.** See GYNECOLOGIC; GYNECOLOGICAL.

**gynaecologist.** See GYNECOLOGIST.

**gynaecology.** See GYNECOLOGY.

**gynecologist.** A specialist in the diseases of women.

**gynecology.** The study of diseases of women.

**gynephobia.** Fear of the female sex.

**gyrus.** One of the folds on the surface of the brain.

**habit.** A constantly repeated action or condition.

**habit spasm.** An involuntary repeated movement of groups of muscles resulting in eye-blinking, shoulder-shrugging, facial grimaces, sniffing, tongue-clucking, coughing, throat-clearing, or sighing. Habit spasms are most often seen in childhood, and when the cause is not due to copying an adult, which is frequently the case, then it is due to nervous tension. Studies in Britain and Scandinavia have revealed that conflict in the home is the main precipitating factor, but even animals suffer from tics or habit spasms. Chickens kept in egg-laying batteries develop a head-shaking movement which disappears when they are allowed to roam free, and bears and other animals confined in cages display head-bobbing or other recurrent movements which stop when the animal is allowed more space. Treatment of habit spasms in children is not easy, for drugs are quite useless and scolding the child only makes the habit worse. The primary fault lies with the parents and the

home environment, and some parents will not accept that it is their own nervous irritability which causes the child to be nervous and insecure. When parents do accept this explanation and submit to treatment for themselves, many habit spasms in children disappear automatically.

**habituation.** 1. Adaptation to a situation. 2. A continued desire for and use of drugs with slight or no increase in dosage and the absence of physical dependence; see also ADDICTION.

**haemangioma.** See HEMANGIOMA.

**haemarthrosis.** See HEMARTHROSIS.

**haematemesis.** See HEMATEMESIS.

**haematherapy.** See HEMATHERAPY.

**haematin.** See HEMATIN.

**haematocrit.** See HEMATOCRIT.

**haematology.** See HEMATOLOGY.

**haematoma.** See HEMATOMA.

**haematometra.** See HEMATOMETRA.

**haematomyelia.** See HEMATOMYELIA.

**haematopericardium.** See HEMATOPERICARDIUM.

**haematoperitoneum.** See HEMATOPERITONEUM.

**haematophobia.** See HEMATOPHOBIA.

**haematopoiesis.** See HEMATOPOIESIS.

**haematosalpinx.** See HEMATOSALPINX.

**haematospermia.** See HEMATOSPERMIA.

**haematothorax.** See HEMATOTHORAX.

**haematuria.** See HEMATURIA.

**haemochromatosis.** See HEMOCHROMATOSIS.

**haemoglobin.** See HEMOGLOBIN.

**haemoglobinometer.** See HEMOGLOBINOMETER.

**haemolysin.** See HEMOLYSIN.

**haemolysis.** See HEMOLYSIS.

**haemolytic.** See HEMOLYTIC.

**haemopericardium.** See HEMOPERICARDIUM.

**haemoperitoneum.** See HEMOPERITONEUM.

**haemophilia.** See HEMOPHILIA.

**haemophiliac.** See HEMOPHILIAC.

**haemophobia.** See HEMOPHOBIA.

**haemopneumothorax.** See HEMOPNEUMOTHORAX.

**haemoptysis.** See HEMOPTYSIS.

**haemorrhage.** See HEMORRHAGE.

**haemorrhagic.** See HEMORRHAGIC.

**haemorrhoid.** See HEMORRHOID.

**haemorrhoidal.** See HEMORRHOIDAL.

**haemorrhoidectomy.** See HEMORRHOIDECTOMY.

**haemosalpinx.** See HEMOSALPINX.

**haemostasis.** See HEMOSTASIS.

**haemostat.** See HEMOSTAT.

**haemostatic.** See HEMOSTATIC.

**haemotherapy.** See HEMOTHERAPY.

**haemothorax.** See HEMOTHORAX.

**half-life.** The period of time in which the activity of a radioactive substance decays to one-half its initial value. The term is useful in calculating dosages in radiotherapeutics.

**halibut liver oil.** An oil rich in vitamins A and D, extracted from halibut liver.

**halitosis.** Foul breath. This may be due to infected tonsils, dirty and tartar-covered teeth, an infected sinus, an inflammatory or purulent condition in the nose and throat, a sour stomach, or swallowing of such food as onions.

**hallucination.** A visual delusion such as seeing relatives who are long dead, or the reptiles, spiders, and various crawling monsters seen by victims of delirium tremens.

**hallucinosis.** A mental disorder in which hallucinations are the main symptom.

**hallux.** The big toe.

**hallux valgus.** Deviation of the big toe towards the other toes, forming a bunion.

**hallux varus.** Deviation of the big toe away from the other toes.

**ham.** The area of the thigh from the buttock to the back of the knee, in which region are the hamstring muscles.

**hamamelis.** Witch hazel, an astringent.

**hamartoma.** A tumorlike mass of cells making up a nodule which arises from faulty development in the embryo. A typical example is the vascular birthmark called a nevus. Strictly speaking, hamartomas are not true neoplasms, but in a few cases they may undergo neoplastic changes.

**hamartophobia.** Fear of making a mistake.

**hammer.** The malleus, a small bone in the middle ear.

**hammer finger.** A deformity of the finger in which the last joint is so flexed that the finger looks like a hammer. Also called *mallet finger.*

**hammer toe.** A flexion deformity at the joint of the toe nearest the foot, in which the soft tissues have contracted and prevent the toe from being straightened. In the majority of cases the cause is ill-fitting shoes that prevent the toe from lying flat, and so is commoner among women. In a few instances hammer toes are found in several members of the same family. The treatment is a surgical operation if the toe is causing crippling pain. Also called *mallet toe.*

**hamstrings.** The tendons of the hamstring muscles in the thigh. They serve to bend the knee and turn the foot.

**Hand-Schüller-Christian syndrome.** A condition in which there is prominence of the eyeballs, diabetes insipidus, and yellow staining of the skin; a disorder seen primarily in children.

**hangnail.** A loose fragment of skin at the root of the nail, which ultimately becomes infected and inflamed and may produce a whitlow; commonly caused by picking at the skin.

**Hansen's disease.** See LEPROSY.

**haptophore.** The specific molecular group by which toxins become "hooked on" to antibodies and so neutralized in the body.

**hard sore.** A syphilitic chancre. Also called *venereal sore.*

**harelip.** A congenital deformity of the upper lip and often associated with cleft palate. During early embyonic development there is failure of nasal and maxillary processes to unite correctly. See also CLEFT PALATE.

**hartshorn.** Ammonia water. In the past the horn of the stag was used for the manufacture of ammonia, which was called Spirit of Hart's Horn.

**harvest fever.** A feverish illness caused by a spirochetal germ and occurring among agricultural workers.

**Hashimoto's disease.** Chronic inflammation of the thyroid gland.

**hashish.** A drug derived from hemp. See CANNABIS.

**haunch bone.** The ilium, part of the pelvis.

**haustus.** A draft of medicine.

**Haverhill fever.** An infectious disease named after a town in Massachusetts; characterized by high temperature, a skin rash in which spots may be flat, raised, or hemorrhagic, and arthritis; possibly transmitted by infectious milk.

**hawking.** Clearing phlegm from the throat.

**hay fever, seasonal.** Strictly speaking this is not a fever but allergic rhinitis. It is due to flower and grass pollens irritating the lining of the eye and nose causing swelling and irritation, a constantly running nose, together with bouts of sneezing that are sometimes uncontrollable. Treatment consists of desensitization by injection and the administration of antihistamine drugs.

**headache.** Any pain in the head.

**heart.** The hollow muscular organ that maintains the circulation of the blood. It is divided into two halves by a septum, each half consisting of two chambers separated by valves. The two upper chambers are called *atria* while the two lower chambers are called *ventricles.* Blood from all over the body enters the right atrium and passes into the right ventricle, which pumps the blood into the lungs to be oxygenated. From the lungs the oxygenated blood passes into the left atrium and then into left ventricle. The left ventricle then contracts, forcing the oxygenated blood into the aorta, which distributes it throughout the body. In the unborn baby the lungs are not in use and the blood is oxygenated by the mother. The baby's blood passes from the right side of the heart to the left through a hole in the septum, thus bypassing the nonactive lungs. At birth, with the baby's first cry, this hole in the septum snaps shut and the lungs inflate. Sometimes, however, the hole persists, leading to a form of congenital heart disease which is now amenable to surgery. The heart muscle is nourished not by the blood in its chambers but by two arteries that arise from the aorta as it leaves the right ventricle. These two arteries form a crown around the heart and are known as coronary arteries. If one of these clots up partly or completely, the condition is known as coronary thrombosis. The wave of contraction in the heart is rhythmical and is controlled by nerve paths which initiate the contraction from atrium to ventricle. The heart of a normal person beats 70 to 80 times a minute, though it is often less than this in trained athletes. The rate is increased by excitement, exercise, and fever, and slowed by diphtheria and some heart diseases.

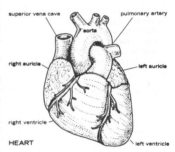

superior vena cava — aorta — pulmonary artery

right auricle — left auricle

right ventricle

HEART — left ventricle

**heart attack.** There are several types of heart attack. *Angina of effort.* This type of heart attack is caused by a spasm of the artery to the heart, not by a blood clot. The sufferer usually knows that exercise brings on chest pain, has usually consulted a doctor about it, and carries with him either trinitrin tablets to chew or amyl nitrite capsules to break and sniff when the pain occurs. He will not be unconscious but will be sitting or standing clutching his chest and complaining of pain. If he has his tablets or capsules they should be administered; he should be kept quiet and still and the doctor sent for. *Coronary thrombosis.*

This is due to a clot of blood in an artery suppplying the heart muscle. The victim is seized with a sudden, fierce, severe constricting pain around the center of the chest. This pain is often thought to be indigestion; it may radiate down either arm or up into the neck. It makes people terrified, and they are usually shocked and look ill. Imperative treatment is not to allow the casualty to move. He should be kept as still as possible, not allowed to help himself, and be laid down just where he is. A doctor should then be summoned. *Stokes-Adams attacks.* This is the rarest form of heart attack. It is caused by the heart beating so slowly (it may be only ten beats to the minute) that insufficient blood is reaching the brain and the person literally faints. First-aid treatment is similar to any ordinary faint; lay the patient down and send for the doctor.

**heart block.** A disturbance in the rhythm of the heart in which the atria beat faster than the ventricles. It is due to an interruption in the conduction of impulses between the atria and ventricles. The normal contractions of the heart start in the atria, which transmit impulses down the nerves (His's muscle bundle) which run through the central dividing wall of the heart, causing the corresponding ventricles to contract, and producing a synchronous pattern of contractions, atrium to ventricle.

**heartburn.** A hot, burning sensation in the esophagus or stomach due to too much acid in those parts. See also ACID-ITY.

**heart murmur.** See MURMUR: CARDIAC MURMUR.

**heat exhaustion.** People not acclimatized to the tropics or to working in a hot atmosphere, such as a foundry, may lose many pints of sweat a day, and lost with it is much of the body's salt. This results in cramplike pains in muscles, headaches, giddiness, vomiting, collapse or unconsciousness, or both. First aid consists of keeping the casualty cool and rapidly replacing the lost fluid and salt by giving copious drinks, consisting of a quarter tablespoonful of salt to a glass of water flavored with fruit cordial. If the casualty has sweated so much he can sweat no more, heat exhaustion may turn into heat stroke.

**heat rash.** See PRICKLY HEAT.

**heat stroke.** The body temperature in heat stroke may reach as high as 108° F. The skin is dry and burning hot, and the casualty rapidly becomes unconscious. First-aid treatment is to get the patient's temperature down by placing him in a cool and drafty place.

If there is no natural draft one should be created by electric fans or other means. He should then be wrapped in a wet, cold sheet and an ice bag applied to his head. The temperature must not be reduced too suddenly, for this will cause shock. It should be taken at intervals and when it has dropped to around 101°F. the wet sheet should be replaced by a dry one, still keeping the casualty in a current of cool air. If the temperature starts to go up again the wet-sheet treatment should be repeated. When the patient becomes conscious he should be treated as a case of heat exhaustion and given copious drinks of flavored salt water.

**Heberden's disease.** See ANGINA PECTORIS.

**Heberden's nodes.** Small, rounded, bony swellings on the fingers which result from osteoarthritis in the fingers. They may or may not cause considerable pain.

**hectic fever.** A daily recurring fever with the highest temperature in the evening, accompanied by bouts of sweating and shivering. It is often seen in tuberculosis.

**hedenophobia.** Fear of pleasure.

**heliotherapy.** Treatment by exposure to sunlight or ultraviolet light.

**helix.** The rounded margin of the external ear.

**helminth.** A general term covering any of several varieties of intestinal and parasitic worms, especially one that parasitizes the intestines of a vertebrate.

**helminthiasis.** The condition of having worms in the intestines or other parts of the body.

**helminthic abscess.** An abscess started by a helminth worm.

**helminthophobia.** Fear of worms.

**hemangioma.** A growth originating in blood vessels. See NEVUS.

**hemarthrosis.** Hemorrhage into a joint, usually the result of an injury.

**hematemesis.** The vomiting up of blood. This may be due either to sudden hemorrhage from an ulcer, when the blood comes up red and in large quantities, or to small bleedings into the stomach, when the blood, being partially digested, is dark in color.

**hematherapy.** The treatment of disease by the use of blood or plasma.

**hematic abscess.** An abscess caused by an infected blood clot.

**hematin.** The iron-containing chemical in hemoglobin, which colors the red blood cells.

**hematocrit.** 1. An apparatus which separates blood cells by centrifugal force. 2. The proportion of the whole blood volume occupied by the blood cells which have been precipitated by centrifuging; also called *hematocrit*

*reading.* 3. The tube in which the blood cells are separated by centrifugal force; also called *hematocrit tube.*

**hematology.** The study of the blood and its diseases.

**hematoma.** A tumor containing blood. It is often the result of a blow causing small veins to bleed under the skin or into the body tissues and forming a swelling. Once bleeding stops the blood clots begin to resolve and become absorbed, leaving a certain amount of fibrous tissue which usually results in a small permanent collection of scar tissue at the site of the hematoma. The first-aid treatment is to apply a cold compress or ice pack to slow down the bleeding during the first 24 hours.

**hematometra.** A collection of blood within the cavity of the womb.

**hematomyelia.** A hemorrhage into the spinal cord.

**hematopericardium.** A hemorrhage into the pericardium.

**hematoperitoneum.** Hemorrhage into the abdominal cavity.

**hematophobia.** Fear of the sight of blood.

**hematopoiesis.** The formation of red blood cells.

**hematosalpinx.** Hemorrhage into the Fallopian tube.

**hematospermia.** Blood-stained seminal fluid.

**hematothorax.** Hemorrhage into the pleural cavity.

**hematuria.** The presence of blood in the urine.

**hemianacusis.** Loss of hearing in one ear.

**hemianaesthesia.** See HEMIANESTHESIA.

**hemianalgesia.** Insensibility to pain down one side of the body.

**hemianesthesia.** Anesthesia of one side of the body.

**hemianopia.** Blindness in one half of the visual field. Also called *hemianopsia.*

**hemiatrophy.** Wasting of one side or one part of the body.

**hemicrania.** A paroxysmal headache affecting one side of the head, associated with nausea, vomiting, or both and sometimes preceded by disturbances of vision, such as seeing flashing lights or colored lights.

**hemiplegia, hemiparesis.** Paralysis of one side of the body.

**hemlock.** A poisonous plant of the parsley family. The poison is quite deadly stuff, and children have been poisoned by using the plant's hollow stems to make musical pipes or pea shooters. In ancient Greece the official form of execution was to make the condemned man drink wine containing hemlock. Socrates died in this manner.

**hemochromatosis.** A disease characterized by cirrhosis of the liver and diabetes, associated with pigmentation due to deposits of the iron-containing pigment hemosiderin. It is due to the abnormal and excessive absorption of iron from the intestinal tract, and since the body is unable to get rid of this iron it is stored in the liver where it causes degeneration of the liver cells. The liver and spleen enlarge and fluid may accumulate in the abdomen. The skin is generally pigmented a slaty color, especially in the exposed parts of the body, and has a wrinkled appearance. In some cases severe diabetes appears suddenly. Atrophy of the sex organs and loss of secondary sexual characteristics are common. The disease rarely affects women since iron is eliminated in the menstrual blood.

**hemoglobin.** The red chemical contained in the red blood cells. Hemoglobin forms a loose chemical combination with oxygen, which it picks up from the lungs and carries round through the arteries to nourish the tissues. After releasing the oxygen, hemoglobin then picks up carbon dioxide, a waste product, which it carries through the veins back to the lungs where the carbon dioxide is expelled with the expired air. Combined with oxygen, hemoglobin is bright red, but when combined with carbon dioxide it is much darker. It is for this reason that arterial hemorrhages are brighter than venous hemorrhages.

**hemoglobinometer.** An instrument for measuring the amount of hemoglobin in the blood.

**hemoglobinuric fever.** A severe form of malaria associated with bloody urine.

**hemolysin.** A substance which liberates hemoglobin from the red blood cells.

**hemolysis.** Destruction of the red blood cells.

**hemolytic.** Pertaining to hemolysis.

**hemopericardium.** Hemorrhage into the pericardium.

**hemoperitoneum.** Hemorrhage into the peritoneal cavity.

**hemophilia.** An inherited familial condition in which there is excessive bleeding from the most trivial injuries due to a defect in the clotting power of the blood. Although transmitted by the female line, the defect almost exclusively affects the male members of a family.

**hemophiliac.** A person suffering from hemophilia.

**hemophobia.** Fear of the sight of blood.

**hemopneumothorax.** A collection of blood and air within the pleural cavity, the space between the lungs and the chest wall.

**hemoptysis.** Spitting up of blood. This may occur in conditions such as bronchitis or a catarrhal cold, or it may be the first sign of a growth in the lung or of active tuberculosis. Sometimes, however, the blood does not come from the lungs but from the back of the throat.

**hemorrhage.** An escape of blood from the blood vessels. The body can afford to lose one or two pints of blood without too much harm, but losses in excess of this will almost certainly cause surgical shock, a grave condition that calls for urgent blood transfusion. Bleeding is not always the result of an accident or blow but may be due to bursting of a diseased blood vessel, such as happens with a stroke. No matter where the bleeding occurs, if it is a large one the body has to manage on short supplies and in order to do this the blood vessels in the skin contract so that the skin becomes cold and clammy. The anemic brain first becomes irritable, causing the casualty to be excitable, restless, and talkative, but later he slumps into a semicomatose state. The heart tries to overcome the blood loss by pushing the remainder round the body faster, so that the pulse becomes more and more rapid and weaker. *External hemorrhage.* All external bleeding can be stopped by pressure and many cases can be controlled by a firm pad and bandage. If the bleeding is not arrested by these, it usually means they have not been properly applied and an even tighter bandage must be placed over the top of the first one. If bleeding is still not controlled, then pressure must be applied with the fingers or thumbs at an arterial pressure point or by a constrictive bandage, which can be made from such things as a roll of bandage, a handkerchief, or a man's tie wound on firmly. The ideal, of course, is a broad rubber elastic bandage which can be bought and kept in the first-aid box. The skin should be protected with something soft, the constrictive bandage placed above the wound, and tied just tight enough to stop the bleeding. Actually it takes very little pressure to arrest bleeding, so there is no need to apply too much for it may do harm. From then until the casualty is handed over to the care of a doctor the bandage should be cautiously loosened every 15 minutes to see if the bleeding has stopped. If it has, the loosened bandage is left in position so that it can be retightened without delay should the bleeding recur. Small superficial cuts cannot lose very much blood however emotional or excitable the patient may become, and it is good first-aid practice to allow these cuts to bleed for a time to wash out the wound before applying a pad and bandage. *Internal hemorrhage.* Bleeding into internal cavities, such as the chest, abdomen, skull, or into the soft tissues around a fractured bone, can be quite large. The patient will be pale, in a state of collapse, and will feel faint or giddy. The body will call for fluid to replace the lost blood volume, so the patient will feel thirsty. The only first aid for these conditions is to reassure the patient and send for medical aid immediately.

**hemorrhagic.** Bloody.

**hemorrhagic abscess.** An abscess containing a mixture of blood and pus.

**hemorrhoid.** A pile. Piles are varicose veins of the anus which may either be internal and bleed frequently producing anemia, or become large and protrude from the anus, causing pain and discomfort. Slight internal piles are treated by injections, and severe ones by surgical removal.

**hemorrhoidal.** Pertaining to hemorrhoids or piles.

**hemorrhoidectomy.** The surgical removal of piles.

**hemosalpinx.** The presence of blood in the Fallopian tube.

**hemostasis.** The arrest of the blood circulation in a part.

**hemostat.** Forceps used for controlling bleeding.

**hemostatic.** Arresting bleeding.

**hemotherapy.** Treatment which uses injections of blood.

**hemothorax.** Blood in the pleural cavity, the space between the lungs and the wall of the chest.

**Henoch's purpura.** A blood disease characterized by abdominal pain, vomiting of blood, the passing of blood in the stools, and a generalized skin rash of small blood spots.

**heparin.** A substance found in the liver and other tissues which prevents clotting of the blood and the formation of blood platelets. It is used as an anticoagulent for such disorders as coronary thrombosis, and is now derived from animal livers and lungs.

**hepatic.** Pertaining to the liver.

**hepatic fever.** A fever associated with inflammation of the membranes of the gall bladder and bile ducts of the liver.

**hepatitis.** Inflammation of the liver.

**hepatolenticular degeneration.** A familial disease starting in adolescence and characterized by liver disease and degenerative changes in the brain which result in defects of speech, swallowing, and mental debility. Also called *Wilson's disease, progressive lenticular degeneration.*

**hepatomegaly.** Enlargement of the liver.

**hereditary.** Transmitted from parents to offspring.

**heredity.** The transmission of mental or physical characteristics from parent to offspring.

**hermaphrodism.** A condition in which the sexual organs and characteristics of both male and female are combined in the same individual.

*In a normal child the presence of a penis denotes a male and a vagina the female. Sometimes, however, a child is born with no obvious penis or with an enlarged clitoris which looks like a penis. The child is then reared in the sex it superficially appears to be until the secondary sexual characteristics (smooth skin, breasts for a female; beard, deep voice, and so on, for a male) develop and throw doubt on the individual's true sex. If the child has both ovarian and testicular tissue, the child is a true hermaphrodite—a rare condition. The true sex can be determined by scraping a few cells from the inside of the cheek and submitting them to a chromosome test.*

**hermaphrodite.** A person affected with hermaphrodism.

**hernia.** Protusion of an organ through the walls of the cavity in which it is contained; a rupture. A hernia can occur in the brain, lungs, and other organs, but most common is the abdominal hernia.

**abdominal hernia.** Hernia in which a portion of an organ protrudes through the muscular walls of the abdomen, forming a swelling. Diagnosis of these hernias is obtained by asking the patient to cough, thus raising the intra-abdominal pressure and transmitting an impulse which can be seen in the swelling. In healthy individuals the best treatment is surgical repair of the tear in the abdominal muscles. Patients with severe bronchitis and coughing are not suitable for operation, as continual post-operative coughing would break down the stitches. Also unsuitable are patients with very poor abdominal muscles, for strong tissue is needed to close the gap. A truss can be used to control a hernia in the groin (inguinal hernia) but all hernias near the top of the inner thigh (femoral hernias) should be operated on, for in these there is a big risk of strangulation causing intestinal obstruction. However, all persons finding a swelling in the lower part of their abdomen or groins should seek medical advice.

**hiatus hernia.** Protrusion of part of the stomach through the esophageal opening in the diaphragm.

**hernial.** Relating to a hernia.

**herniate.** To form a hernia.

**heroic.** Bold or daring measures taken to treat a patient in a parlous condition.

**heroin.** A derivative of morphine, which in turn is made from opium. A powerful pain reliever, but because of the risk of producing drug addiction it is kept in reserve for really desperate or dying patients.

**herpes.** A skin disease practically always caused by a virus and characterized by intense pain and crops of blisters on the skin. There are many varieties of herpes, but used alone the term commonly refers to herpes simplex.

**herpes labialis.** The sores or blisters that sometimes occur around the mouth in association with the common cold.

**herpes zoster.** A disturbance of a spinal nerve in which crops of blisters on the skin are distributed along the course of the nerve as it emerges from the spine and sweeps round the body in a semicircle. If the condition involves a nerve supplying the face, there is a risk of blisters occurring on the surface of the eye producing a scar and blindness. Herpes zoster is probably due to the same virus that causes chickenpox in children, and wherever chickenpox occurs in an area then herpes zoster appears in the adult population. A curious characteristic of herpes zoster is that long after the blisters have healed and the skin has become normal the severe neuralgic pain persists and can become very troublesome and extremely difficult to treat. Also called *shingles.* See also CHICKENPOX.

**herpetic.** Relating to herpes.

**herpetic fever.** A fever occurring with chills, sore throat, and blisterlike eruptions around the mouth.

**herpetiform.** Resembling herpes.

**heterogeneous.** Different in kind or nature.

**heterophoria.** A general term covering any tendency of the eyes to turn away from the position correct for binocular vision. Actual squinting does not occur unless one eye is covered as the desire for binocular vision is sufficient to overcome the imbalance of the eye muscles. There are, however, specific terms for the direction of each deviation. *Esophoria* means an inward squint; *exophoria* an outward squint; *hyperphoria*, an upward squint; *hyperesophoria*, an upward and inward squint; *hyperexophoria*, an upward and outward squint.

**heterophthalmia.** A condition in which each of the two eyes is a different color.

**heteroplasty.** Surgical transfer of grafts of skin, tissue, or organs from one individual to another.

**heterosexual.** Relating to the opposite sex; pertaining to both sexes.

**heterotopia.** Displacement. Usually applied to an organ or tissue cells found in abnormal locations.

**heterotropia.** Inability to have bifocal vision owing to the deviation or squinting of one eye.

**heterozygous.** The offspring resulting from the crossbreeding of two pure but different strains.

**hexamethonium.** A group of chemicals used in the treatment of high blood pressure.

**hexamine.** A drug used to disinfect the urinary tract.

**hiatus.** An empty space or opening.

**hiatus hernia.** A protrusion of part of the stomach through the opening in the diaphragm, which normally contains only the esophagus. In this condition the hole in the diaphragm is not a tight fit around the esophagus and permits a portion of the stomach to push upwards into the chest cavity, producing a special type of indigestion and regurgitation, which is worse when lying down.

**hiccup, hiccough.** A spasmodic contraction of the diaphragm producing the well-known noise or hiccup. Hiccups sometimes occur in epidemic form and affect a whole town, and this form is probably due to a virus infection. Hiccups can also be an indication of serious deterioration in a patient during the course of some severe disease. The remedies "guaranteed" to stop an attack range from oil of peppermint on sugar in the cheaper grade, to sipping ice-cold champagne in the more expensive bracket. There are also numerous other remedies, all of which contain either carminatives or stomach sedatives. The one remedy which should never be employed is the unexpected slap on the back, for in sensitive people this may cause severe shock.

**Higginson's syringe.** A rubber enema syringe.

**Highmore, antrum of.** A sinus in the cheeks that communicates with a nasal passage.

**hilar.** Relating to a hilus.

**hilus, hilum.** The point on the surface of an organ through which the blood vessels, nerves, and other ducts enter or leave.

**Hippocrates.** A Greek physician who was born on the island of Cos about 460 B.C. Hippocrates is known as the "Father of Medicine" and many of his aphorisms have proved to be as true today as when he first made them.

72

**Hippocratic oath.** The ethical code of doctors. Most of the Hippocratic principles are honored as much today as when formulated by Hippocrates.

*I swear by Apollo the physician, and Aesculapius and Health, and Allheal, and all the gods and goddesses, that, according to my ability and judgment, I will keep this Oath and this stipulation—to reckon him who taught me this Art equally dear to me as my parents, to share my substance with him, and relieve his necessities if required; to look upon his offspring in the same footing as my own brothers, and to teach them this Art, if they shall wish to learn it, without fee or stipulation; and that by precept, lecture, and every other mode of instruction, I will impart a knowledge of the Art to my own sons, and those of my teachers, and to disciples bound by stipulation and oath according to the law of medicine, but to none others. I will follow that system of regimen which, according to my ability and judgment, I consider for the benefits of my patients, and abstain from whatever is deleterious and mischievous. I will give no deadly medicines to anyone if asked, nor suggest any such counsel: and in like manner I will not give to a woman a pessary to produce abortion. With purity and with holiness I will pass my life and practice my Art. I will not cut persons laboring under the stone, but will leave this to be done by men who are practitioners in this work. Into whatever houses I enter, I will go into them for benefit of the sick, and will abstain from every voluntary act of mischief and corruption; and, further, from the seduction of females or males, of freemen or slaves. Whatever, in connection with my professional practice, or not in connection with it, I see or hear, in the life of men, which ought not to be spoken of abroad, I will not divulge, as reckoning that all such should be kept secret. While I continue to keep this Oath unviolated, may it be granted to me to enjoy life and the practice of the Art, respected by all men, in all times. But should I trespass and violate this Oath, may the reverse be my lot.*

**Hirschsprung's disease.** A condition found in children in which the lower part of the colon is enormously dilated and may contain a week's accumulation of feces. The presenting symptom is constipation. It is thought to be due to overaction of the sympathetic nerves which paralyzes the colon and increases the tone of the intestinal valves. Cutting the sympathetic nerves produces a cure and, oddly, so does a high spinal anesthetic, for as soon as the anesthetic wears off the improvement in the colon is main-

tained, though why this should be so is not understood. Surgical removal of the dilated colon is seldom performed now, for most cases respond to the measures mentioned above.

**hirsuties.** Excessive or abnormal growth of hair, especially that which occurs on the face and legs of some women.

**His's muscle bundle.** A bundle of nerve and muscle fibers in the heart responsible for the rhythmic contractions of the atria and ventricles. See also HEART BLOCK.

**histamine.** A chemical that naturally occurs inside the body, and which can also be produced synthetically. Histamine has the property of dilating blood vessels, a condition that arises in such allergic disorders as urticaria. Histamine can be neutralized by antihistamine drugs such as Benadryl.

**histologist.** One who practices histology.

**histology.** The science and study of tissue structure and the microscopical appearances of body tissues.

**histoplasmosis.** A usually fatal disease caused by a fungus, and characterized by high temperature, severe anemia, and gross wasting of the body.

**history.** Medical history is an account of the patient's symptoms and previous illnesses; family history is a description of the illnesses or abnormalities that have been suffered by the patient's relatives.

**hives.** Urticaria or nettle rash.

**hoarseness.** Dysphonia.

**hobnail liver.** The popular name for alcoholic cirrhosis of the liver.

**Hodgkin's disease.** A disease principally affecting the lymph glands, which become enlarged and of a rubbery consistency. The enlargement is not associated with pain. Commencing in one group of glands, the condition spreads to other groups and to the lymphoid tissue in the spleen, liver, and other organs, which also become enlarged. Loss of weight, high temperature, and generalized itching may be symptoms and once the disease is established there is increasing generalized weakness, progressive anemia, and shortness of breath. Treatment principally consists of radiotherapy, but a series of drugs now being developed appear to control the disease and it is hoped that they will eventually provide a cure or at least a greater degree of amelioration. Also called *lymphadenoma.*

**homatropine.** A drug used to treat certain eye disorders and to widely dilate the pupil and paralyze the muscles of accommodation to facilitate deep examination of the back of the eyeball. The drug is derived from atropine,

which is used for the same purpose, but its effects wear off sooner than those of atropine.

**homeopath.** A practitioner of homeopathy.

**homeopathic.** Relating to homeopathy.

**homeopathy.** A system of treatment invented by Hahnemann in America, whose motto was "like cures like." He taught that drugs should be tested on normal human beings; that symptoms caused by drugs in healthy persons were cured by the same drugs when present in illness; that the effectiveness of a drug was in inverse proportion to the size of the dose; and that eruptive skin diseases must be allowed to come out and should not be driven in.

*When homeopathy was introduced in about 1796 it gained support from doctors because it appeared that patients derived benefit from it. The truth is that in those days, with no scientific knowledge, doctors and quacks were giving such large doses of poisonous and potent drugs that patients were being made worse, but following Hahnemann's tenet of "the smaller the dose the greater the effect," the doctors reduced their dosages and this obviously contributed to the recovery of their patients. The small doses of drugs used by the homeopaths, in fact, did no good, but on the other hand they did no harm and someone once said, very cynically, "The patients of the homeopaths died of their disease whereas the patients of the doctors died of the cure." The vogue of homeopathy was brief because it was soon replaced by scientific medicine which showed that only a few drugs were of value in treating disease and that these few drugs are indispensable and must be used in their proper effective doses.*

**homicidal mania.** A type of insanity in which the patient has murderous impulses.

**homicide.** A general term meaning the killing of a human being, but it can have the meaning of killing without malice or intent, which distinguishes it from murder.

**homoeopath.** See HOMEOPATH.

**homoeopathic.** See HOMEOPATHIC.

**homoeopathy.** See HOMEOPATHY.

**homogeneous.** Having the same nature or of uniform character.

**homologous.** Belonging to the same type or having a similar structure.

**homosexuality.** Sexual condition in which sexual desire is directed to a member of the same sex. See also SODOMY.

**hookworm disease.** See ANCYLOSTOMIASIS.

**hordeolum.** Latin for a grain of barley, and the old-fashioned term for a sty on the eyelid, which looks like a barley grain.

**hormones.** Chemical substances secreted by the endocrine glands into the bloodstream where they circulate and carry out specific changes in distant organs.

**horn.** A substance mainly composed of keratin, of which hair and nails are composed.

**Horner's syndrome.** Ptosis (drooping of the upper eyelid), enophthalmos, contracted pupil, anhidrosis, and lack of expression of the side of the face affected; caused by paralysis of the cervical sympathetic nerves in the neck due to trauma pressure, growths, disease of the brain or spinal cord, or syphilis.

**horripilation.** Goose flesh; the erection of hairs on the skin. See also GOOSE FLESH.

**horsepox.** A term loosely used to include a number of diseases which occur in horses, such as pseudotuberculosis and contagious pustular stomatitis, which is an infection of the mouth region. The virus appears to be indistinguishable from the causative virus of vaccinia.

**horseshoe kidney.** A congenital defect in which the kidneys, instead of being separate, are joined at their lower ends, forming a horseshoe shape.

**host.** The organism (plant or animal) on which a parasite lives.

**housemaid's knee.** Prepatellar bursitis, a swelling in front of the knee cap due to an effusion into the bursa situated over the knee cap. See also BURSA.

**humanize.** The term applied to viruses which have passed through the human body.

**humanized milk.** Cow's milk which has been reduced in fat and increased in sugar so that it closely resembles human milk.

**humerus.** The upper arm; the bone of the upper arm.

**humidity.** Moisture or the state of being moist.

**absolute humidity.** The amount of water vapor present in the air at any given time.

**relative humidity.** The percentage of water vapor in the air compared with that which would be present if the air was saturated with water vapor.

**humor.** Any body fluid.

*Galen, who was born in Asia Minor in A.D. 131, advanced a theory that the body, like the universe, was composed of four elements—fire, air, water, and earth. He believed fire was hot, air was dry, water was wet, and earth was cold, and that in health heat and cold were balanced and so were dryness and moisture, while disease resulted when the balance between the four humors was disturbed. The drugs Galen employed to restore the balance had the four fundamental qualities of the body, so that a disease with fever was to be treated with cooling drugs and a disease with chills was to be treated with heating drugs. The selection of the proper heating, cooling, moistening, or drying drugs was determined by the character and intensity of the disease. He assessed all the drugs as possessing these fundamental qualities in different degrees; thus bitter almond was heating in the first degree and drying in the second degree, while pepper was heating in the fourth degree and cucumber seeds were cooling in a similar degree, hence the common expression "cool as a cucumber." It is not so long ago that sassafras tea was used to "cool" the blood of children in springtime. Galen also described four dispositions or humors, the choleric, the melancholic, the phlegmatic, and the sanguine. His was a brave and even monumental effort to try to treat disease at least by some system, even if it was unscientific by present-day standards.*

**humoral.** Relating to body fluids.

**humour.** See HUMOR.

**hunchbacked.** Kyphosis.

**Huntington's chorea.** An adult form of St. Vitus's dance; this is a rare disease the symptoms of which are almost identical with those of ordinary rheumatic chorea, comprising involuntary movements, ataxy, paralysis, and slow, slurring speech. It gradually appears in adult life, usually about the age of 40, and is accompanied by progressive mental deterioration, with delusions, and a tendency to suicide. Maniacal outbursts are not uncommon. The disease always progresses slowly to a fatal termination in from five to thirty years and treatment has no effect. It appears to be a familial disease with a tendency to pass from one generation to the next.

**Hutchinson's pupil.** A diagnostic sign of hemorrhage into the brain. The pupil on the side of the hemorrhage is dilated, that on the other side is contracted.

**Hutchinson's teeth.** Peg-shaped incisor teeth, notched at the cutting edge, seen in patients suffering from hereditary syphilis.

**Hutchinson's triad.** Three conditions diagnostic of hereditary syphilis. They are: (1) diffuse inflammation of the eye, especially the cornea; (2) disease of the labyrinth of the ear; and (3) Hutchinson's teeth.

**hyalin.** A clear, homogeneous translucent material occurring normally in cartilage and in the vitreous of the eye; the colloid contained in the thyroid gland, mucin, the umbilical cord, and also seen in tissue degeneration.

**hyaluronidase.** An enzyme preparation used to facilitate the diffusion of injected drugs. It is also found in snake venom.

**hybrid.** The offspring of parents who differ in one or several distinct characteristics.

**hybridism.** Crossbreeding.

**hydatid.** A cyst usually forming in the liver or lungs, due to the growth of the larval stage of the dog tapeworm. The tapeworm larva is introduced into the body by using crockery from which an infested dog has eaten or through the habit of kissing a pet dog.

**hydatidiform.** Resembling a hydatid.

**hydradenitis.** Inflammation of the sweat glands in the armpit.

**hydraemia.** See HYDREMIA.

**hydragogue.** A drug which increases the secretion of water from the kidneys. Also called *diuretic*.

**hydramnion, hydramnios.** Distension of the amnion by an excess of amniotic fluid. The amnion is the membrane surrounding the fetus in the womb. See also LIQUOR AMNII.

**hydrarthrosis.** An accumulation of fluid in a joint.

**hydration.** The action of combining chemically with water.

**hydremia.** A watery dilution of the bloodstream.

**hydroa.** A general term for any skin disease characterized by the formation of little blisters.

**hydrocele.** Any collection of serumlike fluid, but especially one occurring between the two membranes covering the testicle and the spermatic cord. The condition is relieved by puncture and drainage of the fluid, but the ultimate cure is surgical removal of the layers of membrane which form the fluid.

**hydrocephalic.** Relating to hydrocephalus.

**hydrocephalus.** An abnormal collection of cerebrospinal fluid within the cavities or ventricles of the brain, which may be present at birth or develop in early infancy. Cerebrospinal fluid, which is manufactured in the ventricles and bathes the brain and spinal cord, normally drains off into the general circulation, but if an obstruction prevents it from draining away in the normal manner, or if there is an increase in its rate of secretion, it causes a progressive enlargement of the child's head, thinning of the skull, wasting of the brain, mental impairment, and convulsions. Also called *water on the brain*.

**hydrochloric acid.** The acid contained in the gastric juice.

**hydrolysis.** The chemical process by which a substance unites with water and then divides into smaller molecules.

**hydrometer.** An apparatus used for estimating the specific gravity of fluids.

**hydronephrosis.** Distension of the kidney by urine due to an obstruction to its outflow. In time this destroys the kidney substance if not relieved by a surgical operation.

**hydroperitoneum.** The presence of fluid within the abdominal cavity. Also called *abdominal ascites.*

**hydrophobía.** A disease transmitted by the bite of a dog or other mammal suffering from rabies. The name is based on the suffering animal's apparent fear of water. See RABIES.

**hydrophobic.** Relating to hydrophobia.

**hydrops.** Dropsy, an abnormal accumulation of fluid in any tissue or body cavity.

**hydrosalpinx.** Distension of the Fallopian tube with fluid.

**hydrotherapy.** The treatment of disease by medicated baths.

**hydrothorax.** The accumulation of fluid in the pleural cavity, the cavity between the lungs and the wall of the chest.

**hydroureter.** Distension of the ureteric tube of the kidney due to an obstruction at its lower end.

**hydroxybutyric acid.** An organic acid that is an intermediary in fat metabolism, and a member of a group of compounds called acetone bodies or ketone bodies. This acid appears in the blood in disorders such as diabetes, and if it accumulates it acts as an anesthetic and produces diabetic coma. Hydroxybutyric acid is the evil-smelling and evil-tasting compound present in rancid butter and decomposing sweat. See also SWEAT.

**hydruria.** The discharge of large quantities of urine of low specific gravity.

**hygiene.** The science of health. The word is derived from Hygieia, the ancient Greek goddess of health, who was the daughter of Aesculapius, the god of medicine.

**hygienist.** A person trained in hygiene.

**hygrometer.** An instrument for recording the amount of moisture in the air.

**hygroscopic.** Capable of absorbing moisture from the air.

**hymen.** A fold of mucous membrane which partly occludes the external opening of the vagina.

**imperforate hymen.** A hymen which completely occludes the external opening of the vagina. When this occurs the hymen has to be excised (hymenectomy) in order that the menstrual blood can be discharged.

*The hymen used to be considered an indication of virginity, since, if one was present, it ruptured when intercourse took place on the wedding night; in point of fact, many athletic young girls do not have a hymen and are still virginal. In the past after the wedding night of kings and queens, it was the practice of senior courtiers to examine the bottom sheet of the royal marital bed for signs of blood, indicating that the royal couple had consummated the marriage.*

**hyoid.** A U-shaped bone in the front of the neck which acts as the fulcrum for the throat muscles. In cases of strangulation this bone is always examined and almost invariably it is fractured, indicating that severe pressure has been exerted on the neck.

**hyoscine.** A drug derived from hyoscyamus. See SCOPOLAMINE.

**hypengyophobia.** Fear of responsibility.

**hyperacidity.** Excessive acidity.

**hyperacousis.** Abnormal acuteness of the sense of hearing.

**hyperactivity.** An abnormal and excessive activity.

**hyperacuity.** Abnormal perception of sound.

**hyperadrenalism.** See PHEOCHROMOCYTOMA.

**hyperaemia.** See HYPEREMIA.

**hyperaesthesia.** See HYPERESTHESIA.

**hyperalgesia.** Increased sensibility to pain.

**hyperchlorhydria.** An excess of acid in the stomach.

**hyperdistension.** Abnormal distension.

**hyperdiuresis.** Excessive flow of urine.

**hyperemesis.** Excessive vomiting.

**hyperemesis gravidarum.** The excessive morning sickness of pregnancy. This condition must be treated in a hospital, for it has been known to become so severe and dangerous that pregnancy has had to be terminated. See also MORNING SICKNESS.

**hyperemia.** Localized congestion with blood.

**active hyperemia.** Congestion due to increased blood flow from an artery.

**passive hyperemia.** Congestion due to obstruction of the venous flow of blood. Also called *cyanosis.*

**hyperesthesia.** Increased sensitivity.

**hyperexophoria.** An upward and outward squint.

**hyperextension.** Overextension of a joint.

**hyperflexion.** Overflexion of a joint.

**hyperglycaemia.** See HYPERGLYCEMIA.

**hyperglycemia.** An excessive amount of sugar in the blood, as in diabetes.

**hyperhidrosis, hyperidrosis.** Excessive sweating.

**hyperinsulinism.** A deficiency of sugar in the blood, due to an excess of insulin. See also HYPOGLYCEMIA.

**hyperinvolution.** Shrinkage of an organ to smaller than normal size, especially after enlargement. The term usually refers to the womb contracting down to a smaller than normal size after pregnancy.

**hyperkeratosis.** 1. Excessive formation of the horny layer of the skin. 2. Enlargement of the cornea.

**hypermetropia.** Long-sightedness. It is frequently due to the eyeball being shorter than normal from front to back.

**hypermotility.** An increase in activity.

**hypermyotonia.** State of increased muscle tone.

**hypernephroma.** A malignant growth of the kidney. Also called *Grawitz's tumor.*

**hyperparathyroidism.** Overactivity of the parathyroid glands, usually due to a small tumor. The condition is characterized by spontaneous fractures of bone, pain, weakness of bones and muscles, a tendency to stones in the kidneys. It produces osteitis fibrosa cystica and osteomalacia.

**hyperphoria.** A condition in which the level of the eyes is out of line, the visual axis of one eye being above or below that of the other.

**hyperpiesia, hyperpiesis.** Hypertension or high blood pressure.

**hyperpituitarism.** Overfunction of the pituitary gland in the brain, resulting in acromegaly or gigantism. See ACROMEGALY.

**hyperplasia.** The increase in size of a tissue or organ, due to an increase in the number of its constituent cells.

**hyperplastic.** Relating to hyperplasia.

**hyperpnea.** Overbreathing or panting.

**hyperpnoea.** See HYPERPNEA.

**hyperpyretic.** Relating to hyperpyrexia.

**hyperpyrexia.** A very high body temperature.

**hyperresonance.** An abnormally hollow sound heard when the chest is percussed. It may indicate that a lung has collapsed.

**hypersecretion.** An abnormally increased secretion.

**hypersensitiveness.** Abnormally increased sensibility. This term is often confused with allergy and both terms are frequently misused. It is sometimes claimed that a person is "allergic" to a substance when in fact he is hypersenstive to it. For instance, the patient who gets an increased reaction from the normal dose of a drug, is, strictly speaking, hypersensitive to that drug, and allergy does not come into it at all. On the other hand, people who get a reaction, such as a skin rash, when they eat certain foods are sometimes said to be hypersensitive when what is meant is allergic. See also ALLERGY.

**hypertension.** Raised blood pressure.

**benign hypertension.** This term is misleading, for there is little about the condition which is benign. It was so called merely because high blood pressure can be present for many years without producing ill effects. However, in time it causes heart failure, hemorrhage into the retina, or a stroke.

**malignant hypertension.** A disease syndrome consisting of very high blood pressure, transient cerebral attacks, and disease of the retina, and with papilledema occurring in the course of disorders such as kidney disease, eclampsia, and essential hypertension.

**hypertensive.** Characterized by high blood pressure.

**hyperthermia.** A rise of body temperature not due to infection.

**hyperthyroidism.** Overactivity of the thyroid gland. Also called *exophthalmic goiter, toxic goiter, thyrotoxicosis, Graves's disease.* See GOITER.

**hypertonia.** Increased tone or activity, usually of the muscles.

**hypertonic.** Characterized by hypertonia.

**hypertoxic.** Excessively poisonous.

**hypertrichiasis, hypertrichosis.** Superfluous hair or excessive growth of hair on the body.

**hypertrophic.** Pertaining to hypertrophy.

**hypertrophy.** An increase in the size of a tissue or an organ due to an enlargement of its constituent cells.

**compensatory hypertrophy.** The increase in size of an organ in order to increase its function. This occurs if a kidney or lung has been removed, when the remaining organ enlarges to try to assume the function once performed by both.

**simple hypertrophy.** An increase in the number of individual cells of an organ.

**true hypertrophy.** An increase in size of all the component tissues of an organ or msucle, often as the result of excessive use. It occurs, for instance, in the muscles of weight lifters from continually lifting heavy weights.

**hypervitaminosis.** A condition brought about by the taking of excessive amounts of vitamins.

**hyphidrosis.** Too little perspiration.

**hypnolepsy.** An abnormal desire to sleep. Also called *narcolepsy.*

**hypnophobia.** Fear of falling asleep.

**hypnosis.** A form of sleep induced by a hypnotist during which suggestions are made, strengthened by an element of command. Contrary to popular belief, the patient cannot be made to do actions or deeds under hypnosis which he or she would be unwilling to do while awake. If such suggestions are made the patient either wakes up screaming or ignores the instruction. Hypnotism therefore cannot be used to start an unwilling person on a life of crime. On the other hand if a person had a secret ambition to, say, punch a policeman in the nose, then instuctions to do this while under hypnosis would reinforce the previously held desire and the patient, after waking up, might go out and punch a policeman in the nose. Hypnotism is used in the treatment of neurosis because while the patient is asleep the doctor can make powerful suggestions to dispel the symptoms of such conditions as hysterical paralysis, sicknesses and illnesses such as hysteria, nerve rashes, and asthma. In dealing with the emotionally disturbed, hypnotism is used to encourage the patient to speak freely of the experiences that led up to the nervous state, thus producing a mental catharsis.

*Hypnotism has probably been used far back in time, especially among the mystics of the Far East. It came into prominence when Franz Mesmer, a German, went to Paris under the patronage of Marie Antoinette and practiced what he called animal magnestism, later called mesmerism. Later, Phineas Quimby of Maine practiced animal magnetism, or hypnotism, in America. In his early days Quimby's method of treatment consisted of sitting beside the patient, usually a woman, and with his left hand on her bare abdomen, stroking her head with his right and talking her into a hypnotic trance, during which he encouraged her to speak of her troubles. Quimby later founded New Thought, which laid down that disease was a purely mental condition resulting from evil thoughts. This brought great comfort to many neurotic people even if they still contracted organic diseases, and was in fact a form of hypnotic faith healing.*

**hypnotic.** Inducing sleep; relating to hypnotism; a drug that promotes sleep.

**hypnotism.** The science of hypnosis.

**hypnotist.** One trained in the art of hypnotism.

**hypnotize.** To induce hypnosis.

**hypoacidity.** Deficiency of normal acid in the stomach.

**hypoactivity.** A decrease in activity.

**hypochlorhydria.** Deficiency of hydrochloric acid in the gastric juice.

**hypochondriac.** A person suffering from hypochondriasis.

**hypochondriacal.** Pertaining to hypochondriasis.

**hypochondriasis.** A condition of mental depression caused by the patient's belief he is suffering from a grave illness and which may be quite unrelieved by any reassurance that a doctor may give. See also HYPOCHONDRIUM.

**hypochondrium.** The upper lateral regions of the abdomen beneath the ribs. The right hypochondrium contains the liver and gall bladder and the left hypochondrium the spleen. See also ABDOMINAL AREAS.

*In ancient times various organs were alleged to be the seat of certain emotions, and the heros of Homeric poems had their souls in their livers while the heroines had their romantic emotions situated in their hearts. Shakespeare refers to this when Ford asks Pistol "Love my wife?" and he replies "With liver burning hot." The liver was also held responsible for mental depression and other emotional, neurotic, and hypochondriacal symptoms. The term melancholy is derived from two Greek words meaning black bile, which was alleged to cause depression and was manufactured by the liver. There are many forms of organic disease which can be imitated by neurotic symptoms.*

**hypodermic.** Beneath the skin. Commonly refers to an injection under the skin.

**hypodermis.** The layer of tissue beneath the skin.

**hypofunction.** Diminished function.

**hypogastric.** Pertaining to the hypogastrium.

**hypogastrium.** The middle region of the abdomen below the umbilicus.

**hypoglossal.** Situated under the tongue.

**hypoglossal cranial nerve.** The twelfth cranial nerve.

**hypoglycaemia.** See HYPOGLYCEMIA.

**hypoglycemia.** Deficiency of sugar in the blood.

**spontaneous hypoglycemia.** A deficiency of blood sugar due to excessive production of insulin by the pancreas, which may be the result of a growth in the pancreas or of a functional disturbance of the endocrine system. It is characterized by a feeling of hunger, perspiration, muscular shakes, mental confusion, convulsions, and even coma. It is frequently claimed in court that a person accused of being drunk at the steering wheel was, in fact, suffering from spontaneous hypoglycemia.

**hypohidrosis.** Abnormally diminished perspiration.

**hypomenorrhea.** A condition in which the menstrual cycle is prolonged and often irregular due to malfunction of the ovaries. There is scanty loss of blood and the intervals between periods may be months. It may be caused by immaturity of the sexual organs in the adolescent female and in adults it may be due to disease causing depression of ovarian function.

**hypomenorrhoea.** See HYPOMENORRHEA.

**hypoparathyroidism.** Diminished activity of the parathyroid glands. These are situated behind the thyroid gland and control calcium metabolism. The condition sometimes follows surgical removal of part of the thyroid gland and results in spasmodic muscle contractions, a lowering of the calcium content of the blood, and sometimes cataract.

**hypophoria.** A condition in which the vision from one eye is directed below that of the other.

**hypophyseal.** Pertaining to the pituitary gland.

**hypophysectomy.** Surgical removal of the pituitary gland.

**hypophysis.** Any outgrowth, but used without qualification the term refers to the hypophysis cerebri, the pituitary gland.

**hypopituitarism.** Diminished function of the pituitary gland. See SIMMONDS' DISEASE.

**hypoplasia.** Defective or incomplete development of a tissue or organ.

**hypopyon.** The presence of pus in the anterior chamber of the eye. Also called *onyx*.

**hyposecretion.** Deficiency of secretion.

**hypospadias, hypospadia.** A birth deformity in which the opening of the urethra is situated on the undersurface of the penis instead of at the tip.

**hypostasis.** 1. Sediment. 2. The collection of blood in the dependent parts of the body or an organ immediately after death. It is one way by which the pathologist can tell whether a body has been moved after death. For instance, if immediately after death a body was laid on its back, the blood would pool in that part and produce a congested appearance. Therefore, if the body was later found turned on to its face the blood staining on the back would indicate that the body had been moved since death.

**hypostatic abscess.** See WANDERING ABSCESS.

**hypotension.** Low blood pressure.

**hypotensive.** Characterized by hypotension.

**hypothalamus.** A portion of the lower cerebrum beneath the thalamus. It influences the posterior lobe of the pituitary gland and contains important centers that control temperature regulation, water balance, and sleep.

**hypothenar.** The pad of soft tissue on the palm of the hand at the base of the little finger.

**hypothermal.** Having low temperature; tepid.

**hypothermia.** Subnormal temperature of the body. It can now be induced by placing a limb or the whole body in ice. This freezing slows the circulation, reduces pain and shock, and lessens the body's oxygen requirements. It has been used as an adjunct to surgery in brain and heart operations and in the repair and replacement of arteries. Another method of hypothermia is to pass a tube down the patient's throat into the duodenum. This tube is part of a refrigeration circuit to freeze a duodenal ulcer, which it is claimed will then heal without the need of surgery.

**hypothyroidism.** Deficient activity of the thyroid gland. See also MYXEDEMA; CRETINISM.

**hypotonia.** Diminished tone or activity, usually of muscles.

**hypotonic.** Below the normal strength or tension. The converse is hypertonic.

**hypotropia.** A downward squint.

**hypovitaminosis.** The state of being short of vitamins.

**hypsophobia.** Fear of heights.

**hysterectomy.** Surgical removal of the womb. It is indicated when constant and excessive bleeding occurs with such diseases as fibroids or growths of the womb or hemorrhages at the change of life. If the ovaries are removed with the womb an artificial change of life occurs, but if only the womb is removed the woman ceases to menstruate, can no longer become pregnant, but is otherwise normal.

**panhysterectomy.** Removal of the womb, ovaries, and Fallopian tubes.

**subtotal hysterectomy.** Removal of the womb except for the cervix.

**vaginal hysterectomy.** Removal of the womb via the vagina instead of through the abdominal wall.

**Wertheim's hysterectomy.** Removal of the whole of the womb and its surrounding lymph glands.

**hysteria.** Hysterical attacks are usually fairly obvious because of their bizarre character. They usually occur before an audience. In severe cases the attacks may be accompanied by crying, wailing, or screaming, and sometimes by unconsciousness. It is a psychoneurotic condition in which anxiety is converted into temporary physical abnormalities which have no organic basis. There are other manifestations of hysteria. In one form a whole limb appears paralyzed —not only is it limp and helpless but there is complete sensory loss, the patient apparently being insensitive to pinprick. There is no evidence of acci-

dent in these cases. First-aid treatment is not necessary and all forms of fuss should be avoided. The old practice of throwing cold water over the patients or slapping them is to be deprecated. The patient needs medical treatment and later serious investigation by a neuropsychiatrist.

**hysteric, hysterical.** Relating to hysteria.

**hystero-oophorectomy.** Surgical removal of both the womb and the ovaries.

# I-J

**iatrogenic disease.** Disease produced unintentionally by the doctor. For example, in order to correct an overactive thyroid gland part of it is removed. If, however, too much is excised the gland becomes underactive and this condition is referred to as an iatrogenic disease. A further example is the nervous disorder arising in a patient after he has been told the diagnosis of his disease, or perhaps after he has misinterpreted a remark made by the doctor to him or to another person.

**iatrology.** The science of medicine.

**ichor.** The watery fluid escaping from a wound.

**ichthammol.** A thick black substance derived from coal. It is incorporated in ointments as a treatment for eczemas and to relieve pruritus. Also called *ichthyol*.

**ichthyosis.** A congenital condition of the skin which is deficient in grease glands and so is dry and scaly for life. The dryness can be relieved, however, by regularly rubbing in either vegetable oil, such as olive oil, or lanolin. Also called *fishskin disease, porcupine disease*.

**icteric.** Pertaining to jaundice.

**icterogenic.** Producing jaundice.

**icterohemorrhagic fever.** Spirochetal jaundice. See LEPTOSPIROSIS.

**icteroid.** Like jaundice.

**icterus.** See JAUNDICE.

*The word* icterus *derives from the Greek for a yellow bird, and the color of the jaundiced patient was compared to that of the bird.*

**icterus gravis neonatorum.** See JAUNDICE: HEMOLYTIC JAUNDICE.

**icterus neonatorum.** See JAUNDICE: PHYSIOLOGICAL JAUNDICE.

**id.** A term used in psychoanalysis to denote the primitive psychic force which produces the instinctive energy necessary for self-preservation and propagation of the species—in other words, our animal instincts; the subconscious part of the mind.

**ideation.** The formation of ideas.

**idiocy.** A congenital condition of mental deficiency.

*In ancient Greece it was the duty of every citizen to take his turn at certain public duties. Those who did not participate were referred to as the "idiotai," meaning persons ignorant of public affairs, and the term "idiot" is derived from this.*

**amaurotic idiocy.** A congenital, hereditary type of idiocy thought to be associated with a disorder of fat metabolism and characterized by severe mental deficiency, disturbances of motor function, and defective vision..If it appears shortly after birth, it is known as Tay-Sachs's disease; if it appears during later childhood it is called the juvenile type; and if it appears later in life it is called Kufs type.

**Mongolian idiocy.** A form of idiocy in which the face resembles that of a Mongol, with obliquely placed eyes, thick protruding tongue, short broad fingers, and other defects.

**idiopathic.** A term descriptive of a disease which arises spontaneously and not due to or associated with any other disease, as far as is known to medical knowledge. Sometimes a cause is discovered for such diseases which, of course, removes it from the idiopathic category.

**idiopathic abscess.** An abscess of unknown cause.

**idiosyncrasy.** Any peculiar characteristic of body, mind, or temperament. A peculiarity of constitution that makes an individual react differently from most persons to drugs or treatments, such as the individual who cannot take an aspirin tablet without becoming giddy and having a skin rash.

**idiot.** A person suffering from idiocy.

**ileac.** Relating to the ileum, part of the small intestine.

**ileectomy.** Surgical removal of the ileum.

**ileitis.** Inflammation of the ileum, part of the small intestine.

**regional ileitis.** A chronic inflammatory disease usually affecting the last part of the ileum, and characterized by the development of granulomatous tissue in the intestinal walls, which sometimes leads to obstruction. Also called *Crohn's disease, terminal ileitis*.

**ileocaecal.** See ILEOCECAL.

**ileocaecostomy.** See ILEOCECOSTOMY.

**ileocecal.** Relating to the ileum and the cecum.

**ileocecostomy.** A surgical operation in which the ileum is joined to the cecum

after excision of a portion of the terminal ileum, as in the treatment of ileitis.

**ileocolic.** Relating both to the ileum and the colon.

**ileocolostomy.** The surgical formation of a passage between the ileum and the colon to by-pass the diseased cecum.

**ileoileostomy.** A surgical operation in which a diseased piece of the ileum is removed and the ends rejoined.

**ileosigmoidostomy.** An operation in which the ileum is joined to the sigmoid colon to by-pass a diseased portion of the cecum, ascending, or transverse colon.

**ileostomy.** A surgical operation by which the ileum is brought to the surface of the abdominal wall to form an opening for the discharge of its contents. This is used when there is obstruction or disease of the cecum or colon.

**ileum.** The lower half of the small intestine between the jejunum and the cecum.

**ileus.** Paralysis of the intestine which causes an obstruction; sometimes follows surgery on the intestines.

**iliac.** Relating to the ilium, a bone of the pelvis.

**iliofemoral.** Referring to the ilium and femur.

**ilio-inguinal.** Relating to the ilium and the groin.

**iliopectineal.** Referring to the ilium and pubes.

**iliopsoas.** Two muscles which lie together, low in the rear of the abdomen.

**ilium.** The upper broad wing-shaped bone which sticks out from the true pelvis and forms the ridge of bone popularly referred to as the "hip." Since this bone lies so conveniently beneath the skin, many surgeons remove pieces from it to use as grafts to bridge gaps in fractures. Also called *innominate bone*.

**illusion.** A perception which misinterprets the object perceived; a false perception.

**illusional.** Pertaining to illusions.

**image.** 1. A more or less accurate representation of an object. 2. The picture of an object formed by a lens.

**imago.** 1. In psychoanalysis, the childhood conception only partly based on reality of a parent or of some loved person retained in the subconscious mind and carried into adulthood. 2. The sexually mature adult stage of an insect.

**imbalance.** Lack of balance, especially between muscles.

**imbecile.** Affected by imbecility.

**imbecility.** Mental deficiency which is less severe than idiocy.

**immiscible.** Not capable of being mixed together.

**immobility.** The state of fixation.

**immobilization.** Fixing or making immobile, such as applying splints to a limb or the permanent fusion of a joint by surgery.

**immune.** Protected against infectious disease.

**immune body.** See antibody.

**immunity.** The state of being resistant to disease. Most babies have an immunity to infectious disease during the first two or three weeks of life, passed on from the mother. Some people appear to be naturally immune to certain bacteria-caused ailments, but it is difficult to be sure that they have not had at some time a mild dose of the illness and it has passed unrecognized as an attack of "flu."

**active immunity.** 1. Immunity created by recovery from an infection. 2. Immunity acquired by the injection of a small dose of a germ poison or killed germs into the patient, the body immediately responding in the same way to the injected matter as though an invasion of actual germs had taken place, by creating germ antibodies. These antibodies persist in the bloodstream, so that if the germ itself gains entry to the body at a later date it is immediately destroyed by the antibodies circulating in the blood.

**passive immunity.** Immunity created by injecting into the patient serum obtained from a person, sometimes an animal, who has recovered from the disease and who has produced and has circulating in his blood vast quantities of antibodies. These antibodies are then used to produce for the patient a temporary protection which only lasts for a few weeks but which may be sufficient to tide him over until the more permanent active immunity can be created.

**immunization.** The act of rendering immune. There are many varied immunization schedules in use and they vary as advances in knowledge occur, but a current popular scheme is as follows. *Two months*—triple antigen injection against diphtheria, tetanus, and whooping cough. *Three months*—second injection of triple antigen. *Four months*—third injection of triple antigen. *Seven months*—first dose of poliomyelitis vaccine. *Eight months*—second dose of poliomyelitis vaccine. *Twelve months*—vaccination against smallpox. *Fifteen months*—boost dose of triple antigen and third dose of poliomyelitis vaccine. *Five years*—boost dose of triple antigen and fourth dose of poliomyelitis vaccine. *Eight years*—boost dose of triple antigen. *Nine years*—revaccination against smallpox.

*Twelve years*—B.C.G. vaccination against tuberculosis. Immunity can also be given against influenza, yellow fever, typhoid fever, and cholera, and it may soon be possible to immunize against the common cold.

**impacted. 1.** Wedged in tightly, as an embedded tooth. **2.** Applied to a fracture in which the broken ends of a bone are driven into each other. **3.** The condition in which the baby's head becomes wedged in the pelvis during labor.

**impaction.** The state of being wedged or fixed.

**dental impaction.** A condition in which an unerupted tooth becomes wedged against the tooth in front and is unable to grow out of the gum.

**fecal impaction.** Blockage of the bowels by large quantities of hard impassable feces.

**ureteal impaction.** Blockage of a ureter by a calculus, preventing the passage of urine and causing back pressure on the kidney.

**impalpable.** Not capable of being recognized by the sense of touch.

**imperception.** Defective perception.

**imperforate.** Having no opening. See also IMPERFORATE ANUS; HYMEN; IMPERFORATE HYMEN.

**imperforation.** A condition in which an opening is abnormally closed.

**imperforate anus.** A congenital defect in which there is no opening in the anal region. The condition is relieved by surgery.

**impermeable, impervious.** Not permitting passage, especially of fluids.

**impetigo.** A general term for any inflammatory and pustular skin disease.
**Bockhart's impetigo.** See IMPETIGO FOLLICULARIS, below.

**impetigo contagiosa.** An acute inflammation of the skin characterized by the formation of flat vesicles which become pustular and later form crusts. The condition is most commonly seen on the face, and children are affected more often than adults, school outbreaks being common as the disease rapidly spreads from close contact. The cause of the condition is a bacterial invasion by either *Streptococcus pyogenes* or *Staphylococcus aureus.* Itchy skin conditions such as scabies and pediculosis are often complicated by impetigo. Any crusted, infected-looking rash suddenly appearing on the face of a child should be considered impetigo, and medical advice sought. Antibiotics by mouth and applied to the skin are remarkably effective in a few days. Until the condition is controlled the patient should be kept at home and isolated.

**impetigo follicularis.** A pustular inflammatory condition of the hair follicles on any part of the skin. Also called *Bockhart's impetigo.*

**impetigo herpetiformis.** A rare type of impetigo characterized by the formation of superficial pustules that may be discrete but tend to form little round groups. The condition mostly occurs in pregnant women and is sometimes very severe.

**impetigo neonatorum.** A form of impetigo accompanied by blisters and occurring in newborn infants. The germ is carried in the nose of a nurse or a visitor, or by someone suffering from impetigo. Also called *pemphigus neonatorum.*

**implantation.** The act of setting up or of grafting a tissue.

**impotence, impotency.** Lack of power, especially lack of sexual power.

**impregnate. 1.** To fertilize or make pregnant. **2.** To saturate.

**impregnation. 1.** The act of fertilization or making pregnant. **2.** The process of saturating.

**impulse.** A push or communicated force; a sudden mental urge to do an action.

**inactivation.** The process of rendering inactive. For example, a fluid containing bacteria, which has been sterilized by heat and the germs destroyed, is referred to as inactivated. Inactivation of the complement is the process of heating fresh serum to a temperature of 56°C. for 30 minutes to destroy its complement. See also COMPLEMENT.

**inanition.** Exhaustion as the result of starvation.

**inarticulate.** Without joints; disjointed. The term particularly applies to the utterance of vocal sounds which are not capable of being understood. It popularly means speechless or pronouncing indistinctly.

**in articulo mortis.** At the point of death.

**inassimilable.** Refers to substances which cannot be absorbed and used by the body as nutriment.

**inborn.** Congenital.

**incarcerated.** Imprisoned, wedged, confined, unable to escape. The term is often used to describe a hernia which cannot be replaced without resort to surgery.

**incest.** Sexual intercourse between close relatives, such as brother and sister—a criminal offense.

**incidence.** The amount or range of occurrence, as of a disease.

**age incidence.** The age at which a condition may occur.

**angle of incidence.** The angle at which a ray of light strikes a reflecting or refracting surface.

**incidence rate.** The number of cases of a disease appearing per unit of population within a defined time interval.

**line of incidence.** The path of a ray or projectile.

**point of incidence.** The point upon which a ray or projectile strikes a reflecting or refracting surface.

**sex incidence.** The incidence of a condition in each sex.

**incipient.** At the beginning, or about to develop.

**incised.** Cut surgically.

**incision.** A surgical cut or wound. Incisions are named according to their location, shape, direction, after the organ or structure in which they are made, and frequently after the surgeon who first used them.

**buttonhole incision.** A small straight cut made into an organ or cavity.

**crucial incision.** Two cuts made at right angles to ensure adequate drainage.

**exploratory incision.** An incision made for the purpose of diagnosis.

**muscle-splitting incision.** An incision in which the muscles are split in the direction of their fibers in order to secure a better line of closure after the operation.

**paramedian incision.** An incision made to one side of the midline of the body, organ, or structure, being operated on. There are several variations to this type of incision. For instance, one made on the right of the midline of the abdomen below the navel is called a lower right paramedian incision, while if it were made above the umbilicus it would be called an upper paramedian incision.

**rectus incision.** An incision made through a rectus muscle or through the rectus sheath of the abdomen.

**incisive. 1.** Cutting. **2.** Pertaining to the incisor teeth.

**incisor teeth.** The four front teeth of each jaw. See also TEETH.

**inclusion.** The state of being enclosed or included.

**inclusion body.** An object found within the body cells in virus diseases, sometimes representing the virus itself.

**incoherence.** The quality of being incoherent; absence of connection of ideas or of language.

**incoherent.** Not connected or coherent; incomprehensible.

**incompatibility.** The property of being incompatible.

**incompatible.** Usually refers to substances which are incapable of being used or put together because they interact adversely or have opposing qualities. Pharmacists have a very strict list of incompatibles which are never put together in the same medicine. See also COMPATIBLE.

**incompetence.** Insufficiency or inability to perform a function, as in a leaky heart valve. In legal medicine it refers to an incapacity or absence of legal fitness, such as the incompetence of a drunken man to drive a car legally or of an insane person to make a valid will.

**incompressible.** Not capable of being compressed.

**incongruence, incongruity.** 1. The absence of agreement. 2. Lack of harmony; not matching or corresponding; odd, peculiar, or bizarre.

**incontinence.** The inability to control the excretion of urine or feces.

**incoordination.** Inability to bring into harmonious movement or action, such as the inability to move muscles in their proper sequence. See also ATAXIA.

**incorporation.** The complete union of one substance with another.

**incrustation.** The formation of a crust.

**incubation.** The period between the entry of a germ into the body and the appearance of the disease it causes; the process by which microorganisms are cultured in a laboratory.

**incubator.** 1. An apparatus used for the cultivation of microorganisms, eggs, or other living tissues. 2. An apparatus used for rearing delicate or prematurely born infants, in which warmth, moisture, and oxygen content are controlled.

**incubus.** A nightmare.

**incurable.** Not capable of being cured; fatal.

**incus.** The central of the three tiny bones situated in the middle ear, which receives vibrations from the eardrum and transmits them to the organ of hearing where they are interpreted as sound. Also called *anvil.*

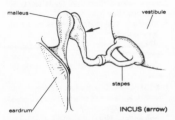

INCUS (arrow)

**index.** The formula expressing the ratio of one dimension of an object to another dimension.

**cardiac index.** The volume of blood which flows per minute per square meter of the body surface. The normal average is nearly four pints.

**cephalic index.** The ratio between the width of the skull multiplied by a hundred, and the skull's length.

**color index.** The ratio between the percentage of hemoglobin in the blood and the first two figures of the number of red blood cells per cubic millimeter; used to identify certain blood diseases.

**index finger.** The forefinger, that finger next to the thumb.

**Indian hemp.** See CANNABIS.

**Indian sickness.** Gangrene of the anus and rectum.

**indication.** A sign. Any symptom, cause, or occurrence in a disease which indicates its course of treatment.

**indigestion.** Any upset of the normal digestive processes resulting in symptoms of discomfort; lack of digestion; imperfect digestion. The symptoms may be pain, flatulence, or a feeling of distension. Temporary indigestion is often due to a dietary indiscretion and is best treated by temporary starvation to rest the stomach and medication. Any indigestion that lasts more than four days or constantly recurs in cycles requires medical attention to determine the cause. Constant taking of proprietary indigestion remedies merely allows the cause to get worse and makes it more difficult for the doctor to effect a cure. Indigestion may have nothing to do with the stomach but be caused by gallstones or chronic appendicitis, so that treatment to the stomach is illogical and useless.

**indole.** One of two chemicals (the second being skatole) which gives odor and color to the feces.

**indolent.** 1. Sluggish. 2. Referring to a painless ulcer that is slow to heal.

**induction.** 1. The act of inducing or causing to occur, such as inducing labor in a pregnant woman either because the birth is overdue or because the baby is becoming too large; see also LABOR. 2. The production of an electric current in a body from another body which is close by but not in contact. This principle is used to control some forms of heart disease, where the heart is not beating rhythmically or at a sufficient speed. An instrument is sewn inside the chest in contact with the heart and the wound closed; a second instrument is then attached to the chest wall to induce an electric current at regular intervals to the first instrument and so stimulate a heartbeat.

**indurated.** Hardened or solidified. The cause may be congestion with blood, inflammation, infiltration by growths, or fibrosis.

**black induration.** Fibrosis of the lung found in miners suffering anthracosis.

**brown induration.** Chronic passive congestion and fibrosis of the lung with pigmentation by an iron-containing blood pigment.

**grey induration.** The diffuse fibrosis of the lung found in chronic pneumonia.

**red induration.** A chronic fibrosis of the lung associated with a deposit of red oxide of iron and also seen in marked passive congestion of the lungs.

**infant.** 1. A child during its first year of life. 2. In law, a person under the age of 21 years.

**infant feeding.** *Baby's requirements.* A baby needs 2½ ounces of breast milk per day for every pound of body weight, thus a ten-pound baby requires approximately 25 ounces of milk per day. Artificial foods are made by reconstituting cow's milk powder with water and adding sugar. It is usual to start with half-cream powder and after some weeks, if the baby is able to take it, transferring gradually to full-cream powder. For convenience, the manufacturers print a table of amounts on each tin and in practice these prove to be approximately correct. *When to feed.* Small, weak, or premature babies may need feeding every three hours, but others can be fed every four hours from 6 a.m. to 10 p.m. Another method, called *demand feeding,* is to feed the baby when he appears to be crying for it, but more often than not he settles down to a schedule of every four hours. The disadvantage of the scheme is that the mother never knows what interval she has before the next demand. A normal baby should not require a routine *night feed* of either milk or water. *Types of bottle.* The *Soxhlet bottle* is a single-ended bottle, and though it is easier to store or stack in a sterilizer, the baby has to suck against a vacuum and this often results in air swallowing, "wind," and colic. The *boat-shaped bottle* is double-ended, one for a nipple and one for a rubber valve. If the valve is left off the baby gets the milk easier and there is less chance of air swallowing. *The nipple flow.* When the bottle is held nipple down, the milk should drip out at one drop per second. If it drips too slowly the nipple hole can be enlarged with a red-hot needle. If the milk emerges in a continuous stream, this is too fast and a fresh nipple should be used. *Sterilization of bottles.* Bottles and nipples, after a thorough cleansing, should be covered with water in a saucepan and boiled for ten minutes. They should then be left in the saucepan, with the lid on, to cool, and not touched until required for the next feed. *Vitamin supplements.* All artificially fed babies and probably most breast-fed ones need extra vitamins. These are obtained from halibut or cod liver oil (vitamins A and D) and fresh fruit juice (vitamin C). For babies who seem upset by the fruit juice, the vitamins can be obtained in glycerinated form. Vitamins should never be put in the bottle with the milk. *Test feeds and weight progress.* If baby is weighed before and after each feed in the day this will give the total daily intake. To determine what a baby should weigh it is necessary to know that a normal infant should gain one ounce per day for the first 100 days of its life, excluding the first ten days during which it loses and regains its birth weight. After that the rate is one pound per month up to the age of one year. The following are two examples of this method of calculation of what baby should weigh. (1) Birth weight 7 pounds. Age 40 days. Baby should have put on 40 ounces less ten ounces for the first ten days equals 30 ounces. Therefore baby should weigh 7 pounds (birth weight) plus 1 pound 14 ounces (progress) equals 8 pounds 14 ounces. (2) Birth weight 8 pounds. Age 7 months. For the first three months the baby should have gained 100 ounces less 10 ounces equals 90 ounces plus one pound per month for months 4, 5, 6 and 7, that is 4 pounds. This baby should have gained 5 pounds 10 ounces plus 4 pounds equals 9 pounds 10 ounces which plus its birth weight totals 17 pounds 10 ounces.

**infantile paralysis.** See POLIOMYELITIS.

**infantilism.** The persistence of childlike characteristics into adult life. Organs which fail to mature and produce an adult function are also described as infantile.

**intestinal infantilism.** See CELIAC DISEASE.

**renal infantilism.** The underdeveloped state which arises in a child suffering with chronic nephritis.

**uterine infantilism.** A condition in which the womb has not developed properly into the adult stage; one of the causes of primary sterility in the female.

**infarct.** A wedge-shaped area of tissue that has died due to the cutting off of its blood supply. Infarcts occur because some parts of the body are supplied by arteries which come to an end point; these areas have no collateral circulation, being entirely dependent on the end artery for their blood supply. Therefore, if the end artery becomes blocked the wedge-shaped portion of tissue which it supplies dies. Infarction can occur in the heart, kidneys, lungs, spleen, and other tissues. It is met with in coronary thrombosis, which produces an infarct in the heart muscle. If the infarct is small the body can replace it with fibrous tissue and

the patient recovers, but if it is a large one it produces a catastrophe which results in death.

**infarction.** The development of an infarct.

**infection.** Invasion of the body by pathogenic microorganisms capable of causing disease; the reaction of the tissues to their presence and the poisons produced by them.

**airborne infection.** Infection transmitted through the air on dust and moisture particles.

**contact infection.** Infections transmitted by direct contact with another person.

**cross infection.** Infection transmitted between patients with different types of germs; a great problem in hospitals.

**direct infection.** See CONTACT INFECTION, above.

**droplet infection.** Infection by droplets of moisture expelled into the air by talking, coughing, and sneezing, and which for a period remain suspended in the atmosphere.

**endogenous infection.** Infection caused by microorganisms which are normally present in the body. For instance, if the coliform bacillus, which normally inhabits the intestine, migrates to the urinary bladder it causes cystitis.

**exogenous infection.** Infection caused by germs which are not normal inhabitants of the body.

**focal infection.** Infection in which germs exist in certain localized areas from where they are distributed into the bloodstream. Common sites, or foci, include bad teeth, tonsils, and nasal passages.

**latent infection.** A condition in which germs, after they have ceased to multiply, remain alive in isolated parts of the body.

**mixed infection.** Infection caused by more than one type of germ.

**pyogenic infection.** Infection by pus-producing germs.

**secondary infection.** Infection following an infection by a different type of germ.

**silent or subclinical infection.** An infection which produces no signs.

**infectious.** Caused by germs.

**infective.** Infectious. Used adjectively to indicate that the causative factor in certain illnesses is a germ process.

**infective endocarditis.** A malignant inflammatory process of the lining of the heart.

**infective mononucleosis.** See GLANDULAR FEVER.

**inferolateral.** Situated below and to one side.

**inferomedian.** Situated below and in the midline.

**inferoposterior.** Situated below and to the rear.

**infested.** The state of having arthropod parasites in or on the body which includes, insects, mites, and ticks.

**inflammation.** A reaction of the tissues to injury; characterized by local heat, swelling, redness, and pain. The causes are innumerable.

**influenza.** An acute infectious virus disease which occurs in epidemic form throughout the world in various guises and in varying severity. Sometimes it occurs as a respiratory disease, with high temperature, shivering, and severe pains of the limbs; at other times it affects the gastrointestinal tract, causing high temperature, shivering, vomiting, and diarrhea. There is no specific treatment, and though antibiotics have no effect on the causative organism, some doctors use them to prevent secondary invading germs getting a grip while the patient's resistance is temporarily lowered by the influenza. It is definitely not a disease which responds to fortitude and perseverance, shrugging off the attack as if it were of no consequence, and continuing to work, for with virus infections there is a great risk of sudden collapse if the patient is active while suffering with the disease. Treatment of the mild attack, therefore, is to rest in bed, which is imperative, and to take every four hours three aspirin tablets with copious drinks. The patient should stay in bed until the temperature has been normal or below normal for at least 24 hours, preferably 48 hours. The influenza vaccines do appear to protect many people and they are given by one or at most two injections, around October or November. The vaccine is only effective for one year and has to be repeated.

**influenzal.** Relating to influenza.

**infra-axillary.** Below the armpit.

**infraclavicular.** Below the collarbone.

**infracostal.** Below the ribs.

**infradiaphragmatic.** Below the diaphragm, the muscular wall dividing the chest and abdomen.

**inframammary.** Below the mammary gland.

**inframandibular.** Below the mandible.

**inframaxillary.** Below the maxilla.

**infraorbital.** Below the eye socket.

**infrapatellar.** Below the patella.

**infrapubic.** Below the pubis.

**infrared.** The heat waves found at one end of the spectrum.

**infrascapular.** Below the scapula.

**infraspinous.** Below any spine, whether of the scapula or a vertebra.

**infrasternal.** Below the sternum.

**infratemporal.** Below the temporal bone, the bone forming the temple part of the skull.

**infratonsillar.** Below the tonsil.

**infraturbinal.** One of the bones which jut out into the nasal space.

**infundibulum.** Any funnel-shaped passage or part, such as the stalk of the pituitary gland or the wide funnel-shaped region of the Fallopian tube at its fringed end.

**infusion.** An extract made by using boiling water on some plant substance, tea for instance.

**inguinal.** Relating to the groin. See also HERNIA.

**inhalation.** The breathing of medicated vapors into the nose or lungs. Various substances can be used for this purpose and are prepared by adding to a quart jug half full of boiling water a teaspoonful of friar's balsam or vapor menthol and eucalyptus compound. The patient places a towel over his head, holds his face close to the jug, closes his eyes to prevent the vapor causing a stream of tears, and inhales the steam deeply either by the nose or mouth, depending on the condition being treated.

**inheritance.** The acquisition of characteristics transmitted from the parents to their children. See also CHROMOSOME, MENDELISM.

**dominant inheritance.** An inherited trait which appears in a hybrid (an organism having one dominant and one recessive gene) and in which only the dominant gene expresses itself and the recessive gene is suppressed—such as brown eyes dominant over blue eyes. The dominant trait will also appear in an individual which is pure (two dominant genes) for the characteristic involved.

**recessive inheritance.** An inherited trait which appears only when the individual has only the genes for the characteristic involved. Thus, in the case of blue eyes, the individual must be carrying two genes for blue eyes.

**sex-linked inheritance.** An inherited characteristic carried by the X-chromosomes.

**inhibit.** To stop or repress.

**inhibition.** The act of stopping or repressing; a restraint.

**inhibitor.** Something which stops or represses.

**injected.** Introduced into the body by means of an injection; congested.

**injection.** The introduction of a liquid into a tissue, cavity, or blood vessel by means of a hypodermic syringe and needle; the liquid so injected.

**innervation.** The nerve supply of a part; the conduction of nervous energy.

**innocent.** Not harmful. Medically used to describe something harmless or benign as opposed to malignant, which may imply cancerous.

**innominate.** Without a name. This term arose in medical language because when the anatomy of the body was first described, by some mischance certain parts were unnamed.

**innominate artery.** The largest branch of the arch of the aorta. Also called *brachiocephalic artery.*

**innominate bone.** The bone forming the front wall and sides of the pelvic cavity.

**innominate veins.** The two brachiocephalic veins which join to form the superior vena cava.

**inoculation.** The introduction into the body of a germ, germ poison, or serum to set up the production of antibodies, which will subsequently protect the individual from an attack of the disease. Also called *preventive inoculation.* See also IMMUNIZATION; VACCINATION.

**inoperable.** Any condition which cannot or should not be operated upon. It commonly refers to a cancerous condition which has spread far beyond the original site, making it pointless to operate on the original growth because of growth deposits in all the surrounding organs.

**inquest.** An enquiry held by a coroner into the cause of violent or sudden death. In the case of sudden death, a doctor cannot issue a death certificate unless he has been treating the patient for a period prior to death, and death was to be expected as the natural sequence of the disease process for which the doctor was giving treatment.

**insanity.** Temporary or permanent derangement of one or more psychical functions.

**insemination.** The deposit of seminal fluid within the vagina. See also A.I.; A.I.D.; A.I.H.

**insenescence.** The process of growing old.

**insertion.** 1. The act of implanting. 2. The point at which a muscle is attached to the bone it moves.

**insidious.** The stealthy and unseen progress of an illness or disorder.

**in situ.** In a given or natural position; undisturbed.

**insomnia.** Sleeplessness. Apart from pain or discomfort, insomnia may be produced by nervous excitement preventing the normal relaxation which enables sleep to develop, or by extensive daytime catnapping. The taking of purgatives at bedtime provokes wakefulness, and so do stimulating drinks such as coffee. Drinks like cocoa may dilate the kidneys, and the resulting urge to urinate will wake the patient; this also applies to a large intake of beer during the evening. In many cases of temporary insomnia sleeping pills are not required because much of the distress is more due to a feeling of self-pity than to the insomnia, and a hot drink or toddy at bedtime and a warm bed are all that is necessary to induce sleep. Insomnia may, however, be a significant symptom of a threatened nervous breakdown.

**inspiration.** 1. Breathing in. 2. A bright thought or idea.

**inspiratory.** Pertaining to inspiration.

**inspissated.** Rendered dry, thick, or less fluid by inspissation.

**inspissation.** The process of rendering dry by evaporation or absorption of the liquid contents of a substance. For example, inspissated pus is the dried solid part of the pus after the liquid has been withdrawn.

**instep.** The arched part of the upper side of the human foot.

**instinct.** The faculty of performing for the most part useful or beneficial acts without reason and without previous experience.

**instinctive.** Prompted by instinct.

**insufflation.** The blowing of a powder or a liquid into a cavity.

**insufflator.** An instrument used for insufflation.

**insulin.** A hormone manufactured in the pancreas by little areas of tissue called the islands of Langerhans, and then secreted into the blood where it controls the digestion of carbohydrates. A deficiency of insulin produces diabetes mellitus, popularly called sugar diabetes. There are a number of insulin preparations, two of which are protamine zinc insulin and globulin zinc insulin. Both have a very slow rate of absorption after injection, exerting their effect for 24 hours so that the patient needs only one injection a day. See also DIABETES.

**insulin reaction or shock.** A condition due to an excess of insulin in the blood. It may occur spontaneously, but is mostly due to overdosage of insulin. See also COMA; HYPOGLYCEMIA.

**insusceptibility.** Immunity.

**integument.** A covering. The term most often refers to the common integument, the skin.

**integumentary.** Pertaining to the skin.

**integumentum commune.** The skin or common integument.

**intelligence.** The faculty or ability for comprehending, and reasoning with facts and propositions. See also I.Q.

**interalveolar.** Between alveoli, small cavities, or cells.

**interarticular.** Situated between joints or joint surfaces.

**interatrial.** Between the atria.

**interauricular.** Between the auricles (upper chambers of the heart). These chambers are more correctly known as atria.

**intercarpal.** Between the carpal bones, the small bones of the hand.

**intercellular.** Between cells.

**interchondral.** Between cartilages.

**interclavicular.** Between the clavicles, the collarbones.

**intercondylar.** Between condyles, the rounded prominences or knuckles on the end of some bones that usually form part of a joint.

**intercostal.** Between the ribs.

**intercostohumeral.** Between the arm and the ribs.

**intercranial.** Relating to the inner part of the skull.

**intercrural.** Between the legs.

**intercurrent.** Intervening within time, or between events.

**intercurrent disease.** An illness occurring in a patient already suffering from another disease. For instance, if a patient suffering from chronic heart disease then contracts pneumonia, the pneumonia is the intercurrent disease.

**interdental.** Between the teeth.

**interdiction.** A legal process by which the control of the affairs of an insane person is placed in the hands of a relative or some other person.

**interdigital.** Between the fingers or toes.

**interfemoral.** Between the thighs.

**interference.** The phenomenon by which two waves of light or sound meet and cancel each other out.

**intergluteal.** Situated between the buttocks, which are composed of the gluteal muscles.

**interlobar.** Situated between two lobes, the lobes of the lungs, for example.

**interlobar abscess.** An abscess occurring between two lobes of the lungs.

**interlocking of twins.** A complication of labor in which twins become fixed one to the other, such as chin under chin, preventing natural birth and necessitating delivery by cesarean section.

**intermammary.** Between the breasts or the mammary glands.

**intermenstrual.** Occurring between menstrual periods.

**intermenstruum.** The interval between two consecutive menstrual periods.

**intermittent fever.** See MALARIA.

**interosseous.** Situated between two bones.

**interosseous muscles.** The small muscles between the main bones of the hands and feet.

**interpalpebral.** Between the eyelids.

**interpolation.** Surgical transfer of tissue to a new situation.

**interscapular.** Between the shoulder blades or the scapulae.

**interspinal.** Between two vertebral spines.

**interstices.** Small spaces within a structure, something like lattice work.

**interstitial.** Situated between two important parts; occupying the interspaces or interstices of a part; or pertaining to the finest connective tissue of an organ.

**interstitial keratitis.** Inflammation of the layers composing the cornea.

**interstitial pregnancy.** See PREGNANCY: ECTOPIC PREGNANCY.

**intertriginous.** Relating to intertrigo.

**intertrigo.** A form of moist eczema which occurs where two folds of skin touch each other. It is due to the skin being constantly moist with perspiration, which causes it to break down and become inflamed. The commonest sites for intertrigo are beneath a pendulous breast or in a groin, or armpit.

**interventricular.** Between two ventricles, particularly the cardiac ventricles, the two lower chambers of the heart. The term also refers to the ventricles in the brain, the spaces containing cerebrospinal fluid.

**intervertebral.** Between two vertebrae.

**intervertebral disc.** The disc of cartilage located between the spinal vertebrae and which acts as a form of shock absorber. If this disc ruptures or presses on one of the spinal nerves, which emerge in pairs between the vertebrae, it causes pain along the distribution of that nerve, giving rise to the characteristic symptoms and signs of the condition commonly called disc trouble. Also called *slipped disc.*

**intestinal.** Relating to the intestine.

**intestinal infantilism.** See CELIAC DISEASE.

**intestinal juice.** A secretion from glands in the duodenal wall containing digestive enzymes that complete digestion started in the mouth and stomach.

**intestine.** The general name for that part of the digestive tract extending from the lower end of the stomach to the anus, and which, in the average adult male, is approximately 28 feet long. The first part, called the small intestine because it has a smaller diameter than the large intestine, is about 23 feet long with a diameter of about 1½ inches. It starts at the outlet of the stomach and comprises the duodenum, jejunum, and ileum, which joins with the beginning of the large intestine at the cecum. The second part, the large intestine, is about 5 feet long with a diameter of about 3 inches and comprises the cecum and appendix, ascending colon, transverse colon,

descending colon, pelvic colon, and rectum. The small intestine is concerned in the digestion of food and its absorption into the body, and the large intestine with the absorption of water from the waste products of digestion and their excretion.

**intima.** The tunica intima, the innermost of the three coats forming the wall of a blood vessel.

**intimal.** Relating to the intima.

**intra-abdominal.** Within the abdominal cavity.

**intra-arterial.** Within an artery.

**intra-articular.** Within a joint.

**intra-atrial.** Within an atrium (one of the two upper chambers of the heart).

**intra-aural.** Within the ear.

**intra-auricular.** Within an auricle, one of the two upper chambers of the heart. These chambers are more correctly called atria.

**intrabuccal.** Within the cheek or mouth.

**intracapsular.** Within a capsule, but usually referring to the capsular ligament of a joint.

**intracardiac.** Within the heart.

**intracellular.** Within a cell.

**intracranial.** Within the skull.

**intradermal.** Within the dermal layer of the skin.

**intradural.** Within the dura mater, the outermost of the three membranes covering the brain and spinal cord.

**intragastric.** Within the stomach.

**intraglandular.** Within a gland.

**intrahepatic.** Within the liver.

**intra-intestinal.** Within the gut.

**intramammary.** Within the breast, the mammary gland.

**intramedullary.** Within the medullary region of the brain, or within the marrow cavity of a bone.

**intramembranous.** Within a membrane.

**intramural.** Within the walls of an organ.

**intramuscular.** Within a muscle.

**intranasal.** Within the nose.

**intraneural.** Within a nerve.

**intraocular.** Within the eye.

**intra-oral.** Within the mouth.

**intra-orbital.** Within the eye socket.

**intra-osteal.** Within a bone.

**intra partum.** During birth or delivery.

**intrapelvic.** Within the pelvis.

**intrapericardial.** Within the pericardium, the sac surrounding the heart.

**intraperitoneal.** Within the peritoneal cavity of the abdomen. Since the whole abdomen is lined with peritoneum, the term literally means intra-abdominal.

**intrapleural.** Within the pleural cavity of the chest. The pleural membrane lines the chest wall and covers the lungs, and the pleural cavity is the space between the two layers of membrane.

**intrathoracic.** Within the chest cavity.

**intratracheal.** Within the trachea, the main air passage from throat to lungs.

**intratympanic.** Within the tympanic cavity, the cavity of the middle ear situated between the eardrum on the outside and the organ of hearing on the inside and into which opens the Eustachian tube running from the back of the nose.

**intra-urethral.** Within the urethra, the tube which carries urine from the urinary bladder to the outside.

**intra-uterine.** Within the uterus.

**intravaginal.** Within the vagina.

**intravascular.** Within a blood vessel.

**intravenous.** Within a vein, such as intravenous injection, the injection of a fluid into a vein.

**intraventricular.** Within a ventricle, one of the two lower chambers of the heart. The term may also refer to the ventricles of the brain, the spaces containing cerebrospinal fluid.

**intravesical.** Within the urinary bladder.

**intravitreous.** Within the vitreous, the substance which fills the globe of the eyeball.

**intrinsic.** 1. Situated within. 2. The inherent characteristics of an object occurring within itself.

**intrinsic factor.** A substance normally contained in gastric juice and absent in pernicious anemia. Also called *Castle's factor.*

**introitus.** Any entrance or inlet; usually refers to the vaginal opening.

**introversion.** 1. A turning inward of an organ. 2. The introspective attitude of mind in which the individual is primarily concerned with himself rather than with other people and the outside world.

**introvert.** An introspective person.

**intubation.** The passing of a tube into a part, especially the introduction of a tube into an opening made into the trachea at the front of the neck to relieve obstructed breathing in certain conditions.

**intumescence.** A swelling or the process of swelling.

**intussusception.** A condition in which a piece of the intestine becomes ensheathed within an adjacent piece in a manner similar to the tuck some housewives put above the elbow of a shirt sleeve to shorten it. The normal muscular movement of the intestine then attempts, ineffectually, to propel the ensheathed portion as though it were part of the intestine's normal contents; this causes intestinal obstruction. Intussusception is seen most commonly among children, usually males about nine to twelve months

old. There is sometimes a history of intestinal disturbance, either constipation or diarrhea, but usually the patient is a healthy infant who is suddenly seized with acute attacks of colicky abdominal pain. The pain passes off, leaving the child white and listless, only to return a few minutes or even, sometimes, hours later. There is frequently vomiting, sometimes the child has its bowels open, and at first the stool appears normal but later consists of only blood and mucus. The pain gradually becomes increasingly frequent and more and more blood and mucus are passed. If unrelieved, the abdomen distends and the child sinks into a state of collapse. Although some cases have recovered spontaneously, the patient is nearly always admitted to a hospital for treatment. Efforts have been made to treat intussusception by such bloodless methods as abdominal manipulation, and injection of air and fluids into the bowel, and some success has been claimed for enemas which have pushed the trapped piece of intestine out of the gut. The only certain way to reduce an intussusception, however, is a simple operation in which the surgeon gently milks the two pieces of intestine apart without cutting it. Delay in treatment may result in the trapped portion becoming gangrenous and this involves a more serious operation to remove the gangrenous part and to rejoin the cut ends.

**intussusceptum.** The piece of intestine which receives the intussuscipiens and which together form an intussusception.

**intussuscipiens.** The piece of intestine which enters the intussusceptum to form an intussusception.

**inunction.** The rubbing of ointment into the skin.

**inundation fever.** A disease of the typhus group transmitted to man by the bite of a mite carried by field mice and rats. It is characterized by a high temperature of two or three weeks' duration, a primary sore, inflamed glands, a skin rash, with deafness and symptoms of lung congestion. Also called *Japanese river fever, Kedani fever, scrub typhus, rural typhus, tropical typhus, pseudotyphoid of Delhi, Sumatra mite fever, Tsutsugamushi disease.*

**in utero.** Within the uterus or womb.

**invaginated.** The process of becoming ensheathed; the state of burrowing or infolding to form a hollow space within a solid structure. Typical examples are invagination of the lining membrane of the nose into the skull bone in order to form a nasal sinus, and the invagination by one piece of intestine into another.

**inversion.** 1. A turning inward; upside down. 2. Reversal of a normal relationship.

**sexual inversion.** Homosexuality.

**visceral inversion.** A condition in which an organ is on the opposite side to normal. See also TRANSPOSITION.

**invert.** A homosexual.

**invertase.** An enzyme which catalyzes sucrose to glucose and levulose. Also called *sucrase.*

**invertebrate.** An animal without a backbone.

**in vitro.** Refers to actions taking place in test tubes as opposed to those which take place in the body (in vivo). In many cases, in vitro tests prove successful but when applied to the body the same result is not obtained.

**in vivo.** Occurring within the body. See also IN VITRO.

**involuntary.** Something which occurs independently of the will.

**involuntary muscles.** Those muscles not under the control of the conscious will and which act without the individual making any conscious effort. They include those in the heart, intestines, and the bladder.

**involution.** 1. A turning inwards. 2. The return of the womb to normal size and shape following childbirth or its regression after the change of life.

**involution melancholia.** A profound depression that occurs in people of advanced age due to a form of fibrosis of the brain, popularly called, "softening of the brain."

**iodine.** A nonmetallic element with a metallic luster and a peculiar smell; the iodine normally used for antiseptic purposes is a 2 percent solution in alcohol. It is important that iodine solution should be stored in glass-stoppered bottles and the stopper must always be reinserted after use, for if it is not the alcohol will evaporate until the solution is 40 percent strong, when it is known as pigment of iodine, and if applied to the skin it will cause a burn. Iodine has been used as an ointment or as a tincture for the treatment of fungus infections, and because of its liquefying action on thick sputum is included in cough mixtures to "cut the phlegm." Iodine is also a normal constituent of the thyroid gland and essential for its proper functioning. In areas where iodine is lacking in the diet this deficiency results in the production of goiters and cretinism and in some countries, Switzerland, for example, ordinary table salt must contain iodine by law to prevent this occurring. So-called colorless iodine consists of potassium iodide with little free iodine present and has little or no antiseptic action. It is useless for treating wounds. See also GOITER; CRETINISM.

**ipsilateral.** Situated on the same side.

**I.Q.** The abbreviation for intelligence quotient. It is calculated by using a series of intelligence tests and dividing the person's test-determined mental age by his chronological age and multiplying by 100. See also INTELLIGENCE.

**iridectomy.** Surgical removal of part of the iris, the colored part of the eye.

**iridochoroiditis.** Inflammation of the iris of the eye and the choroid, the middle membrane of the eye.

**iridocyclitis.** Inflammation of the iris and the ciliary body of the eye.

**iridotomy.** Surgical cutting of the iris of the eye without removing any part.

**iris.** The colored circular portion surrounding the black pupil of the eye. It separates the front and back chambers of the eyeball and rests against the front of the crystalline lens, and its color is determined by the presence of pigment bodies known as melanophores. The iris contains two sets of muscles; one set circularly arranged to contract the pupil and the other set arranged radially to dilate it. Normally the pupil opens or closes in proportion to the strength of light present, dilating at twilight and contracting in bright sunlight. Cerebral irritation causes the pupil to contract, and morphine and other narcotics contract it to pinpoint size. Paralyzing damage to the brain causes the pupil to dilate and so do belladonna and allied drugs, as do anesthetics and fear. At death the iris is widely dilated.

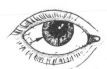

IRIS (arrow)

**iritis.** Inflammation of the iris of the eye.

**irradiation.** The passage of x-rays, gamma rays, ultraviolet rays, or infrared rays through patients for treatment or diagnosis.

**irreducible. 1.** Not capable of being restored to a normal position. **2.** A hernia which cannot be returned within the abdomen and becomes a fixed, painful swelling that may produce the signs of intestinal obstruction which can only be relieved by surgery.

**irritability. 1.** The attribute of living organisms to become aroused to distinctive action following a certain stimulus. **2.** The state of being excessively responsive to slight stimuli; overly sensitive.

**ischaemia.** See ISCHEMIA.

**ischaemic.** See ISCHEMIC.

**ischemia.** Without blood.

**ischemic.** Relating to ischemia.

**ischemic heart disease.** Coronary thrombosis or severe angina.

**ischial.** Relating to the ischium.

**ischiorectal abscess.** An abscess situated near the opening of the anus. Also called *anorectal abscess, marginal abscess, perirectal abscess*.

**ischium.** The lower part of the innominate bone of the pelvis, upon which the body rests when in a sitting position.

**isoagglutination.** The clotting of blood caused by the action of the blood serum of one animal upon the red cells of another animal of the same species, and the basis of all tests performed to check a specimen of blood before it can be transfused to a patient.

**isoagglutinin.** The substance in the blood serum which causes isoagglutination.

**isomer.** One of two substances, both of which have the same percentage composition but which differ from each other in atomic arrangement of the molecule. Thus both substances have different physical and chemical properties, but are broadly speaking the same; for example red and yellow phosphorous.

**isomeric.** Having the qualities of an isomer.

**isomerism.** The quality of being isomeric.

**isometric.** Having similar dimensions.

**isometropia.** The same kind and degree of refraction in both eyes.

**isophoria.** The condition in which both eyes lie in the same horizontal plane.

**isothermal.** Of equal temperature.

**isotonia, isotonic.** Of equal tone.

**isotonic solution.** A solution which has the same concentration as that of another solution with which it is being compared.

**isotope.** A chemical element with the same atomic number as another but a different atomic weight. Many common elements consist of several isotopes, the apparent atomic weight of the element actually representing the average weight of all the isotopes.

**radioactive isotopes.** Elements which have been rendered radioactive by being placed in an atomic pile. Chemicals known to migrate specifically to certain parts of the body can be used as tracers which can be followed by a Geiger counter for investigating bodily processes; or they can be used for the effect their radioactive rays exert on the part to which they migrate. For instance, because iodine in the body goes direct to the thyroid gland, radioactive iodine is employed to treat overactivity of that gland. Also called *tracer elements*. See also TRACER.

**itch.** Scabies.

**itching.** Pruritus.

**Jacksonian epilepsy.** A form of epilepsy in which the convulsions are confined to certain muscles; due to specific diseased areas of the brain. See also EPILEPSY.

**jactitation.** Severe restlessness that at times appears in gravely ill patients.

**jaundice.** A condition in which the body is discolored yellow by the presence of bile salts and pigments in the blood. Jaundice may be caused by a disease of the liver with obstruction of the bile ducts, by changes in the blood, or by the swallowing of poisonous substances such as arsenic. There are many types, and only those most common are given below. See ICTERUS.

**acholuric jaundice.** A chronic type of jaundice which is more or less mild and either persistent or intermittent. It is accompanied by anemia, enlargement of the spleen, and an increased tendency for the red blood cells to be destroyed. Abnormal amounts of bile pigments are not found in the urine. It may be an inherited condition, or it may be acquired. Sometimes it is cured by removal of the spleen.

**black jaundice.** A fatal disease of newborn infants characterized by hemorrhaging, jaundice, and bloody urine. Also called *Winckel's disease.*

**catarrhal jaundice.** An acute disease characterized by jaundice coming on a few days after what appears to be a gastrointestinal upset, and accompanied by loss of appetite, diarrhea, and sometimes a raised temperature. The urine is colored an orange-yellow by the presence of bile pigments, and the absence of bile pigments in the feces leaves them a light yellow color. It sometimes occurs in epidemic form and is caused by a bacterium or a virus which produces inflammation and blockage of the bile ducts in the liver. It is the commonest type of jaundice.

**hemolytic jaundice.** A jaundice due to the excessive destruction of red blood cells. When it occurs in a newborn baby it is frequently due to incompatibility of the mother's and baby's blood, known as the Rhesus factor, and is treated by the total replacement of the baby's blood. Also called *icterus gravis neonatorum.* See also KERNICTERUS; RHESUS FACTOR.

**homologous serum jaundice.** Jaundice associated with inflammation of the liver. It is thought to be transmitted by injecting a patient with a syringe and needle previously used on a patient who carried the causative factor of this type of jaundice. This factor is resistant to boiling, the ordinary means of syringe sterilization, but is destroyed by high-pressure steam sterilization.

**obstructive jaundice.** A form of jaundice due to mechanical obstruction of the bile ducts by gallstones, a growth, or by narrowing of the ducts.

**physiological jaundice.** The mild yellowing that occurs at birth in the baby and passes off in a few days. Also called *icterus neonatorum.*

**jaws.** The bones bearing the teeth. The upper jaw consists of two bones called maxillae, and each maxilla forms half of the roof of the mouth, part of the wall of the nose, and part of the eye socket. The lower jaw also consists of two halves, which unite at the chin in infancy to form a single bone called the mandible.

**jejunal.** Pertaining to the jejunum.

**jejunectomy.** Surgical removal of all or a portion of the jejunum.

**jejunitis.** Inflammation of the jejunum.

**jejunocolostomy.** A surgical operation by which the jejunum is joined to the colon.

**jejunoileitis.** Inflammation of both jejunum and ileum.

**jejunoileostomy.** A surgical operation in which the jejunum is joined to the ileum and a part of the intestine between them removed.

**jejunojejunostomy.** An operation in which a portion of the jejunum is removed and the cut ends rejoined.

**jejunostomy.** An operation in which a loop of jejunum is brought to the surface and opened so that the intestinal contents emerge through the abdominal wall.

**jejunotomy.** Surgical opening of the jejunum, usually to remove a foreign body such as a small toy swallowed by a child.

**jejunum.** The portion of the small intestine between the duodenum and the ileum.

**jerk.** A sudden involuntary movement of a muscle. See ANKLE; KNEE.

**joint.** The place of union between two or more bones of the body and functioning to promote motion and flexibility.

**jugular.** Pertaining to the neck or throat.

**jugular veins.** Veins carrying blood from the head and neck to the heart. If such veins are severed, rapid loss of blood ensues. First aid consists of a compress with pressure. In no case should a tourniquet be applied.

**juice.** 1. Fluid of plant and animal tissues. 2. A digestive secretion; see also GASTRIC JUICE, INTESTINAL JUICE, PANCREATIC JUICE.

# K-L

**Kahn's test.** A blood test for syphilis.

**kakorrhaphiophobia.** Fear of failure.

**kala-azar.** A disease of tropical and subtropical countries caused by the protozoan *Leishmania donovani,* and transmitted by sandflies. The incubation period is from one to four months, but cases have occurred as long as two years after exposure. It is associated with enlargement of the spleen and liver, great wasting of the body, and irregular fever of long duration. Also called *black disease, black fever, dumdum.*

**kaolin.** Aluminium silicate or china clay. A purified form is used as a coating for pills and is incorporated in ointments, lotions, and poultices. It is also given internally for disorders of the intestinal tract, such as enteritis, dysentery, and diarrhea, because it combines with germ poisons and traps them.

**Kedani fever.** See INUNDATION FEVER.

**Kelly-Paterson syndrome.** See PLUMMER-VINSON SYNDROME.

**keloid.** The excessive formation of scar tissue in a wound, producing a raised, hard, growthlike structure. It can be treated by plastic surgery. Though there is a possibility of it recurring in the operation scar, the risk is well worth taking if an ugly keloid is producing cosmetic anxiety. Also spelled *cheloid.*

**Kenny method.** A method of treating poliomyelitis, named after the Australian nursing sister who introduced it. The method consists of wrapping the patient's back and limbs in woolen cloths wrung out in hot water. As soon as the limb pains cease, passive exercise is given and the patient is taught to exercise his muscles without assistance.

**kenophobia.** Fear of large empty spaces.

**keratalgia.** Pain in the cornea of the eye.

**keratectasia.** Protrusion of the cornea.

**keratectomy.** Surgical removal of part of the cornea of the eye. Also called *kerectomy.*

**keratiasis.** The occurrence of multiple warts on the skin.

**keratin.** The protein substance which forms horny tissues, hair, and nails.

**keratinization.** The process of converting into keratin or of becoming horny.

**keratinous.** Relating to keratin.

**keratitic.** Pertaining to keratitis.

**keratitis.** Inflammation of the cornea of the eye. There are many types.

**keratocentesis.** Puncture of the cornea of the eye.

**keratoconjunctivitis.** Inflammation of both the cornea and the conjuctival membrane of the eye.

**keratoderma.** A horny skin.

**keratodermatosis.** Any skin disease characterized by thickening.

**keratodermia.** A thickening of the skin. Also called *hyperkeratosis.*

**keratogenesis.** The development of horny growths.

**keratogenous.** Pertaining to the formation of horny growths.

**keratoid.** Hornlike.

**kerato-iritis.** Inflammation of both the cornea and the iris of the eye.

**keratoleukoma.** A white opacity in the cornea of the eye.

**keratoma.** A callosity; a horny tumor.

**keratomalacia.** Softening of the cornea of the eye due to a deficiency of vitamin A in the diet.

**keratoplasty.** Surgical repair of the cornea of the eye.

**keratosis.** Any skin disease characterized by overgrowth of the horny skin, or any condition of a lining membrane characterized by cornification.

**keratosis arsenical.** A patchy thickening of the skin occurring after long-continued ingestion of arsenic.

**keratosis blennorrhagica.** A disease characterized by horny outgrowths, chiefly of the hands and feet, and occurring during the course of gonorrhea.

**keratosis follicularis.** A rare hereditary disease characterized by horny projections occurring in and about the hair follicles. They are firmly adherent and produce a rough texture to the skin. Also called *Darier's disease.*

**keratosis nigricans.** A generalized pigmentation of the skin, accompanied by wartlike growths, usually associated with malignant disease of the internal organs.

**keratosis palmaris et plantaris.** A marked congenital thickening of the palms of the hand and soles of the feet.

**keratosis pharyngeus.** A rare disorder in which there is a hornlike outgrowth from the crypts of the tonsils in the back of the throat.

**keratosis pilaris.** A chronic skin disease marked by hard, conical elevations around the hair follicles usually of the arms and thighs.

**keratosis seborrheica.** Flat areas of skin with greasy scales which thicken up.

**keratosis senilis.** A skin disease appearing in old people and characterized by brownish warty growths, occurring chiefly on the face, backs of the hands and feet, and surfaces exposed to the wind and sun.

**keratotomy.** The surgical incision of the cornea of the eye.

**kerectomy.** Surgical removal of part of the cornea of the eye. Also called *keratectomy.*

**kernicterus.** Jaundice of the brain, occurring in babies suffering from hemolytic neonatal jaundice. It is the most severe and gravest form of jaundice in childhood because it causes degeneration of parts of the brain. See also JAUNDICE: HEMOLYTIC JAUNDICE.

**Kernig's sign.** A test performed in the diagnosis of meningitis and irritation of the meninges. If, with the thigh flexed upon the abdomen, pain is produced by extending the lower leg, or if there is marked resistance, the sign is positive.

**ketogenesis.** The production of ketone or acetone bodies.

**ketogenic.** Pertaining to ketogenesis.

**ketone.** An organic chemical compound containing the carbonyl group, CO.

**ketone bodies.** Substances formed by the liver when the digestion of fats is disturbed, such as occurs in diabetes.

**ketonuria.** The presence of ketone bodies in the urine.

**ketosis.** The condition in which ketone bodies are present in the blood, as occurs in states of acidosis.

**ketosteroids.** Steroids, a group of compounds which chemically resemble cholesterol, in which ketone groups are attached to carbon atoms. When the ketone is in the No. 17 position of the nucleus it is known as a 17-ketosteroid. These substances are normally present in the urine, 10-25 milligrams being excreted in the urine in 24 hours by a male and 4-15 milligrams by a female. Below average values occur in hypopituitarism, Addison's disease, and hypogonadism, and the value may be doubled in Cushing's disease and adrenal tumors. Testosterone and other androgens, which have male sex hormone characteristics, are 17-ketosteroids.

**kidney.** Either of the two bean-shaped glandular organs whose function is to extract from the blood certain waste products and water, which is passed to the bladder as urine by means of a tube called the ureter. They also salvage substances from the urine and return them to the body. Each kidney is about four inches long, two inches wide and one inch thick, and weighs from four to six ounces. Embedded in fat, the kidneys are situated on the back wall of the abdomen, one on each side of the spinal column, in the lumbar region. They are not, however, on exactly the same level, the one on the right being a little lower owing to the presence of the liver. The kidneys are essential to life, but should one become diseased or injured, the other is capable of enlarging to twice its size and performing the function of both, and one can survive on one-third of one kidney.

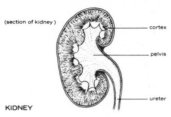

(section of kidney)

— cortex

— pelvis

— ureter

KIDNEY

**amyloid kidney.** The state of amyloid or waxy degeneration of the kidney seen in amyloid degeneration. Also called *lardaceous kidney, waxy kidney.*

**artificial kidney.** An apparatus through which the patient's blood is circulated outside the body in order to remove its poisonous and waste products. It is used in cases where kidney function is defective.

**confluent kidney.** A congenital abnormality in which the two kidneys are fused into one organ. See also HORSESHOE KIDNEY, below.

**contracted kidney.** The final stage of chronic glomerulonephritis, arteriolar nephosclerosis, or chronic pyelonephritis.

**cystic kidney.** A kidney containing cysts.

**floating kidney.** A kidney which has become detached from its normal position. Its ability to move results in kinking of the ureter, causing Dietl's crisis, which produces paroxysms of pain and, when the ureter becomes unkinked, the sudden production of a large volume of urine. Also called *wandering kidney, movable kidney.*

**horseshoe kidney.** Partial fusion of the two kidneys at birth, usually at the lower end. See also CONFLUENT KIDNEY, above.

**lardaceous kidney.** See AMYLOID KIDNEY, above.

**large white kidney.** An enlarged and pale kidney which may be due to amyloid disease, nephrosis, chronic lipoid nephrosis, or chronic nephritis.

**movable kidney.** See FLOATING KIDNEY, above.

**primitive kidney.** The pronephros of the embryo.

**red granular kidney.** A description of the kidney seen in cases of very high blood pressure.

**sacculated kidney.** The advanced stage of hydronephrosis.

**small white kidney.** A description of the kidney seen in chronic glomerulonephritis.

**surgical kidney.** A kidney affected with suppuration or tuberculosis.

**wandering kidney.** See FLOATING KIDNEY, above.

**waxy kidney.** See AMYLOID KIDNEY, above.

**king's evil.** An old name for scrofula. *It was once thought that scrofula could be cured by the touch of a king's hand. The superstition began during the reign of Edward the Confessor and thousands of people attended great ceremonies in order to have their affliction touched by the monarch, but since he also hung round each patient's neck a gold coin suspended on ribbon, it is probable that the patients' enthusiasm for the gold outweighed their belief in the cure. Charles II was the busiest of the royal touchers, but it is alleged that more people died of scrofula during his reign than at any other time in English history. In the fifteenth century, the practice became an elaborate church ceremony, and the ritual was included in the Church of England's Book of Common Prayer until 1719, when it was quietly removed. William of Orange was accused of cruelty when he refused to practice the royal touch, and on the only occasion he was induced to lay hands on a patient he said: "God give you better health and more sense." When Queen Anne succeeded William she revived the practice and one of those she is reported to have touched for scrofula was Dr. Samuel Johnson. Anne was, however, the last English monarch to perform the royal touch, but the French kings practiced it until 1775, and Louis XVI is reputed to have touched 2,400 sick persons on his coronation day.*

**kleptomania.** A morbid desire to steal; obsessive stealing; a mental disorder marked by a desire to steal. The objects stolen are usually worth little and have a symbolic value only.

**kleptomaniac.** A person affected with kleptomania.

**Klinefelter's syndrome.** A congenital abnormality characterized by underdevelopment of the testicles, sterility, and mental retardation.

**Klumpke's paralysis.** Paralysis of the wrist and fingers, resulting from damage to nerves in the region of the neck, due to strain on the baby's head and neck during childbirth.

**knee.** The joint between the femur and the tibia, or the front of the leg in the region of this joint.

**knee cap.** The patella, the roughly circular bone lying in front of the knee joint.

**knee jerk.** A jerk forward of the lower leg produced by the doctor's tapping the ligament below the knee cap when the leg hangs loosely flexed at right angles. The sign is normally present, but when it is absent it is indicative of a disorder of the central nervous system. The sign may be difficult to elicit in some nervous people because they hold the leg rigid and refuse to allow it to kick out.

**knock-knee.** A condition in which the knees touch while the ankles are far apart. Also called *genu valgum*.

**knuckles.** The joints of the fingers, especially those connecting the palm of the hand with fingers and thumb.

**Koplik's spots.** Small red spots surrounded by quite white areas which appear on the inner side of the cheek, near the back teeth, some days before the rash of measles is seen.

**Korsakow's (or Korsakov's) psychosis.** A severe form of mental derangement characterized by loss of memory, hallucinations, often severe agitation, and polyneuritis produced by excessive drinking of alcohol, and an inadequate intake of food. The disorder results as much from the deficient diet and the chronic gastritis commonly found in alcoholics as from the direct poisonous effect of the alcohol. The polyneuritis causes a variety of symptoms apart from muscular weakness in the arms and legs. The patient cannot feel light touches on the skin but cries out with pain if the deeper structures are pressed. These patients are usually confined to a hospital, where they are given a diet with a high vitamin content, especially of vitamin B complex, and then weaned from their usually high intake of alcohol. Also called *Korsakow's syndrome*. See also ALCOHOLIC PSYCHOSIS.

**kraurosis.** A dry, shriveled condition of some part of the body.

**kraurosis vulvae.** A shriveling up of the vulva. See also LEUKOPLAKIA VULVAE.

**krebiozen.** A controversial substance alleged to be effective in the treatment of cancer.

**kwáshiorkor.** A nutritional disease of babies and young children, mostly in Africa, caused by a diet deficient in protein and vitamins. It is literally a starvation disease. The child is apathetic, retarded in growth, and has muscular wasting and dropsy, with alterations in pigmentation of the skin and hair and in the hair texture. Also known as *malignant malnutrition*, *nu-tritional dystrophy*, *fatty liver disease*, *infantile pellagra*.

**kyphoscoliosis.** A curvature of the spine both backwards and sideways.

**kyphosis.** A backwards curvature of the spine producing the humpbacked appearance.

**kyphotic.** Pertaining to kyphosis.

**labia.** The lips; the plural of labium.

**labial.** Pertaining to the lips, to a labium, or to lip sounds.

**labia majora.** The two folds of hair-bearing skin situated one on each side of the vulva.

**labia minora.** The two folds of mucous membrane situated one on each side of the vulva within the labia majora.

**labile.** Unstable. For example, labile high blood pressure is the type of reading a doctor obtains in a highly nervous and emotional person. It is not a true record of the normal blood pressure.

**labium.** A lip; the singular of labia.

**labor.** The act of childbirth. The onset of labor may be indicated in one of three ways. (1) Painful contractions of the womb may commence and be felt either in the abdomen or back. The "pains" recur at regular intervals, and proof that they are labor pains can be obtained by placing a hand on the abdomen where the womb can be felt to harden with each pain. (2) The bag of water lying in front of the baby may rupture, producing a flood of liquid from the birth canal. (3) Slight bleeding may occur from the vagina. This is popularly known as a "show." Labor is described as having three stages. *First stage.* This is the period during which the womb contracts and its neck or cervix opens. *Second stage.* The passage of the baby down the birth canal. *Third stage.* The extrusion of the placenta. Also called *accouchement, confinement, parturition, travail.*

**dry labor.** A birth in which, because of the poor fit of the baby's head to the birth canal, the liquor amnii, the fluid in which the baby floats in the womb, has drained away.

**induced labor.** Labor started artificially by either the obstetrician rupturing the membranes, or by giving intravenously a drug which stimulates the womb to contract.

**instrumental labor.** The extraction of the baby by midwifery forceps.

**premature labor.** The onset of labor after the 28th week and before the 40th week of pregnancy. After the 28th week there is a chance, however small, that the baby will survive, but if labor starts prior to the 28th week the baby has little chance and this is called a miscarriage or abortion.

**labour.** See LABOR.

**labyrinth.** The inner ear. It contains both the organ of hearing and that which controls the sense of balance. See also EAR.

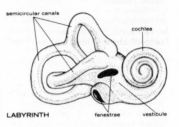

LABYRINTH

**labyrinthine nystagmus.** The nystagmus seen in disorders of the labyrinth.

**labyrinthine vertigo.** Vertigo associated with disorders of the labyrinth.

**labyrinthitis.** Inflammation of the labyrinth. See also MÉNIÈRE'S DISEASE.

**laceration.** A tear or irregular wound produced by tearing or crushing.

**lacrima.** A tear.

**lacrimal.** Pertaining to the tears.

**lacrimal abscess.** An abscess in a tear gland or tear duct.

**lacrimal gland.** The gland that produces tears. It lies in a dent of the bone which forms the brow in the upper outer region of the eye socket.

**lacrimation.** The normal or excessive production of tears; watering of the eye.

**lactagogue.** A substance which stimulates the breasts to produce milk.

**lactalbumin.** The milk protein.

**lactate.** A salt of lactic acid.

**lactation.** The production of milk from the breasts or the act of suckling by the baby.

**lactational.** Relating to lactation.

**lacteal.** 1. Pertaining to milk. 2. A lymphatic duct in the small intestine which takes up chyle.

**lactic.** Pertaining to milk or milk derivatives.

**lactic acid.** An acid found in some milk and in muscle tissue. It is used to aid digestion.

**lactic acid milk.** Milk to which lactic acid has been added to make the curds of cow's milk more flocculent and more easily digestible by the child.

**lactiferous.** Secreting or conveying milk.

**lactiferous ducts.** The 16 milk ducts in the breast, which open at the tip of the nipple.

**lactin.** Lactose.

**lactose.** Milk sugar, found in the milk of mammals. Also called *lactin*.

**lactosuria.** The presence of lactose in the urine.

**Laennec's disease.** Alcoholic cirrhosis of the liver.

**Laennec's pearls.** Small gelatinous bodies found in the sputum of asthmatic patients.

**laevulose.** See LEVULOSE.

**laevulosaemia.** See LEVULOSEMIA.

**laevulosuria.** See LEVULOSURIA.

**lagophthalmos.** Inability to completely close the eyelids.

**lamella.** 1. A medicated disc or tiny tablet which is inserted inside the lower eyelid in the treatment of eye infections. 2. A lamina or layer. 3. A basement membrane in an organ.

**lamina.** A thin plate or layer as of bone, or a thin membrane.

**laminated.** Composed of laminae.

**lamination.** Arranged in layers.

**laminectomy.** Surgical removal from a vertebra or vertebrae of the arches of bone over the spinal cord.

**laminitis.** Inflammation of a lamina.

**lancet.** A knife with a two-edged blade.

**lancinating.** Descriptive of a pain which is shooting or stabbing in character.

**Landry's paralysis.** A form of paralysis which creeps up the body. See also PARALYSIS: LANDRY'S PARALYSIS.

**Langerhans's islands.** Small islands of cells which manufacture insulin; found in the pancreas.

**lanolin.** The fat or grease derived from processing sheep's wool and used as an ointment base.

**lanugo.** Properly, the downlike hair which covers the human fetus between the fifth and ninth months of pregnancy. The term is, however, generally accepted as applying to any downlike hair.

**laparoscopy.** A diagnostic procedure in which a tiny incision is made into the abdominal wall and a laparoscope (an instrument containing a light) is passed through it to enable the surgeon to inspect the interior of the abdomen and organs contained therein.

**laparotomy.** Any abdominal surgical operation performed to discover the cause of the patient's complaint and with the intention of performing the appropriate corrective operation at the same time.

**lardaceous.** Lardlike.

**lardaceous degeneration.** See AMYLOID DEGENERATION.

**laryngeal.** Pertaining to the larynx or voice box.

**laryngeal crises.** Attacks of acute laryngeal spasm, producing choking fits. They may be due to irritating gases, foreign bodies, inflammation, ulceration, tumors in the larynx, irritation of the recurrent laryngeal nerve from tumors, aneurysms in the chest, tabes dorsalis, or hysteria.

**laryngectomy.** Surgical removal of the larynx.

**laryngismus.** Spasm of the larynx.

**laryngismus stridulus.** Spasm of the larynx which causes the child to hold the breath and go blue in the face; this gradually subsides and the first intake of breath is described as a crowing noise. It occurs in children suffering from tetany and is often due to a disturbance of the calcium content of the blood associated with the presence of rickets and always in association with adenoids. It is commonest between the ages of six months and two years.

**laryngitis.** Inflammation of the larynx. Laryngitis may be acute or chronic in character, and catarrhal, suppurative, diphtheritic, tuberculous, or syphilitic in type. The acute catarrhal type, which accompanies a heavy cold, is most common, and is characterized by hoarseness and sometimes by complete loss of voice. The less common variety is chronic catarrhal laryngitis, which consists of persistent hoarseness, pain and dryness of the throat, sometimes pain and difficulty on swallowing, and an irritable cough. See INHALATION.

**laryngocentesis.** Surgical puncture of the larynx.

**laryngofissure.** A surgical operation on the larynx to remove growths.

**laryngological.** Pertaining to laryngology.

**laryngologist.** A specialist in laryngology.

**laryngology.** The science of the diseases of the larynx.

**laryngoparalysis, laryngoparesis.** Paralysis of the muscles of the larynx.

**laryngopharyngeal.** Pertaining to both the larynx and the pharynx.

**laryngopharyngitis.** Inflammation of the larynx and the pharynx.

**laryngopharynx.** The lower portion of the pharynx; it opens into the larynx and esophagus.

**laryngophony.** The sound of the voice as heard through a stethoscope when the endpiece is placed over the larynx.

**laryngoplasty.** Surgical operation on the larynx to make good a defect.

**laryngoplegia.** Paralysis of the muscles of the larynx.

**laryngoscope.** A surgical instrument consisting of a long-handled mirror which is placed at the back of the throat to inspect the inside of the larynx.

**laryngoscopy.** Inspection of the interior of the larynx with a laryngoscope.

**laryngospasm.** A spasm of the interior of the larynx and vocal cords.

**laryngostenosis.** Constriction of the larynx.

**laryngotomy.** Surgical incision of the larynx.

**laryngotracheitis.** Inflammation of both the larynx and the trachea.

**laryngotracheotomy.** The surgical operation of making an artificial airway by incising through the cartilaginous rings of the upper portion of the trachea and inserting a metal tube, so that the patient will breathe through the tube instead of through the mouth.

**larynx.** The cartilaginous boxlike voice organ situated in the neck behind the Adam's apple and betwen the trachea and the pharynx.

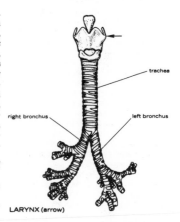

LARYNX (arrow)

**lassitude.** Exhaustion or weakness not due to exertion.

**lateral.** At or belonging to the side or away from the midline of the body.

**lateroflexion.** A tendency to lurch to one side when walking forwards; a sign of Parkinson's disease.

**laterotorsion.** A twisting to one side.

**lateroversion.** Turning to one side.

**laudanum.** Tincture of opium.

**laughing gas.** Nitrous oxide, the "gas" sometimes used for dental anesthesia.

**Laurence-Moon-Biedl syndrome.** Fröhlich's syndrome, complicated by retinitis pigmentosa (hardening, pigmentation, and wasting of the retina), mental deficiency, and the presence of more than the normal number of fingers and toes.

**lavage.** The washing out of an organ, such as the stomach or bowel.

**lead.** A soft bluish-grey malleable metal, occurring in nature chiefly as a sulphide. Its soluble salts are violent irritant poisons.

**lead poisoning.** This occurs in acute and chronic forms. *Acute lead poisoning.* This form is characterized by an immediate metallic taste, a burning sensation in the throat, and severe abdominal pain with paralysis, followed by collapse and even death. If the poison has just been swallowed and the casualty has not vomited, then this should be induced by giving two teaspoonfuls of Epsom salts in a cup of water. If the poison has been swallowed one-half to one hour previously, then it is a waste of time to induce vomiting, for the poison will have already passed into the intestine. The burning pain in the stomach can be relieved by giving the patient milk to drink. All cases should, however, be rushed to hospital for treatment. *Chronic lead poisioning.* This type of lead poisoning occurs in persons long exposed to repeated absorption of small amounts of the metal. There is lack of appetite, general lassitude, various symptoms of indigestion, and obstinate constipation associated with attacks of violent abdominal pain, and a blue line may appear on the gums just where the teeth emerge. Various nervous symptoms may develop, such as the characteristic dropping of the wrist due to a lead palsy; epileptic fits, acute mania, delirium, and coma may also appear. Research has shown that chronic lead poisoning may sometimes be the cause of a form of mental defect in children, caused by sucking objects containing lead. It is recommended that all mentally retarded children should have a blood test for lead.

*Accidental outbreaks of lead poisoning have been caused by using lead pipes to convey fluids such as cider or beer, resulting in the acid content of the fluids dissolving lead off the lining of the pipes. Nowadays lead is not used in the glazing of earthenware, but it was at one time; therefore ancient glazed earthenware pots should not be used to ferment wine or to hold food or drink which has an acid content.*

**lead, electrocardiographic.** One of the wires which are attached to various parts of the body and then to an electrocardiogram to record the minute electrical currents generated by the heart muscle when it contracts. They are used by heart specialists to detect cardiac disorders. Some patients become nervous when these wires from the machine are attached to their body. Their fears are quite groundless, however, for the only electricity which passes through these wires are the very minute electrical currents generated inside the patient's body. In any event, the modern electrocardiograph is transistorized and often works from small batteries.
**lead sugar.** Acetate of lead, a virulent poison.

**leather-bottle stomach.** The descriptive term applied to a stomach that has become considerably thickened from infiltration by cancer.
**leg.** The lower extremity, especially that part from knee to ankle.
**leiomyoma.** A tumor arising in smooth muscle.
**leiomyosarcoma.** A malignant tumor containing smooth-muscle cells.
**Leishman-Donovan bodies.** Small bodies found in the liver and spleen of patients suffering with kala-azar.
**leishmaniasis.** Infection caused by protozoa of the genus *Leishmania.* There are several species, each having different clinical manifestations. See also KALA-AZAR.
**lens.** A transparent piece of glass, crystal, or plastic, shaped so as to converge or scatter rays of light. Lenses are described according to the shape of their surfaces, the purpose for which they are employed, or the tint used to cut out certain parts of the light spectrum.
**contact lens.** A thin, curved lens placed directly over the eyeball.
**Crookes' lens.** A lens which stops the passage of ultraviolet and infrared rays.
**crystalline lens.** The eye lens situated behind the pupil. When this becomes opaque and milky in appearance it is called a cataract.
**lenticular.** Pertaining to or resembling a lens, to the crystalline lens of the eye, or to the lenticular nucleus of the brain.
**progressive lenticular degeneration.** A rare progressive disease of the nervous system of unknown cause, usually affecting children of the same family. There is always disease of the liver, and the first nervous sign is usually involuntary movement of the hands and feet, which may be of several kinds. There may also be tremors which increase on voluntary movement, and these may be followed by rigidity of the face, the muscles of the neck, and later of the trunk. The rigidity increases steadily until the patient becomes helpless. Progressive muscular weakness and general emaciation follow, and the patient becomes facile, docile, and childish. No curative treatment is known. Also called *Wilson's disease.*
**lentigo.** A freckle or a small circumscribed pigmented spot, occurring on the face and backs of the hands; usually caused by exposure to the sun, but sometimes of congenital origin.
**leontiasis ossea.** This is not a disease entity but a term descriptive of a single symptom—the enlargement of one or more of the facial bones, which in

extreme instances results in the whole face becoming distorted until there is some slight resemblance to that of a lion. Typically, the condition starts in childhood, when the bony enlargement is caused either by a diffuse inflammation of the bone due to gross dental sepsis, or by some other disease of bone. In adults, a similar appearance can be caused by Paget's disease, bone syphilis, and tumors of the nose and air sinuses. The condition is sometimes seen in leprosy. Also called *Virchow's disease.*
**leper.** A person affected with leprosy.
**leprosarium.** A hospital or colony where lepers are isolated and treated.
**leprosy.** A chronic contagious disease occurring almost exclusively in tropical and subtropical countries; characterized by lesions of the skin or nerves with resulting deformities and mutilations. It is caused by the bacterium, *Mycobacterium leprae.* It is of low infectivity and the mode of spread is unknown, but intimate contact with a leper is essential. Only 3 percent of people living with lepers contract the disease, children being more susceptible than adults. The prognosis in advanced cases is not good, but if treated early, the life expectancy is increased and some cases are completely cured. Patients are not discharged until they have been germ-free for at least two years, and even then it is not possible to say whether they are cured or only having a remission for which leprosy is notorious. Also called *Hansen's disease.*
**leprous.** Affected with or pertaining to leprosy.
**leptomeningitis.** See PIARACHNITIS.
**leptospirosis.** A group of infections caused by a species of spirochete widely distributed among rodents. Human contact with the urine of these rodents can produce a febrile condition characterized by jaundice, muscle pains, and hemorrhages. Also called *leptospira icterohemorrhagica, Weil's disease.*
**lesbianism.** Homosexuality between women.
**lesion.** Any damage to living tissue caused by disease or injury.
**lethargy.** A state of drowsiness or stupor.
**leucaemia.** See LEUKEMIA.
**leucemia.** See LEUKEMIA.
**leucocyte.** See LEUKOCYTE.
**leucocythaemia.** See LEUKOCYTHEMIA.
**leucocytic.** See LEUKOCYTIC.
**leucocytogenesis.** See LEUKOCYTOGENESIS.
**leucocytolysis.** See LEUKOCYTOLYSIS.
**leucocytopenia.** See LEUKOCYTOPENIA.
**leucocytosis.** See LEUKOCYTOSIS.

**leucoderma, leucodermia.** See LEUKO-
DERMA; LEUKODERMIA.

**leucoerythroblastosis.** See LEUKOERY-
THROBLASTOSIS.

**leucokeratosis.** See LEUKOKERATOSIS.

**leucoma.** See LEUKOMA.

**leucopenia.** See LEUKOPENIA.

**leucoplakia.** See LEUKOPLAKIA.

**leucorrhoea.** See LEUKORRHEA.

**leucotomy.** See LEUKOTOMY.

**leukaemia.** See LEUKEMIA.

**leukaemic.** See LEUKEMIC.

**leukemia.** A disease of the blood-forming organs characterized by the uncontrolled proliferation of the white
cells and by the drawing into the
bloodstream of immature white cells
in large numbers. Several varieties
are described, and their differentiation
is important because each has its own
prognosis.

**acute leukemia.** This variety occurs
most frequently in children up to the
age of five years, though it can occur in
the young adult. The onset is abrupt
with the rapid development of anemia,
weakness, loss of weight, sore throat,
headache, and pains in the bones. The
temperature becomes high and blood
spots show on mucous membrane and
skin surfaces. Hemorrhages occur in
various parts of the body and some are
severe enough to kill. The average duration of life is about six months, but
some cases assume more chronic form
and live for about a year. The extreme
pallor and enlargement of the lymph
glands, especially those of the neck,
are the first signs to attract attention.
The spleen may be small or greatly
enlarged and the liver may be enlarged as well. The lungs may show
bronchitis or patches of pneumonia or
pleurisy, and inflammation of the
heart may set in. Treatment consists
of blood transfusions, hormone therapy with cortisone, and the administration of drugs which tend to slow up
the progress of the disease.

**chronic lymphatic leukemia.** This
disease occurs in the middle or later
part of life and is hardly ever seen in
children. It affects males twice as often
as females, and is characterized by enlargement of the liver, the spleen, and
all the body's lymphatic tissue, and it
is accompanied by the presence of an
enormous number of lymphocytes in
the blood. The disease is usually fatal,
the average duration of life being only
three to four years from the onset, or
about one and a half years after coming under treatment. In exceptional
cases life may be prolonged for 10, 15,
or 20 years.

**chronic myeloid leukemia.** Characterized by an enormously enlarged
spleen, anemia, and hemorrhages, the
early symptoms are fatigue, loss of
weight and strength, upset digestion,
and enlargement of the abdomen, due
to the increasing size of the spleen. It
is invariably fatal, the average duration of life being just over three years
from the onset. There is no evidence
that treatment prolongs life, though it
greatly increases the comfort of the
patient. Sometimes a temporary remission can be induced by injections of
drugs which slow down the production
of white cells. Also called *melocytic
leukemia, splenomedullary leukemia,
chronic leukemic myelosis.*

**leukemic.** Pertaining to leukemia.

**leukocyte.** A white blood corpuscle.
There are various kinds of leukocytes,
which are distinguished from each

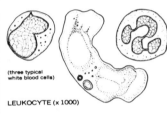

(three typical
white blood cells)

LEUKOCYTE (x 1000)

other under the microscope by their
different staining reactions.

**polymorphonuclear      leukocyte.**
This type of white cell is part of the
body's protective mechanism against
infections, for its function is to destroy
any germ it meets. The leukocytes
themselves become casualties in their
attack on the germs, and pus in a
wound is in fact a collection of thousands of dead germs and dead leukocytes.

**leukocythemia.** See LEUKEMIA.

**leukocytic.** Pertaining to leukocytes.

**leukocytogenesis.** The formation of
leukocytes.

**leukocytolysis.** The destruction of leukocytes.

**leukocytopenia.** See LEUKOPENIA.

**leukocytosis.** An increase in the number of leukocytes in the blood. Leukocytes are normally found to be increased during pregnancy and also in
many infections and toxemias. Leukocytosis can be diagnostic of an inflammatory condition, and the body's response to treatment can be checked by
a daily leukocyte count, which becomes lower as the patient's condition
improves. This is a simple procedure
for the patient, the blood usually being
collected from a pinprick in a finger.

**leukoderma, leukodermia.** A chronic,
congenital skin condition in which
patches devoid of pigment are usually
surrounded by areas with increased
pigmentation. There is no treatment,
but the pale areas can be masked by
staining with suntan lotions and other
cosmetics. Also called *lichromia, piebald skin, vitiligo.*

**leukoerythroblastosis.** A condition
characterized by either anemia, the
presence of immature red and white
cells in the blood caused by deposits of
cancer in bone, osteosclerosis due to
marble bone disease, or by myelos-
clerosis. Also called *osteosclerotic anemia.*

**leukokeratosis.** See LEUKOPLAKIA.

**leukoma.** A white opacity of the cornea
of the eye.

**leukopenia.** A decrease in the normal
number of white cells in the blood.

**leukoplakia.** A disease characterized
by a whitish thickening of the surface
of a mucous membrane that becomes
hypertrophied and sometimes undergoes cancerous changes.

**leukoplakia buccalis.** Leukoplakia
affecting the mucous membranes of
the cheeks.

**leukoplakia lingualis.** Leukoplakia
affecting the tongue. It is sometimes a
manifestation of syphilis.

**leukoplakia vulvae.** Leukoplakia of
the vulva. Also called *kraurosis vulvae.*

**leukorrhea.** A whitish vaginal discharge popularly known as "the
whites." There are two main varieties:
one is dead white and due to a fungus;
the other is more yellowish and is due
to a bacterium. Neither is caused by
dirt, venereal disease, or by anything
of which a woman need be ashamed,
and both are promptly cured by sup-
positories placed inside the vagina for
two or three weeks. Leukorrhea is not
only a disease of adult women but can
be seen in quite young girls, and is so
commonplace as almost to be normal
in the female. See also DÖDERLEIN'S BA-
CILLUS.

**leukotomy.** A surgical operation to divide some of the nerve fibers coming
from the front of the brain that carry
the impulses of thought. It is performed when mental conditions, especially extreme agitation, do not respond to other forms of treatment.
However, as better methods of treating mental disorders are discovered,
leukotomy is falling into disuse.

**Levi-Loraine syndrome.** Infantilism;
a form of dwarfism.

**levulose.** Fruit sugar.

**levulosemia.** The presence of levulose
in the blood.

**levulose test.** A test performed to
check the liver's efficiency.

**levulosuria.** The presence of levulose
in the urine.

**libido.** Sexual desire.

**lichen.** A term applied to a large group of skin disorders which exhibit solid papules with exaggerated skin markings. The two most commonly seen are lichen planus and lichen simplex.

**lichen planus.** A skin condition characterized by an eruption of small lilac-tinted, flat-topped, shiny papules, which are polygonal in outline, on the front of the wrist, lumbosacral area, external genitals, inner side of the thighs, shins, calves, and ankles, and sometimes on the lining of the mouth. The cause is not known, but it may be due to either a bacterium or a virus. The disease occurs most commonly between the ages of 30 and 60 years, in women more frequently than in men; children are seldom affected. At first the papules may be discrete, but usually they collect together to form irregular rounded areas covered with fine adherent scales. Itching is usually a prominent feature and it can be so distressing as to prevent sleep and cause frantic scratching, but in some cases it may be slight, or even absent. No specific treatment is known, though large doses of vitamin B have been thought to be helpful and so has the administration of cortisone or similar drugs. X-ray treatment to some areas has brought relief. It is a difficult disorder to treat, for while one case may respond dramatically to treatment, another case may be resistant to all the doctor's efforts.

**lichen simplex.** A skin disorder of psychogenic origin. The onset is acute, one attack may last for weeks, months, or years, and recurrences are often seasonal. The itching is continuous, always worse at night, and intense scratching may cause reddening or even a type of nettle rash. This is soon followed by a papular eruption, the papules being pale or red, small, and ill-defined. The affected skin may become deeply pigmented with obvious damage from scratching and later secondary infection by germs. The disease is sometimes associated with asthma, hay fever, bronchitis, and general disorders of health. Also called *common prurigo.*

**licheniasis.** The formation of lichen; the condition of a person suffering with lichen.

**lichenification.** The development of thickened skin from long, continued scratching.

**lichenoid.** Resembling lichen.

**lien.** Latin for spleen.

**lienteric.** Relating to lientery.

**lientery.** A form of disturbed bowel action, in which the swallowing of food causes evacuation of the bowel a short time afterward. It is usually due to overexcitement of the bowel, and may be nervous in origin. The condition can also occur when the gastric juice has an abnormally low acid content, and many of these cases are cured by the patient taking extra acid mixed in fruit juice at each meal. Also called *lienteric diarrhea.*

**ligament.** A band of flexible, tough, dense, white, fibrous tissue connecting the articular (joint) ends of the bones and sometimes enveloping them. The term is also applied to certain folds of the peritoneum.

**ligamental, ligamentary, ligamentous.** Having the function of or pertaining to a ligament.

**ligate.** To apply a ligature.

**ligation.** The operation of tying a ligature.

**ligature.** A cord or thread for tying blood vessels; or, the act of tying or binding. Such cords are manufactured from silkworm gut, nylon, kangaroo tendon, and even from steel or silver wire. See also SUTURE.

**absorbable ligature.** This type of ligature is used in deep structures, where, after a set time, it is absorbed.

**nonabsorbable ligature.** A ligature, which cannot be absorbed by the tissues and is employed either where it is required permanently or in sites from which it is easily removed.

**limb.** An arm or leg.

**limbus.** A border or edge.

**limen.** A threshold or boundary.

**liminal.** Relating to a threshold, especially pertaining to the lowest limit of perception.

**linctus.** A thick, sweetened liquid medicinal preparation, usually compounded with sugar syrup.

**lingua.** The tongue.

**lingua geographica.** A condition of the tongue characterized by soreness and patchy shedding of the tongue's surface producing reddening areas which slowly change their distribution. Treatment consists of bland mouthwashes, such as salt water. If the soreness is severe, highly spiced foods, condiments, highly acid foods, sharp-tasting drinks, and excessive smoking—all of which tend to sting the tongue and aggravate the soreness—should be avoided. The condition is harmless and a patient's fears of cancer of the tongue can be allayed. It does, however, tend to persist indefinitely in spite of treatment and doctors sometimes advise patients to regard the condition as a "normal" abnormality.

**lingual.** Pertaining to, or shaped like, a tongue.

**liniment, linimentum.** A liquid preparation for massaging into the skin to produce counterirritation and relief by drawing to the part an increased supply of blood. The action of the massage provides a soothing effect. The commonest in use is linimentum album, a turpentine preparation popularly called "horse liniment" which is used by athletes for massaging stiff muscles. Liniments should not be used on broken skin.

**lint.** Thick, loosely woven, absorbent material, smooth on one side and fluffy on the other. The smooth side should always be applied to the skin, for the fluffy side will leave little bits of cotton in the wound. White lint is used to apply poultices or ointments, and pink lint, so colored to indicate that is has been impregnated with boracic, for applying hot fomentations. See FOMENTATION.

**lip. 1.** Either of two fleshy parts or folds forming the margins of the mouth. **2.** The edge of an opening or cavity.

**lipaemia.** See LIPEMIA.

**lipase.** An enzyme occurring in the pancreas, liver, and certain seeds, which is capable of breaking down fats into fatty acids and glycerin.

**lipemia.** An increase in the fat content of the blood.

**lipid.** See LIPOID.

**Lipiodol.** An oily, proprietary preparation containing iodine and used as a contrast medium.

**lipodystrophy.** Any disturbance of fat metabolism.

**progressive lipodystrophy.** A curious disorder in which there is great loss of subcutaneous fat from face, neck, upper limbs, and trunk, whereas the buttocks and legs may be entirely normal. There is a superficial appearance of wasting, but closer inspection reveals that the muscles are normal in size. About 80 percent of reported cases have been in females. The onset tends to occur in early life—in about half of the cases before the age of ten years, and in about three-quarters before the age of twenty years. There are no real symptoms and the patient appears to be in good health, but in some cases resentment at the peculiar physical appearance results in psychological anxieties. A few cases have been associated with either overactivity of the thyroid gland or even diabetes. There is no treatment for the condition once established and it remains more or less stationary.

**lipofibroma.** A tumor composed of fat and fibrous tissue.

**lipogenesis.** The formation of fat.

**lipogenic.** Pertaining to lipogenesis.

**lipoid.** A term applied to a mixed group of substances related to fats, which are insoluble in water but soluble in such fat solvents as chloroform and benzine. One such lipoid is cholesterol, which, it is believed, may be a factor in causing such conditions as coronary thrombosis. See also CHOLESTEROL.

**lipoidosis.** A disturbance of the metabolism of the lipoids.

**lipoiduria.** A condition in which lipoids are found in the urine.

**lipolysis.** The decomposition or splitting up of fats.

**lipolytic.** Pertaining to lipolysis.

**lipoma.** A fatty tumor.

**lipomatosis.** The excessive formation of fat under the skin.

**lipomatous.** Relating to a lipoma.

**lipuria.** The presence of fat droplets in the urine.

**liquefacient.** Possessing the power to liquefy.

**liquefaction.** The change, usually of a solid tissue, to a fluid or semifluid state, due to occlusion of the blood supply, the action of bacteria, or chemical corrosive action. The term is also used in chemistry to indicate the condensation of gases into a liquid.

**liquescent.** Tending to become liquid.

**liquid paraffin.** A colorless, oily mixture of liquid hydrocarbons derived from the fractional distillation of crude oil. Medically, it is used either to lubricate instruments or to treat constipation. However, though liquid paraffin has long been considered an entirely safe and harmless method of treating constipation, it has now been discovered that it has certain effects on the intestine. Constant and regular administration of liquid paraffin to small children can cause them to lose weight. This occurs because the oil coats the inner surface of the intestine and prevents the passage of water-soluble food into the intestinal walls, where it is normally absorbed. It is also thought that large doses of liquid paraffin taken regularly for several years may possibly irritate the lining of the intestine and cause disease changes. There are now many other and better ways of treating chronic constipation. Ready-made enemas for self-administration can now be bought.

**liquor amnii.** The fluid in which the fetus floats within its membranes inside the womb. Its function is mainly protective, acting as a buffer against external injury, assisting to maintain the baby at an even temperature, and allowing it free movement. During la-

bor the fluid-filled membranes in front of the baby (the bag of waters) act as a wedge to dilate the neck of the womb. The fluid is produced partly from the mother's blood, in part from the membranes, and partly from the baby's urine. It has also been claimed to have nourishing value, for the baby swallows it during the later months of gestation. At the time of delivery there is an average of from one to two pints, though there may be as little as half a pint. In the condition called hydramnios, however, it exceeds four pints. Also called *amniotic fluid.*

**lithiasis.** The formation of calculi in the body.

**lithic. 1.** Pertaining to calculi. **2.** Pertaining to lithium.

**lithium.** A metal belonging to the group of alkalis and with the chemical symbol of Li. Its various salts are used in the treatment of gout, rheumatism, and urinary disorders.

**lithocenosis.** The extraction from the bladder of fragments of a stone which has been previously crushed.

**lithoclast.** See LITHOTRITE.

**lithoclasty.** See LITHOTRITY.

**lithosis.** See SILICOSIS.

**lithotomy.** Surgical incision into the bladder for the removal of a stone.

**lithotripsy.** See LITHOTRITY.

**lithotrite.** An instrument which is passed into the urinary bladder to crush a stone.

**lithotrity.** The operation of crushing a stone in the urinary bladder, and washing out the powdered remains.

**lithuresis.** The passage of small stones in the urine.

**Little's area.** The area of mucous membrane on the forward part of the nasal septum. It is frequently the site of a small erosion and the commonest site from which nosebleeding occurs.

**Little's disease.** See DIPLEGIA: CEREBRAL DIPLEGIA.

**liver.** The largest glandular organ in the body, the liver is situated below the arch of the right side of the chest in the upper abdominal cavity. It is about 12 inches wide, 6 inches thick,

and 6 inches from top to bottom at its longest part; it weighs about 3½ pounds. The liver produces bile and manufactures glucose, which it stores as glycogen. This is the body's fuel store which is released in an emergency and reconverted into glucose. Although the liver is essential to life, a large part of it can be diseased without causing death.

**livid.** Bluish colored.

**lividity.** The condition of being livid.

**lobar.** Relating to a lobe.

**lobate.** Possessing lobes.

**lobe.** A part of an organ separated from the surrounding part by a cleft.

**lobectomy.** Surgical removal of a lobe, as, for instance, from the brain or lung.

**lobitis.** Inflammation of a lobe, especially the lobe of a lung.

**lobular.** Pertaining to or resembling lobules.

**lobulated.** Consisting of lobes or lobules.

**lobule.** A small lobe.

**lochia.** The discharge of blood from the womb, which occurs during the first week or so after childbirth.

**lochial.** Pertaining to the lochia.

**lochiometra.** An accumulation of the lochia within the womb.

**lochiorrhagia.** Excessive flow of lochia.

**lochiorrhea.** See LOCHIORRHAGIA.

**lochiorrhoea.** See LOCHIORRHEA.

**lockjaw.** An infectious disease caused by the bacterium, *Clostridium tetani.* It is a fallacy that cuts between the index finger and thumb are more prone to produce lockjaw than any other wound. Also called *trismus.* See TETANUS.

**locomotor.** Pertaining to movement.

**locomotor ataxia.** The uncertain gait of someone suffering with tabes dorsalis, a condition arising in untreated syphilis.

**locular.** Loculated or divided into loculi.

**loculation syndrome.** A condition in which there is spinal obstruction preventing the communication of the cerebrospinal fluid with the cerebral ventricles so that the fluid stagnates. In this syndrome, the fluid is yellow-colored, there is an increase in globulin content, and coagulation takes place immediately upon withdrawal of the fluid.

**loculus.** A small space.

**logagnosia.** A disorder of the brain involving aphasia or other word defects of the central nervous system.

**logagraphia.** Inability to express ideas in writing.

**logaphasia.** Loss of ability to express one's ideas in speech or writing.

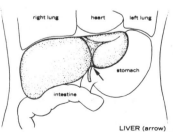

right lung    heart    left lung

stomach

intestine

LIVER (arrow)

**logoclonia.** A disorder in which there is a repetition of the end syllables of words. Also called *logoklony.*

**logomania.** Excessive talkativeness, a symptom of certain psychotic states.

**logoneurosis.** Any mental disorder accompanied by a speech disorder.

**logorrhea.** Excessive talkativeness.

**logorrhoea.** See LOGORRHEA.

**loin.** The part of the back between the thorax and the pelvis.

**long-sightedness.** See HYPERMETROPIA.

**loose body.** An object floating more or less freely in a joint cavity. It may be a piece of cartilage, bone, or a loosened part of the joint.

**lordosis.** Excessive development of the lumbar curve, the hollowed-out curve in the lumbar region.

**lordotic.** Pertaining to lordosis.

**loss of memory.** Amnesia.

**louping ill.** A form of brain inflammation in sheep caused by a virus and capable of being transmitted to man.

**louse.** See PEDICULUS.

**louse fever.** See FAMINE FEVER.

**lucid interval.** The recovery of consciousness for a short spell. This occurs in accidents involving damage to the skull and brain. The casualty, unconscious from concussion, recovers consciousness for a time, then goes into a coma as cerebral compression arises. The term also applies to the transitory return to normal of patients in certain mental or psychotic states.

**Ludwig's angina.** A severe form of inflammation of the floor of the mouth which spreads to the throat and other parts.

**lues.** Syphilis.

**Lugol's solution.** A mixture of iodine and potassium iodide in water. A treatment used for overactivity of the thyroid gland.

**lumbago.** Fibrositis affecting the lumbar muscles in the small of the back. While many cases are due to a combination of fibrositis and the muscular pain such as results from a heavy bout of digging, others, especially if recurrent, are associated with a prolapsed intervertebral disc.

**lumbar.** Pertaining to the loins or lumbar region.

**lumbar puncture.** The operation of passing a needle into the spinal canal. The procedure is used to measure the pressure of the cerebrospinal fluid; to obtain samples of the fluid for testing; to inject drugs for the treatment of certain conditions; or to introduce anesthetics. It is performed by first anesthetizing the skin and then inserting the needle between the third and fourth lumbar vertebrae and into the spinal canal. The spinal cord divides into a sheaf of nerves at the level of the third lumbar vertebra, therefore by inserting the needle below this level there is no danger of puncturing the cord.

**lumbocostal.** Pertaining to the loins and the ribs.

**lumbodorsal.** Pertaining to both lumbar and dorsal regions.

**lumboinguinal.** Pertaining to both lumbar and inguinal regions.

**lumbosacral.** Pertaining to both lumbar and sacral vertebrae (situated between the hip bones at the back of the pelvis).

**lumbricalis muscles.** Small muscles in the hand and foot.

**lumen.** The bore or cavity of a tube, such as an artery or the intestine.

**lunacy.** Insanity. The term is derived from *luna*, the Latin for moon, since it was formerly thought that the moon's rays caused insanity. It was also believed, and still is by some superstitious people, that those afflicted with insanity reached the height of their madness at full moon.

**lunar caustic.** Solid silver nitrate. It is held in the metal jaws of a stick and used to touch excessive granulation tissues forming in a wound.

**lung.** Either of the two respiratory organs by which the blood obtains oxygen from the atmosphere. The right lung consists of three lobes while the left has only two. They occupy the cavity on each side of the chest, being separated from each other by the heart and mediastinum. Each lung develops

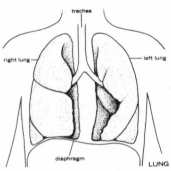

LUNG

from a branch of the trachea called a bronchus, which divides and redivides into smaller and smaller branches called bronchioles, eventually terminating in almost innumerable air-containing sacs called alveoli. Blood is brought to the lungs by the pulmonary arteries, where it picks up oxygen and releases carbon dioxide in the walls of the alveoli and then returns to the heart by way of the pulmonary veins. Each lung is enclosed in a double layer of membrane called the pleura, the space between the layers being called the pleural cavity. One layer covers the lung itself and is called the visceral pleura, while the other layer, called the parietal pleura, lines the cavity of the chest. It is claimed that if the respiratory surface of a lung was laid flat it would cover an area of 70 square meters. See also RESPIRATION.

**lunula.** The white half-moon-shaped area at the base of a nail.

**lupoid.** Resembling lupus.

**lupoma.** The primary nodule of lupus vulgaris.

**lupus.** A term applied to two quite distinct forms of skin disease, lupus erythematosus and lupus vulgaris. However, used without qualification it refers to lupus vulgaris. Other terms prefixed by lupus are descriptive of the stages in development of both the aforementioned diseases.

**lupus erythematosus.** A nontuberculous skin disease occurring in chronic discoid, subacute, and acute varieties. It is usually chronic but occasionally acute, and characterized by red scaly patches of various sizes, which produce scar formation. It is a capricious disease, which in its acute form can be fatal. The chronic form occurs on exposed areas such as the face, scalp, and hands, the skin follicles becoming plugged with a horny material.

**lupus vulgaris.** This form is true tuberculosis of the skin. Diverse and variable, it is a slowly developing, scarring, and deforming disease which often involves the face, and is characterized by the appearance of nodules resembling jelly.

**luteal.** Relating to lutein.

**lutein.** A yellow pigment present in the corpus luteum, in egg yolk, and fat cells.

**luteinization.** The development of lutein into the egg space (the Graafian follicle).

**luteoma.** A tumor arising from the corpus luteum.

**luxation.** A dislocation.

**lymph.** The fluid in the lymphatic vessels and lymph spaces.

**lymphadenitis.** Inflammation of a lymphatic gland.

**lymphadenoid.** Resembling or having the character of a lymph gland or lymphatic tissue.

**lymphadenoma.** 1. An enlarged lymph node. 2. A lymphoma.

**lymphangioma.** A tumor composed of dilated lymph vessels or of newformed lymph channels.

**lymphangitis.** Inflammation of a lymphatic vessel. Lymphangitis causes the red lines that are seen to run up a limb from an infected wound, and are an indication that the infection is both severe and beginning to spread. See also LYMPHATIC SYSTEM.

**lymphatic.** Pertaining to or characterized by lymph.

**lymphatic abscess.** An abscess occurring in a lymph gland.

**lymphatics.** The lymph-conveying capillary tubes or vessels.

**lymphatic system.** A system of vessels and glands, including the thoracic duct, which drains lymph from the various body tissues and returns it to

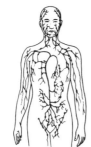

LYMPHATIC SYSTEM (simplified)

the bloodstream. Lymph is an almost colorless fluid derived from the blood and it passes through the capillaries into the spaces around the body cells to provide the cells with nutriment. The lymph is then carried away partly by the veins and partly by minute tubes, the lymphatic vessels, both containing valves to ensure that the lymph passes in one direction only. At intervals along the course of the lymphatic vessels are glands, sometimes called lymph nodes, which filter the lymph before it reenters the venous system via the thoracic duct. This duct is situated at the base of the neck on the left side. Infection from a particular area passes through the local groups of lymph glands which, in their struggle to obstruct the passage of infection into the circulation, may become inflamed and swollen, sometimes breaking down into abscesses.

**lymphocyte.** A type of white blood cell.

**lymphocytic.** Pertaining to lymphocytes.

**lymphocytoma.** A malignant lymphoma containing predominately mature lymphocytes.

**lymphocytopenia.** See LYMPHOPENIA.

**lymphedema.** A form of edema due to blockage of the lymphatic vessels. See

also ELEPHANTIASIS.

**lymphoedema.** See LYMPHEDEMA.

**lymphocytosis.** An increase in the number of lymphocytes in the blood.

**lymphodermia.** A disorder of the lymphatic vessels in the skin.

**lymphodermia perniciosa.** The enlargement of lymph glands due to leukemia.

**lymphogranuloma.** See HODGKIN'S DISEASE.

**lymphogranuloma inguinale.** A venereal disease of virus origin characterized by a hard sore in the genital area, followed by enlargement of the lymph glands in the groin. Also called *venereal lymphogranuloma*.

**lymphoid.** Having the appearance of lymph, lymphatic cells, or lymphoid tissue.

**lymphoma.** A general term applied to neoplasms of the lymphoid tissue including Hodgkin's disease.

**lymphopenia.** Decrease in the number of lymphocytes in the blood. Also called *lymphocytopenia*.

**lymphosarcoma.** A cancerous disease affecting lymphatic structures.

**lysin.** An antibody which has the power to cause the dissolution of cells.

**lysis.** 1. The gradual decline in the manifestations of a disease. 2. The gradual fall of a high temperature; also called *defervescence*. 3. The solution of a tissue by the action of a lysin.

**lyssophobia.** Morbid fear of rabies.

# M

**maceration.** The process of softening a tissue by the action of a fluid.

**macrocephalia, macrocephaly.** Abnormal enlargement of the head.

**macrocephalous.** Having an abnormally large head.

**macrocheilia.** Excessive size of the lips.

**macrocheiria.** Congenital overdevelopment of the hands.

**macrocolon.** An abnormally long colon.

**macrocornea.** An abnormally large cornea.

**macrocyte.** An extra large-sized red blood cell found in certain forms of anemia, such as pernicious anemia.

**macrodactylia.** Congenital enlargement of fingers or toes.

**macrodontia.** Abnormally large teeth.

**macrodystrophia.** See LIPODYSTROPHY; PROGRESSIVE LIPODYSTROPHY.

**macrogastria.** Abnormal enlargement of the stomach.

**macroglossia.** Abnormal enlargement of the tongue.

**macromastia, macromazia.** Abnormally large breasts or breast.

**macromelia.** An abnormal enlargement of any member of the body.

**macrophage.** A cell concerned with attacking and ingesting germs and which is found wandering in the blood in areas where there is great activity against germ invasion. It is not a true white cell, but is produced in the reticuloendothelial system.

**macropodia.** Congenital enlargement of the feet.

**macrorhinia.** Abnormal enlargement of the nose.

**macroscopic.** Capable of being seen with the naked eye.

**macroscopy.** The examination of objects with the naked eye.

**macula.** An unelevated spot or a circumscribed discoloration of the skin. There are many types.

**macula caeruleae.** A bluish grey spot on the skin caused by the body louse.

**macula corneae.** Opacities seen in the cornea of the eye.

**macula lutea.** The yellow spot (the area of clearest vision) seen in the retina of the eye.

**maculate.** Spotted.

**maculation.** The condition of being spotted; the formation of maculae.

**macule.** A macula; a spot.

**maculopapular.** Descriptive of a skin rash consisting of both macules and papules.

**maduromycosis.** A fungus most commonly found in the foot with necrosis, swelling, pus discharge, and formation of nodules. Also called *mycetoma*.

**magnetism.** The attraction or repulsion produced by magnetic forces.

**maidenhead.** The hymen.

**main-en-griffe.** French for claw hand.

**mal.** Disease.

**grand mal.** Major epilepsy.

**mal de Cayenne.** Elephantiasis.

**mal de mer.** Seasickness.

**mal de pinta.** A disease of the skin, probably of venereal origin, characterized by alterations in pigmentation and patchy thickening. Also called *carate, azul, spotted sickness*.

**mal de rosa.** Pellagra.

**mal des bassines.** An inflammation of the skin affecting those working in the silkworm industry; due to hypersensitivity to silkworm cocoons.

**mal perforant.** A perforating ulcer of the foot seen in tabes dorsalis.

**petit mal.** Minor epilepsy.

**mala.** The cheekbone or the cheek.

**malacia.** Softening of the tissues.

**malar.** Pertaining to the cheekbones or to the cheeks.

**malaria.** An infectious disease characterized by periodic paroxysms which consist of a hot stage, a cold stage, and a sweating stage occurring in this order; enlargement of the spleen; and the presence of the causative organism in the blood. The disease is caused by several species of protozoans belonging to the genus *Plasmodium*, transmitted to man by the bite of an infected mosquito of the genus *Anopheles*. Several types are known and they are named according to the interval between paroxysms, this being determined by the time it takes the particular species of organism to develop in the body. Prevention and treatment are now carried out by the use of synthetic chemicals, although quinine, the original treatment, is still occasionally used. See also CINCHONA.

**benign tertian malaria.** Malaria caused by *Plasmodium vivax*, with paroxysms occurring at intervals of 48 hours.

**quartan malaria.** Malaria caused by *Plasmodium malariae*, the paroxysms occurring every 72 hours.

**subtertian malaria.** Malaria caused by *Plasmodium falciparum*, the paroxysms in this type being either continuous or irregular and remittent. Also called *malign tertian fever, aestivo-autumnal fever.*

*The old-fashioned name for malaria was ague, the enlarged spleen being called the ague cake. Among tribal peoples in malarial countries the spleen is often so enormously enlarged that it can be easily fractured by a blow, the result of which is often a fatal hemorrhage. This knowledge has, on occasion, been put to use as a method of attack, the victim being struck, usually with a short, stout stick, on that part of the abdomen overlying the spleen.*

**malarial.** Pertaining to malaria.

**malarial hemoglobinuria.** See BLACK-WATER FEVER.

**malarial treatment.** The treatment of certain types of paralysis by infecting the patient with benign tertian malaria.

**malassimilation.** Defective absorption; usually refers to inability to absorb certain kinds of food from the intestine.

**malignancy.** The quality of being malignant; often refers to a cancerous condition.

**malignant.** Severe, evil, or threatening to life. The term is applied to any virulent condition which tends to go from bad to worse.

**malignant edema.** Gas gangrene.

**malignant endocarditis.** An ulcerative, infective condition of the lining of the heart. See also ENDOCARDITIS.

**malignant malaria.** Subtertian malaria. See GANGRENE: GAS GANGRENE.

**malignant pustule.** The skin pustule of anthrax.

**malingering.** To feign illness in order to avoid duty or work, or to attain some other consciously desired result.

**malleal, mallear.** Pertaining to the malleus, a bone in the middle ear. Also called *hammer.*

**malleolar.** Pertaining to a malleolus.

**malleolus.** A rounded knob of bone on each side of the ankle joint. That on the inner side is the end of the tibia and is called the internal malleolus; the one on the outer side is the end of the fibula and is called the lateral malleolus.

**mallet finger.** See HAMMER FINGER.

**mallet toe.** See HAMMER TOE.

**malleus.** One of the small bones in the middle ear which conduct sound from the eardrum to the organ of hearing. Also called *hammer.*

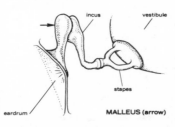

MALLEUS (arrow)

**malocclusion.** Any variation in the normal bite of the teeth, one set upon the other; the normal being with the upper front teeth slightly over the bottom teeth.

**malposition.** Out of normal position; refers especially to the position of the baby in the uterus when it assumes an attitude unsuitable for easy delivery, or to the bad position of a tooth.

**malpresentation.** Any position of the baby during childbirth which impedes delivery.

**Malta fever.** See ABORTUS FEVER.

**Malthus doctrine.** The doctrine advanced by Malthus in the nineteenth century which claimed that the increase in the world's population was proportionately greater than that of food supplies. Malthus advocated that this should be prevented by late marriage and the teaching of contraception.

**mamilla.** The breast nipple or a nipple-like prominence.

**mamillary.** Strictly, pertaining to a breast nipple, but now commonly used to indicate anything pertaining to the female breast.

**mamma.** The breast; the mammary gland.

**mammalgia.** Pain in the breast.

**mammary.** Pertaining to the breast.

**mammary abscess.** An abscess of the breast usually connected with breast feeding, the infection entering through a cracked nipple. Also called *milk abscess.*

**mammate.** Possessing breasts.

**mammectomy.** Surgical removal of a breast. Also called *mastectomy.*

**mandible, mandibula.** The lower jawbone. See also JAW.

**mandibular.** Pertaining to the lower jaw.

**Mandl's paint.** A mixture of iodine and oil of peppermint in glycerine, commonly used for painting inflamed throats prior to the discovery of antibiotics.

**mandragora.** The mandrake plant. It has narcotic and sedative properties.

*The mandrake has a very long history with many legends centering around it. The ancients believed it to be an aphrodisiac as well as a narcotic and the Bible records (Genesis 30, 14) that Rachel sought the mandrakes of Leah as a cure for barrenness. The plant derives its name from its fork-shaped roots which bear a crude resemblance to a man, and it was believed that if the plant was uprooted the man in the roots shrieked in agony and that anybody who heard this would go mad. Shakespeare had Juliet say: "And shriek like mandrakes torn out of the earth, that living mortals, hearing them, run mad" (Act 4, sc. 3). So, in order to avoid hearing the shriek, either a dog was tied to the roots and made to pull up the plant or the gatherer stuffed his ears and blew a horn.*

**mange.** An infectious disease of domestic animals which affects their skin and causes bare patches in their fur. It is caused by itch mites belonging to the family *Sarcoptidae*, and is occasionally transmissible to man.

**camel mange.** This type is a curse to those who ride camels, and caused a big epidemic among the Camel Corps in Palestine in 1919.

**cat mange.** This type is also transmissible to man. The female mite burrows into the patient's skin to lay its eggs, just as in scabies. The eggs germinate in eight days and the young mites emerge from and run about the skin, causing intense itching.

**dog mange.** This type occurs especially in women who cuddle pets up to their necks. It rarely produces a widespread rash, and is quickly cured by sulfur ointment.

**horse mange.** This occurs in stable lads and others in contact with horses, and was prevalent in mounted units during the First World War.

**mania.** 1. Tremendous enthusiasm or overexcitement; any excessive desire or passion. 2. A mental disorder, characterized variously by emotional excitement, flight of ideas, hallucinations, delusions, disturbance of orientation, extreme muscular restlessness, and incessant talking. The whole picture represents a very obvious mental disturbance, often of a violent nature. The term also refers to a syndrome due to some organic cause, such as chronic alcoholism or poisoning by certain drugs causing mental excitement or dementia paralytica.

**maniac.** A person affected with mania.

**manic.** Pertaining to mania.

**manic-depressive insanity.** A mental derangement occurring at intervals, either as an acute mania or as a profound depression, not leading to mental deterioration of the faculties during the intervening periods.

**Mantoux reaction.** A skin test for tuberculosis in which a minute amount of dead tubercle bacteria is injected into the skin. A positive test shows at the injection site after 48 hours, being an edematous swelling surrounded by a pink zone. This means only that a tuberculous infection has occurred in the patient, and, except in small children, is not evidence that the infection is active at the time of the test. A negative test shows no skin reaction and is evidence that the patient is not suffering from tuberculosis.

**manubrium.** A handle-shaped structure, particularly the manubrium sterni, the upper portion of the sternum.

**marasmus.** General wasting of the body.

**marble bones.** See OSTEOPETROSIS.

**marginal abscess.** See ISCHORECTAL ABSCESS.

**marihuana.** A drug of habituation obtained from the plant, Indian hemp, *Cannabis sativus*, and usually smoked in cigarettes. Research on the nature of the intoxication report the following transitory effects: reddening of the eyes, slight increase in pulse rate, fuzziness of memory, irritation of lung tissue, and a slight lessening on performance tests of a psychomotor nature. Users of marihuana report such effects as euphoria, beauty, distortions of vision and space, etc. Further scientific studies are needed to learn the long-term effects. Also called *cannabis, hashish, marijuana, grass, weed, pot, Indian hemp.*

**marrow.** The soft substance filling the cavities of the long bones which manufactures the red blood cells.

(section of bone)

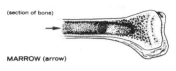

MARROW (arrow)

**marsh fever.** Malaria.

**masochism.** A sexual perversion in which pleasure is obtained in receiving cruel treatment, pain, and humiliation; named after Leopold von Sacher-Masoch, an Austrian novelist, who both indulged in and wrote about these practices.

**massage.** Therapeutic manipulation of tissues, as stroking, kneading, or tapping either with the hand or an instrument such as a vibrator.

**masseter.** The large jaw muscle on the side of the face, which hardens and can be felt when the jaws are clenched.

**mastadenitis.** Inflammation of the breast tissue.

**mastadenoma.** A harmless tumor of the breast. See also ADENOFIBROMA.

**mastalgia.** Pain in the breast.

**mastectomy.** Surgical removal of a breast. Also called *mammectomy*.

**mastitis.** Inflammation of a breast.

**mastodynia.** Pain in the breast.

**mastoid.** The mastoid process; the air cells situated behind and above the ear, which communicate with the middle ear.

**mastoidal.** Pertaining to the mastoid.

**mastoidalgia.** Pain in the mastoid area.

**mastoid antrum.** The cavity in the region of the mastoid bone behind the ear.

**mastoidectomy.** Surgical removal of mastoid air cells behind the ear which have become inflamed by middle-ear disease. Since the introduction of antibiotics for the treatment of middle-ear infections, the operation is less frequently performed.

**mastoiditis.** Inflammation of the mastoid air cells behind the ear.

**mastoidotomy.** Incision of the mastoid air cells behind the ear.

**mastopexy.** A plastic surgical operation on the breast.

**mastorrhagia.** Bleeding from the breast.

**masturbation.** Production of sexual orgasm by self-manipulation of the genitals. Also called *self-abuse, chiromania.*

*Masturbation can be seen in small babies who rub their thighs together for the pleasurable sensation it evokes,* *not, of course, for sexual gratification. Infantile masturbation passes off quickly, but the habit may recur in two to four-year olds and again in the school years, when, inevitably, it is linked with some fantasy. In children, the harm done by masturbation is more due to the guilty feeling it induces than to the actual incident, and as a rule it is a cold, lonely, and frightened child who masturbates itself to sleep—not a sex maniac. The act is a compulsive, nervous habit related to nail-biting, head rolling, sucking, chewing and biting habits, and sometimes stammering. The essential quality common to them all is the repetition of an act to which there is a strong, compulsive urge, a feeling of tension until the act is performed, followed by a temporary sense of relief. Many mothers naturally link masturbation in a child with the adult sex act and they must overcome their own feelings of anxiety and repugnance before they can successfully deal with the habit in their child. It is useless to increase the child's sense of shame, for all these activities are, to some extent, fired off by anxiety, and if the symptom is driven in to a more primitive mental level, the habit will certainly be more likely to be indulged in secretly. If the sense of shame can be excluded, the child can be more readily freed to play with things other than his own body. A certain amount of petting, alternative outlets, and free social activity, all go far to counteract this pull-back into fantasy, and if the child can talk about his imaginations, so much the better. However, any detailed treatment of the symptom is better dealt with in a child guidance clinic.*

**matter.** Pus.

**maxilla.** The upper jaw. See also JAW.

**maxillary.** Pertaining to the upper jaw.

**M.B.** The abbreviation for *medicinae baccalaureus*, the Latin for bachelor of medicine.

**McBurney's point.** The point of maximum tenderness in acute appendicitis. It is about one-third of the way along an imaginary line drawn between the navel and the anterior superior iliac spine (front part of the hipbone). This only applies when the appendix lies in its usual position, but if it is curled underneath the colon, the tender point may be in the flank.

**M.D.** 1. The abbreviation for *medicinae doctor*, the Latin for doctor of medicine. 2. An abbreviation for mental defective.

**measles.** A highly infectious virus disease characterized by fever, catarrh of the upper respiratory tract, a distinctive rash, with a liability to complications, such as inflammation of the middle ear and pneumonia. One attack usually confers immunity. An effective vaccine has been developed which probably gives immunity for life. The vaccine is usually given to nine- or ten-month old infants. If the child has already been exposed, gamma globulin rather than the vaccine is recommended. Gamma globulin injection may prevent the child from contracting measles, but if not, the disease will usually take a milder course and with fewer complications. Also called *morbilli, rubeola*. See also GERMAN MEASLES.

*Measles occurs in epidemic form every two or three years, 85 percent of all cases being in children between the ages of six months and ten years. More than half of these cases are in children up to the age of five years, though babies under six months of age are rarely affected, for it would seem they have an inherited immunity. Nine or ten days after becoming infected the child develops what appears to be a severe head cold, with sore eyes, running nose, a hard cough, and a temperature which may reach 103 F. For the next two or three days all the symptoms become aggravated; the temperature rises to 104 - 105 F., and small spots which look like a grain of salt on a pink base, or Koplik spots, appear on the inside of the cheeks. The rash appears two or three days after the Koplik spots, starting about the brows, behind and below the ears, and around the mouth, and spreading rapidly, sometimes after a short hesitation, over the face, neck, trunk, and extremities. It is usually fully out by the fifth or sixth day.*

**meatal.** Pertaining to a meatus.

**meatus.** Any passage, channel, or orifice.

**external auditory meatus.** The ear opening and ear passage.

**urethral meatus.** The opening of the urethra, the tube through which urine is discharged from the body.

**Meckel's diverticulum.** The blind end of what was the yolk sac in the embryo, situated from one to three feet above the ileocolic valve. It is present in some form in about only 2½ per cent of individuals. Many forms of acute abdominal trouble have been caused by this vestigial structure and even inflammatory attacks similar to acute appendicitis. Occasionally gallstones have lodged within it and caused perforation and peritonitis.

**meconium.** The dark green feces discharged from the bowels of a newborn baby. It is a normal phenonenon, but unless the mother is previously warned, it can produce profound maternal anxiety.

**media. 1.** The middle coat of a vein, artery, or lymph vessel. **2.** The transparent parts of the eye. **3.** Substances used for culturing microorganisms.

**mediastinal.** Pertaining to the mediastinum.

**mediastinitis.** Inflammation of the mediastinum.

**mediastinum.** The space between the lungs, or more accurately that between the sacs of pleural membrane containing the lungs. It is divided into anterior, middle, posterior, and superior mediastinum.

**anterior mediastinum.** This area contains blood vessels to the breasts.

**middle mediastinum.** This area contains the heart, the aorta, the vena cava, the division of the trachea, and the pulmonary arteries and veins.

**posterior mediastinum.** This area contains part of the aorta, the esophagus, and other veins and nerves.

**superior mediastinum.** This area lying above the heart contains the origins of various muscles, the transverse portion of the arch of the aorta, the left carotid and subclavian arteries, and other blood vessels and nerves, as well as the trachea, esophagus, and remains of the thymus gland.

**medicine. 1.** Any substance used in treating disease or relieving pain. **2.** The art or science of restoring or preserving health.

**Mediterranean fever.** See ABORTUS FEVER.

**medium. 1.** An intervening substance or space in which anything moves or through which it acts. **2.** A substance used to cultivate bacteria. **3.** A halfway stage.

**medulla. 1.** The bone marrow or anything resembling marrow in structure or in relationship to other parts, such as a fatty substance occupying certain cavities; the central part of an organ as distinguished from the cortex or outside. **2.** The medulla oblongata, a portion of the brain continuous with the spinal cord.

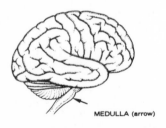

MEDULLA (arrow)

**medullar, medullary.** Pertaining to the marrow or a medulla.

**medullated.** Containing or surrounded by a medulla.

**megacaecum.** See MEGACECUM.

**megacardia.** A large heart.

**megacecum.** An abnormally large cecum.

**megacephaly.** A large head. Also called *macrocephaly, megalocephaly*.

**megacolon.** A large, distended colon. Also called *Hirschsprung's disease*.

**megalocephaly.** A large head. Also called *macrocephaly, megacephaly*.

**megalomania.** A mental condition characterized by delusions of grandeur.

**meibomian cyst.** A cyst caused by blockage of a meibomian gland. These glands, similar to the sebaceous glands of the skin, are on the inner surface of the eyelids, with openings emerging on the free margins of the lids. When these glands become inflamed and swollen, they look like styes, but whereas a stye occurs in an eyelash follicle on the free edge of the eyelid, a meibomian cyst occurs in the substance of the eyelid and can only be seen by everting the eyelid.

**meiosis. 1.** Excessive contraction of the pupil of the eye. **2.** A special type of cell division in which there is a reduction in chromosome numbers.

**melaena.** See MELENA.

**melanaemia.** See MELANEMIA.

**melancholia.** A mental disorder characterized by extreme depression, fear, brooding, painful delusions, and a disinclination to undertake any mental or physical activity. In one variety, however, there is gross agitation. The term is derived from the Greek for black bile, which was considered by the ancient Greek physicians to be the cause of this mental disturbance.

**melanemesis.** Also called *black vomit, coffee-ground vomit*. See HEMATEMESIS.

**melanemia.** A condition in which black pigment is found in the blood.

**melaniferous.** Containing melanin.

**melanin.** A black pigment occurring normally in the coats of the eye, skin, hair, and muscles. It may be increased in the skin and lining membranes of the body in Addison's disease and in melanotic tumors. It is also the basis of sun tan.

**melanism.** The abnormal presence of melanin in an organ.

**melanocarcinoma.** Melanoma.

**melanoderma.** Abnormal pigmentation of the skin.

**melanodermatitis toxica lichenoides.** Tar worker's dermatitis.

**melanogen.** The substance which is the forerunner in the production of melanin.

**melanoid.** Dark colored; resembling melanin.

**melanoma.** Any tumor characterized by the presence of melanin pigment. Strictly speaking this is a harmless tumor, such as a pigmented mole.

**melanoma sarcoma.** A pigmented mole that has become cancerous. Also called *melanotic carcinoma, melanosarcoma.*

**melanomatosis.** The presence of multiple melanomas.

**melanosarcoma.** A melanoma.

**melanosis.** Abnormal pigmentation of the skin.

**melanosis coli.** Black pigmentation of the lining of the colon, which may be caused by purgatives.

**melanotic.** Containing melanin.

**melanuria.** The presence of melanin in the urine.

**melena.** The passage of dark, black stools, due to hemorrhage inside the intestinal tract, the blood having been altered by digestive processes. The possibility of this condition should always be borne in mind when a person known to suffer from a duodenal or gastric ulcer or longstanding, severe indigestion suddenly becomes pale, faint, and ill and does not recover within a few minutes, as happens with a simple faint. In cases of severe bleeding the patient may show signs of surgical shock and collapse; this indicates the need for urgent medical advice. The black stools may not be seen until 12 or 24 hours after the hemorrhage.

**melissophobia.** Fear of bees.

**melitensis.** Undulant fever.

**melitococcic fever.** See ABORTUS FEVER.

**melon-seed bodies.** Small objects found within a joint cavity or in a cyst attached to a tendon sheath.

**melts.** Animal spleen sold as pet food.

**membrane.** A thin layer of tissue surrounding a part, separating adjacent cavities, lining a cavity, or connecting adjacent structures.

**membranoid.** Like a membrane.

**membranous.** Relating to, having the nature of, or characterized by the formation of a membrane.

**menagogue.** An agent to promote the menstrual flow.

**menarche.** The appearance of the first monthly period.

**mendelism.** The laws of inheritance propounded by the Bohemian monk Mendel. An offspring inherits from his parents characteristics not as a blending of qualities from both of them but as separate units. Traits are described as either dominant or recessive. For example, brown eyes are dominant and blue eyes are recessive. If the two genes inherited, one each from each parent, are both dominant, the offspring will have brown eyes and will be pure for brown; if the two genes are brown and blue, the offspring will

again be brown-eyed and will be hybrid for brown; and if the two genes are blue, the offspring will be blue-eyed. The above example illustrates the Law of Dominance. In the plant world, red is dominant to white in sweet pea flowers. If a red flower is crossed with a white flower, all the first generation will be red-flowered, but hybrids for red. However, if these red hybrid flowers are self-fertilized, then the next generation will produce red flowers in the ratio of three to one. The union of the genes in the hybrid red flowers was only temporary, and when sperms and eggs are produced they are either carrying the gene for red color or for white color. This is called the Law of the Purity of Gametes. This separation of traits in the gametes and a new combination of traits in the next generation illustrates the Law of Segregation. There are some exceptions where the Law of Dominance does not operate.

**Ménière's disease.** A condition characterized by the sudden onset of vertigo, accompanied by nausea, vomiting, and increasing deafness, with noises in the ear. Also called *labyrinthitis.*

**meningeal.** Pertaining to the meninges.

**meninges.** The three membranes covering the brain and spinal cord. The outer membrane is called the dura mater, the middle one the arachnoid mater, and the innermost the pia mater.

**meningioma.** A tumor usually situated in the coverings of the brain, but occasionally found in other parts of the central nervous system. It grows by expansion but may be invasive and therefore malignant.

**meningism.** A state indicating irritation of the brain characterized by headache and neck stiffness, but without the signs of true meningitis. The term is also applied to a hysterical state simulating meningitis. Also called *pseudomeningitis.*

**meningitis.** Inflammation of the coverings of the brain, and practically always due to a germ arising in some part of the body other than the central nervous system. When it affects the dura mater it is called pachymeningitis; when it involves the pia mater and arachnoid mater it is called leptomeningitis. There are also many subdivisions classified according to the causative organism, the mode of onset, or clinical course of the disease.

*The germ may be blood-borne from some other part of the body or be produced from an extension of infection within the skull, such as an inward extension of ear disease. The clinical features of acute meningitis vary in in-*

*tensity from case to case, but the commonest are intense headache, pain in the back or neck, with rigidity of the spine, especially in the neck. There is a characteristic combination of irritability with drowsiness, in some cases passing on to coma. The patient often lies curled up on his side in a stuporous condition, becoming irritable and refractory if disturbed. There may be bouts of restlessness and periodical inarticulate cries. The nonpassage of urine is a common and sometimes early sign, which together with a raised temperature, severe headache, and neck stiffness are sufficient to arouse the suspicion of meningitis. The withdrawal of some cerebrospinal fluid by lumbar puncture to determine both diagnosis and cause is usually the first medical investigation. Antibiotics and cortisone have completely altered the outlook for nearly all cases of meningitis, irrespective of their cause. Since many of these cases arise in children the anxious mother frequently arrives at a diagnosis of meningitis on the most flimsy grounds, such as a headache and vomiting. Unless, however, there is also neck stiffness, indicated by the child's reluctance to have his neck lifted from the pillow and flexed, or inability to draw up his knee and touch it with the mouth, then the condition is unlikely to be meningitis.*

**meningocele.** A rare, congenital deformity in which the cerebral or spinal coverings protrude through a bony defect in the skull or vertebral column. The defect can be closed by surgery.

*The human embryo commences as a flat plate which turns on itself and joins to form a tube, but on rare occasions a slight defect in the join allows the meningeal membranes to protrude.*

**meningococcus.** The germ that causes cerebrospinal fever.

**meningoencephalitis.** Inflammation of the brain and its coverings.

**meningoencephalocele.** A protrusion of the brain and its coverings through a bony defect in the skull. See also MENINGOCELE.

**meningoencephalomyelitis.** Inflammation of the coverings of the brain and the spinal cord.

**meningomyelitis.** Inflammation of the spinal cord and its coverings.

**meningomyelocele.** A protrusion of a part of the spinal cord and its membranes through a bony defect in the spinal column. See also MENINGOCELE.

**meniscectomy.** Removal of a cartilage from within a joint, usually the knee joint.

**meniscotomy.** Surgical removal of a meniscus.

**meniscus.** 1. Any crescent-shaped structure. 2. A disc of gristle found inside a joint. **3.** A type of lens. **4.** The crescentic surface of liquids in narrow tubes.

**meniscus lateralis.** The outer of the two cartilages of the knee joint.

**meniscus medialis.** The internal cartilage of the knee joint.

*The meniscus lateralis and medialis are often damaged by athletes and football players. The injury is caused by turning sharply while running at speed, and grinding off a piece of cartilage which lodges between the bones of the joint and locks it solid so that the patient is unable to straighten the leg. The first aid for these injuries is to support the knee on one or two pillows, to keep it flexed, and then seek medical aid.*

**menopausal.** Pertaining to the change of life in a woman.

**menopause.** That time in a woman's life at which her childbearing period is coming to an end. It usually occurs between the ages of 40 and 50 years, and in most women is characterized only by the cessation of menstruation. In other women there is a heightened emotional change which causes irritability, attacks of depression, and hot flushes all over the body. These can be controlled by sedatives and hormone treatment. Some of the depression arises because the woman fears she will no longer be able to respond to the sexual advances of her husband. This is, of course, a complete myth. Any sexual frigidity that occurs is due purely to the psychological depression and upset that this fear promotes, for even women in their sixties can still be sexually excitable and responsive. It is a curious fact that often there is a sudden increase in some women's fertility during the menopause and, not having had a child for many years, they find themselves pregnant at a time when it is unwelcome. It is therefore unsafe to abandon contraceptive practices until a woman has reached the age of 48 and has not menstruated for the previous two years, for then she is quite unlikely to conceive. Also called *change of life, climacteric.*

**artificial menopause.** A menopause caused by surgical removal or irradiation of the ovaries.

**menorrhagia.** Excessive loss of blood at the menstrual periods. It can only be estimated in relation to the previous history of the woman's menstrual flow and whether the blood loss is excessive enough to produce anemia. If the loss is excessive then the womb will have to be scraped, for not only is this procedure a diagnostic test for menorrhagia but it is frequently curative.

**menorrhea.** Properly, the normal flow of the menstrual periods, but commonly applied to describe an excessive menstrual flow. Strictly speaking excessive flow should be called hypermenorrhea or menorrhagia.

**menorrhoea.** See MENORRHEA.

**menses.** The monthly discharge of blood from the uterus. The mechanism of menstruation is quite simply this: Each monthly cycle starts with an egg rupturing from the ovary and passing into the Fallopian tube, where it awaits fertilization. If fertilization fails to take place, the lining of the womb or the endometrium, under the influence of the ovary, breaks down, splits off, and causes bleeding from small blood vessels. This blood then mingles with the broken-down endometrium to form the menstrual discharge. A new endometrium then commences to grow in preparation for a possible pregnancy the following month. There is a popular fallacy that menstruation is a monthly loss of "bad blood." This is nonsense, for if the womb fails to bleed there is, of course, no blood to go anywhere and as it is normal blood anyway it cannot do harm. Normally, if a woman who has had regular periods fails to menstruate, it means that she is pregnant, though certain emotional strains can interfere with the menstrual cycle and cause suppression of the monthly period. However, this is less common than pregnancy. Those women who have always been irregular with periods, and sometimes go months without one, usually have a defect of the womb or ovaries which is frequently amenable to hormone treatment.

**menstruation.** The menses.

**menstruum. 1.** Latin for monthly. **2.** A solvent; the term arose in pharmacy because at one time some extracts were left to "work" for several weeks to get the maximum extraction from the chemical or herb into the solvent.

**mensuration.** The process of measuring.

**mental.** Pertaining to the mind.

**mentum.** The chin.

**mesal.** Relating to or lying in the middle line.

**mesarteritis.** Inflammation of the middle coat of an artery.

**mesencephalon.** The midbrain.

**mesenteric.** Relating to a mesentery.

**mesenteritis.** Inflammation of mesentery.

**mesenterium.** A mesentery.

**mesentery.** A fold of peritoneum attaching the intestines to the back wall of the abdomen. Lying within the folds

of the mesentery are the mesenteric glands.

**mesial.** Related to or lying in the middle line of the body.

**mesmerism.** Animal magnetism or hypnotism. See ANIMAL MAGNETISM.

**mesoappendix.** The mesentery of the appendix.

**mesocolic.** Pertaining to the mesocolon.

**mesocolon.** The peritoneal fold connecting the colon with the back wall of the abdomen.

**mesoderm.** The middle layer of the three germinal layers of the embryo. It lies between the ectoderm and the entoderm, and produces connective tissue, bone, cartilage, muscle, sex organs, urinary organs, the heart, and blood vessels.

**metabolic.** Pertaining to metabolism.

**metabolism.** The complex phenomena by which the body builds foodstuffs up into complex tissue elements (anabolism) and also converts complex substances into simple ones for the use of body energy (catabolism).

**basal metabolism.** The minimum amount of energy expenditure necessary to maintain essential body life when the body itself is at complete rest in a warm room, 12 to 18 hours after the intake of food.

**metabolite.** Any product of metabolism.

**metacarpal.** Pertaining to the metacarpus.

**metacarpectomy.** Surgical removal of any of the metacarpal bones.

**metacarpophalangeal.** Pertaining to the metacarpus and the phalanges (finger bones).

**metacarpus.** The five metacarpal bones which form the palm of the hand.

**metal fume fever.** A feverish reaction following the inhalation of finely divided particles of metallic oxides. Also called *brass chills, brass founders' ague, metal ague, zinc chills, smelters' shakes.*

**metaphrenia.** A mental state in which the patient directs all his energies to personal gain or aggrandisement and completely neglects or ignores his family.

**metaphyseal, metaphysial.** Relating to a metaphysis.

**metaphysis.** The growing end of a bone situated between the epiphysis and the diaphysis of a long bone.

**metaphysitis.** Inflammation of a metaphysis.

**metaplasia.** The transformation of one tissue into another.

**metaplastic.** Pertaining to metaplasia.

**metastasis.** The transfer of disease from a primary focus to a distant one by conveying the causal agent or cells through blood vessels or lymph channels. This is the mode by which cancer spreads.

**metastatic.** Pertaining to metastasis.

**metastatic abscess.** An abscess caused by an infected embolus, as a blood clot, usually in the lung or liver, arising in cases of pyemia, caused by pus-producing organisms in the blood, or by subacute bacterial endocarditis.

**metatarsal.** Relating to any of the five bones constituting the metatarsus region of the foot.

**metatarsalgia.** A sudden burning cramp in the front portion of the foot, in the region of the fourth metatarsal bone. The pain, the source of which is obscure, usually occurs in one foot only, and is agonizing, requiring removal of the shoe and massage of the foot to get relief. Metatarsalgia is frequently due to wearing shoes which are too short, or it may be associated with a dropping of the front arch of the foot.

*Any factor which throws the major weight of the body on to the outside of the foot, instead of transmitting it to the bones of the big toe and first metatarsal, can produce this type of pain. The condition is met with in women who wear shoes which, irrespective of the height of the heel, have no internal platform on which the heel can rest, so that the continuous sharp slope forwards from the heel compels the foot to slide downwards, crushing the heads of the metatarsal bones together and curling up the toes.*

**metatarsectomy.** Surgical removal of a metatarsal bone.

**metatarsophalangeal.** Pertaining to metatarsus and the phalanges of the toes.

**metatarsus.** The five metatarsal bones situated between the bones of the instep and the toes.

**meteorism.** Gaseous distension of the abdomen. Also called *tympanites.*

**methaemoglobin.** See METHEMOGLOBIN.

**methaemoglobinaemia.** See METHEMO-GLOBINEMIA.

**methaemoglobinuria.** See METHEMO-GLOBINURIA.

**methemoglobin.** An altered form of hemoglobin, chocolate-brown in color, found in the blood after poisoning by chemicals like potassium chlorate, nitrates, nitrobenzol, acetanilid, and phenacetin. Since phenacetin and other of these chemicals are included in popular headache and pain-relieving remedies, the danger of taking such remedies without medical advice is clearly evident.

**methemoglobinemia.** The presence of methemoglobin in the blood.

**methemoglobinuria.** The presence of methemoglobin in the urine.

**metra.** The womb (uterus).

**metralgia.** Pain in the womb.

**metrectomy.** Surgical removal of the womb. Also called *hysterectomy.*

**metritis.** Inflammation of the womb.

**metrocarcinoma.** Cancer of the womb.

**metropathia, metropathy.** Any disease of the womb.

**metropathia hemorrhagica.** Painless excessive bleeding from the womb, associated with alterations in the ovaries and probably caused by a hormone defect.

**metropathic.** Pertaining to disorders of the womb.

**metroperitonitis.** Inflammation of the womb and peritoneum; peritonitis resulting from inflammation of the womb; inflammation of the peritoneal covering the womb.

**metroptosis.** Dropping of the womb.

**metrorrhagia.** Bleeding from the womb, not connected with menstruation.

**metrorrhea.** Any discharge from the womb.

**metrorrhexis.** Rupture of the womb.

**metrorrhoea.** See METRORRHEA.

**metrosalpingitis.** Inflammation of the womb and the Fallopian tube.

**metrosalpinx.** The uterine or Fallopian tube.

**metrostaxis.** Continuous bleeding from the womb.

**Michel's clips.** Metal clips used as an alternative to stitches for closing a skin wound.

**micrencephalon.** 1. An abnormally small brain. 2. The cerebellum.

**micrencephalous.** Pertaining to micrencephalon.

**micrencephalus.** A person with an abnormally small brain.

**microbe.** A living organism of minute size, usually microscopic; applied especially to microscopic forms of life capable of causing disease.

**microbial, microbic.** Pertaining to a microbe.

**microbiology.** The science of microorganisms.

**microcephalic.** Pertaining to microcephaly.

**microcephalism.** The condition of having an abnormally small head.

**microcephalous.** Relating to an abnormally small head.

**microcephalus.** A person with an abnormally small head.

**microcephaly.** Abnormal smallness of the head.

**micron.** A unit of measurement and equal to a one-thousandth part of a millimeter. A conventional microscope will reveal objects of this size, while the ultraelectronic microscope will reveal objects as small as one-millionth part of a millimeter.

**microorganism.** Any animal or plant organism so small that it is visible only through a microscope.

**microscope.** An instrument used to obtain an enlarged view of small objects and reveal details not seen by the unaided eye.

**microscopic.** Of such extremely small size as to be visible only by the use of a microscope.

**microtome.** An instrument used to cut tissue into extremely thin sections for microscopic examination.

**miction.** Micturition.

**micturate.** To pass urine.

**micturition.** The act of passing urine.

**midbrain.** The mesencephalon.

**migraine.** A condition characterized by paroxysysmal intense pain in the head, preceded or accompanied by disturbances of sensation or muscle movement, or both, with various other phenomena. The headache is usually confined to one side and is often followed by vomiting. The attack is sometimes heralded by alterations in vision, such as inability to focus the eyes for reading, or the presence of dancing colored lights. Less common features are confusion of speech, inability to read words, or even loss of speech. Other phenomena sometimes experienced include: a feeling that insects are crawling across the skin, which, although harmless, is alarming to the patient; numbness of various parts of the body, such as the lips and tongue; and, very rarely, paralysis of the sixth and sometimes of the third and fourth cranial nerves, or a combination of all three, resulting in severe double vision which passes off in a few days, or, at most, in a few weeks. Unfortunately, once this does occur it is apt to recur with subsequent attacks. Migraine subjects are commonly energetic and highly intelligent, and many have a meticulous standard of thoroughness and precision, almost amounting to obsession. The malady may originate in early childhood, but commonly appears at puberty and tends to persist, with fluctuations in severity and frequency, throughout adult and middle life. Women often have migraine attacks associated with their monthly periods, only to remain entirely free during pregnancy, and ceasing altogether at the change of life. Its persistence into old age in either sex is exceptional. Many patients become morbidly depressed, fearing they have a brain disease, but a history of migraine from childhood is a strong indication that this is unlikely. However, the sudden onset of migraine in an adult does require complete investigation by a nerve specialist. One form which can produce diagnostic difficulties is that in which the pain occurs not in the head but in the abdomen; this is called abdominal migraine. Nothing is known with certainty as to the essential cause of migraine, and even though there is a strong belief that it is due to the spasm of a blood vessel in the brain, absolute proof is lacking. Many authorities are firmly convinced that it is an allergic disorder associated with familial diseases such as asthma, hay fever, and urticaria. Errors of visual refraction, digestive disorders, upsets of endocrine function, and psychological disturbances have all been blamed as responsible causes, but it is probable that they are never more than precipitating factors in susceptible individuals. Fatigue, anxiety, and frustration do play an important part, as do overexertion, indiscretions or irregularities of food, exposure to excessive light or noise, and prolonged eyestrain. Treatment consists in the patient trying to take a calmer approach to life, and the correction of any abnormality, especially the wearing of spectacles if these are needed. Combinations of sedative and antispasmodic drugs, taken regularly in small doses over a very long period, reduce the number of attacks and, sometimes, may even effect a cure. Ergotamine tartrate, if taken early, will frequently cut short an attack, and for mild attacks a long sleep in bed will often free the patient of headache. Apart from these measures, there have been almost as many remedies guaranteed to cure as there are patients with migraine! Also called *hemicrania*.

**migrans.** Wandering.

**mil. 1.** A thousandth part of a liter, one cubic centimeter. **2.** A thousandth part of an inch.

**miliaria.** A severe inflammatory condition of the sweat glands.

**miliaria rubra.** See PRICKLY HEAT.

**miliary.** A descriptive term applied to conditions in which the lesions are about the size of millet seeds—one-half to one millimeter. For example, in miliary tuberculosis, a blood-transmitted form of tuberculosis, there are tiny lesions in many parts of the body.

**miliary abscess.** A minute tuberculous abscess.

**milieu.** Environment.

**milium.** A small, pearly, noninflammatory elevation, situated mainly on the face. These milia often become quite hard and last for years.

**colloid milium.** A form of skin degeneration, usually affecting persons of middle or advanced age, characterized by the presence, especially on the face, of minute, shining, flat or slightly raised lesions of a pale or bright lemon color.

**milk. 1.** The whitish fluid secreted by the breasts for the nourishment of the young. **2.** Any whitish fluid resembling milk, such as coconut milk. **3.** A suspension of chemicals, such as milk of magnesia.

**adapted milk.** Milk modified to suit the digestive capacity of a child.

**after-milk.** The stripping or the last milk obtained at a milking.

**buttermilk.** Milk which remains after churning butter.

**certified milk.** Cow's milk obtained and bottled according to regulations designed to minimize milk-borne infection.

**citric acid milk.** A milk preparation to which citric acid has been added.

**condensed milk.** Milk that has been partially evaporated and enriched by sugar.

**evaporated milk.** Milk treated by heat to lose about half of its water content. It is then canned, sterilized, and sometimes fortified by ultraviolet irradiation.

**fore-milk. 1.** The milk first withdrawn at each milking. **2.** Colostrum, the thickened secretion obtained from the breasts before proper lactation starts.

**fortified milk.** Milk enriched by ingredients such as albumin, cream, or vitamins.

**homogenized milk.** Milk so treated that the fat globules are very minute and emulsification so complete that the cream does not separate when the milk is allowed to stand.

**hydrochloric acid milk.** Milk acidified by the addition of dilute hydrochloric acid.

**humanized milk.** Cow's milk altered in composition to closely resemble human milk.

**lactic acid milk.** Cow's milk treated with lactic acid to make it more digestible. It is used to feed babies with a weak digestion.

**lemon juice milk.** Milk to which ¾ ounce of lemon juice has been added per quart.

**modified milk.** See HUMANIZED MILK, above.

**pasteurized milk.** Milk that has been heat-treated to destroy germs.

**skimmed milk.** Milk from which the cream has been removed. Also called *separated milk.*

**vegetable milk.** A synthetic milk derived from vegetables such as the soya bean.

**witch's milk.** The milk that sometimes appears in the breasts of newborn babies. See also BREAST.

**milk abscess.** See MAMMARY ABSCESS.

**milk crust.** A crusty mass seen on the scalps of very young babies. It is a form of seborrhea which rapidly responds to the following ointment: Hydrarg. Ammon. Chlor. 15 grains, Liquor Picis Carb. 30 minims. Paraffin Molle Flav. to one ounce; apply night and morning.

**milk fever.** See CHILDBED FEVER.

**milk leg.** A swelling and inflammation of the leg caused by phlebitis of the femoral vein and sometimes associated with childbirth.

**milk pox.** A mild form of smallpox.

**milk sickness. 1.** An acute disease accompanied by weakness, loss of appetite, and vomiting, due to drinking milk or eating flesh of animals which have contracted a disease called trembles. **2.** Milk sickness is also a popular name for brucellosis, which is contracted by drinking milk from animals infected with the germ of brucellosis.

**milk teeth.** The first or deciduous teeth. See also TEETH.

**Miller-Abbott tube.** A double-tubed nasal catheter, used for the relief of intestinal distensions due to obstruction in the small intestine. It is passed down the nose and the smaller tube is inflated to produce a small balloon at its tip which the normal movement of the intestine then takes down to the desired location. The larger tube is then used to aspirate intestinal contents.

**miner's asthma.** See SILICOSIS.

**miner's elbow.** Inflammation of the bursa over the elbow. Also called *student's elbow.* See also BURSA.

**miner's nystagmus.** A condition seen in coal miners in which the eyes are in a state of constant movement.

**miner's phthisis.** See SILICOSIS.

**miner's spit.** The black spit of the coal miner which contains particles of coal dust.

**miosis.** Constriction of the pupil of the eye. Also called *meiosis.*

**miotic.** Pertaining to miosis.

**mirror speech.** Speech in which the syllables are spoken backwards.

**mirror writing.** Writing in which the words are written backwards, as they would appear in a mirror.

**misandry.** A dislike of men.

**misanthrope.** A person who hates the society of other people and wants to be a recluse.

**miscarriage.** See ABORTION.

**misce.** The Latin for mix; used on a doctor's prescription as an instruction to the chemist to mix the ingredients.

**miscible.** Refers to substances which can be mixed together.

**misogamy.** Hatred of marriage.

**misogyny.** Hatred of women.

**mistura.** The Latin for a medical mixture.

**mithridatism.** Immunity to poison acquired by its administration in gradually increasing doses. See also SULFUR.

**mitosis.** The normal process of cell reproduction by which a cell divides—both cytoplasm and nucleus—into two daughter cells. Each daughter cell receives a full complement of the chromosomes present in the original cell. Also called *karyokinesis*.

1. parent cell at rest    2. chromosomes condense

3. nuclear wall disintegrates    4. chromosomes align and split

5. chromosomes separate    6. nuclei begin to organize

7. two halves of cell separate    8. two identical daughter cells

MITOSIS

**mitral.** Resembling a bishop's miter in shape.

**mitral valve.** The valve situated between the left atrium and left ventricle of the heart, which, when open, resembles a bishop's miter. It is frequently affected by rheumatic fever. Also called *atrioventricular valve*.

**mittelschmerz.** German for middle pain. The term is applied to abdominal pain occurring regularly halfway between two menstrual periods. It is thought to be due to changes in the maturing egg cell and probably marks the time at which it ruptures out of the ovary and begins to make its way towards the Fallopian tube.

**mobilization.** 1. The act of reestablishing mobility in a fixed or stiffened part, a joint for example. 2. The freeing of an organ to make it accessible during surgery. 3. The liberation of a substance stored in the body, such as mobilization of the glycogen stored in the liver.

**molar.** A grinding tooth. One of the large double back teeth, of which there are three on each side of both jaws.

**mole.** 1. A mass formed in the womb when a pregnancy dies and degenerates. 2. The term is loosely applied to any blemish of the skin; see NEVUS.

**blood mole.** A mass of clotted blood, membranes, and placenta sometimes found in the womb after an abortion.

**carneous mole.** See FLESHY MOLE, below.

**cystic mole.** See HYDATIDIFORM MOLE, below.

**fleshy mole.** 1. A blood mole which has become more solid and assumed a fleshy appearance. 2. The almost shapeless remains of a dead fetus retained within the womb.

**hairy mole.** A pigmented mole on the skin, from which hairs are growing.

**hydatidiform mole.** A tumorlike growth in parts of the placenta within the womb. It grows rapidly and there is cystic degeneration which leads to undue enlargement of the pregnant womb with bloody discharge and often spontaneous abortion.

**pigmented mole.** A pigmented spot found in the skin.

**true mole.** A mole, found within the womb, which contains the remains of a fetus or fetal membranes.

**tubal mole.** The remains of a fetus which has grown in a Fallopian tube, died, and become infiltrated with blood.

**vesicular mole.** See HYDATIDIFORM MOLE, above.

**molluscous.** 1. Pertaining to molluscum. 2. Pertaining to the mollusca—slugs, snails, oysters, and the like.

**molluscum.** A term applied to certain chronic skin diseases characterized by pulpy nodules.

**molluscum contagiosum.** A chronic skin disease, probably of viral origin, characterized by small pearly, round, flat-topped tumors, sometimes with a central depression, containing a cheeselike substance arising from one of the layers of the skin.

**molluscum fibrosum.** See NEUROFIBROMATOSIS.

**molluscum sebaceum.** A skin tumor occurring mostly on the face and limbs. It grows rapidly for several weeks and then, if left alone, withers and disappears in two or three months.

**monarthric.** Pertaining to one joint.

**monarthritis.** Inflammation of one joint.

**monarticular.** Pertaining to one joint.

**monaural.** Pertaining to one ear.

**mongolian idiocy, mongolism.** See IDIOCY: MONGOLIAN IDIOCY.

**Monilia.** A group of fungi. Also called *Candida*.

**moniliasis.** A fungus infection which may affect the skin, mucous membranes, nails, bronchi, lungs, vagina,

or intestinal tract. Rarely, septicemia may occur.

**moniliform.** Shaped like a necklace or a string of beads.

**monobrachius.** Congenital absence of an arm.

**monocular.** Pertaining to one eye or to a microscope with a single eyepiece.

**monocyte.** A type of white blood cell.

**monocytic.** Pertaining to a monocyte.

**monocytopenia.** An abnormal decrease in monocytes in the blood.

**monocytopoiesis.** The process whereby monocytes are formed.

**monocytosis.** An abnormal increase of the monocytes in the blood.

**monodactylism.** A congenital malformation characterized by the presence of only one finger or one toe on the hand or foot.

**monodactylous.** Having only one finger or toe on a hand or foot.

**monomania.** A neurosis characterized by a fixed idea.

**monomaniac.** A person suffering from monomania.

**mononuclear.** Having a single nucleus.

**mononucleosis.** A condition of the blood or tissues in which there is an increase in the number of large monocytes.

**infectious mononucleosis.** A communicable disease of unknown origin, with fever, sore throat, generalized swollen lymph glands, especially those of the back of the neck, and an increase in abnormal mononuclear cells in the blood. There may be a rash similar to that of German measles, and enlargement of the spleen. Complete recovery is the rule and complications are rare. The disease may be of virus origin, it often occurs in mild epidemic form, and usually attacks children and young adults. The incubation period varies from five to twelve days and if the diagnosis is in doubt it is usually confirmed by the Paul-Bunnell blood test. There is no specific treatment apart from bed rest during the feverish stage but the condition produces so much debility that a long convalescence is required. Also called *glandular fever*.

**monoparaesthesia.** See MONOPARESTHESIA.

**monoparesis.** Paralysis of a single limb.

**monoparesthesia.** Numbness and tingling in a single limb.

**monophasia.** A condition characterized by limitation of speech to a single syllable, word, or phrase.

**monophobia.** Fear of being alone.

**monoplegia.** Paralysis of one limb or one group of muscles.

**monospasm.** The spasm of a single muscle or a group of muscles.

**monosymptomatic.** Having only one presenting symptom.

**mons pubis.** The rounded eminence of fatty tissue situated beneath the skin in front of the symphysis pubis (the region just above the external genital organs). It becomes covered with hair at puberty. Also called *mons veneris.*

**monthly sickness.** Menstruation.

**moral imbecile.** A person with inherent criminal tendencies, but who may or may not have a mental defect.

**moral insanity.** Insanity in which there is complete absence of moral values. The term is now rarely used.

**morbid.** Pertaining to disease or diseased parts.

**morbidity. 1.** The quality of disease or of being diseased; the conditions inducing disease. **2.** The ratio of sick individuals to the total population of a community.

**morbilli.** See MEASLES.

**morbilliform.** Resembling measles. Usually refers to a rash resembling that of measles.

**moria.** A morbid determination to make supposedly witty remarks.

**moribund.** In a dying state.

**morning sickness.** The nausea of pregnant women. It mainly occurs during the first three months but may continue throughout the pregnancy. A simple sedative or eating dry toast before getting out of bed in the morning may alleviate the condition. If these methods fail, many doctors prescribe Ancoloxin tablets or one of the many antiemetic tablets available. Antihistamine tablets, such as Anthisan and Benadryl, are also effective in some cases. See also HYPEREMESIS: HYPEREMESIS GRAVIDARUM.

**morphea.** A skin disease which may occur as bands or as small spots. These areas of skin become indurated and hard and are at first a pink color, which slowly tints into an ivory color. The areas lose their hair cells and sweat glands. Also called *white spot disease.* See also SCLERODERMA.

**morphoea.** See MORPHEA.

**morphogenesis, morphogeny.** The development of the form and structure of an organ.

**morphological.** Pertaining to morphology.

**morphology.** A branch of biology dealing with the form and structure of organisms.

**mortality. 1.** The death rate. **2.** The quality of being mortal.

**motile.** Capable of movement.

**motility.** Spontaneous movements; ability to perform voluntary movements.

**motion sickness.** Nausea, vertigo, and vomiting, due to the unaccustomed motion of a ship, airplane, train, or motor car affecting the organ of balance in the ear. Treatment consists in either using the form of transport which causes the sickness often enough to become acclimatized to the movement, and/or taking drugs which sedate the labyrinth of the ear and stomach and so limit the production of symptoms. There are several drugs for this purpose, but the most commonly used and probably the most effective is hyoscine.

**motor.** Pertaining to or that which causes movement, such as a motor nerve cell.

**motor aphasia.** Difficulty in articulation, producing retarded, scanty speech, usually associated with defects in writing and understanding and other processes not directly concerned with the production of speech. It is usually due to a lesion of the left cerebral hemisphere.

**motor area.** That part of the brain's surface which controls the movement of muscles.

**motor points.** Those places on the surface of the body from which stimulation of single muscles or motor nerves by electric current can best be obtained.

**motor syndrome.** Flaccidity of muscles with loss of power and sometimes exaggerated tendon reflexes due to a lesion of the cerebral cortex.

**mountain fever.** An infectious form of fever transmitted to man by some varieties of ticks, characterized by high temperature, headache, pains in bones and muscles, a red, spotty rash, and mental symptoms. Formerly thought to be limited to the Rocky Mountain area, the disease occurs throughout the Western Hemisphere. Also called *Rocky Mountain spotted fever.*

**mountain sickness.** A condition due to a deficiency of oxygen intake brought about by reduced air pressure and characterized by shortness of breath, rapid pulse, vomiting, headache, and a slowing up of mental functions. Also called *altitude sickness.*

*Before it was realized the condition was caused by lack of oxygen to the brain and oxygen-breathing apparatus supplied, it produced some curious results. For example, during the Second World War, prior to the installation of oxygen apparatus in high-flying aircraft, a bomber crew sent out on a raid returned and bombed their own airdrome, thinking they were over the enemy target.*

**movement. 1.** A change of position. **2.** Evacuation of the bowels; the feces, the matter evacuated from the bowels.

**mucilage.** A watery solution of a gum or of starch.

**mucilaginous.** Pertaining to the nature of mucilage.

**mucin.** The principal constituent of mucus. It is insoluble in water but soluble in dilute alkali, and it is for this reason that nasal catarrh is often treated by the sniffing of weak alkaline solutions, such as a teaspoonful of bicarbonate of soda to a pint of water, which dissolves the mucus and relieves some of the catarrh.

**mucocele.** The collection of mucus in a cavity.

**mucocutaneous.** Relating to the mucous membrane and the skin.

**mucoid. 1.** Resembling mucus. **2.** A group of proteins found in ligaments and cartilage. Mucoids differ from mucins mainly in solubility.

**mucolytic.** Destroying mucus.

**mucomembranous.** Pertaining to mucous membranes.

**mucopurulent.** Consisting of mucus and pus.

**mucopus.** A combination of mucus and pus.

**mucosa.** A mucous membrane.

**mucosal.** Pertaining to mucous membrane.

**mucosanguineous.** Composed of mucus and blood.

**mucous.** Containing or resembling mucus.

**mucous colitis.** See COLITIS: MUCOUS COLITIS.

**mucus.** The thick liquid secreted by mucous glands. It consists of water, mucin, inorganic salts, and epithelial cells held in suspension.

**mule spinner's disease.** A condition occurring among operators of spinning mules in cotton mills and characterized by warts or ulcers of the skin, which have a strong tendency to become malignant.

**müllerian duct.** The duct in the developing embryo from which, in the female, is formed the Fallopian tubes, womb, and vagina. In the male it atrophies, leaving a small, blind recess called the prostatic utricle, which is in effect the remnant of the womb in the male.

**multicellular.** Having many cells.

**multigravida.** A pregnant woman who has been pregnant on a previous occasion.

**multilobular.** Having many lobes.

**multilocular.** Containing many cavities; polycystic.

**multinuclear, multinucleated.** Having more than one nucleus. Also called *polynuclear.*

**multipara.** A woman, not necessarily a pregnant woman, who has previously had one or more children.

**multiparity.** The state of being multiparous.

**multiparous.** Having produced several children.

**multiple sclerosis.** See SCLEROSIS: MULTIPLE SCLEROSIS.

**mummification.** Dry gangrene, or the shriveling up in the womb of a dead fetus.

**mumps.** An acute, infectious, virus disease, characterized by swelling and inflammation of one or more of the salivary glands. Also called *epidemic parotitis, infectious parotitis.*

*The salivary glands are six in number; the two parotid glands, one situated on each side of the face just in front of the ears, produce the thin saliva of the mouth; the two submaxillary glands, lying beneath the jaw, and the two sublingual glands lying below the tongue, supplying a thicker type of saliva. The disease sometimes affects one gland at a time; two glands may swell, giving the characteristic swollen face; or one gland may enlarge and as it goes down another gland may swell up. The incubation period is about three weeks, after which there is fever, headache, and pain beneath the ear. A painful swelling soon develops in the parotid region which causes pain on eating and swallowing. The symptoms gradually disappear after about a week. The general constitutional disturbance is usually slight and the patient seldom feels very ill. One attack usually confers immunity. The only complication to be feared is that the mumps virus has a predilection for the ovaries and the testicles, and if these swell up it may cause sterility. In view of this disastrous, though rare, complication, it is advisable to keep all cases of mumps at rest in bed until the swellings have subsided, for this is known to greatly lessen the risk. There is no specific treatment for mumps apart from good nursing care and rest in bed. As during the attack the mouth is lacking in saliva it is important that it should be washed out and the teeth cleaned after every meal. The diet should not contain much meat or food which is acid or tart in taste, as this only causes the glands to produce saliva which cannot get into the mouth and thus only serves to increase the size of the mumps. A very rare complication called cerebral mumps appears in the form of an attack of meningitis.*

**mural.** Pertaining to a wall.

**mural fibroid.** A tumor situated within the wall of the womb.

**mural pregnancy.** A pregnancy occurring just inside the Fallopian tube as it enters the womb.

**murmur.** A blowing or whistling sound heard over the heart or a blood vessel.

**cardiac murmur.** An abnormal sound heard over and produced within the heart. These murmurs, or added sounds, have been clearly classified as either innocent or a sign of a disorder. There are many types and each is diagnostic of the disorder present.

**muscle.** A structure composed of bundles of fibers whose power to contract effects bodily movement. There are over 500 muscles in the body and they vary in length from less than an inch to more than 24 inches, their shapes being circular, tubular, or sheathlike. Broadly, they are of two types: (1) involuntary, or smooth muscles, found in the skin, bladder, blood vessels, and the walls of the digestive organs, which cannot be controlled by the will; and (2) voluntary, or striated muscles, such as those controlling the limbs or facial expression, which are under the control of the will. The cardiac muscle, however, is different from the types above for, although it is involuntary muscle, it is composed of a modified striated muscle tissue. Muscles exert their pull in only one direction; therefore, a joint requires two sets: one to flex it and the other to straighten it. The points of attachment of a muscle are called its origin and insertion. The attachment to the bone to be moved by the muscle is the insertion, while the more or less fixed end is called the origin.

skeletal (voluntary) muscle fiber

cardiac (involuntary) muscle fiber

smooth (involuntary) muscle fiber

MUSCLE

**muscular.** Pertaining to muscles; possessing well-developed muscles.

**muscular dystrophy.** A disease of familial incidence and unknown cause, usually beginning in the third or fourth decade of life and characterized by muscle wasting of peculiar distribution quite unlike that of any other disease. There is also a peculiar difficulty in relaxing the muscles after effort, a feature which at once separates it from all other forms of muscular wasting.

**muscular rheumatism.** See FIBROSITIS.

**musculature.** The muscular system of the body.

**mutation.** A change in form or characteristic. In biology, it refers to changes occurring in chromosomes or genes, which result in detectable changes in the characteristics of the individual, and which are inherited and thus may represent a definite stage in the gradual evolution of a species. Mutations may be natural or may be induced artificially by means of x-rays or radioactivity.

**mute.** Dumb.

**mutism.** Dumbness.

**myalgia.** Pain in the muscles. Also called *fibrositis, muscular rheumatism.*

**myasthenia.** Muscular debility.

**myasthenia gravis.** A chronic malady predominantly affecting the 20-30 year age-group and characterized by excessive fatigability of the muscles. This leads to a variable paralysis which is brought on or rapidly increased by exertion and tends to improve with rest, but which may ultimately become permanent. The causative factor is unknown but there appears to be an association with overactivity of the thyroid gland, since it has been known to follow that condition.

*The muscles first affected are those supplied by one of the twelve cranial nerves, but sometimes the muscle weakness is general from its commencement. In the early stages, the disease may present itself in a variety of ways. For instance, a clerk may find that near the end of the day he sees double or that one or both upper eyelids droop, or a lecturer may notice that his voice gradually grows weaker, is husky, and acquires a nasal quality. In both cases the conditions disappear after a night's rest, only to reappear during the succeeding day. Another patient may start to eat a meal normally but then find he has increasing difficulty in swallowing until, by the end of the meal, swallowing is no longer possible; or there may be inability to smoke a cigarette or whistle, because the lip muscles cannot maintain a sustained pressure. In severe cases, the eyelids can only be closed with difficulty and the patient may sleep with the eyes wide open. In all instances the sustained muscular effort results in increasing weakness so that the action or movement has to be abandoned. Dramatic relief from some symptoms can be obtained by taking Neostigmine, but the dose has to be repeated every four to six hours.*

**myatrophy.** Muscle wasting. Also called *amyotrophia.*

**mycelium.** The lacework filaments of a fungus.

**mycetes.** The fungi.

**mycetismus.** Mushroom poisoning. Also called *mycetism.*

**mycology.** The study of fungi and the diseases that they cause.

**mycosis.** Any disease caused by a fungus. It may be a superficial mycosis, as in tinea capitis, tinea barbae, or tinea cruris, when the fungus invades the skin; or it may be a deep mycosis, where the infection is essentially or potentially spread through the system as in actinomycosis, mycetoma, and coccidioidomycosis.

**mycosis fungoides.** A malignant disease, running a slow course, and characterized by patches of eczema, infiltration, nodules, tumors, and ulcerations. Although usually a fatal illness, cases do occur where, for some inexplicable reason, there has been a spontaneous remission.

**mycotic.** Pertaining to mycosis.

**mycotoxin.** A poison produced from a fungus.

**mydriasis.** Dilation of the pupil of the eye.

**mydriatic.** Relating to mydriasis, or a drug which dilates the pupil.

**myectomy.** Surgical removal of part or the whole of a muscle.

**myelencephalitis.** Inflammation of the brain and spinal cord.

**myelencephalon.** Part of the afterbrain.

**myelin.** The white sheath which forms the protective covering of a nerve fiber.

**myelination.** The formation of a myelin sheath.

**myelitis.** Inflammation of the spinal cord or of the bone marrow.

**acute ascending myelitis.** A form of inflammation of the spinal cord which ascends towards the brain, usually occurring as a manifestation of poliomyelitis or of diphtheria, and can even originate from the poisonous effect of tick bites. Also called *Landry's paralysis.*

**acute myelitis.** An acute inflammation of the spinal cord.

**disseminated myelitis.** See ENCEPHALOMYELITIS.

**transverse myelitis.** Inflammation extending across the spinal cord at a specific level, which results in paralysis and anesthesia of that part of the body supplied with nerves from the spinal cord below the level of the inflammation.

**myelocele.** See MYELOMENINGOCELE.

**myelocyte.** One of the red bone marrow cells from which are developed leukocytes. They are sometimes present in severe infections, and present in large numbers in the blood in cases of myeloid leukemia.

**myelocytic.** Characterized by the presence of myelocytes.

**myelocytosis.** The presence of myelocytes in the blood.

**myelo-encephalitis.** Inflammation of the spinal cord and the brain.

**myelogenic, myelogenous.** Produced by myeloid cells of the blood-forming tissues.

**myelography.** X-ray examination of the spinal cord after introducing, by lumbar puncture, substances opaque to x-rays.

**myeloid.** Resembling bone marrow; derived from bone marrow; relating to myelocytes.

**myelomalacia.** Morbid softening of the spinal cord.

**myelomatosis.** A very rare and fatal disease of unknown origin, characterized by the development in the skeleton of multiple tumors which arise from the bone marrow. The bones affected are in the following order of frequency: spine, ribs, sternum, skull, scapula, pelvis, clavicle, humerus, and femur. Death usually occurs within six months of the onset of symptoms, but occasionally a patient has survived for one or two years. Also called *hematogenous myeloma, Kahler's disease, plasmacytoma.*

**myelomeningitis.** Spinal meningitis.

**myelomeningocele.** Protrusion of part of the spinal cord with its membranes through a hole in a vertebra. Also called *myelocele.*

**myelopathic.** Relating to disease of the spinal cord.

**myelopathy.** Any disease of the spinal cord or of myeloid tissues.

**myeloplegia.** Paralysis of the spine.

**myelorrhagia.** Bleeding into the spinal cord.

**myelosis.** Myeloid leukemia. See LEUKEMIA: CHRONIC MYELOID LEUKEMIA.

**myelotomy.** Surgical cutting of the spinal cord.

**myelotoxic.** Destructive to bone marrow.

**myenteric.** Pertaining to the muscular coat of the intestines.

**myocarditis.** Inflammation of the myocardium.

**myocardium.** The muscular walls of the heart.

**myocele.** The protrusion of a muscle through a tear in its sheath.

**myoclonus.** A sudden contraction of the muscles. See also EPILEPSY.

**myoglobinuria.** The presence in the urine of a muscle protein which colors the urine red. Physical exertion or a feverish illness are predisposing causes and the muscles involved become swollen and painful prior to the appearance of the red urine. Also called *idiopathic paroxysmal myoglobinuria.* See also RHABDOMYOLYSIS.

**myoma.** A tumor composed of muscle tissue. Also called *leiomyoma, rhabdomyoma.*

**myomalacia.** A degeneration and softening of muscle tissue.

**myomatous.** Resembling a myoma.

**myomectomy.** Excision of a myoma. The term commonly refers to the removal of a fibroid tumor from the wall of the womb.

**myometritis.** Inflammation of the walls of the womb.

**myometrium.** The muscular wall of the womb.

**myoneural.** Relating to both muscle and nerve.

**myoneural junction.** The termination of a nerve in a muscle. Also called *neuromyal junction.*

**myopathia, myopathy.** 1. Any disease of muscles. 2. The muscular dystrophies, a group of muscular disorders, often familial, characterized by progressive muscular weakness with either wasting or the false appearance of swelling of the muscles.

**myopathic.** Pertaining to any disease of muscles.

**myope.** A person suffering with myopia.

**myopia.** Short-sightedness.

**myopic.** Affected with short-sightedness.

**myosis.** See MEIOSIS.

**myositis.** Inflammation of muscles.

**myositis ossificans.** A condition characterized by the deposit of bony tissue in muscles.

**myospasm.** A muscular spasm or cramp.

**myosteoma.** A bony tumor in muscle tissue.

**myotenotomy.** Surgical incision into muscles or tendons.

**myotomy.** Surgical division of a muscle.

**myotonia, myotonus.** Muscular tone (the state of slight tension normally present in a muscle) or muscular spasm.

**myotonia acquisita.** Muscular spasm developing after injury or disease.

**myotonia atrophica.** A familial disease usually beginning between the ages of 30 and 50 years, characterized by a wasting of muscles unlike that of any other disease and affecting those of the face and neck, extending to the trunk and limbs. Associated with this wasting is a peculiar difficulty in relaxing the muscles after effort. Also called *dystrophia myotonica.*

**myotonia congenita.** A very rare hereditary and familial illness of unknown cause, commencing in early childhood, characterized by a striking slowness in the relaxation of the muscles after voluntary effort. Cold, heat, fatigue, and hunger make the condition worse. It has no tendency to shorten life and tends to become more marked from infancy to puberty and then less marked as age increases. It has never been known to recover spontaneously. Also called *Thomsen's disease.* See also AMYOTONIA CONGENITA.

**myringa.** The eardrum.

**myringitis.** Inflammation of the eardrum.

**myringoplasty.** Surgical repair of the eardrum.

**myringoscope.** An instrument for examining the inside of the ear. Also called *auriscope.*

**myringotome.** An instrument for incising the eardrum.

**myringotomy.** Surgical cutting of the eardrum.

**myrinx.** The eardrum.

**mysophobia.** Fear of dirt.

**mythophobia.** Fear of telling lies.

**myxedema.** A condition due to underactivity of the thyroid gland, associated with low basal metabolism and increased sensitivity to cold.

**congenital myxedema.** See CRETINISM.

**myxoedema.** See MYXEDEMA.

**myxofibroma.** A tumor composed of fibrous and myxomatous tissue.

**myxoid.** Resembling mucus.

**myxoma.** A tumor arising from connective tissue, containing large quantities of mucoid material.

**myxomatosis.** The presence of numerous myxomas.

**infectious myxomatosis.** An infectious virus disease in rabbits, with widespread tumors resembling myxomas.

# N

**naevocarcinoma.** See NEVOCARCINOMA.

**naevoid.** See NEVOID.

**naevous.** See NEVOUS.

**naevus.** See NEVUS.

**nail.** The horny plate on the end of each finger and toe.

**ingrowing toenail.** This is due to cutting the nail down into the flesh. Toenails should always be cut squarely across so that the sides of each nail sit in the full length of the fleshly groove provided for them

**narcism, narcissism.** Love of self. In psychoanalysis, the persistence in the adult of a condition that is a normal stage in the infant's psychosexual development, in which the child's love object is its own person. The term derives from Narcissus, the character in Greek mythology who fell in love with his own reflection.

**narcoanalysis.** Psychoanalysis while the patient is under the influence of drugs and narcotics. This procedure is the basis of the so-called "truth drugs," and what in effect happens is that the critical powers of the brain are dulled by drugs so that the answer to a question is likely to be the truth because the higher centers are not working sufficiently to be able to fabricate a lie.

**narcolepsy.** An uncontrollable desire to sleep for short periods during the day. It has been observed in cases of epilepsy, inflammation of the brain, and in some cases of brain tumors, though in many patients no cause can be found. The condition is treated by brain stimulants such as amphetamine.

**narcoleptic.** Relating to narcolepsy.

**narcosis.** A state of profound stupor, unconsciousness, or arrested activity induced by drugs.

**narcotic.** Producing or related to narcosis; colloquially, a drug producing narcosis.

**narcotism.** Narcosis.

**narcotize.** To induce narcosis.

**nares.** The nostrils.

**nascent.** 1. Characterized by the liberation of gaseous substances from a chemical combination. 2. Just born or just coming into existence.

**nasolabial.** Pertaining to the nose and lips.

**nasolacrimal.** Pertaining to the nose and lacrimal apparatus.

**nasopalatine.** Pertaining to the nose and palate.

**nasopharyngeal.** Pertaining to the nose and pharynx or to the nasopharynx.

**nasopharyngitis.** Inflammation of the nasopharynx.

**nasopharynx.** That part of the throat above the soft palate and behind the nose.

**natal.** 1. Pertaining to birth. 2. Pertaining to the buttocks.

**natality.** The birth rate.

**nates.** The buttocks.

**natural selection.** The theory expounded by Darwin and others that nature tends to maintain and perpetuate those species having particular genetic characteristics that best fit them for survival in their environment. Darwin considered natural selection to be of fundamental importance in the process of evolution.

**nausea.** A sensation of sickness, frequently a prelude to vomiting.

**navel.** See UMBILICUS.

**navicular.** 1. Boat-shaped. 2. Referring to the scaphoid bone, a boat-shaped bone in the hand or foot.

**near-point.** The point nearest the eye at which an object can be seen distinctly.

**near-sighted.** Myopic; short-sighted.

**nearthrosis.** The production of a false joint due to the nonunion of a broken bone.

**nebula.** 1. A faint greyish opacity of the cornea of the eye. 2. A spray or a liquid intended for use in an atomizer.

**nebulae.** The plural of nebula.

**nebulizer.** An instrument used for spraying.

**necrobiosis.** Physiological death of a cell or cell groups. Necrobiosis is seen in the death of cells of the epidermis and blood, which are constantly being replaced This is in contrast to necrosis, which is death of cells due to a disease process, and to somatic death, which is death of the entire organism.

**necrobiosis lipoidica diabetica.** A skin disease mostly occurring in diabetic women and characterized by many yellow to red plaques.

**necrophobia.** A morbid fear of dead bodies or of death.

**necropsy.** Autopsy or post-mortem.

**necrosis.** Pathological death of a cell or cell groups, which are still in contact with living tissues.

**caseation necrosis.** The necrosis seen in tuberculosis, with the formation of a cheeselike substance.

**coagulation necrosis.** A type of necrosis characterized by cell death with preservation of the cell outlines. Seen most frequently in infarction (death of tissue due to the loss of its blood supply). Also called *embolic necrosis, ischemic necrosis.*

**colliquative necrosis.** See LIQUEFACTIVE NECROSIS, below.

**diphtheritic necrosis.** Necrosis of mucous membrane characterized by the formation of a tough, leathery membrane, composed of coagulated cells and fibrin.

**embolic necrosis.** See COAGULATION NECROSIS, above.

**fat necrosis.** Necrosis in the fatty tissues around the pancreas, due to acute destructive disease of the pancreas and caused by the liberation of pancreatic enzymes, which attack fat.

**ischaemic necrosis.** See COAGULATION NECROSIS, above.

**liquefactive necrosis.** Necrosis in which the tissues liquefy. Also called *colliquative necrosis.*

**phosphorus necrosis.** A necrosis of bone, especially of the lower jaw, occurring in people exposed to the fumes of phosphorus. Also called *phossy-jaw.*

**necrospermia.** A condition in which the semen contains only dead spermatozoa.

**necrotic.** Pertaining to necrosis.

**necrotomy.** 1. Autopsy or necropsy. 2. The surgical removal of a sequestrum.

**negativism.** A behavior disorder characterized by a propensity not to do what is asked or to do the opposite.

**nematode.** A roundworm or threadworm belonging to the class *Nematoda*.

**nematosis.** Infestation with threadworms.

**neonatal.** Pertaining to the newborn.

**neonate, neonatus.** A newborn child.

**neophobia.** Fear of newness.

**neoplasia.** The formation of a neoplasm.

**neoplasm.** A new and abnormal growth of tissue, such as a tumor.

**neoplastic.** Relating to neoplasm.

**neoplasty.** Plastic surgery for the restoration of lost tissue.

**nephralgia.** Pain in a kidney.

**nephrectomy.** Surgical removal of a kidney.

**nephric.** Pertaining to the kidney.

**nephritic.** Pertaining to nephritis.

**nephritis.** Inflammation of the kidney.

**nephrocapsulectomy.** Surgical removal of the kidney capsule.

**nephrocapsulotomy.** Surgical incision of the kidney capsule.

**nephrogenic.** Arising from a kidney.

**nephrolith.** A stone in the kidney.

**nephrolithiasis.** The presence of stones in the kidney.

**nephrolithotomy.** Surgical removal of a stone in the kidney.

**nephroma.** A kidney tumor.

**nephromalacia.** Softening of the kidney.

**nephromegalia, nephromegaly.** Enlargement of the kidney.

**nephron.** The filtering mechanism of the kidney.

**nephropathy.** Any disease of the kidney.

**nephropexy.** Surgical fixation of a dropped kidney.

**nephrophthisis.** Tuberculosis of the kidney.

**nephroptosis.** Downward displacement of the kidney. Also called *floating kidney*.

**nephro-.** A combining form meaning kidney.

**nephrosclerosis.** Involvement of the kidney in a blood vessel disease associated either with hardening of the kidney arteries or general hardening of the arteries of the body, causing disturbance in kidney function and providing a clinical picture identical with that of chronic nephritis, plus high blood pressure. There are various classifications of nephrosclerosis associated with conditions such as arteriosclerotic kidney, ischemic nephritis, malignant hypertnesion, chronic interstitial nephritis, and red granular

kidney. The ultimate result is kidney failure, heart failure, or both, as well as other complications due to high blood pressure.

**nephrosis.** Any degeneration of the kidney without signs of inflammation. It is characterized by gross edema and the passage of albumin in the urine.

**nephrostomy.** The surgical formation of a fistula leading to the kidney pelvis.

**nephrotic.** Relating to nephrosis.

**nephrotomy.** Surgical incision into the kidney.

**nephrotuberculosis.** Tuberculosis of the kidney. Also called *nephrophthisis*.

**nephro-ureterectomy.** Surgical excision of the kidney and a whole or part of the ureter.

**nerve.** A collection of bundles of nerve fibers which convey either motor impulses from the brain to the muscles of the body or sensory impulses from all parts of the body back to the brain.

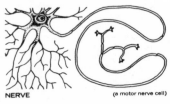

NERVE　　　　　　　　(a motor nerve cell)

**nervous.** Pertaining to a nerve, nerves, or nervousness.

**nervous exhaustion.** A state of fatigue and discomfort due to emotional causes. Also called *neurasthenia*.

**nervousness.** Excessive excitability of the nervous system characterized by shaken mental poise and stability, muscle tremors or weakness, and an uncomfortable awareness of self.

**nettle rash.** Urticaria.

**neural.** Pertaining to a nerve or to the nervous system.

**neuralgia.** Severe pain along the course of a nerve. The pain is sharp, stabbing, and comes in paroxysms, lasting usually for a short time; tenderness is often present at the points of exit of the nerve, and the paroxysms can be produced by contact with specific areas called trigger zones.

**intercostal neuralgia.** Neuralgia occurring in the course of the nerves running round the chest. Often associated with herpes zoster.

**postherpetic neuralgia.** Neuralgia following an attack of herpes zoster. It persists in the area concerned long after the shingles blisters have healed.

**trigeminal neuralgia.** Severe pain in the trigeminal nerve radiating over the side of the face and the scalp. The scalp is so exceedingly tender that even brushing the hair can become impossible. Treatment in the severest cases is to destroy the nerve with an alcohol injection, and although this cures the pain it also leaves the side of the face without any skin sensation. Also called *tic douloureux*.

**neuralgic.** Pertaining to neuralgia.

**neurasthenia.** A group of symptoms formerly ascribed to debility or exhaustion of the nerve centers. The symptoms include fatigue, lack of energy, various aches and pains, and disinclination to join in any activity. It is a diagnosis fast becoming obsolete, because the disorder is due either to disease which needs active treatment or to a neurosis which needs psychiatric treatment. It became fashionable to make this diagnosis in the past to avoid having to tell a patient pointblank that he was neurotic.

**neuraxis.** The slender nerve fiber that emerges from a nerve cell, properly called an axis cylinder. That part of the nervous system represented by the brain and spinal cord.

**neuraxon.** An axis cylinder. See NEURAXIS.

**neurectasis.** Surgical stretching of a nerve.

**neurectomy.** Surgical removal of part of a nerve.

**neurectopia.** The abnormal position of a nerve.

**neurilemma.** The deicate sheath encasing a nerve fiber.

**neurinoma.** A tumor arising from the sheath covering a nerve. Also called *neurofibroma, neurilemmoma*.

**neuritis.** Degeneration or inflammation of a nerve or nerves, accompanied by pain, hypersensitivity, loss of skin sensation, muscular paralysis, muscle wasting, and loss of nerve reflexes in the part concerned. The condition is frequently confused wih neuralgia.

**adventitial neuritis.** Neuritis caused by an infection of the nerve sheath.

**ascending neuritis.** Neuritis which extends from the periphery of the body and ascends the nerve towards the brain or spinal cord.

**axial neuritis.** A form of neuritis affecting the axis of a nerve.

**degenerative neuritis.** Neuritis involving nerve fibers. See MULTIPLE NEURITIS, below.

**descending neuritis.** Neuritis which starts in the nerves leaving the brain and descends through the spinal cord to the periphery of the body.

**disseminated neuritis.** See SEGMENTAL NEURITIS, below.

**endemic neuritis.** Neuritis associated with beriberi, which occurs in starvation and diets lacking in vitamin B; extensively seen during the Second World War in Japanese prison camps.

**infectious neuritis.** An acute multiple neuritis, probably due to a virus.

**interstitial neuritis.** Neuritis involving the connective tissue of a nerve.

**mononeuritis.** Neuritis in a single nerve.

**multiple neuritis.** Also called *peripheral neuritis*. See POLYNEURITIS, below.

**optic neuritis.** Swelling of the optic disc at the back of the eyeball, which makes its outline indistinct, with narrowing of the arteries and dilation of the veins, which is of great diagnostic importance because it can be so readily seen by the doctor with an ophthalmoscope.

**parenchymatous neuritis.** A form of degenerative neuritis.

**peripheral neuritis.** See POLYNEURITIS, below.

**polyneuritis.** Neuritis affecting several nerves simultaneously, especially those in the limbs, producing paralysis and wasting of muscles, with disturbances in sensation. Commonly caused by alcohol, lead, and arsenic poisoning; diabetes, beriberi, and sometimes due to a virus infection. It may also occur in diphtheria, typhoid fever, or syphilis. Also called *multiple neuritis, peripheral neuritis.*

**retrobulbar neuritis.** Inflammation of the optic nerve behind the eyeball.

**segmental neuritis.** Neuritis affecting a segment of a nerve.

**toxic neuritis.** Neuritis due to poisoning. See also POLYNEURITIS, above.

**traumatic neuritis.** Neuritis developing following nerve damage.

**neurodermatitis.** A skin disorder of nervous origin, usually accompanied by severe irritation that causes scratching, which in turn provokes a thickening and roughening of the skin called lichenification. Broadly speaking, when a person of highly emotional and nervous temperament is getting to the limit of his nervous stability, he will either suffer from a nervous breakdown or neurodermatitis. Apart from relief of the itching, the doctor has to make a complete review of the patient's anxiety problems, and once these have been solved the skin automatically recovers.

**neurodermatosis.** See NEURODERMATITIS.

**neurofibroma.** A tumor arising from nerves and nerve tissue, essentially fibrous in nature. Also called *neuri-*

*lemmoma, neural fibroblastoma, schwannoma.*

**neurofibromatosis.** A condition characterized by the presence of neurofibromas in the skin or along the course of nerves. These painless, multiple tumors may appear in hundreds, gradually increasing in both number and size. The condition has an hereditary tendency and is often associated with such congenital abnormalities as spina bifida, meningocele, syringomyelia, mental deficiency, and epilepsy. In many cases the condition is compatible with a long and relatively normal life, although there is always a tendency towards slow progression. Danger to life results only from tumors occurring in the brain or spinal cavities or from the rare malignant degeneration in the tumors. The treatment, if anything, is surgical removal of the tumors. Also called *molluscum fibrosum, molluscum pendulum, von Recklinghausen's disease, Smith-Recklinghausen's disease.*

**neurogenous.** Arising from some part of the nervous system.

**neuroglia.** A general term for the fibrous and cellular supporting tissues of the central nervous system.

**neuroglioma.** A tumor composed of neuroglial tissue.

**neurology.** Study of the nervous system and its diseases.

**neurolymph.** Cerebrospinal fluid.

**neurolysis.** Exhaustion of a nerve by overstimulation; nerve tension; the loosening of adhesions binding a nerve; disintegration of nerve tissue.

**neuroma.** A tumor arising from a nerve.

**amputation neuroma.** A neuroma occurring in the stump of an amputated limb. It forms a tender, sensitive area, which can make the wearing of an artificial limb difficult.

**neuromalacia.** Softening of the nerves.

**neuromuscular.** Relating to both nerves and muscles.

**neuron, neurone.** A nerve cell and its nerve fibers.

**lower motor neuron.** A neuron which has its cell body in the brain or spinal cord and an axon which passes peripherally to end on muscle.

**upper motor neuron.** A neuron originating in the motor area of the brain and terminating in the motor nuclei of a cerebral nerve or in the central grey column of the cord.

**neuronal, neuronic.** Relating to a neuron.

**neuroparalysis.** Paralysis due to a disorder of the nervous system.

**neuropathic.** Relating to neuropathy.

**neuropathology.** The study of the intrinsic causes of disorders of the nervous system.

**neuropathy.** Any disease of the nervous system.

**neurophysiology.** The study of the physiology of the nervous system.

**neuroplasty.** Surgical repair of a nerve, such as nerve grafting.

**neuropsychiatry.** The branch of medicine which deals with both nervous and mental disorders.

**neurosis.** A term applied to a large group of emotional disorders not due to organic disease of the nervous system and resulting only in partial disorganization of the patient's personality. All neuroses are characterized by an emotional state, anxiety or fear, or by preoccupation, obsession, and a concentration on the functions of the body and its organs. Common to most neuroses is an underlying inability to have normal relationships with other people, which may originate far back in childhood. In most cases there is an unconscious repression of an idea or wish connected with a past incident, on which the anxiety state and its symptoms are built. It is unfortunate that neurosis is generally interpreted by the uninformed as malingering—a totally different condition. Although all neuroses basically spring from the same mental disturbance, nevertheless they have been classified, because for varying reasons so many patients fall into one or other category. Also called *psychoneurosis*.

**anxiety neurosis.** A neurosis characterized by overwhelming anxiety for no obvious reason.

**cardiac neurosis.** A form characterized by complaint of pain near the heart, accompanied by severe palpitations and not due to heart disease. Also called *effort syndrome*.

**conversion neurosis.** A neurosis in which the patient converts his anxiety into a positive physical symptom not connected with the real cause of the anxiety. See also TRANSFERENCE NEUROSIS, below.

**obsessional neurosis.** A neurosis in which compulsive acts or ideas dominate the patient's life. For instance, such patients may have to confirm that they have shut a door perhaps ten or more times before they are satisfied, or they may be obsessed with a compulsion to count the tea leaves they are putting into a teapot or the number of peas they have shelled.

**occupational neurosis.** A neurosis due to the patient's employment and occurring in such people as manual workers, typists, telegraphists, musicians, seamstresses, and in some craftsmen. In effect, the symptom becomes the excuse to avoid performing a job which may be frustrating or uncongenial, especially if the instrument or tool used is of bad design. Taking writer's cramp as a general example, the onset is gradual, writing becomes inexplicably more difficult and tends to be irregular, the strokes extending too high or too low. The subject grasps the pen with excessive force, correct adjustment of the fingertips becomes hard and apt to fail, with the index finger slipping off the pen. This the patient tries to correct by a still firmer grip, so that the hand begins to ache and feels heavy and tired. With time, the symptoms increase, the writing becomes increasingly irregular, and eventually the nib is driven through the paper. As the condition grows worse, the cramp appears even more readily, so that ultimately just to take up the pen may cause it, and yet at the same time other fine and repetitive movements of the hand and its muscles may be performed with normal ease and facility. Treatment consists in first excluding organic disease of the nervous system as a cause of the symptoms, with attention to general physical well-being. Psychological treatment may be valuable in determining from what the patient is really trying to escape, in relieving underlying anxiety and tension, and in enabling him to make a better adaptation to his surroundings. Careful selection of occupation is important .

**transference neurosis.** A neurosis which usually has a sex basis, and typically it is a very tense, worried, and anxious patient who constantly complains of, say, a sore throat for which the doctor can find no obvious cause. Investigation elicits that the real problem is one connected with the sex organs but the patient feels it is more respectable to seek aid for a sore throat than to admit the real site of the trouble.

**traumatic neurosis.** A neurosis occurring after an accident, very often a quite trivial accident, in a person disposed to react in such a way.

**war neurosis.** Neurosis caused by an experience connected with warfare in an emotionally unstable person so disposed to react in such a way, as the so-called "shell shock" of the First World War.

**neurosurgery.** Surgery of the brain, spinal cord, and nervous system.

**neurosuture.** The sewing together of the ends of a divided nerve.

**neurosyphilis.** Syphilis involving the central nervous system.

**neurotic.** Relating to or suffering from neurosis.

**neurotomy.** The cutting of a nerve.

**neurotoxin.** A toxin peculiarly destructive to nervous tissue.

**neurotripsy.** The crushing of a nerve. For instance, in the treatment of duodenal ulcers the nerve to the duodenum is, on occasion, crushed to provoke relaxation of coats of the intestine. This alleviates the irritability, and permits the ulcer to heal.

**neurotrophic.** Relating to the influence of nerves upon the nutrition and maintenance of the normal condition in tissues.

**neurotropic.** Turning towards or having an affinity for nervous tissue.

**neurovascular.** Pertaining to both nervous and vascular structures.

**neutropenia.** A deficiency of neutrophil cells in the blood.

**neutrophil, neutrophile.** A leukocyte containing granules stainable with neutral dyes, the commonest of which is the polymorphonuclear leukocyte. See also LEUKOCYTE.

**neutrophilia.** An abnormal increase of neutrophil cells in the blood.

**nevocarcinoma.** Cancer developing from a mole.

**nevoid.** Resembling a nevus.

**nevous.** Spotted with moles.

**nevus.** A growth composed of blood vessels arising in the skin. Also called *birthmark, mole.* There are many types.

**blue nevus.** A buttonlike, firm, slaty-blue nodule usually found in the lower part of the back. It is harmless and does not grow. No treatment is necessary, but excision can be performed if the patient wishes it.

**caverno-capillary nevus.** See NEVUS VASCULOSUS, below.

**nevus flammeus.** A growth of blood vessels in the skin, present at birth and often persisting throughout life. Also called *port-wine stain.*

**nevus pigmentosus.** The dark-colored spot or mole so frequently seen on the skin.

**nevus vasculosus.** A bright red, or slightly raised, tiny nodule that may be present from birth or appear within the following two weeks. It steadily enlarges until about the age of nine months, when it begins to gradually disappear, finally disappearing without trace or with slight scarring at about the age of five years.

**senile hemangioma.** A pinhead-sized or larger red spot occurring on the face and trunk often after the age of 40 years. These spots have no significance as regards general health and they need no treatment. Also called *Campbell de Morgan spots.*

**spider nevus.** A small, red spot with faint pink lines radiating from it. See also STELLATE HEMANGIOMA, below.

**stellate hemangioma.** A spider nevus, so called because the pink lines of the blood vessels run out as a web over the skin. Spider nevi may become more numerous during pregnancy and in liver disorders. They respond to treatment with the cautery needle.

**strawberry nevus.** See NEVUS VASCULOSUS, above.

**newborn.** An infant during the first four weeks of life. At birth, the average baby is 20 inches long, has a head circumference of 13½ inches, and weighs between 6 and 8½ pounds with a general average of 7¼ pounds. Infants weighing 5½ pounds or less are classified as premature, irrespective of the period of gestation, and require special care. The further the birth weight is below this arbitrary level, the more precarious is the infant's chance of survival. The newborn infant normally loses weight during the first four or five days—large infants tending to lose more than smaller ones. The birth weight is normally regained by the seventh to tenth day, except in infants who have lost more than 8 ounces, when recovery takes longer. The skull bones are not closed at birth and one of the areas where the scalp covers the brain with no bone intervening is called the anterior fontanelle. It tends to bulge when the child cries (this is normal), and to be sunken when the child is dehydrated from diarrhea, vomiting or both. Enlargement of one or both breasts, due to the influence of female sex hormone derived from the mother, is common in the newborn, and sometimes the breasts secrete a fluid which has been called "witch's milk." No treatment is required and the condition subsides within a few weeks. In the past there was a curious practice, described as "breaking the nipple strings," of attacking these swellings by forcible kneading and manipulation—a senseless and cruel procedure that sometimes led to violent inflammation and abscess formation. In female infants, during the first two weeks of life, there may be transient swelling of the vulva associated with a whitish, and sometimes blood-stained, mucoid discharge which, like the breast enlargement, is due to the female sex hormone derived from the mother. Both swelling and discharge subside spontaneously without treatment. In the male infant, the foreskin is adherent to the penis and cannot be retracted. This is normal and should not be misconstrued as a reason for circumcision. The small red birthmarks so commonly found on the skin over the front and back of the skull are popularly known as "marks of the stork's beak." They require no treatment and usually clear spontaneously during the first year. The abdomen appears to be larger than normal and moves freely with respiration, which is frequently quite irregular in the first few weeks. Apart from the normal nerve reflexes involved in crying, swallowing, sucking, breathing, digestion, defecation, and urination, the newborn infant should show other well-defined reflexes, which if absent indicate prematurity, birth injury, or abnormality. The grasp reflex is very vigorous and may be so strong that if the infant grabs the examiner's fingers it can actually be lifted off the bed. The pupils react to strong light, the normal response of the infant being to close the eyes firmly. Sometimes there is a vague attempt to follow a strong light with the eyes, even during the first month of life. Other reflexes are also present but are usually difficult to demonstrate. As a rule, a newborn infant acquires an immunity to infectious diseases from the mother, but as the child approaches the age of three months its immunity is very low and it is for this reason that many doctors then start inoculations, especially against whooping cough.

**newgrowth.** See NEOPLASM.

**news bell.** See TINNITUS.

**nidus.** A nucleus, or the point of origin or focus of infections.

**night blindness.** Subnormal vision in half-light or dim light.

**nightmare.** A violent dream producing anxiety. The term is derived from Mara, the Norse God, who was supposed to strangle sleeping people. Some children suffer from low blood sugar during sleep and the nightmare reaction is a hypoglycemic attack. The remedy consists in giving extra sugar with the supper meal. Also called *incubus.*

**night screaming, night terror.** A state of deep anxiety due to a disturbing dream, from which the patient does not awake and for which he later has complete loss of memory. The condition occurs very commonly in children who have enlarged adenoids and nasal obstruction and may disappear when the adenoids have been removed.

**night sweat.** Excessive sweating during the night, sufficient to soak the night clothes, associated with either a toxic state, such as tuberculosis or a violent anxiety state.

**nightwalking.** Noctambulation, somnambulism, sleepwalking.

**nipple.** The pigmented, conical elevation on the breast, to which converge the 14 to 16 milk ducts from the lobes of the breast.

**nit.** The popular name for the egg or larva of the louse.

**niter.** Saltpeter, potassium nitrate.

**noctambulation.** Nightwalking.

**nocturia.** Nocturnal enuresis, nycturia, bed-wetting.

**nocturnal enuresis.** Bed-wetting.

**nocturnal pollution.** See POLLUTION: NOCTURNAL POLLUTION.

**nocuous.** Noxious, poisonous, harmful.

**nodding spasm.** A shaking movement of the head. It is seen in several complaints and commonly met with in infants, when it is known as spasmus nutans. In this instance, it is quite normal, harmless, and passes off within the first year. In older children, involuntary head movements may be due to St. Vitus's dance or to habit spasms of nervous origin. Involuntary movements of the head are also seen in the tremors of old age and Parkinson's disease, and in cases of alcohol and tobacco poisoning.

**node.** 1. A knob or protuberance; a point of constriction. 2. A small rounded organ. 3. A lymph gland.

**atrioventricular node.** A structure in the heart which assists in the control of orderly heartbeats, starting in the atria and followed by contraction of the ventricles. Also called *auriculoventricular node.*

**Heberden's nodes.** Knobby deformities of the fingers seen in osteoarthritis.

**Keith and Flack node.** See SINOATRIAL NODE, below.

**lymph nodes.** Lymphatic glands.

**Parrot's nodes.** Bony swelling on the skull of babies with congenital syphilis.

**Ranvier's node.** The region in a nerve where there is a local constriction of the nerve sheath.

**sentinel nodes.** A lymph gland situated above the left collarbone, which may be the site of spread from cancer of the stomach, from other abdominal areas, or from within the chest. Also called *signal node.*

**signal node.** See SENTINEL NODE, below.

**singer's node.** Inflammatory nodules occurring on the vocal cords of singers.

**sinoatrial node, sinoauricular node.** The structure situated at the mouth of the large superior vena cava vein which enters the right atrium of the heart and which is the starting point of the heart's conducting system, by which an orderly arrangement of the heart's contractions is instituted. It has been called the pacemaker of the heart. Also called *Keith and Flack node.*

**syphilitic node.** A localized swelling on bones due to syphilis.

**nodose.** Pertaining to nodes.

**nodosity.** The condition of having nodes or a node.

**nodular.** Composed of or characterized by the presence of nodules.

**nodule.** A small node.

**aggregate nodules.** Groups of lymph nodules massed together in the walls of an organ, such as those in the walls of the small intestine, where they are called Peyer's patches.

**Aschoff nodules.** The specific lesion of rheumatic fever, located around the blood vessels in the heart muscle, and occasionally found elsewhere.

**juxta-articular nodules.** Nodules found beneath the skin in patients suffering with syphilis or yaws. The tumors are hard in consistency and are found above the joints of the upper extremities, especially the elbow, and on the legs.

**lymph nodule.** A small mass of dense lymphatic tissue.

**rheumatic nodule.** A nodule, especially near the wrist or elbow, which can be felt through the skin, occurring in limited numbers in the graver cases of rheumatic fever in childhood. It is nearly always an indication that the heart has been involved in a rheumatic process.

**Schmorl's nodule.** The projection of the center of an intervertebral disc into the soft, spongy substance of an adjoining vertebra. When extensive, it produces wedge-shaped vertebrae and causes severe curvature of the spine.

**sideritic nodules.** Nodules, found in some organs, which are the result of a local hemorrhage, the nodule being formed of blood clot which is changing to fibrous tissue.

**typhoid nodules.** Characteristic lesions found in the liver of patients with typhoid fever.

**nodulus.** A nodule.

**nodus.** A node.

**noma.** A very rare, severe, inflammatory, gangrenous condition which starts in the mouth of severely debilitated children and often precipitated by an infectious disease such as measles. It has also been known to attack the vulva. Also called *cancrum oris, gangrenous stomatitis.*

**nonunion.** The failure of a broken bone to join.

**nonviable.** Not capable of living.

**nosebleed.** See EPISTAXIS.

**nosomania.** The delusion of being ill.

**nosomycosis.** Any disease caused by a fungus.

**nosophilia.** A neurotic determination to be ill.

**nosophobia.** A neurotic fear of being ill.

**nosotoxicosis.** Any disease caused by poisoning.

**nostrum.** A quack remedy.

**notifiable.** Referring to diseases that are required by law to be reported to the board of health.

**notochord.** The rod-shaped embryonic tissue around which the vertebral column forms.

**nubile.** Of marriageable age, or of an age at which it is possible for the female to bear a child.

**nubility.** The state of sexual development at which it is possible for sexual intercourse to take place.

**nucleus pulposus.** The semifluid central area of an intervertebral spinal disc. One theory about spinal disc pains is that this structure can be pushed out sideways and press on a spinal nerve, producing pain.

**nullipara.** A woman who has never borne a child.

**nulliparity.** The condition of being nulliparous.

**nulliparous.** Never having borne a child. Also called *nonparous.*

**numb.** Defective sensibility.

**numbness.** Local anesthesia; insensibility to touch.

**nummiform.** Nummular.

**nummular.** Coin-shaped, or resembling rolls of coins.

**nummulation.** 1. The formation of nummular structures. 2. The condition in which the red blood cells collect together in so-called rouleaux formation (resembling rolls of coins).

**nutans.** Nodding.

**nutation.** Nodding of the head. See NODDING SPASM.

**nutmeg liver.** A term descriptive of a congested liver having a mottled appearance.

**nutrition.** The process by which living organisms take in food materials and use them for energy, general maintenance of the body, and growth. Nutrition involves digestion, absorption, assimilation, etc.; and is concerned with foods that promote health.

**nyctalgia.** Pain occurring chiefly at night.

**nyctalope.** A person who sees better in dim light than by daylight.

**nyctalopia.** Properly, night blindness.

**nyctophilia.** The neurotic preference of night to day.

**nyctophobia.** Neurotic fear of the dark.

**nycturia.** Nocturnal enuresis, nocturia, bed-wetting.

**nympha.** A labium minus pudendi (one of the two smaller lips at the vaginal opening).

**nymphectomy.** Surgical removal of one or both nymphae.

**nymphomania.** Excessive sexual desire in women.

**nystagmiform.** Resembling nystagmus.

**nystagmus.** An involuntary oscillatory movement of the eyeball.

*True nystagmus can be caused in the early months of life by conditions which affect the vision, such as ophthalmia neonatorum, congenital cataract, total color blindness, albinism, and cases in which there is an unusual distribution of pigment in the retina. The nystagmus associated with spasmus nutans (nodding movements of the head) occurs in the first year of life and disappears spontaneously. It is believed to be due to defective illumination. Nystagmus developing in later life is caused by various factors. It may be due to constant strain imposed by peculiar occupational conditions— miner's nystagmus, for instance, is probably caused by continued work in dim light. As a rule, however, this type improves once the causative factor is removed. Nystagmus occurs in some general nervous diseases—disseminated sclerosis, syringomyelia, Friedreich's ataxia; in any disease affecting the cerebellum; in cases of peripheral neuritis and myasthenia gravis; and one form, called myoclonic nystagmus, is associated with spasmodic movements of the head and body and increased knee jerk reflexes. Internal ear diseases involving the semicircular canals produce the condition (labyrinthine nystagmus), and so can excessive syringing of the ear with hot or cold water. Poisons such as manganese and lead can also cause the condition.*

# O

**obesity.** An excessive increase of fat in the body; overweight.

**obstetrician.** A physician in obstetrics.

**obstetrics.** That section of medicine which deals with pregnancy, childbirth, and the health of the mother during the six to eight weeks after childbirth.

**obstipation.** Intractable constipation.

**obturator.** A structure, natural or artificial, which closes an opening. Many structures lying within an opening take their name from it, such as the obturator foramen of the innominate bone.

**occipital.** Relating to the occiput.

**occipito-anterior.** A term descriptive of the position of the baby's head prior to birth in which the back of the skull faces towards the front of the mother's abdomen.

**occipitocervical.** Relating to the occiput and the neck.

**occipitofacial.** Pertaining to the occiput and the face.

**occipitofrontal.** Pertaining to the occiput and the forehead, or to the occiput and the frontal lobes of the brain.

**occipitomental.** Relating to the occiput and the chin.

**occipitoparietal.** Relating to the occiput and the parietal bones, or to the occiput and the parietal lobes of the brain.

**occipitoposterior.** A term descriptive of the position of the baby's head prior to birth in which the back of the skull faces towards the mother's spine.

**occipitotemporal.** Pertaining to the occiput and the temporal bones of the skull, or to the occiput and the temporal lobes of the brain.

**occiput.** The back of the skull.

**occluding.** Closing or shutting up.

**occlusion.** 1. The act of closing or shutting up. 2. The absorption, by a metal, of gas in large quantities, as of hydrogen by platinum. 3. The full meeting or contact in a position of rest, of the masticating surfaces of the upper and lower teeth; also called *the bite.*

**buccal occlusion.** The position of a premolar or molar tooth which is outside the line of occlusion.

**centric occlusion.** The relation of the incisal edges and the inclined planes of the teeth, when the jaws are closed in a position of rest.

**coronary occlusion.** Coronary thrombosis; a heart attack in which the coronary artery, which supplies the blood to the heart muscle, is blocked.

**distal occlusion.** The position .of a tooth when it is more posterior than normal.

**eccentric occlusion.** The relation of the inclined planes of the teeth when the jaws are closed in any of the excursive movements of the lower jaw.

**labial occlusion.** The position of an incisor or canine tooth which is outside the line of occlusion.

**lingual occlusion.** The position of a tooth inside the normal line of occlusion and therefore nearer the tongue than it should be.

**mesial occlusion.** The position of a tooth when it is more anterior than normal.

**puerperal tubal occlusion.** Blockage of the Fallopian tubes following labor. It is usually due to an inflammatory reaction, and is a cause of what is called one-child sterility. Once the inflammation has been treated, the tube can usually be opened up by inflation with gas under pressure.

**torso-occlusion.** The position of a tooth turned on its own axis.

**traumatic occlusion.** An abnormal occlusal stress, leading to injury of the teeth.

**tubal occlusion.** See PUERPERAL TUBAL OCCLUSION, above.

**occlusive.** Closing or shutting up.

**occlusive pessary.** A rubber contraceptive appliance used either to cover the neck of the womb or to block the upper end of the vagina.

**occult.** Hidden or secret.

**occult blood.** Blood which is not apparent to the naked eye.

**occupational disease.** Disease produced by the patient's occupation.

**occupational neurosis.** See NEUROSIS: OCCUPATIONAL NEUROSIS.

**occupational therapy.** Specialized employment designed for remedial purposes, such as sawing wood or carpentry to exercise a shoulder joint.

**ochlophobia.** Fear of crowds.

**ocular.** Pertaining to the eye, or to the eyepiece of an optical instrument.

**oculenta.** Eye ointments.

**oculist.** An ophthalmologist.

**oculogyral, oculogyric.** Refers to movements of the eyeball.

**oculogyral attacks.** A sudden upward movement of the eyeballs, which appear to be locked in that position, accompanied by wrinkling of the forehead, extension of the neck, and by all the muscular activity associated with looking upwards. These attacks occur as a complication of encephalitis lethargica. The attacks may occur several times a day or at intervals of several months; they may be precipitated by emotion, fatigue, or watching movies, and often pass off after a night's sleep. There is commonly a degree of mental depression and while this lasts the patient may be subjected to obsessional thoughts or indulge in feelings of persecution. The attacks often gradually grow less frequent over a period of years and may even cease completely. Their frequency and duration, in many cases, can be considerably reduced by the regular administration of such drugs as amphetamine sulphate. Also called *oculogyric spasms*.

**oculomotor.** Pertaining to the movement of the eye or to the oculomotor nerve (the third cranial nerve).

**oculomycosis.** Any eye disease caused by a fungus.

**oculus.** The eye.

**odontalgia.** Toothache.

**odontinoid.** 1. Toothlike. 2. A tumor composed of tooth substance.

**odontitis.** Inflammation of a tooth.

**odontoma.** A tumor arising from tooth structures.

**oecology.** See ECOLOGY.

**Oedipus complex.** The abnormal erotic attachment of a male child to his mother; named after the mythological Greek hero who killed his father and married his mother.

**oesophageal.** See ESOPHAGEAL.

**oesophagectasis.** See ESOPHAGECTASIS.

**oesophagectomy.** See ESOPHAGECTOMY.

**oesophagismus.** See ESOPHAGISMUS.

**oesophagitis.** See ESOPHAGITIS.

**oesophagocele.** See ESOPHAGOCELE.

**oesophagoduodenostomy.** See ESOPHAGODUODENOSTOMY.

**oesophagoenterostomy.** See ESOPHAGOENTEROSTOMY.

**oesophagogastrostomy.** See ESOPHAGOGASTROSTOMY.

**oesophagojejunostomy.** See ESOPHAGOJEJUNOSTOMY.

**oesophagomycosis.** See ESOPHAGOMYCOSIS.

**oesophagoplasty.** See ESOPHAGOPLASTY.

**oesophagoscope.** See ESOPHAGOSCOPE.

**oesophagospasm, oesophagismus.** See ESOPHAGOSPASM; ESOPHAGISMUS.

**oesophagostenosis.** See ESOPHAGOSTENOSIS.

**oesophagostomy.** See ESOPHAGOSTOMY.

**oesophagotomy.** See ESOPHAGOTOMY.

**oesophagus.** See ESOPHAGUS.

**oestradiol.** See ESTRADIOL.

**oestrin.** See ESTRIN.

**oestrogen.** See ESTROGEN.

**oestrone.** See ESTRONE.

**oestrum, oestrus.** See ESTRUM; ESTRUS.

**olecranal.** Pertaining to the olecranon.

**olecranoid.** Pertaining to or resembling the olecranon.

**olecranon.** The upper end of the ulna at the elbow joint. On the inner side of the olecranon runs the ulnar nerve which, when struck, causes the sensation of "pins and needles." Also called *funny bone*.

**olfactory.** Pertaining to the sense of smell.

**oligemia.** A deficiency in blood volume. Also called *oligohemia*.

**olighidria, oligidria.** A deficiency of sweating.

**oligocholia.** Deficiency in the production of bile.

**oligocythaemia.** See OLIGOCYTHEMIA.

**oligocythemia.** A deficiency of the red cells in the blood.

**oligogalactia.** Deficiency in the production of milk.

**oligohaemia.** See OLIGOHEMIA.

**oligohemia.** A deficiency in blood volume. Also called *oligemia*.

**oligohydramnios.** A deficiency in amniotic fluid.

**oligomelus.** Congenital absence of a limb.

**oligomenorrhea.** A below-normal blood loss at menstruation.

**oligopnea.** Diminution in the rate of breathing.

**oligopnoea.** See OLIGOPNEA.

**oligospermia.** A deficiency in the number of spermatozoa in the semen.

**oligotrichia.** Scanty hair.

**oliguria.** The passage of too little urine in relation to the fluid intake.

**olophonia.** Abnormal speech caused by malformation of the vocal organs.

**omental.** Pertaining to the omentum.

**omentectomy.** Surgical removal of part of the omentum.

**omentitis.** Inflammation of the omentum.

**omentopexy.** Surgical fixation of the omentum to a nearby part; usually done to promote extra blood circulation.

**omentum.** Folds of peritoneal membrane which extend between the stomach and the other abdominal organs.

**omentumectomy.** Surgical removal of the omentum.

**omphalectomy.** Surgical removal of the umbilicus.

**omphalitis.** Inflammation of the umbilicus.

**omphalocele.** An umbilical hernia.

**omphalophlebitis.** Inflammation of the umbilical vein.

**omphalos.** The umbilicus.

**omphalotomy.** Cutting of the umbilical cord, as at birth.

**onchocerciasis.** Infestation with a type of filarial worm which produces tumors of the skin, dermatitis, and eye complications.

**onco-, oncho-.** A prefix denoting a tumor.

**oncogenesis.** The process of tumor formation.

**oncogenic.** Pertaining to oncogenesis.

**oncology.** Study of the factors governing tumor growth.

**onychatrophy.** Atrophy of the nails.

**onychauxis.** Hypertrophy of the nails.

**onychectomy.** Surgical removal of a nail.

**onychia, onychitis.** Inflammation of the matrix (the tissue under the nail) of the nail, or of the nail substance.

**onychocryptosis.** Ingrowing nails.

**onychogryposis, onychogryphosis.** Hypertrophy of the nails, usually resulting in a clawlike deformity.

**onychoid.** Resembling a nail.

**onycholysis.** Loosening of a nail from its bed.

**onychomadesis.** A condition in which one or more nails are shed at intervals.

**onychomalacia.** Abnormal softening of the nails.

**onychomycosis.** Any fungus disease of the nails.

**onychophagy.** Nail-biting.

**onychorhexis.** Brittleness of the nails.

**onychoschisis.** Partial or complete separation of the nails from the nail bed.

**onychosis.** Any nail disease.

**onyx.** 1. A finger nail or toe nail. 2. A hypopyon.

**onyxis.** Congenitally ingrowing nails.

**oophorectomy.** Surgical removal of an ovary. Also called *ovariectomy.*

**oophoritis.** Inflammation of an ovary. Also called *ovaritis.*

**oophorohysterectomy.** Surgical removal of the womb and ovaries. Also called *ovariohysterectomy.*

**oophoromalacia.** Softening of an ovary.

**oophoron.** The ovary.

**oophoropathy.** Any disease of the ovary.

**oophoropexy.** Surgical fixation of a dropped ovary.

**oophoroplasty.** Surgical repair of the ovaries.

**oophorosalpingectomy.** Surgical removal of the ovary and Fallopian tube.

**oophorosalpingitis.** Inflammation of the ovary and Fallopian tube. Also called *salpingo-oophoritis.*

**operable.** Refers to a condition in which surgery offers a reasonable hope of improvement. For instance, in cases of cancer it infers that the cancer has not spread and is so localized that it can be removed completely.

**ophidiophobia.** Fear of reptiles.

**ophthalmalgia.** Pain in the eye.

**ophthalmia.** Inflammation of the eye, especially one in which the conjunctiva is involved.

**catarrhal ophthalmia.** Simple conjunctivitis, usually with a mucopurulent discharge.

**Egyptian ophthalmia.** An obsolete name for trachoma.

**ophthalmia neonatorum.** The inflammatory condition causing profuse discharge from the eyes, occurring in a newborn baby which has contracted gonorrhea of the eyes from its mother.

**ophthalmitis.** Inflammation of the eye.

**ophthalmologist.** A specialist in eye disorders.

**ophthalmology.** The study of disorders of the eye.

**ophthalmopathy.** Any disease of the eye.

**ophthalmophobia.** Fear of being stared at.

**ophthalmoplegia.** Paralysis of the eye muscles.

**ophthalmoscope.** An instrument containing a light and various lenses and used to examine the inside of the eye and retina.

**ophthalmoscopy.** Examination of the inside of the eye with an ophthalmoscope.

**opiate.** 1. A preparation of opium. 2. Any medicine that induces sleep.

**opisthotonoid.** Resembling opisthotonos.

**opisthotonos.** A violent muscular spasm, which so arches the back that the patient is literally resting on the back of his skull and his heels. It sometimes occurs in cerebrospinal fever, epilepsy, rabies, tetanus, and strychnine poisoning.

**opsonin.** A substance normally present in blood serum, and which can be increased by immunization, which makes bacteria attractive to the white blood cells. This phenomenon is part of the body's defense against bacteria, and it is as though opsonin acts like a piquant sauce on cold meat, encouraging the white cells to engulf large numbers of bacteria.

**optic.** Pertaining to the eye or vision.

**optic atrophy.** Wasting of the optic nerve.

**optic disc.** The small area at the back of the eyeball where the retinal blood vessels and the optic nerve enter. It is insensitive to light, and changes in its appearance may assist in the diagnosis of certain disease conditions.

**optic nerve.** The second cranial nerve, which supplies the retina with its pathway for transmitting visual impressions to the brain.

**optimum.** The set of conditions at which vital processes are carried out with the greatest activity and success.

**oral.** Pertaining to the mouth.

**orbicular.** Circular. The term is applied to circular muscles, such as the orbicular muscle of the eye (orbicularis oculi) and the orbicular muscles of the mouth (orbicularis oris).

**orbit.** The bony socket which contains the eye.

**orchectomy.** Surgical removal of a testicle. Also called *orchidectomy, orchiectomy.*

**orchialgia.** Pain in the testicle.

**orchidotomy.** Surgical incision into a testicle. Also called *orchiotomy.*

**orchiepididymitis.** Inflammation of both testicles and epydidymis. The epididymis is a small structure, lying behind and above the testicle, composed of tubes which carry spermatozoa from the testicle.

**orchiopexy.** See ORCHIORRHAPHY.

**orchioplasty.** Surgical repair of the scrotum.

**orchiorrhaphy.** Surgical fixation of the testicle in the scrotum.

**orchiotomy.** Surgical incision of a testicle.

**orchis.** The testicle.

**orchitic.** Relating to orchitis.

**orchitis.** Inflammation of a testicle. See also MUMPS.

**orchotomy.** The surgical operation of castration.

**organ.** A structurally coherent and identifiable portion of the body consisting of a group of closely associated tissues all contributing to the performance of a specific function or functions, as the stomach functions in digestion.

**orgasm.** The culmination point of the sexual act or of sexual excitement.

**orolingual.** Pertaining to the mouth and the tongue.

**oronasal.** Pertaining to the mouth and nose.

**oropharyngeal.** Relating to the mouth and pharynx.

**oropharynx.** The back part of the throat behind the tongue.

**orthodiagram.** The record made in orthodiagraphy.

**orthodiagraphy.** A method for checking the outer edges and exact size of an organ, usually the heart, by using parallel x-rays to outline the edges of an organ on a special screen.

**orthodontia.** The correction of irregularities in the teeth.

**orthodontic.** Relating to orthodontia.

**orthodontics.** The science of orthodontia.

**orthodontist.** One skilled in orthodontia.

**orthognathism.** A condition in which the jaws, especially the upper jaw, have little or no forward projection.

**orthognathous.** Having jaws with little or no forward projection. See ORTHOGNATHISM.

**orthopaedics.** See ORTHOPEDICS.

**orthopaedist.** See ORTHOPEDIST.

**orthopedics.** That branch of surgery concerned with the corrective treatment of deformities, diseases, and ailments of muscles, bones, ligaments, and joints.

**orthopedist.** A specialist in orthopedic surgery.

**orthopnea.** Inability to breathe except in an upright position. It usually occurs in heart failure and some other forms of heart disease.

**orthopnoea.** See ORTHOPNEA.

**orthoptic.** Pertaining to normal vision with both eyes.

**orthoptics, orthoptic training.** The science of promoting efficient vision with both eyes, usually by exercise or training, and including the treatment of partial blindness and of muscle imbalances and squints.

**orthostatic.** Pertaining to or caused by standing upright.

**orthostatic albuminuria.** The appearance of albumin in the urine when the patient stands up or takes muscular exercise, but disappearing after a rest in bed. Albumin is an abnormal constituent of urine and its appearance is usually a sign of bodily disease. Orthostatic albuminuria, however, is not an indication of a disease process, but is frequently present in young healthy adults.

**orthotonus.** A form of muscular cramp which compels the patient to lie rigid and stretched out.

**Osgood-Schlatter's disease.** See SCHLATTER'S DISEASE.

**Osler-Libman-Sacks syndrome.** Disseminated lupus erythematosus. See LUPUS: LUPUS ERYTHEMATOSUS.

**Osler's disease.** Also called *Osler-Vaquez disease.* See POLYCYTHEMIA VERA.

**Osler's nodes.** Small painful nodules found in the pulp of the finger tips in subacute infectious endocarditis, an infection invariably occurring in a heart which is already damaged. In 80 percent of cases the infecting germ is a hemolytic streptococcus.

**osmidrosis.** A condition in which the sweat has an abnormally offensive odor. Also called *bromidrosis.*

**osmosis.** The passage of a fluid through a semipermeable membrane from a more concentrated solution into a more dilute one.

*This phenomenon is of the greatest importance in the functioning of the body, because it governs many processes, such as the separation of lymph and blood, and the absorption of fluid by cells. For example, if a teaspoonful of Epsom salts mixed with one or two tablespoonfuls of water is swallowed, the osmotic pressure of this solution draws fluid out of the body and into the bowels, resulting in liquid stools, diarrhea, and dehydration of the body. This effect of osmosis can be put to good account in cases of edema, such as patients being given a concentrated Epsom salt solution to rid their tissues of excess fluid. On the other hand, if a teaspoonful of Epsom salts in a full tumbler of water is swallowed, the osmotic pressure of this weaker solution, although it causes a watery stool, does not draw fluid out of the body and the Epsom salts prevent the body from absorbing the water, which passes through unchanged in volume.*

**ossa.** Bones.

**osseous.** Bony.

**ossicle.** A small bone, especially one of the three small bones in the middle ear.

**ossicula auditus.** The auditory ossicles in the middle ear.

**ossiculectomy.** Surgical removal of one of the small bones in the middle ear.

**ossiferous.** Producing or containing bone tissue.

**ossific, ossificans.** Producing bone, or being converted into bone.

**ossification.** Being converted into bone.

**ossiform.** Bonelike.

**ossify.** To convert into bone.

**osteal.** Bony.

**ostealgia.** Pains in the bones.

**ostectomy.** Surgical removal of a piece or the whole of a bone.

**ostectopy.** Displacement of a bone.

**osteitis.** Inflammation of a bone.

**condensing osteitis.** A form of inflammation usually involving the whole of a long bone and resulting in the marrow cavity filling with a dense bony mass, so that the bone becomes heavier and denser.

**deformans osteitis.** A chronic condition characterized by excessive deposits of bony tissue on the bone surface and within its marrow, which later solidifies, causing curving and enlargement. It chiefly affects skull, spine, pelvis, and lower leg bones. Also called *Paget's disease.*

**dento-alveolar osteitis.** Osteitis occurring in the jaw bones in association with pyorrhea.

**fibrosa osteitis.** The occurrence in bones of cysts and tumorlike masses caused by a disturbance in calcium and phosphorus metabolism. Also called *hyperparathyroidism, von Recklinghausen's disease.*

**gummatous osteitis.** A type of inflammation characterized by the formation of syphilitic growths in or on bones.

**osteoarthritis.** Strictly, this condition is not an inflammation of the bone of joints but a degeneration of tissues characterized by thickening of the joint region with bony outgrowths which lead to roughening and joint deformity, limiting movement, and causing pain. In complete contradiction to most popularly held beliefs, osteoarthritis is NOT caused by acid, infection, poisons, drugs, food, constipation, cold, or damp, but is "old age" of the joints. Neither should it be confused with gout or rheumatoid arthritis and many people would suffer far less if they disregarded the wonderful claims made for patent medicines and "certain cures." A joint affected with osteoarthritis should not be overexercised or strained in an effort to "work it off," as this only makes the pain worse. If the joint is painful, the patient should not stand or walk for long periods; on the other hand he should not remain in one position for too long or be afraid of simple movements to prevent stiffness. Severe pain not amenable to sim-

ple measures can be relieved by various surgical means.

**osteoarthropathy.** Any disease of the joints.

**pulmonary osteoarthropathy.** A disease characterized by bulblike enlargement of the tips of the fingers (called "clubbing") and toes, with thickening of the ends of long bones and a peculiar curvature of the nails. The disease is usually associated with conditions of the lungs or chest which result in circulatory congestion, and sometimes occurs in congenital heart disease. Also called *hypertrophic pulmonary osteoarthropathy.*

**osteoarthrotomy.** Surgical excision of the end of a long bone.

**osteochondritis.** Although the term implies inflammation of both bone and cartilage, the changes most frequently found are degeneration and regeneration of bone (particularly at the growing ends of long bones), and for this reason many doctors prefer to use the term osteochondrosis. When this degeneration occurs in the bony area below the kneecap it is called Osgood-Schlatter disease, and this is commonly met with in adolescent boys as a form of chronic pain below the kneecap, especially after exercise. Recovery always occurs with rest and attention to the general health.

**osteochondritis deformans juvenilis.** A disease of the upper end of the thigh bone affecting children between five and ten years of age. See PERTHES' DISEASE.

**osteochondritis dissecans.** A joint affection characterized by partial detachment of fragments of cartilage and underlying bone from the joint surface and frequently resulting in so-called "loose bodies" within the joint. The knee joint is most commonly affected.

**vertebral osteochondritis.** A change occurring during growth, in which the joint surfaces of a spinal vertebra appear roughened, irregular, and the bone appears to be less dense. It occurs in young people, with complaint of chronic backache, frequently in the upper part of the spine. Also called *Scheuermann's disease.*

**osteochondroma.** A growth composed of bone and cartilage.

**osteochondromatosis.** The presence of multiple osteochondromas.

**osteochondrosarcoma.** A cancerous growth arising from bone and cartilage cells.

**osteochondrosis.** See OSTEOCHONDRITIS.

**osteoclasia, osteoclasis.** Surgical fracture of a long bone, without opening the tissues, to correct a deformity. The term is also applied to the destruction of bony tissue and to the resorption of bone.

**osteoclastoma.** A giant-cell tumor arising in bone, regarded as harmless, but may recur after removal.

**osteodermia.** The conversion of a portion of skin into bony tissue.

**osteodiastasis.** The separation of a bone or of two bones.

**osteodystrophia.** Defective bone formation. It includes such bone defects as are seen in rickets, dwarfism, and the like.

**osteodystrophia deformans.** A disease of late life, affecting one or more bones, with deformity from abnormal growth. No cause is known. Also called *osteitis deformans, Paget's disease.*

**osteodystrophia fibrosa.** A rare condition occurring only in females in which a patchy pigmentation is associated with cysts in the bones. Also called *Albright's disease.*

**osteoectomy.** Surgical excision of a bone or part of a bone.

**osteoectopy.** Displacement of a bone.

**osteo-epiphysis.** A bony epiphysis.

**osteofibroma.** A tumor of bone and fibrous tissue.

**osteogenesis.** The development of bony tissue.

**osteogenesis imperfecta.** An hereditary condition characterized by abnormal fragility of the bones, resulting in spontaneous fractures, associated with striking blueness of the whites of the eyes, and sometimes with deafness. These young, unfortunate people, by the time they reach school age, may have fractured many bones, some several times, with only the slightest amount of force. Also called *osteopsathyrosis, Lobstein's disease, fragilitas ossium.*

**osteogenetic.** Relating to osteogenesis.

**osteogenetic sarcoma.** A malignant growth arising from the deep layers of periosteum.

**osteogenic.** Osteogenetic.

**osteoid.** Resembling bone. Also the young matrix (layer) of true bone in which calcium salts are deposited to form proper bone.

**osteoid chondroma.** A form of growth arising beneath the periosteum and composed of cells from which true bone may be formed.

**osteoid sarcoma.** A malignant growth of noncalcified bony tissue.

**osteology.** The study of bones.

**osteoma.** A tumor arising in bony tissue.

**cancellous osteoma.** An outgrowth of bone derived from cancellous or spongelike bone.

**compact osteoma.** A compact and solid outgrowth of bone derived from the compact layer of bone which lies near the surface.

**osteomalacia.** A disease due to vitamin D deficiency in adult life, characterized by softening of the bones, a low concentration of calcium and phosphorus in the blood, together with an increased secretion of calcium and phosphorus in the urine. The bones become curved and deformed and there is a liability to spontaneous fractures.

**osteomyelitic.** Pertaining to osteomyelitis.

**osteomyelitis.** Inflammation and abscess formation in the cavity of a bone.

**osteonecrosis.** Death of bone.

**osteopaedion.** See OSTEOPEDION.

**osteopath.** One skilled in osteopathy.

**osteopathic.** Pertaining to osteopathy.

**osteopathy.** 1. Any disease of bone. 2. The term is also applied to a school of healing which teaches that the body is a vital mechanical organism whose structural and functional integrity are coordinate and interdependent, the perversion of either constituting disease. Its major effort in treatment is manipulation.

**osteopedion.** The calcified remains of a fetus within the womb. Also called *lithopedion.*

**osteoperiostitis.** Inflammation of both the bone and the periosteum.

**osteopetrosis.** A congenital disease characterized by increased density of the bones, spontaneous fractures, enlargement of the spleen, and anemia. Symptoms usually begin in childhood, with fractures following injury, and general backwardness. The anemia is mainly due to a narrowing of the bone marrow cavity, which stores the blood-forming mechanism, so that the total "blood factory space" throughout the body is significantly reduced. Also called *Albers-Schonberg disease, marble bones, osteosclerosis.*

**osteophyte.** A small local outgrowth of bone from the periosteum commonly seen in osteoarthritis.

**osteoplastic.** Pertaining to the formation of bone, or to osteoplasty.

**osteoplasty.** Repair operations on bone.

**osteopoikily.** A congenital and quite painless disease of bone characterized by the presence of small dense areas which are liable to occasional spontaneous fractures. Also called *osteopoikilosis, osteosclerosis fragilitas.*

**osteoporosis.** Abnormal porousness of bone. The loss of bony substance results in brittleness or softness of the bones involved, but they are not changed in shape and the condition is only recognized in an x-ray picture. The condition occurs in such diseases as osteoporosis congenita, hyperparathyroidism, rickets, Still's disease, sy-

ringomyelia, Cushing's syndrome, and in bones which have long been encased in plaster casts.

**osteopsathyrosis.** See OSTEOGENESIS IMPERFECTA.

**osteosarcoma.** Malignant disease arising in bone.

**osteosclerosis.** See OSTEOPETROSIS.

**osteoseptum.** The bony part of the wall between the nostrils.

**osteosis.** The formation of bone.

**osteotomy.** Surgical division or removal of part of a bone.

**osteotrite.** A surgical instrument used for scraping away diseased bone.

**ostial.** Pertaining to an opening.

**ostitis.** See OSTEITIS.

**ostium.** A mouth or opening.

**otalgia.** Earache.

**otectomy.** Removal of the auditory ossicles (three little bones in the middle ear).

**othaematoma.** See OTHEMATOMA.

**othaemorrhagia.** See OTHEMORRHAGIA.

**othaemorrhoea.** See OTHEMORRHEA.

**othematoma.** A hematoma (blood-filled swelling) of the outer ear.

**othemorrhagia.** Hemorrhage from the ear.

**othemorrhea.** A blood-containing discharge from the ear.

**otic.** Pertaining to the ear.

**otitic.** Pertaining to otitis.

**otitis.** Inflammation of the ear. See also EAR DRUM.

**otitis externa.** Inflammation of the external ear.

**otitis interna.** Inflammation of the internal ear.

**otitis media.** Inflammation of the middle ear.

**otogenous.** Originating in the ear.

**otolith.** A stone formed within the membranous labyrinth of the ear.

**otologist.** A specialist in otology.

**otology.** The study of diseases of the ear.

**otomycosis.** Fungus infection of the ear.

**otopharyngeal.** Pertaining to the ear and pharynx.

**otopharyngeal tube.** The tube which runs from the back of the nose to the middle ear and equalizes the atmospheric pressure on both sides of the ear drum. Also called *otosalpinx, auditory tube.* See TUBE: EUSTACHIAN TUBE.

**otopiesis.** Deafness resulting from abnormal pressure on the labyrinth of the ear.

**otoplasty.** Surgical repair of the external ear.

**otopyorrhea.** Any discharge of pus from the ear opening.

**otopyorrhoea.** See OTOPYORRHEA.

**otorhinolaryngology.** The study of diseases of the ear, nose, and throat.

**otorrhagia.** A discharge of blood from the ear opening.

**otorrhea.** A discharge from the ear opening.

**otorrhoea.** See OTORRHEA.

**otosalpinx.** The Eustachian tube of the ear. Also called *otopharyngeal tube.*

**otosclerosis.** A condition in which there is progressive deafness due to abnormal bone formation in the hearing apparatus interfering with the conduction of sound.

**ovarian.** Relating to the ovary.

**ovarian pregnancy.** The development of a fertilized egg cell within the ovary. Also called *ovariocyesis.*

**ovariectomy.** Surgical removal of an ovary. Also called *oophorectomy, ovariotomy.*

**ovariocentesis.** Surgical puncture of an ovary or of a cyst within it.

**ovariocyesis.** A pregnancy occurring within the ovary.

**ovariohysterectomy.** Surgical removal of the ovaries and womb. Also called *oophorohysterectomy.*

**ovariotomy.** Surgical removal of an ovary; surgical removal of a large ovarian cyst.

**ovaritis.** Inflammation of an ovary. Also called *oophoritis.*

**ovarium.** An ovary.

**ovary.** One of the two glandular organs situated on the back wall of the female pelvis. Together the ovaries contain at birth enough ova (eggs) in embryo form to last a female all her productive life. Each month a ripe ovum escapes

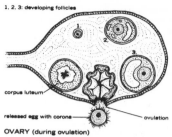

1, 2, 3: developing follicles

corpus luteum

released egg with corona

ovulation

OVARY (during ovulation)

body, together with the unfertilized ovum, as a bloody discharge—the menstrual period. The womb then grows a new lining in preparation for a possible pregnancy the following month.

**overstrain.** Fatigue produced by physical exertion, not amounting to complete exhaustion.

**oviduct.** See FALLOPIAN TUBE.

**ovular.** Pertaining to an ovum.

**ovulation.** The discharge of an egg from the ovary.

**ovum.** An egg. The human ovum is just visible to the naked eye.

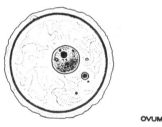

OVUM

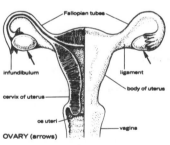

Fallopian tubes

infundibulum

ligament

body of uterus

cervix of uterus

oe uteri

vagina

OVARY (arrows)

from one of the ovaries and finds its way into the Fallopian tube where it awaits fertilization by a spermatozoan, which has traversed the womb (or uterus) and passed into the Fallopian tube. The fertilized ovum then passes into the womb, embeds itself into the lining and commences to grow. If the ovum does not become fertilized, then under the hormone influence of the ovary the lining of the womb splits off and passes out of the

**oxalaemia.** See OXALEMIA.

**oxalemia.** An excess of calcium oxalate in the blood.

**oxaluria.** An excess of calcium oxalate in the urine. Calcium oxalate crystals may cause irritability of the bladder and an increased desire to pass water, with occasionally the passage of albumin and blood in the urine. Oxalates may be a constituent of stones in the kidney, and the crystals may arise from foods high in oxalates, such as rhubarb, spinach, asparagus, sorrel and, to a lesser extent, strawberries.

**oxycephaly.** A high-pointed skull. See ACROCEPHALY.

**oxygen.** A colorless, tasteless, odorless gas, constituting one-fifth of the atmosphere, eight-ninths of water and about one-half of the world's crust. It supports combustion, is essential for life, combines with most elements, and is carried by the blood from the lungs

to the tissues. The air we breathe in is 20 percent oxygen while that we breathe out is 15 percent. This fact is the basis of mouth-to-mouth or mouth-to-nose methods of artificial respiration, for the first-aider breathes in to the casualty air which still contains 15 percent of oxygen.

**oxygenation.** The saturation of a substance with oxygen.

**oxyhaemoglobin.** See OXYHEMOGLOBIN.

**oxyhemoglobin.** The combination of oxygen and hemoglobin in the red blood cells. This combination gives arterial blood its bright red color, compared with the darker red of venous blood in which the hemoglobin is deficient in oxygen.

**oxyopia.** Increased visual perception.

**oxytocia.** Rapid or precipitate childbirth.

**oxytocic.** Hastening childbirth, or a drug that hastens childbirth.

**oxytocin.** A hormone secreted by the pituitary gland in the brain. It can be produced synthetically, and in minute doses is sometimes used to stimulate labor pains and hasten childbirth or to stimulate the womb to contract and prevent it bleeding after childbirth.

**oxyuriasis.** Harboring thread worms.

**Oxyuris.** A genus of threadworms.

**ozaena.** See OZENA.

**ozena.** A chronic disease of the nose, accompanied by a foul discharge.

**ozone.** A modification of oxygen. Oxygen is represented chemically by $O_2$, whereas ozone is represented by three atoms of oxygen as $O_3$. Ozone is used as a disinfectant.

# P

**pacemaker.** A structure that influences the rate of a reaction or a process such as the sinoatrial node, a small mass of muscle tissue which controls the rate of contraction of the heart.

**artificial pacemaker.** A heart-regulating instrument with built-in batteries which has been surgically installed with increasing frequency in recent years.

**pachycephaly.** Abnormal thickness of the skull.

**pachyderma, pachydermia.** Thickening of the skin.

**pachyderma laryngis.** Thickening of the vocal cords due to chronic laryngitis.

**pachydermatous.** Thick-skinned.

**pachylosis.** Thick, dry skin.

**pachymenia.** Thickening of a membrane.

**pachymeningitis.** Inflammation of the dura mater, the outermost of the three membranes covering the brain.

**pachymeningitis externa.** Inflammation of the external layer of the dura mater.

**pachymeningitis hemorrhagica interna.** A collection of blood beneath the dura mater, either from an accident or disease. Also called *subdural hematoma.*

**pachymeningitis interna.** Inflammation of the internal layer of the dura mater.

**pachymeningitis spinalis hypertrophica.** A form of inflammation leading to fibrosis, commonly in the neck region of the spinal cord producing compression of the nerve roots of the spine.

**pachyonychia.** Abnormal thickening of the nails.

**pachytic.** Thick or fat.

**pachytrichous.** Thick-haired.

**pachyvaginitis.** Inflammation resulting in thickening of the vaginal wall.

**packing.** Treating a wound by filling or covering it with gauze or other material.

**paediatrician, paediatrist.** See PEDIATRICIAN; PEDIATRIST.

**paediatrics.** See PEDIATRICS.

**Page's disease.** A form of neurosis which develops in a casualty who is consciously or subconsciously determined to obtain compensation. Also called *Erichsen's disease, railway spine.*

**Paget's disease.** See OSTEITIS: OSTEITIS DEFORMANS.

**Paget's disease of the nipple.** A malignant growth arising in the skin of the nipple of the female breast.

**Paget's recurrent fibroid.** A form of malignant disease of the skin.

**painted sickness.** A skin disease of tropical America characterized by thickened patches of skin and color changes caused by a spirochete. Also called *carate, azul, spotted sickness, mal del pinto, pinta.*

**painter's colic.** Lead poisoning in painters.

**palate.** The roof of the mouth. The front part, mostly composed of bone, is called the hard palate, and the back part, which is soft and muscular, is referred to as the soft palate. See also CLEFT PALATE.

**palatiform.** Shaped like a palate.

**palatine.** Relating to the palate.

**palatitis.** Inflammation of the palate.

**palatoglossal.** Relating to the palate and the tongue.

**palatognathus.** See CLEFT PALATE.

**palatomaxillary.** Relating to both the palate and the maxilla.

**palatonasal.** Relating to the palate and the nose.

**palatopharyngeal.** Relating to the palate and the pharynx.

**palatoplasty.** Surgical repair of the palate.

**palatoplegia.** Paralysis of the soft palate.

**palatorrhaphy.** Surgical suturing of the palate. Also called *staphylorrhaphy.*

**palatoschisis.** See CLEFT PALATE.

**palatum.** The palate.

**palilalia.** A speech defect, in which the last word or words of a phrase are repeated several times.

**palindromia.** The recurrence of a disease.

**palingraphia.** A condition in which the last word or words are repeated when writing.

**palinphrasia.** A disturbance of speech in which words or phrases are repeated.

**palirrhea.** The recurrence of a discharge; regurgitation.

**palirrhoea.** See PALIRRHEA.

**pallaesthesia.** See PALLESTHESIA.

**pallesthesia.** The sensation of vibration.

**palliate.** To soothe.

**palliative.** Something which soothes and relieves but does not cure.

**pallid, pallida, pallidus.** Pale.

**pallor.** Paleness.

**palma.** The palm of the hand.

**palmar, palmic.** Relating to the palm of the hand.

**palmar abscess.** An abscess in the palm of the hand.

**palpable.** Capable of being felt.

**palpate.** To examine by touch.

**palpebra.** The eyelid.

  **palpebra inferior.** The lower eyelid.

  **palpebra superior.** The upper eyelid.

**palpebral.** Relating to the eyelid.

**palpebration.** Winking.

**palpitate.** To flutter or beat fast.

**palpitation.** The sensation of fluttering or a rapid beating of the heart.

**palsy.** Paralysis.

**paludism.** An infrequently used term for malaria.

**pamplegia.** Generalized paralysis.

**panacea.** A remedy alleged to cure all disease.

**panarthritis.** Strictly, inflammation of all the structures forming a joint, but frequently applied to inflammation of all the joints.

**pancarditis.** Inflammation of all the layers of the heart, that is, endocardium, myocardium, and pericardium.

**pancreas.** A gland lying transversely across the back of the abdominal cavity with its right extremity, or head,

lying in contact with the duodenum and its left extremity, or tail, in close proximity to the spleen. It is from six to eight inches long and about an inch thick, weighs some three ounces, and manufactures both an external and an internal secretion. The external secretion, the pancreatic fluid or juice, passes into the duodenum by way of the pancreatic duct. The internal secretion, insulin, is produced in special cells called the islets of Langerhans and passes directly into the circulation. Failure in the production of insulin produces diabetes mellitus.

**pancreatalgia.** Pancreatic pain.

**pancreatectomy.** Surgical excision of all or part of the pancreas.

**pancreatic.** Relating to the pancreas or due to disease of the pancreas.

**pancreatic juice.** A secretion from the pancreas containing three digestive enzymes: amylase, which digests carbohydrate; lipase, which digests fat; and trypin, which digests protein.

**pancreaticoduodenal.** Pertaining to both pancreas and duodenum.

**pancreaticoduodenectomy.** Surgical removal of the whole of the duodenum and part of the pancreas; performed for malignant disease involving the head of the pancreas.

**pancreatico-enterostomy.** A surgical operation in which the pancreatic duct is implanted into the wall of the intestine during pancreaticoduodenectomy.

**pancreaticojejunostomy.** Surgical joining of the pancreatic duct to the jejunum.

**pancreatin.** A preparation of the pancreatic enzymes: trypsin, diastase and lipase.

**pancreatitis.** Inflammation of the pancreas. The acute form may be hemorrhagic, suppurative, or gangrenous, and the onset is usually sudden, with severe abdominal pain, distension, and acute tenderness of the abdomen. It is an acute and severe surgical catastrophe.

**pancreatogenous.** Originating in the pancreas.

**pancreatolipase.** The fat-splitting enzyme produced by the pancreas.

**pancreatolith.** A stone in the pancreas.

**pancreatotomy.** Surgical incision of the pancreas.

**pancreolytic.** Destructive to the pancreas.

**pancreopathy.** Any disease of the pancreas.

**pandemic.** A widespread epidemic; not localized.

**pangenesis.** Darwin's comprehensive theory of hereditary development, according to which all parts of the body give off "gemmules" which collect in the germ cells of the egg. During development they are sorted out one from another, and give rise to parts similar to thcse of their origin.

**panhidrosis.** A condition of prolonged sweating of the whole body. Also called *panidrosis.*

**panhysterectomy.** Surgical removal of the whole of the womb or uterus. The term is especially used to indicate that both the body and the neck of the womb have been removed, whereas when the body of the womb only is removed it is referred to as subtotal hysterectomy. See HYSTERECTOMY.

**panidrosis.** See PANHIDROSIS.

**panmyelophthisis.** General aplasia of the bone marrow.

**panniculitis.** Inflammation of the fatty layer of tissue beneath the skin.

**pannus.** A form of granulation tissue which grows from the conjunctiva into the cornea of the eye.

**panophthalmia, panophthalmitis.** Inflammation of all the eyeball tissues.

**panoptosis.** A drooping of all the abdominal organs.

**pansinusitis.** Simultaneous inflammation of all the sinuses of the head. See also SINUS; SINUSITIS.

**pantalgia.** Pain occurring through the entire body.

**papilla. 1.** The breast nipple. **2.** The optic disc. **3.** Any small nipple-shaped growth, such as those on the tongue which are concerned with touch and taste. These are of two kinds: tall and slender ones called papillae filiformis, and low, broad ones known as papillae fungiformis.

**papillary. 1.** Pertaining to the breast nipple. **2.** Containing papillae; resembling a papilla.

**papillectomy.** Surgical excision of a papilla.

**papilledema.** Swelling of the optic disc with narrowing of the arteries and dilation of the veins. Also called *choked disc, optic neuritis, papillitis.*

**papilliferous.** Bearing papillae.

**papilliform.** Shaped like a papilla.

**papillitis.** Papilledema.

**papilloedema.** See PAPILLEDEMA.

**papilloma.** A growth arising from the surface of skin or mucous membrane. The skin papilloma is benign, harmless, and readily removed by tying its neck tightly with a silk thread to cut off the blood supply so that it becomes necrotic and drops off. Those arising from mucous membranes, such as the lining of the milk ducts of the nipple, the lining of the urinary bladder or intestine, may bleed regularly.

**papillomatosis.** A condition characterized by the presence of multiple papillomas.

**papillose.** Having papillae.

**papillous.** Characterized by the presence of papillae.

**pappataci fever.** A febrile disease of short duration resembling dengue, caused by a virus, and associated with the bite of sandflies. Also called *three-day fever, sandfly fever.*

**papular.** Characterized by the presence of papules.

**papulation.** The formation of papules.

**papule.** A small nodular elevation of the skin, as opposed to a macule, which is a spot flat and level with the skin.

**papulonecrotic tuberculide.** See TUBERCULID.

**papulopustular.** A condition characterized by the presence of both papules and pustules or papules which are turning into pustules.

**papulopustule.** A papule surmounted by a pustule.

**papulovesicle.** A papule surmounted by a vesicle.

**papulovesicular.** A condition characterized by the presence of both papules and vesicles.

**papyraceous.** Like paper.

**para-anaesthesia.** See PARA-ANESTHESIA.

**para-anesthesia.** Loss of sensation in both arms or both legs.

**parablepsis.** Incorrect vision.

**paracanthoma.** A growth arising from the so-called prickle-cell layer of the skin.

**paracardiac.** Near the heart.

**paracentesis.** Surgical puncture of a cavity, usually performed to withdraw fluid.

**parachroia.** Abnormal coloration.

**parachromatism.** Incorrect perception of color; color blindness.

**paracolpitis.** Inflammation of the tissues around the vagina.

**paracusia, paracusis.** A defect of hearing.

**paracusia acris.** Hearing so acute that it is beyond a person's endurance.

**paracusia duplicata.** Hearing double sounds.

**paracusia imaginaria.** See TINNITUS.

**paracusia localis.** Inability to estimate the direction of sounds, usually when one ear is partially deaf.

**paracusia obtusa.** Deafness.

**paracusia willisii.** A deaf condition in which the person hears best in noisy surroundings.

**paracyesis.** A pregnancy occurring outside the uterus or womb, such as in the abdominal cavity, ovary, or Fallopian tube.

**paracystitis.** Inflammation of the tissues surrounding the urinary bladder.

**paradoxia sexualis.** Sexual excitement which occurs independently of the period of the sexual development of the generative organs; the abnor-

mal exhibition of sexual instincts in childhood, prior to puberty, or occurring in the senile years.

**paraesthesia.** See PARESTHESIA.

**paraganglioma.** See PHEOCHROMOCYTOMA.

**paraganglion.** A collection of pheochromocytes alongside certain arteries.

**parageusia, parageusis.** Perversion of the sense of taste.

**paragonimiasis.** Infestation with flukes of the genus *Paragonimus.*

**Paragonimus.** A genus of flatworms; flukes, transmitted from animals to man.

**paragrammatism.** A condition marked by inability to speak grammatically, or by the use of incorrect words. See also SENSORY APHASIA.

**paragraphia.** A condition characterized by the use in writing of wrong or misplaced words.

**parahepatic.** Adjacent to the liver.

**parakeratosis.** A skin condition usually associated with an inflammation of one of its layers resulting in a disturbance of keratinization so that the skin forms soft masses and scales.

**paralalia.** Inability to utter certain sounds.

**paralambdacism.** A disturbance of speech in which the sound of the letter L is replaced by other letters.

**paralexia.** Disturbance in reading, marked by the substitution or transposition of words or syllables.

**paralgesia.** An abnormal painful sensation; painful paresthesia.

**paralogia.** False reasoning.

**paralysis.** Loss of function in a muscle or group of muscles, usually caused by injury to the nerves or nerve centers which control them. A slight loss of muscular function is called a palsy, muscular weakness, or loss of power.

**acute ascending paralysis.** Paralysis of the lower limbs or lower trunk, progressing upwards towards the brain. Usually seen in poliomyelitis, postvaccinal myelitis, and polyneuritis.

**paralysis agitans.** A chronic disease characterized by rigidity of muscles, muscular weakness, slowness of movements, tremor, flexion of the head, trunk, and limbs, and often with a masklike face which registers little or no emotion. Also called *Parkinson's disease.*

**amyotrophic paralysis.** Paralysis due to muscle wasting.

**anapeiratic paralysis.** A neurosis in which the subject believes he is paralyzed due to excessive use of his limbs.

**anterior spinal paralysis.** Poliomyelitis.

**arsenical paralysis.** Paralysis developing in the late stages of arsenical poisoning.

**Bell's paralysis.** Paralysis of the facial nerve. Also called *Bell's palsy*.

**bulbar paralysis.** A condition affecting speech, chewing, swallowing, and breathing, due to disturbances of the brain centers which control the nerves to the muscles of these parts.

**cerebral spastic infantile paralysis.** Also called *spastic diplegia.* See DIPLEGIA: CEREBRAL DIPLEGIA.

**compression paralysis.** Paralysis caused by pressure on a nerve.

**crossed paralysis.** Paralysis of the arm and leg of one side associated with paralysis of the face on the opposite side.

**crutch paralysis.** Paralysis of the arm, due to pressure of a crutch against nerves in the armpit.

**diver's paralysis.** Paralysis occurring in caisson disease.

**Erb-Duchenne paralysis.** Paralysis of the fifth and sixth cervical spinal nerve routes, causing paralysis of the upper arm.

**general paralysis of the insane.** A disease due to syphilis of the brain and nervous system, producing progressive dementia, delusions, inability to speak properly, seizures, tremors, the absence of light reflexes in the pupil, and a generalized wasting of the brain cells. Also called *dementia paralytica.*

**hysterical paralysis.** Muscle weakness or paralysis, without loss of reflex activity, in which no organic nerve lesion can be demonstrated.

**infantile paralysis.** Poliomyelitis.

**infantile spastic paralysis.** See DIPLEGIA: CEREBRAL DIPLEGIA.

**jake paralysis.** Paralysis due to a peripheral neuritis, caused by the excessive eating of Jamaica ginger.

**Landry's paralysis.** Acute ascending paralysis. Some cases are due to polyneuritis, some to poliomyelitis, and others have no known cause.

**mimetic paralysis.** Paralysis of the facial muscles.

**obstetrical paralysis.** Paralysis occurring in the arm of a newborn baby, due to damage to the arm nerves during delivery.

**occupational paralysis.** Muscular weakness and wasting due to nerve compression and overexertion in certain occupations.

**ocular paralysis.** Paralysis of the eye muscles, of the optic nerve, or of the ciliary muscle in the eye.

**oculophrenicorecurrent paralysis.** Paralysis of the recurrent laryngeal and phrenic nerves and associated with Horner's syndrome, such as may occur in cancer of the lung with cancer deposits in the middle of the chest, pressing on the two nerves.

**periodic familial paralysis.** A familial disease, starting in early life and characterized by periodic temporary paralysis with paresthesia and associated with a disturbance of potassium in the body.

**peripheral paralysis.** Paralysis due to any disease of a peripheral nerve.

**phonetic paralysis.** Paralysis of the vocal cords.

**pressure paralysis.** Paralysis due to pressure on a nerve.

**pseudobulbar paralysis.** A condition affecting speech, mastication, and swallowing, due to disease of the nerve pathways.

**Saturday night paralysis.** Paralysis of the arm due to compression of the radial nerve of the arm against the back of a hard chair, occurring during sleep or drunken stupor.

**Volkmann's paralysis.** Paralysis of a hand due to constriction of the blood supply and nerve injury following the application of tight splints to the arm.

**writer's paralysis.** Writer's cramp. See NEUROSIS: OCCUPATIONAL NEUROSIS.

**paralytic.** Pertaining to paralysis; a person affected with paralysis.

**paramammary.** In or around the breast.

**paramastitis.** Inflammation of the tissues around the breast.

**paramastoid.** Situated near the mastoid process behind the ear.

**paramedian.** Close to the central line of the body.

**paramenia.** Painful menstrual periods. Also called DYSMENORRHEA.

**parametric.** Pertaining to tissues around the womb.

**parametric abscess.** An abscess situated at the side of the womb, usually within the folds of the broad ligament.

**parametritis.** Inflammation of the tissues around the womb. Also called *pelvic cellulitis.*

**parametrium.** The connective tissue around the womb.

**paramnesia.** Illusions of memory. See also DÉJÀ VU.

**paramyoclonus multiplex.** A rare disease of unknown cause, occurring in adults and manifested by irregular, rapid muscular twitchings. It is presumed the seat of the disease is in the nerve centers in the brain.

**paramyotonia congenita.** A rare and hereditary form of myotonia congenita characterized by persistent contraction of the muscles of the neck, face, and extremities when the body is exposed to cold. Also called *Eulenberg's disease.*

**paranaesthesia.** See PARANESTHESIA.

**paranephric.** Situated near the kidney.

**paranephritis.** Inflammation of the tissues near the kidney.

**paranephros, paranephrus.** The adrenal gland which is situated on top of a kidney.

**paranesthesia.** Anesthesia of the lower part of the trunk and both legs.

**paraneural.** Near a nerve.

**paranoia.** Delusional insanity. The delusions are often of persecution and are frequently accompanied by hallucinations of an auditory nature. For instance, the patient may be convinced that somebody is trying to poison him, or claim to hear the voices of relatives long since dead.

**paranoiac.** One affected with paranoia.

**paranoic.** Relating to paranoia.

**paranoid.** Resembling paranoia, particularly that form of schizophrenia mainly characterized by delusions and hallucinations.

**paraomphalic.** Situated near the umbilicus.

**paraphasia.** A form of aphasia characterized by the use of wrong words. Also called *jargon aphasia, paraphrasia.*

**paraphimosis.** Constriction of the penis by a retracted and too narrow foreskin.

**paraphonia.** Abnormal condition of the voice.

**paraphrasia.** See PARAPHASIA.

**paraphrenia.** A form of schizophrenia.

**paraplectic.** Affected with paraplegia.

**paraplegia.** Paralysis of both upper or both lower limbs, but usually denotes paralysis of the lower limbs.

**paraplegic.** Related to or affected with paraplegia.

**parapsoriasis.** A group of rare skin diseases characterized by red, scaly lesions resembling lichen planus or psoriasis. All types are resistant to treatment and usually present no subjective symptoms, such as pain or irritation.

**parapyloric.** Around the pylorus.

**pararectal.** Around the rectum.

**pararenal.** Around the kidney.

**pararhotacism.** Inability to sound an R, such as is met with in the child's recitation of "wound and wound the wugged wock the wagged wascal wan."

**pararthria.** Imperfect pronunciation of words.

**parasacral.** Near the sacrum.

**parasalpingitis.** Inflammation of the tissues around a Fallopian tube.

**parasigmatism.** Inability to pronounce S or Sh sounds.

**parasite.** An organism, a plant or an animal, which lives either upon or within, and at the expense of another organism.

**parasitic.** Pertaining to or caused by parasites.

**parasiticide.** Something which destroys parasites.

**parasitism.** See PARASITE.

**parasitotrope, parasitropic.** Acting upon parasites.

**paraspadias.** A congenital malformation in which the opening of the urethra is on the side of the penis instead of at its tip.

**parasternal.** Beside the sternum. Commonly refers to an imaginary line running down the body halfway between the center of the sternum and the nipple.

**parastruma.** Enlargement of the parathyroid gland.

**parasympathetic nerves.** The parasympathetic nerves, together with the sympathetic nerves, form the autonomic nervous system, which passes nerve impulses to tissues other than voluntary muscles. Its function cannot be influenced at will and it supplies such organs as the heart, which beats under its influence without any conscious effort by the individual.

**parasynovitis.** Inflammation of the tissues around a joint.

**parathormone.** See PARATHYROID HORMONE.

**parathyroid.** Any one of the four small endocrine glands situated at the back of the thyroid gland in the neck.

**parathyroid hormone.** The hormone secreted by the parathyroid glands into the bloodstream. It promotes the passage in the urine of phosphates, a decrease of phosphates in the blood plasma, and an increase in blood calcium.

**parathyroidal.** Pertaining to the parathyroid glands.

**parathyroidectomy.** Surgical removal of the parathyroid gland or glands.

**paratrichosis.** The growth of hair in unusual places.

**paratyphoid fever.** An acute infectious fever due to infection with a paratyphoid germ, and resembling in its clinical course either typhoid fever or acute gastroenteritis.

**paravertebral.** Alongside the spinal column.

**paravesical.** Close to the urinary bladder.

**paraxial.** Beside the central axis of the body.

**paregoric.** Camphorated tincture of opium; used as a cough linctus and the essential ingredient of Gee's linctus.

**parencephalitis.** Inflammation of the cerebellum.

**parencephalocele.** A hernia of the cerebellum.

**parencephalon.** The cerebellum.

**parencephalus.** A person with congenital malformation of the brain.

**parenchyma.** The essential tissue of an organ, as distinguished from the connective tissue, blood vessels, and nerves.

**parenchymatous.** Pertaining to the parenchyma.

**parenchymitis.** Inflammation of the parenchyma.

**parenteral.** Outside the intestinal tract. It commonly refers to medications which are not swallowed but given by subcutaneous, intravenous, or intramuscular injection.

**parenteral diarrhea.** Diarrhea in infants caused by some disease outside the intestinal tract, for example, inflamed eardrums or pneumonia.

**paresis.** Slight paralysis.

**pareso-analgesia.** Incomplete paralysis accompanied by inability to feel pain.

**paresthesia.** The presence of an abnormal sensation, such as tingling or pricking on the skin.

**paretic.** Pertaining to or affected with paralysis.

**pareunia.** Sexual intercourse. Dyspareunia is painful sexual intercourse, usually in the female.

**paridrosis.** Any abnormal condition of sweating.

**parietal.** Forming or situated on a wall, such as the parietal layer of the peritoneum; pertaining to or in relation with a parietal bone, for instance, an opening in a parietal bone is called a parietal foramen.

**parietal bones.** Two bones forming the middle region of the top of the skull.

**parietes.** The walls of any cavity.

**parietofrontal.** Relating to both the parietal and frontal bones of the skull.

**parietooccipital.** Relating to both the parietal and occipital bones of the skull.

**parietotemporal.** Relating to both the parietal and temporal bones of the skull.

**Parkinson's disease.** See PARALYSIS: PARALYSIS AGITANS.

**parkinsonism.** The condition of suffering from Parkinson's disease.

**paroccipital.** Around the occipital region.

**paradontitis.** Inflammation of a tooth socket.

**paromphalocele.** A rupture occurring near the navel.

**paronychia.** Inflammation around the nail. Also called *whitlow, felon.*

**paropsis.** Disordered vision.

**parorexia.** Perversion of appetite.

**parosmia.** Perversion of the sense of smell or an hallucination of smell.

**parostosis.** Formation of bony tissue outside the periosteum.

**parotic.** Situated near the ear.

**parotid.** Relating to the parotid gland.

**parotid gland.** The salivary glands situated in front of the ear. It is this gland which enlarges to form the facial swelling in mumps.

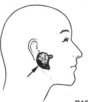

PAROTID GLAND (arrow)

**parotidectomy.** Surgical removal of a parotid gland.

**parotis.** The parotid gland.

**parotitis.** Inflammation of the parotid gland.

**parous.** Having borne one or more children.

**paroxysm.** The periodic increase or crisis in the progress of a disease; a sudden attack; a sudden reappearance of symptoms; a sudden increase in the intensity of existing symptoms; a spasm, fit, or convulsion.

**paroxysmal.** Occurring in paroxysms.

**paroxysmal auricular tachycardia.** A sudden increase in the heartbeat to about 160-180 per minute. It is regular in rhythm and unaffected by exertion or by injections of atropine and is started by impulses arising in the region of the auricle.

**paroxysmal hypertension.** Attacks of high blood pressure due to sudden secretions of adrenaline from a growth of the suprarenal gland.

**paroxysmal rhinorrhea.** The sudden discharge of mucus from the nose. It may be due to allergy, such as hay fever, or to some other disturbance of the lining of the nose.

**paroxysmal ventricular tachycardia.** A rapid beating of the heart which originates in the ventricle.

**parrot disease.** See PSITTACOSIS.

**Parrot's atrophy of the newborn.** Apparent loss of muscle power in the limbs due to congenital syphilis. Also called *arthrepsia, primary infantile wasting.*

**Parrot's nodes.** Outgrowths of bone seen on the frontal and parietal bones of the skull in hereditary syphilis.

**Parrot's sign.** Dilation of the pupil when the skin is pinched. Observed in cases of meningitis.

**Parrot's ulcers.** Whitish or yellowish patches seen in cases of thrush.

**parthenogenesis.** The development of an organism from an unfertilized egg.

**parturient.** In labor or in the act of giving birth.

**parturifacient.** Something which promotes childbirth.

**parturition.** Childbirth.

**parulis.** An abscess beneath the membrane of an alveolar process (tooth socket); a gumboil.

**P.A.S.** An abbreviation for para-aminosalicylic acid. See AMINOSALICYLIC ACID.

**passive.** Not active.

**passive congestion.** Congestion due to the inability of blood to escape from a part.

**passive immunity.** A form of immunity produced without the body taking an active part. See also IMMUNITY: PASSIVE IMMUNITY.

**passive movements.** Movements produced by a doctor moving a part without the patient's help. They are frequently employed in physiotherapy to exercise muscles and joints.

**pasteurellosis.** A disease caused by bacteria belonging to the genus *Pasteurella*, carried by cats and dogs, and transmitted to man by bites, producing an infected wound. Various species of this genus attack animals, producing fowl cholera, animal plague, and tularemia, all of which can be passed on to humans.

**pasteurization.** A method usually applied to preserving milk by heating it to 60-70°C., a temperature sufficient to destroy many germs.

**patella.** The knee cap.

**patellar.** Relating to the knee cap.

**patellar clonus.** Persistent knee jerks produced by drawing the knee cap downwards and keeping it in this position. A sign of increased muscle tone due to a disorder of the nerve paths called the pyramidal tracts.

**patellar reflex.** The jerk of the lower leg produced by tapping just below the kneecap with a patellar hammer. Also called *knee jerk*.

**patency.** The condition of being open.

**patent.** Open.

**pathetic.** Pertaining to the emotions.

**pathic.** Pathological.

**pathogen, pathogenic.** Producing disease.

**pathogenesis.** The mode of development of a disease. Also called *pathogeny*.

**pathogenicity.** The state of being pathogenetic.

**pathogeny.** Pathogenesis.

**pathognomonic.** A sign or symptom so characteristic of a disease as to make diagnosis certain.

**pathological.** Pertaining to the causes of disease.

**pathology.** That branch of medical science which deals with the study of the changes which occur from disease.

**clinical pathology.** The study of pathology which pertains to the diagnosis and care of individual patients.

**patulous.** Open or distended. The term is commonly applied to the opening of the womb when it is suspected that an abortion is about to occur. If the cervix is patulous, abortion is probably inevitable. In the absence of a threatened abortion a patulous cervix indicates that there has been a previous pregnancy.

**Paul-Bunnell test.** A blood test to diagnose infective mononucleosis.

**peccant.** Unhealthy; causing illness or disease.

**pectoral.** Pertaining to the chest; any remedy for diseases of the chest.

**pectoriloquy.** The transmission through the patient's chest of ordinary or whispered voice sounds that can be heard through a stethoscope.

**pedal.** Pertaining to the foot.

**pedialgia.** Pain in the foot.

**pediatrician, pediatrist.** A specialist in children's disorders.

**pediatrics.** The study of diseases of children.

**pedicle.** A slender process or stem.

**pedicular.** 1. Relating to a pedicle. 2. Relating to pediculosis.

**pediculation.** The process of forming a pedicle.

**pediculosis.** Infestation with lice.

**Pediculus.** The louse, a small parasitic insect belonging to the genus *Pediculus*.

**Pediculus capitis.** The head louse.

**Pediculus corporis.** The body louse.

**Pediculus pubis.** The louse found on pubic hair.

**peduncle.** A narrow process serving as a support or a stalk. The term is mostly descriptive of types of tumors hanging free on a stalk, and of certain features of brain anatomy.

**peduncular.** Relating to a peduncle.

**pedunculated.** Having a peduncle.

**pegged tooth.** A term applied to the permanent teeth of those suffering with congenital syphilis, from the peg-like aspect of the tops of the teeth. Also called *Hutchinson's tooth*.

**Pel-Ebstein's disease.** A curious phenomenon in which the patient's temperature rises for three days, stays raised for three days and then falls to normal for three days and then repeats the cycle. The three-day intervals may extend to as long as 10 or 14 days for each element of the cycle. It is associated with Hodgkin's disease.

**pellagra.** A chronic vitamin deficiency disease occurring especially in maize-eating peoples and associated with dietary lack of riboflavin (vitamin $B_2$), pyridoxin ($B_6$) and nicotinic acid ($B_7$). The early stages are characterized by debility, pain in the spine, and digestive disturbances. Later a rash develops, with the skin becoming dry and scaly. In severe cases various nervous manifestations arise, such as spasms, paralysis of both legs, and mental disturbances. Also called *mal de la rosa, mal de sole, maidismus, psilosis pigmentosa, Asturian leprosy, Alpine scurvy*.

**infantile pellagra.** See KWASHIORKOR.

**pellagrin.** One affected with pellagra.

**pellagrous.** Pertaining to pellagra.

**pellicle.** A small, thin, transparent membrane or cuticle; a delicate film on the surface of a liquid.

**pellucid.** Transparent.

**pelma.** The sole of the foot.

**pelohaemia.** See PELOHEMIA.

**pelohemia.** Abnormal thickness of the blood.

**pelotherapy.** The use of medicated mud in the treatment of disease.

**pelveoperitonitis.** Inflammation of the peritoneal membrane lining the pelvis. Also called *pelvioperitonitis*.

**pelvic.** Pertaining to the pelvis.

**pelvic abscess.** A collection of pus in the pelvic cavity which may break into the rectum or vagina.

**pelvic cellulitis.** Inflammation of the connective tissue in the pelvis.

**pelvic index.** The ratio of the measurements of the pelvis from the front to the back compared with the transverse diameter; used as a measurement of adequacy for a baby to pass through the pelvis.

**pelvimeter.** An instrument for measuring pelvic dimensions.

**pelvimetry.** Measurement of the pelvis.

**pelvioperitonitis.** See PELVEOPERITONITIS.

**pelvirectal.** Pertaining to the pelvis and the rectum.

**pelvis.** 1. A basin or basin-shaped cavity, such as the pelvis of the kidney. 2. The bony ring formed by the two innominate bones and the sacrum and coccyx. 3. The cavity bounded by the bony pelvis. This consists of the true pelvis below and the false pelvis above what is called the iliopectineal line. The entrance of the true pelvis, corresponding to this line, is known as the inlet of the pelvis. The outlet of the pelvis is bounded by the pubis in front, the tip of the coccyx behind and the two bony processes called the tubera ischii—these last two bones can be felt in the cheeks of the buttocks.

**android pelvis.** A female pelvis with a deep cavity and conical shape similar to the normal male pelvis and one which is undesirable for easy passage of a baby during labor.

**anthropoid pelvis.** A female pelvis that is long, narrow and oval resembling that of the great ape. This type may cause obstruction to labor.

**beaked pelvis.** A pelvis in which the pubic bones in the front are compressed so as to approach each other and pushed forward. A condition seen in osteomalacia.

**contracted pelvis.** A pelvis having one or more of its major diameters reduced in size, thus making it difficult or impossible for a baby to pass through.

**flat pelvis.** Deformity of the pelvis in which all the front to back measurements are shortened but the transverse measurements are normal.

**funnel pelvis.** A deformity of the pelvis in which the outlet is contracted, the transverse diameter being eight centimeters or less.

**generally contracted pelvis.** A pelvis in which all diameters are shortened.

**gynecoid pelvis.** A female pelvis in which the inlet is round instead of oval.

**obliquely contracted pelvis.** A deformed pelvis with unequal oblique diameters.

**osteomalacic pelvis.** A distorted pelvis characterized by a lessening of the transverse and oblique diameters with great increase in the measurements from front to back.

**transversely contracted pelvis.** A pelvis having a reduced transverse diameter.

**true pelvis.** That part of the pelvic cavity situated below the iliopectineal line.

**pemphigoid.** Resembling pemphigus.

**pemphigus.** An acute or chronic skin disease characterized by irregularly distributed bullae arising off either normal skin or slightly inflamed skin, and sometimes associated with severe general symptoms of ill health.

**pemphigus foliaceus.** A chronic affection characterized by the eruption of flat bullae, followed by universal redness and scaling of the skin, leaving denuded, raw areas.

**pemphigus neonatorum.** A condition seen in newborn infants and usually due to a streptococcal germ affecting the skin. Frequently the contamination is from an attendant who is carrying the germ in the throat.

**pemphigus syphiliticus.** This type of infection occurs in newborn babies with congenital syphilis and is seen on the palms of the hands and soles of the feet.

**pemphigus vegetans.** A form of pemphigus occurring mainly about the armpits, between the thighs, and over the perineum.

**pemphigus vulgaris.** Chronic pemphigus. In this type, bulbous lesions of the mucocutaneous surfaces and the skin occur, and it is often fatal if untreated.

**pendulous.** Hanging down.

**penicillin.** An antibiotic drug which can be injected, taken by mouth, or applied in ointment and which destroys many germ organisms.

**penile.** Relating to the penis.

**penis.** The male sex organ.

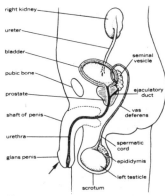

right kidney
ureter
bladder
pubic bone
prostate
shaft of penis
urethra
glans penis
seminal vesicle
ejaculatory duct
vas deferens
spermatic cord
epididymis
left testicle
scrotum

PENIS (arrow)

**pennyroyal.** The popular name for the herb *Mentha pulegium*, which for hundreds of years has been used by women to bring on menstruation when they suspected they were pregnant. It is quite unreliable and probably totally ineffective for this purpose, and not without its dangers.

**peotomy.** Surgical removal of the penis.

**pepsin.** The enzyme secreted by certain glands in the walls of the stomach to break down and digest protein.

**peptic.** Relating to pepsin or to digestion.

**peptic ulcer.** Any ulcer occurring in the region of the stomach or duodenum—a collective term covering gastric ulcer, duodenal ulcer, and pyloric ulcer.

**peptone.** An intermediate product in the digestion of proteins to amino acids.

**per acute.** Very sharp.

**per anum.** Through the anus.

**percuss.** To perform percussion.

**percussion.** Tapping the surface with the finger to elicit a sound which would indicate whether the underlying part is hollow or solid.

**percutaneous.** Performed through the skin; pertaining to a procedure wherein a substance is rubbed into the skin, whether as a treatment or a test.

**perflation.** The blowing of air into or through a cavity to expel its contents.

**perforans.** Perforating.

**perfusion.** A pouring of fluid into or through, or the forcing of a liquid through organs by way of blood vessels.

**periadenitis.** Inflammation of the area around a lymph gland.

**perianal.** Around the anus.

**periangiitis.** Inflammation of the tissues around an artery.

**periapical.** Around an apex.

**periappendicitis.** Inflammation of the tissues around the appendix.

**periarteritis.** Inflammation of the outer sheath of an artery.

**periarteritis nodosa.** A disease in which widespread acute necrosis occurs in the arteries, leading to a variety of disturbances involving the nervous system, heart, kidney, lungs, blood, and abdominal viscera. Also called *polyarteritis nodosa*.

*The condition may occur at any age, although the maximum incidence is between 20 and 30 years, males being affected three times as often as females. The clinical manifestations are varied and all the body systems may be involved, so that the general picture is complicated and difficult to evaluate. It may appear as continued, irregular, and unexplained fever with malaise, loss of weight, progressive anemia, muscle pains, and general misery; as polyneuritis, with nerve pains and paralysis, such as wrist drop or foot drop, associated with fever and anemia; as bleeding within the abdomen due to a ruptured aneurysm, as cerebral bleeding or bleeding from the kidney; or as paroxysmal attacks of asthma and transient attacks of pneumonia. Occasionally the mode of onset resembles some other disease, such as the many inflamed joints suggestive of rheumatoid arthritis, a typical attack of acute nephritis, or the development of very high blood pressure. Treatment is cortisone in fairly large doses.*

**periarthritis.** Inflammation of the tissues around a joint.

**periarticular.** Around a joint.

**periaxillary.** Around an armpit.

**peribronchial.** Around a bronchus.

**peribronchitis.** Inflammation of the tissues around the bronchi.

**pericaecal.** See PERICECAL.

**pericanalicular.** Occurring around small ducts or passages.

**pericapsular.** Surrounding a capsule.

**pericardiac, pericardial.** Relating to the pericardium.

**pericardiectomy.** Surgical removal of part of the pericardium.

**pericardiocentesis.** Surgical puncture of the pericardium by a needle, either to withdraw or to introduce fluid.

**pericardiotomy.** Surgical opening of the pericardium.

**pericarditis.** Inflammation of the pericardium. It may produce adhesions between the sac and the heart, which may disturb the heart's action; a fibrinous exudate, which causes high temperature, shortness of breath, and pain; or an effusion which may be bloody, serous, or purulent. The signs and symptoms include shortness of breath, inability to feel the apex beat of the heart, muffled heart sounds as heard through the stethoscope, low blood pressure, and signs of lung collapse.

**pericardium.** The double-layered membranous sac surrounding the heart. The layer adjacent to the heart, called the visceral pericardium, is a serous membrane while the outer layer, called the parietal pericardium, is a fibrous membrane.

**pericecal.** Around the cecum.

**pericellular.** The tissues surrounding a cell.

**pericementitis.** Inflammation of the periodontium.

**pericholangitis.** Inflammation of tissues around the bile ducts.

**pericholecystitis.** Inflammation of tissues surrounding the gall bladder.

**perichondral.** Relating to the perichondrium.

**perichondritis.** Inflammation of the perichondrium.

**perichondrium.** The tissue covering the surface of cartilage.

**periclasis.** A comminuted fracture.

**periconchal.** Around the ear cavity.

**pericorneal.** Around the cornea of the eye.

**pericoxitis.** Inflammation around the hip joint.

**pericranium.** The membrane covering the skull bones.

**pericystium.** 1. The outer wall of a cyst. 2. The tissue surrounding the urinary bladder.

**pericystitis.** Inflammation of the tissues around the urinary bladder.

**peridental.** Around a tooth.

**peridentine.** The bony layer covering the root of a tooth.

**peridentitis.** Periodontitis.

**perididymis.** The membrane covering each of the testicles.

**periductal.** Around a duct; usually applied to conditions in and around the breast and milk ducts.

**periduodenitis.** Inflammation around the duodenum, often leading to adhesions.

**perifolliculitis.** Inflammation around a hair follicle.

**perigastric.** Around the stomach.

**perigastritis.** Inflammation of the tissues around the stomach.

**perihepatic.** Around the liver.

**perihepatitis.** Inflammation of the membrane covering the liver.

**perilaryngitis.** Inflammation of the tissues around the larynx.

**perilymphadenitis.** Inflammation of the tissues around lymphatic glands.

**perilymphangitis.** Inflammation of the tissues surrounding a lymphatic vessel.

**perilymphatic.** 1. Pertaining to the perilymph (a fluid in the labyrinth of the ear). 2. Around a lymph vessel.

**perimastitis.** Inflammation of the tissues around the breast.

**perimetritis.** Inflammation of the perimetrium.

**perimetrium.** The peritoneal membrane covering the womb.

**perimetry.** Measurement of the visual field.

**perimyositis.** Inflammation of the tissues around a muscle.

**perineal.** Relating to the perineum.

**perineocele.** A rupture in the perineal area.

**perineoplasty.** Surgical repair of the perineum.

**perineorrhaphy.** The sewing up of a wound in the perineum, whether caused by childbirth or surgery.

**perineotomy.** Surgical incision into the perineum. Frequently done at childbirth to allow the baby's head to emerge without it tearing the vulva and causing possible damage to the rectum and other important structures.

**perinephric.** Around the kidney.

**perinephric abscess.** An abscess around the kidney.

**perinephritis.** Inflammation of the tissues around the kidneys.

**perinephrium.** The tissues surrounding the kidney.

**perineum.** The region between the anus and the vulva or between the anus and the scrotum.

**perineural.** Around a nerve.

**perineuritis.** Inflammation around a nerve.

**perineurium.** A nerve sheath.

**periocular.** Surrounding the eye.

**period.** The menstrual period.

**periodic.** Recurring at more or less regular intervals.

**periodicity.** Recurrence at regular intervals.

**periodontal.** Surrounding a tooth; pertaining to the periodontium.

**periodontitis.** Inflammation of the periodontal tissues.

**periodontium.** The membrane lining the cement of a tooth.

**perionychia.** Inflammation around a nail.

**perioophoritis.** Inflammation of the peritoneal covering of the ovary.

**periorbit, periorbita.** The periosteum lining the eye socket.

**periorbital.** Surrounding the eye socket; relating to the periorbita.

**periorchitis.** Inflammation of the tissues around the testicle.

**periost.** Periosteum.

**periosteal.** Pertaining to the periosteum.

**periosteitis.** Periostitis.

**periosteotomy.** Surgical incision of the periosteum.

**periosteum.** The fibrous membrane covering the surfaces of all bones, except at joint surfaces.

**periostitis.** Inflammation of the periosteum.

**periotic.** Around the ear.

**peripachymeningitis.** Inflammation of the outer of the layers of membrane covering the brain. Also called *pachymeningitis externa.*

**peripancreatitis.** Inflammation of the tissues around the pancreas.

**peripapillary.** Around a papilla; around the optic disc.

**peripheral, periphic.** Pertaining to or situated near the periphery.

**peripheral nerves.** The peripheral nerves are those which connect the central nervous system (the brain and spinal cord) to the rest of the body. There are 12 pairs of cranial nerves and 31 pairs of spinal nerves. Some of these are sensory nerves carrying various sensations from the body or the outside world to the central nervous system. Some are motor nerves which carry impulses from the central nervous system to muscles causing them to contract, or to glands activating them. Most peripheral nerves contain both sensory and motor components.

**periphlebitis.** Inflammation of the outer coat of a vein and of the tissues surrounding a vein.

**periportal.** Around the portal vein.

**periproctitis.** Inflammation of the tissues around the rectum or anus.

**periprostatitis.** Inflammation of the tissues around the prostate gland.

**perirectal.** Around the rectum.

**perirectal abscess.** See ISCHIORECTAL ABSCESS.

**perirenal.** Around the kidney.

**perirhinal.** Around the nose.

**perisalpingitis.** Inflammation around the Fallopian tube.

**perisigmoiditis.** Inflammation of the tissues around the sigmoid colon.

**perisinusitis.** Inflammation of the tissues around a sinus.

**perisplanchnic.** Around an abdominal organ.

**perisplanchnitis.** Inflammation of the tissues around an abdominal organ.

**perisplenitis.** Inflammation of the tissues around the spleen.

**peristalsis.** A progressive wave of contraction occurring in the alimentary tract within the body which has longitudinal and transverse muscle fibers. There is a narrowing and shortening of a portion of the tube, which then relaxes while a lower portion becomes shortened and narrowed so that the tube's contents are forced onwards. By this means food is propelled from one end of the digestive tract to the other.

**peristaltic.** Pertaining to peristalsis.

**peristole.** Peristalsis or an individual peristaltic movement.

**perisystole.** The interval between two systoles.

**peritendineum.** The fibrous covering of a tendon.

**peritendinitis.** Inflammation of the peritendineum.

**peritenonitis.** Inflammation of the covering of a tendon.

**perithelial.** Relating to the perithelium.

**perithelioma.** A malignant tumor originating in the perithelium.

**perithelium.** The connective tissue surrounding the capillaries and smaller vessels.

**perithyroiditis.** Inflammation of the tissues surrounding the thyroid gland.

**peritomy.** Surgical removal of a strip of conjunctival membrane around the cornea of the eye.

**peritoneal.** Relating to the peritoneum.

**peritoneotomy.** Surgical incision into the peritoneum.

**peritoneum.** The membrane lining the abdominal cavity and covering the organs contained within it.

**peritonioscopy.** A diagnostic examination of the interior of the abdomen by means of a surgical instrument passed through the abdominal wall.

*The tip of the instrument, which contains a light, is passed through a small incision made in the anesthetized abdominal wall, and the surgeon examines abdominal organs through magnifying lenses at the external end of the instrument. Such an examination may save the patient an unnecessary major operation.*

**peritonitic.** Relating to peritonitis.

**peritonitis.** Inflammation of the peritoneum, the serous membrane lining the abdominal cavity and its organs.

**acute peritonitis.** A form sudden in onset and characterized by intense abdominal pain, tenderness, and board-like rigidity, with vomiting and leukocytosis.

**chronic adhesive peritonitis.** A form characterized by fibrous adhesions between the abdominal organs; it may be localized to one area of the abdomen.

**gonococcal peritonitis.** A form of peritonitis due to the germ of gonorrhea. It is more common in females from gonorrheal infection in the vagina ascending through the womb into the Fallopian tube and abdominal cavity.

**pneumococcal peritonitis.** A type of peritonitis due to the germ of pneumonia, occurring usually in girls between five and ten years of age and characterized by diarrhea, high temperature, with signs of acute peritonitis, and of pneumonia.

**puerperal peritonitis.** A form of peritonitis following childbirth.

**tuberculous peritonitis.** Peritonitis due to the tuberculosis germ.

**peritonsillitis.** Inflammation of the tissues surrounding the tonsil. See also QUINSY.

**peritonsillar.** Around the tonsil.

**peritonsillar abscess.** 1. An abscess behind the tonsil. 2. A quinsy. Also called *circumtonsillar abscess.*

**periureteritis.** Inflammation of the tissues around the ureter.

**periurethritis.** Inflammation of the tissues surrounding the urethra.

**periuterine.** Around the womb.

**perivascular.** Around a blood vessel.

**pernicious.** Deadly, fatal, very severe. See also ANEMIA; MALARIA; VOMITING.

**pernio.** A chilblain.

**perone.** The fibula.

**peroneal.** Relating to the fibula.

**peroneal muscular atrophy.** A distinct and peculiar form of muscular atrophy with a tendency to occur in several members of a family. It usually commences in middle childhood, progresses for some 20 years, and then ceases. The condition starts in the feet, affects the muscles of the lower leg and the lower third of the thigh, after which it stops. A similar condition may start in the hands and progress towards the middle of the forearms but arrest itself at any stage of spread. The muscle wasting is accompanied by partial or complete paralysis and even sensory loss, but the peculiar feature of this condition is the comparatively slight disability which results from what appears to be a profound muscular disturbance of the parts affected. Also called *Charcot-Marie-Tooth mus-*

*cular atrophy, neuritic muscular atrophy.*

**peroral, per os.** Via the mouth.

**per osseous.** Through bone.

**perseveration.** Persistent repetition of words or an activity for no apparent reason, and often associated with disease of the brain.

**perspiration.** Sweat; the secretion of sweat.

**insensible perspiration.** Loss of body weight due to loss of water through both the skin and breathing out water vapor. See also SWEAT.

**Perthes' disease.** A fairly common condition occurring in young people in which the growing bone center in the head of the femur first becomes necrotic and is then absorbed and replaced by new bone. It is probably the result of a disorder of the blood vessels in the part, possibly due to an injury cutting off the blood supply to the growing center, which then dies. The disease appears to run a definite course of about two years, and is two or three times as common in boys as in girls. The onset may be at any age from four to sixteen years, with a maximum from four to nine years. The first complaint is usually a limp, and although pain may be present it is not a marked feature. Examination shows muscle spasm and limitation of movement at the hip, which disappear rapidly with rest but return if weight-bearing is resumed. The treatment is rest until the x-ray pictures show that the bone is no longer soft. However, this does not necessarily mean rest in bed but rest of the joint by the use of a surgical appliance. The condition may be mild, with subsequent full recovery, or severe, with marked deformity of the bone followed by osteoarthritis of the hip joint. Also called *pseudocoxalgia, Legg - Calve - Perthes' disease, coxa plana, osteochondritis deformans juvenilis, quiet hip disease.*

**pertussis.** See WHOOPING COUGH.

**perversion.** A turning away from the normal.

**sexual perversion.** A preference for obtaining sexual gratification by practices other than the usual sexual act.

**pervert.** A perverted individual, especially one who indulges in other than the usual sexual practices.

**per vias naturales.** By natural ways.

**pervious.** Capable of being passed through.

**pes.** A foot; a footlike part. See also TALIPES.

**pes anserinus.** The goose's foot; a term applied to the weblike terminal divisions of the facial nerve.

**pes cavus.** A foot with an unnatural increase in the curvature of the arch.

**pes planus.** Flat-foot.

**pessary.** An instrument placed in the vagina to support the uterus; an instrument, usually made of rubber, placed in the vagina to prevent conception; a bullet-shaped suppository containing chemicals inserted into the vagina to treat infections.

**pest.** See PLAGUE.

**pestiferous.** Causing pestilence.

**pestilence.** Any deadly disease of epidemic origin, such as the plague.

**petechia,** A minute, rounded spot of blood on a surface such as skin, mucous membrane, or cross-section surface of an organ. A rash of petechiae can arise in the skin in diphtheria, heatstroke, plague, spirochetosis icterohemorrhagica, subacute bacterial endocarditis, whooping cough, yellow fever, scarlet fever, typhus, measles, lead, mercury, and arsenic poisoning, and certain blood diseases.

**petechial.** Characterized by the formation of petechiae.

**petit mal.** A minor fit of epilepsy.

**petrification.** Conversion to a stonelike hardness.

**petrissage.** A kneading action in physiotherapy, in which the soft tissues are carefully lifted from the deeper structures and gently squeezed.

**petrolate, petrolatum.** Soft paraffin; used as an ointment base.

**petromastoid.** Pertaining to the petrous and mastoid parts of the temporal bones in the skull.

**petrosphenoid.** Pertaining to the petrous part of the temporal bone and the sphenoid bone.

**petrous.** As hard as stone.

**pexis.** Any surgical operation to fix a part.

**peyerian fever.** See TYPHOID FEVER.

**pH.** A symbol representing the hydrogen ion concentration of a fluid in terms of 14 divisions; pH7 is the neutral point; above seven represents alkalinity in an aqueous solution; below seven represents acidity.

**phaeochromocyte.** See PHEOCHROMOCYTE.

**phaeochromocytoma.** See PHEOCHROMOCYTOMA.

**phagedaena.** See PHAGEDENA.

**phagedena.** Gangrenous ulceration.

**phagocyte.** A blood cell capable of ingesting germs. It is part of the body's protective mechanism against infection.

**phagocytic.** Pertaining to phagocytosis.

**phagocytosis.** Destruction of bacteria by phagocytes.

**phagomania.** Uncontrollable craving for food.

**phagophobia.** Neurotic fear of eating.

**phalangeal.** Pertaining to the phalanges.

**phalanges.** The bones of the fingers and toes.

**phalangitis.** Inflammation of the phalanges.

**phalanx.** A finger or toe bone.

**phallectomy.** Surgical removal of the penis.

**phallic.** Pertaining to the penis.

**phallitis.** Inflammation of the penis.

**phallus.** The penis.

**phantom.** 1. An apparition. 2. A dummy used for practicing surgical operations.

**phantom limb.** The sensation that an amputated limb is still present. Most amputation patients experience this, and often claim the missing limb can be moved at will, while a few complain of severe pain in it. The pain appears to be psychologically determined and is invariably accompanied by other psychiatric disturbances, but with time the phantom usually becomes less prominent in the patient's mind.

**phantom tumor.** An artificial swelling produced by gaseous distension of the intestine or contraction of a muscle; usually evidence of a neurotic personality. Also called *pseudotumor*.

**phantom tumour.** See PHANTOM TUMOR.

**pharmacology.** The science dealing with the action of drugs on living organisms.

**pharmacopoeia.** A book containing methods and formulas for the preparation of drugs. See also BRITISH PHARMACOPOEIA.

**pharyngeal.** Relating to the pharynx.

**pharyngectomy.** Surgical excision of the pharynx.

**pharyngismus.** Spasm of the muscles of the pharynx.

**pharyngitis.** Inflammation of the pharynx.

**pharyngocele.** A protrusion of the pharynx through a gap in the muscular wall of the throat.

**pharyngokeratosis.** Irregular thickening of the lining of the pharynx.

**pharyngolaryngitis.** Inflammation of the pharynx and larynx.

**pharyngomycosis.** Any fungus disease of the pharynx.

**pharyngoparalysis.** Paralysis of the pharynx.

**pharyngopathy.** Any disease of the pharynx.

**pharynx.** The cavity and area behind the nose, mouth, and larynx, extending for about five inches from the base of the skull to a point opposite the sixth cervical vertebra, where it becomes continuous with the esophagus. The upper portion, the *nasopharynx*, is situated at the back of the nose, communicates with the middle ear by means of the Eustachian tube, and forms part of the respiratory tract.

The lower portion is divided into two sections: the *oropharynx*, at the rear of the mouth; and the *laryngopharynx* behind the larynx. These two sections form part of the digestive tract.

**pheochromocyte.** A type of cell present in the sympathetic nerve ganglia and in the medulla of the adrenal gland. Pheochromocytes have the property of being stained yellow by chromic acid salts.

**pheochromocytoma.** A tumor, arising in the suprarenal gland, which causes hyperadrenalinism resulting in excessive production of adrenaline. The disorder is characterized by paroxysms of high blood pressure, chest pain, pallor, perspiration, nausea, vomiting, agonizing headaches, cold clammy hands which are sometimes a congested blue color, shivering, cramps of the calf muscles, contraction of the pupils, high temperature, anxiety, and fear of death. The paroxysms may occur at any time and with variable intervals. They last from five to thirty minutes, the patient being left in a state of utter exhaustion from which it may take hours or days to recover. The treatment consists in surgical removal of the tumor. Also called *paraganglioma*.

**phimosis.** Excessive narrowing of the foreskin in front of the penis so that it cannot be withdrawn over the glans. This is normal in the infant but in the adult it may cause distress and pain during coitus and necessitate circumcision.

**phlebitis.** Inflammation of a vein.

**pelvic phlebitis.** An inflammation of the veins of the pelvis following childbirth. Also called PELVIC THROMBOPHLEBITIS.

**pyelophlebitis.** Inflammation of the veins of the renal (kidney) pelvis.

**suppurative phlebitis.** This is due to infection spreading from adjacent tissues. It leads to the formation of a clot within the vein, called thrombophlebitis, which may break down and distribute infective pieces or emboli to other parts of the body. When not due to a suppurative process it may obliterate the vein by blocking it with a blood clot. Symptoms are pain and edema of the affected part, with redness along the course of the vein, which appears as a hard, tender cord.

**varicose vein phlebitis.** This is usually a very low-grade infection. If it does not rapidly subside with simple treatment, the offending vein can be tied to stop the spread.

**phlebothrombosis.** The formation of a blood clot in a vein as a sequel to inflammation of a vein.

**phlebotomy.** Opening of a vein to extract blood. Also called *venesection*.

---

**phlegmasia.** Inflammation.

**phlegmasia alba dolens.** A rare complication affecting the legs following childbirth. The limb becomes tense, white, glistening and extremely swollen, the edema being very hard and not pitting on pressure. It is probably due to infection and inflammation of the lymphatic vessels setting up a deep, low-grade cellulitis. Also called *white leg, milk leg.*

**phlegmon.** An inflammation characterized by a spreading cellulitis.

**phlegmonous.** Like or pertaining to phlegmon.

**phlogogen.** Something capable of producing inflammation.

**phlogogenic.** Causing inflammation.

**phlogosis.** An obsolete term for inflammation.

**phlyctena.** 1. A blister following a burn. 2. A small bladderlike vesicle containing lymph.

**phlyctenoid.** See PHLYCTENULAR.

**phlyctenula.** A small phlyctena. Also called *phlyctenule.*

**phlyctenular.** Relating to a phlyctenula.

**phlyctenule.** A phlyctenula.

**phobia.** An irrational fear.

**phonation.** The production of voice sounds; speech.

**phonatory.** Relating to phonation.

**phonetic.** Relating to sounds, or to the voice.

**phonic.** Relating to the voice.

**phonic spasm.** Spasm of the throat muscles when attempting to speak.

**phonophobia.** A fear of speaking or a morbid dread of sound.

**phosphaturia.** An excess of phosphates in the urine.

**phosphorism.** Chronic phosphorus poisoning.

**photalgia.** Pain caused by great intensity of light. Also called *photodynia.*

**photic.** Relating to light.

**photoactinic.** Giving forth both luminous and actinic rays. Actinic rays are those which cause chemical changes in tissues.

**photodermia.** Skin disorders caused by exposure to light, sunburn for instance.

**photodynia.** Photalgia. The term is also applied to severe photophobia.

**photodysphoria.** See PHOTOPHOBIA.

**photoophthalmia.** Inflammation of the eye caused by intense light, such as that produced in oxyacetylene welders who forget to wear goggles.

**photophobia.** Intolerance of light, such as is seen in measles; the child's eyes being red, sore, and irritable. Severe photophobia is called photodynia. Also called *photodysphoria.*

**photopsia.** The sensation of flashes of light, occurring in certain disorders of the optic nerve, retina, or brain.

**phototherapy.** Treatment of disease by light rays, such as sunray baths.

**phren-.** A combining form meaning either a relationship to the diaphragm or to the mind.

**phrenalgia.** 1. Depression, melancholia. 2. Pain in the diaphragm.

**phrenasthenia.** 1. Paralysis of the diaphragm. 2. Feebleness of mind.

**phrenasthenic.** 1. Relating to phrenasthenia. 2. A feeble-minded person.

**phrenesthesia.** Idiocy.

**phrenesis.** Delirium, insanity.

**phrenetic.** Maniacal.

**phrenic.** 1. Relating to the diaphragm. 2. Relating to the mind.

**phrenicectomy.** Surgical removal of a portion of a phrenic nerve. It was once commonly done to paralyze the diaphragm and to help collapse a tuberculous lung, but with the advent of more effective antituberculous drugs it is now rarely performed.

**phrenicotomy.** Surgical division of the phrenic nerve. See PHRENICECTOMY.

**phrenitis.** 1. Inflammation of the brain; delirium. 2. Inflammation of the diaphragm.

**phrenohepatic.** Relating to the diaphragm and the liver.

**phrenology.** The theory that the various faculties of the mind occupy distinct and separate areas in the brain cortex, and that the predominance of certain faculties can be predicted from modifications of the parts of the skull overlying the areas where these faculties are located. The theory has absolutely no basis in established fact.

**phrenopathy.** Any mental disease.

**phrenoplegia.** 1. Failure of the mental powers. 2. Paralysis of the diaphragm.

**phrenoptosis.** Prolapse of the diaphragm.

**phrenospasm.** Spasm of the diaphragm.

**phthinoid.** Resembling tuberculosis.

**phthisis.** An almost obsolete term for tuberculosis (especially tuberculosis of the lungs) and for any disease characterized by loss of weight and strength, especially in the presence of lung disease.

**phygogalactic.** Stopping the secretion of milk, or an agent that does so.

**phylactic.** Relating to phylaxis.

**phylaxis.** The activity of the body in defending itself against infection.

**physiological.** Pertaining to physiology.

**physiological compensation.** The enlargement of one organ in an attempt to compensate for a deficiency caused by the failure of another organ. For instance, in defects of the circulation,

the heart can enlarge in order to maintain an adequate blood supply to the body. This specific condition is called cardiac hypertrophy.

**physiologist.** One who studies physiology.

**physiology.** The science that studies the normal functioning of living organisms or their parts.

**physiotherapy.** The use of physical agents, such as heat, electricity, massage, and special exercises in the treatment of disease. Also called *physical medicine.*

**physohaematometra.** See PHYSOHEMATOMETRA.

**physohematometra.** An accumulation of blood and gas or air in the womb, such as happens when the womb contents decompose.

**physometra.** Distension of the womb with gas.

**physopyosalpinx.** The presence of pus and gas in the Fallopian tube.

**phytosis.** Any disease caused by plant parasites.

**phytotoxin.** A poison originating from plants.

**pia, pia mater.** The innermost of the three membranes covering the brain and spinal cord.

**pial.** Relating to the pia.

**pianist's cramp.** An occupational disorder characterized by painful spasm of the fingers or hand. See NEUROSIS: OCCUPATIONAL NEUROSIS.

**piarachnitis.** Inflammation of the pia mater and arachnoid mater membranes of the brain. Also called *leptomeningitis.*

**pica.** A craving for unnatural articles of food; a depraved appetite. The connotation depends on whether the condition affects adults or children.

*In adults pica is a symptom encountered in some forms of insanity and hysteria, in which the individual desires unnatural and unusual food. It also sometimes occurs in the first few months of pregnancy, when the expectant mother refuses to eat normal food but insists, for instance, on a diet of ginger ale and radishes. In children, for instance, some will constantly pluck out and eat hairs, devour fluff drawn from blankets, or eat such things as earth, sand, mud, or dirt of any sort—including cigarette ends and pieces of coal. In early childhood, the habits are of little account, or at most suggest a certain nervousness, which may be due to faults of parental management that must be corrected. Because of that curious spirit of opposition characteristic of little children, and because of their susceptibility to suggestion, the habits, which are usually only a transient phase, will become ingrained if attention is called to*

127

them. *The best treatment is not to comment on the habit but divert the child's attention to a more interesting occupation.*

**Pick's disease.** A disease, complex in character, marked by inflammation of one or more internal membranes. In a few cases the cause is tuberculosis. When the condition affects several membranes simultaneously it is called *Concato's disease* or *polyserositis;* when it mainly affects the pericardium it is called *Pick's disease, chronic constrictive pericarditis;* or *pericarditic pseudo-cirrhosis of the liver.* The last condition, however, is usually tuberculous in origin. The inflammation of the pericardium so disturbs the heart action that it produces congestion of veins as far back as the liver, which becomes involved. The disease runs a long, chronic course with gradually increasing venous congestion, and increasing interference with heart action and liver function. Treatment consists in surgical removal of the pericardium and treatment of the tuberculosis, if present.

**pigmentary.** Relating to or forming pigment.

**pigmentation.** The laying down of pigment; coloring or discoloring caused by pigment.

**pigmented.** Stained by a deposit of pigment.

**pilary.** Relating to the hair.

**piles.** See HEMORRHOIDS.

**piliation.** The formation and production of hair.

**pilomotor.** The muscles which, when they retract, move the hair; the nerves which carry impulses to these muscles.

**pilonidal.** Containing hair. The term usually refers to cysts, which it is thought occur when surface skin has been embedded deep in the tissues as a congenital error, where it manufactures grease, sweat, and hairs, which accumulate to form the cyst. The cyst eventually discharges to the skin surface, producing a pilonidal sinus. The commonest site of these is the lower back, just above the cleft between the buttocks, and is represented by a small pit which constantly discharges a liquid that calls attention to its presence. The treatment is surgical removal.

**pilosis.** Abnormal growth of hair.

**pimple.** A small pustule.

**pineal.** Relating to the pineal body, or pineal gland, a structure in the brain.

**pinguecula.** A small, yellowish-white patch of connective tissue, situated between the cornea and the inner corner of the eye. It occurs in old age.

**pink disease.** A condition occurring in infants and so named because the skin of the entire body is pink from erythema. Also called *acrodynia, erythredema polyneuropathy, infantila erythhredema, Feer's disease, Selter's disease.*

*The hands and feet look raw; there is sleeplessness, depression, agitation, excessive sweating; the child resents strong light; the muscles are slack, and the skin itches unmercifully, causing the child to scratch almost to the point of an hysterical condition. The disease most commonly occurs between the ages of four months and two years, but the onset can be as early as the third week and as late as the eighth year. It runs a chronic course, often with periods of partial remission, and commonly lasts for several months to over a year. The cause has not been definitely established. Treatment is on general grounds: good nursing, high vitamin intake, alleviation of irritation and other symptoms, adequate rest and sleep.*

**pinkeye.** A vague term covering any eye condition in which the "white" of the eye is colored pink by congestion, thus including both conjunctivitis and iritis. In conjunctivitis the iris is clear, whereas in iritis it is cloudy. The conditions must not be confused because, whereas conjunctivitis runs a mild course, iritis can be dangerous, requiring expert medical attention. Also called *acute contagious conjunctivitis.*

**pinna.** The external flap of the ear. Also called *auricle.*

**pinnal.** Relating to the pinna.

**pinta.** A tropical skin disease characterized by the appearance of colored patches on the skin. It is caused by a fungus.

**pinworm.** A threadworm.

**Pirquet's reaction.** A test for tuberculosis in which tuberculin is rubbed into an abrasion made on the skin. Also called *von Pirquet's test.*

**pisiform.** Pea-shaped.

**pisiform bone.** A small bone on the inner front aspect of the wrist.

**pitocin.** A hormone produced by the pituitary gland (situated in the brain), which causes smooth muscles to contract—the womb muscle, for instance. See also PITUITARY GLAND.

**pitressin.** A hormone of the pituitary gland, which raises blood pressure and controls the output of urine by the kidney. See also PITUITARY GLAND.

**pitting.** The formation of pits, as is seen in edema of the skin, when pressure of the finger leaves behind small pits.

**pituitary.** 1. Secreting mucus or phlegm. 2. Pertaining to or designating the pituitary gland.

**pituitary basophilism.** See CUSHING'S SYNDROME.

**pituitary cachexia.** See SIMMOND'S DISEASE.

**pituitary gland.** The human pituitary gland is a small, rounded, reddish-grey gland about 0.57 of a gram in weight, which lies in a bony cradle called the sella turcica, and attached by a stalk to the floor of the brain. Anatomically the gland is described as consisting of a large anterior lobe (*pars glandularis*) and a smaller posterior lobe (*pars neuralis*), of a *pars intermedia*, and a *pars tuberalis.* The name pituitary was originally given to this organ because it was erroneously thought to secrete the mucus of the nose. It is now recognized as probably the most important of the endocrine glands. It is quite fantastic that this tiny gland should have such a widespread control over the functioning of the body. The hormones produced by its frontal lobe regulate the growth of all bodily tissues, control the development and functioning of the thyroid gland, the suprarenal glands, the sex organs, and probably the parathyroid glands. It controls the production of milk in the breast. The hormone secreted by its posterior lobe affects blood pressure and kidney function, and can produce contraction of smooth muscle, such as that of the womb. Also called *hypophysis cerebri.*

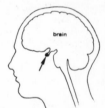

PITUITARY (arrow)

**pituitary gonadotropin.** The hormone of the anterior pituitary lobe, which has a special effect on the function of the sex organs.

**Pituitrin.** A proprietary preparation of the posterior lobe hormone of the pituitary gland.

**pityriasis.** A group of skin diseases characterized by a branny desquamation of the skin and the absence of inflammation.

**pityriasis capitis.** Seborrheic dermatitis of the scalp, popularly called dandruff or scurf. Dandruff usually first appears about the age of six to ten years, many members of the same family may be affected, and the tendency appears to be hereditary. In the dry, scaly stage numerous spores can be found; later, the condition becomes secondarily infected with germs. Occasionally the condition is associated with blepharitis, which only clears up after the scalp condition has been treated. Treatment consists of applying preparations to kill the germs followed by measures to degrease the skin of the scalp. This, together with vigorous brushing and massage to the scalp, will keep it clear.

**pityriasis circinata.** See PITYRIASIS ROSEA.

**pityriasis corporis.** Flannel rash. A skin rash of small pink areas covered with greasy scales. The spots tend to spread to become larger ovals, which usually clear in the middle, thus forming a ring. Itching is not a common feature. The complaint is often associated with dandruff of the scalp, and, in fact, some experts consider that it is the dandruff scales that produce the condition on the rest of the body. The dandruff therefore has to be cleared up at the same time as the body rash is treated.

**pityriasis lichenoides et varioliformis acuta.** A skin disease characterized by small vesicles and pustules that form crusts and leave scars; usually runs a course of one to three months. It is not contagious.

**pityriasis linguae.** Transitory, harmless plaques seen on the tongue.

**pityriasis pilaris.** A chronic affection of the skin marked by hard, conical elevations in the openings of the sebaceous glands of the skin of arms and thighs.

**pityriasis rosea.** A skin disease of the trunk characterized by pale red patches with fawn-colored centers. The cause is unknown. It usually recovers spontaneously in from three to six weeks, with or without treatment. Also called *pityriasis circinata, herpes tonsurans maculosus.*

**pityriasis rubra.** A chronic inflammatory skin disease, usually involving the whole body. The skin is red and covered by whitish scales. The disease varies in duration from months to years and has a grave outlook.

**pityriasis rubra pilaris.** A chronic, mildly inflammatory skin disease in which firm papules with central horny plugs form at the mouths of the hair follicles. The papules tend to coalesce into scaly patches.

**pityriasis simplex.** See SEBORRHEIC DERMATITIS.

**pityriasis steatoides.** A form of seborrheic dermatitis marked by the formation of large waxy scales and often by severe itching and loss of hair.

**pityriasis versicolor.** A chronic fungus disease of the skin, characterized by the presence of yellowish-brown desquamating spots involving principally the trunk. Also called *tinea versicolor.*

**placebo.** A medicine having no pharmacological effect but given to please or humor the patient.

**placenta.** The organ on the wall of the womb to which the developing embryo is attached by the umbilical cord and through which it receives its nourishment. The placenta develops fully about the third month of pregnancy, and transfers food and oxygen from the mother to the embryo and, in the reverse direction, passes waste materials from the embryo into the mother's bloodstream, which she then filters off via her own kidneys. At birth the placenta weighs about one pound, is an inch thick at its center and about seven inches in diameter. In a normal pregnancy, the placenta is attached to the upper part of the uterus so that during labor the baby emerges first; the cord is then cut and tied and subsequently the placenta is extruded. Sometimes, however, the placenta is not inserted into the top of the womb but in the lower part in front of the baby, resulting in a condition called placenta praevia. This is dangerous, for the moment labor starts the placenta begins to bleed. Since the bleeding can take on serious proportions, placenta praevia may be an indication for a cesarean section, an operation in which the baby is removed through an abdominal incision. Also called *afterbirth.*

**abruption of placenta.** Premature detachment of the placenta.

**accessory placenta.** An extra piece of placenta situated apart from the main structure.

**adherent placenta.** A placenta that fails to separate from the wall of the womb after childbirth.

**annular placenta.** A placenta extending around the interior of the womb in the form of a belt.

**battledore placenta.** A placenta in which the umbilical cord is inserted at the outside edge of the placenta.

**bipartite placenta.** A placenta with two divisions.

**circumvallate placenta.** A placenta with an irregular elevation all round its edge on the side facing the baby.

**discoid placenta.** A placenta shaped like a disc.

**duplex placenta.** See BIPARTITE PLACENTA.

**fundal placenta.** A placenta attached at the upper end of the womb, the normal position.

**horseshoe placenta.** A condition in twin pregnancy, in which two placentas are joined together.

**incarcerated placenta.** A placenta retained within the womb because the womb outlet is in spasm and has closed down, leaving too small an opening for the placenta to pass through.

**placenta accreta.** A placenta which has grown into the wall of the womb so thoroughly that there is no longer a line of cleavage, so that it cannot be separated from the womb in the normal way.

**placenta cirsoides.** A placenta in which the umbilical blood vessels have a varicose appearance.

**placenta fenestrata.** An irregular four-sided placenta with an opening near the middle.

**placenta membranacea.** A placenta that is abnormally thin.

**placenta praevia.** A placenta situated in any position in front of the baby. See PLACENTA, above.

**placenta praevia centralis.** A placenta situated directly above the womb opening.

**placenta praevia marginalis.** A condition in which, although the placenta is in front of the baby, the lowest edge of the placenta comes down near to, but does not cover, the opening of the womb.

**placenta praevia partialis.** A condition in which the edge of the placenta overlies, but does not completely obstruct, the opening of the womb.

**placenta reflexa.** A placenta which, instead of being thick in the middle and thinner towards the edges, is thicker at the edges and gives a rolled-back appearance.

**placenta succenturiata.** A placenta which has one or more accessory lobes, which are developed at a greater or lesser distance from the margins of the main placenta.

**retained placenta.** A placenta that is not expelled immediately after or within half an hour of the birth of the baby.

**velamentous placenta.** See BATTLEDORE PLACENTA, above.

**placental.** Relating to the placenta.

**placentation.** The formation and mode of attachment of the placenta.

**placentitis.** Inflammation of the placenta.

**placentoid.** Like a placenta.

**plague. 1.** A specific contagious disease, endemic in Eastern Asia and in former times occurring as epidemics throughout Europe and Asia Minor. It is an acute febrile disease characterized by inflammation of the lymphatics, with the production of buboes, pneumonia, petechial and diffused hemorrhages, and a high mortality. Primarily a disease of rodents, such as rats, it is transmitted to man by the bite of fleas which migrate from the rodent. It is a disease of insanitary conditions, where light and air in the homes are at a minimum, and where rats and mice abound. The incubation period is from three to eight days. The disease begins with fever, pain, and swelling of the lymph glands, followed by delirium, vomiting, diarrhea, and collapse. The recurrent epidemics in London were not finally eradicated until the Great Fire of London rid the city of its rats and insanitary conditions. 2. The term is also applied to any malignant epidemic disease.

**black plague.** The plague which decimated Europe in the 14th century, and so called because of the high incidence of hemorrhages.

**bubonic plague.** The usual form of plague, characterized by bubo formation; formerly prevalent in many parts of the world.

**cattle plague.** A contagious, epidemic, virus disease of cattle, sometimes affecting sheep and goats and occasionally transmitted to man. It is characterized by high temperature and ulceration of the intestinal tract. Also called *rinderpest.*

**fowl plague.** An acute form of septicemia which attacks domesticated birds and is sometimes transmitted to man. It is characterized by fever, profound weakness, prostration, and profuse diarrhea.

**hunger plague.** See FAMINE FEVER.

**levantine plague.** A type of plague occurring in Eastern Europe.

**lung plague.** A mixture of pleurisy and pneumonia in cattle, but occasionally transmitted to man.

**plague sore.** A sore resulting from an attack of the plague.

**plague spot.** The bloody spots seen in the tissues, especially the skin, and characteristic of the plague.

**plague vaccine.** A vaccine used to create immunity against plague.

**pneumonic plague.** An extremely virulent form of the plague characterized by severe pneumonia and a high mortality rate.

**Siberian cattle plague.** See ANTHRAX.

**swine plague.** A hemorrhagic septicemia occurring in pigs and sometimes transmitted to man. It is characterized by pleurisy and pneumonia, with areas of necrosis, and occasionally by a severe septicemia. Also called *hog cholera.*

**planomania.** A morbid tendency to wander.

**plants.** The sole of the foot.

**plantar.** Pertaining to the sole of the foot.

**plantar wart.** A viral growth of the skin located on the sole of the foot. This type of wart is usually sensitive to pressure and thus painful during walking. Also called *verrucca plantaris.*

**plantaris.** A small muscle at the back of the calf of the leg. It is very thin and weak and is frequently ruptured by athletes. When this happens the patient feels as though he has been hit over the calf with a heavy stick. He falls and is unable to rise or walk.

**plaque.** A patch.

**opaline plaques.** White spots scattered over the tonsils, palate, and the inside of the cheeks. They are an early manifestation of syphilis.

**plasma.** The fluid portion of the blood.

**citrated normal human plasma.** Sterile plasma obtained by pooling approximately equal amounts of citrated whole blood from eight or more healthy persons. The plasma is separated from the blood cells, sterility tests are made, a preservative is added, and the plasma is bottled. It may then be kept as a liquid at a temperature between 2° and 5°C., frozen by rapid freezing, or dried in a high vacuum at temperatures below freezing point. All three forms can be stored for a very long time. Plasma can be used for all the purposes for which whole blood is employed, except the restoration of hemoglobin. Since human plasmas are rarely incompatible with each other, they can be used in an emergency to restore the blood volume very rapidly and without much preliminary blood testing, as opposed to blood transfusion, which requires special tests to insure that the blood to be administered is compatible with that of the patient.

**platelet.** Small discs found in the blood which are essential to blood-clot formation. There are 250,000 to 500,000 in each cubic millimeter as well as 6,000 to 8,000 white cells and 5,000,000 red cells. Also called *thrombocyte.*

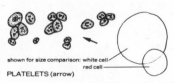

shown for size comparison: white cell
red cell
PLATELETS (arrow)

**platycephalic, platycephalous.** Having a skull of considerable width but excessively flattened from top to bottom.

**Platyhelminthes.** A phylum of flat-bodied, elongated worms.

**platyhieric.** Having a wide sacrum.

**platypelic.** Having a wide pelvis.

**platypodia.** Flatfeet.

**platyrrhine.** Having a broad, flat nose.

**plethora.** The state of being overfull, as of blood.

**plethoric.** Overloaded.

**pleura.** The membrane covering the lungs (visceral pleura) and lining the inside of the chest (parietal pleura), and completely enclosing a potential space known as the pleural cavity. There are two plurae, right and left, entirely distinct from each other.

**pleural.** Relating to pleura.

**pleuralgia.** Pain arising in the pleura.

**pleurectomy.** Surgical removal of part of the pleural membrane.

**pleurisy.** Inflammation of the pleura. Also called *pleuritis.*

**acute pleurisy.** Pleurisy with a sudden onset, high temperature, and pain on breathing. The pain is due to the two layers of inflamed pleura rubbing together, creating a sound which can be heard through the stethoscope like the rubbing together of two pieces of dry brown paper. After a variable time, from hours to days, the pain ceases because there is an outpouring of fluid (pleural effusion), which may be a clear fluid, pus, or blood. The condition may follow an ordinary cold, pneumonia, or influenza.

**adhesive pleurisy.** Pleurisy in which there are adhesions between the two layers of pleural membrane, the one covering the lungs and the other lining the chest cavity.

**chronic pleurisy.** A slowly developing type of pleurisy, usually with adhesions, occurring in such diseases as tuberculosis. See also ADHESIVE PLEURISY, above.

**diaphragmatic pleurisy.** Inflammation of the pleura covering the surface of the diaphragm. It causes intense pain on the slightest attempt at breathing.

**encapsulated pleurisy.** A walled-off pocket of exudate in the pleural space.

**interlobar pleurisy.** Inflammation of the pleura between two lobes of the lungs.

**purulent pleurisy.** A form of pleurisy in which there is much pus and abscess formation. Also called *empyema, pyothorax, suppurative inflammation of the pleura.*

**serous pleurisy.** A form of pleurisy accompanied by a clear pleural effusion.

**pleuritic.** Relating to pleurisy.

**pleuritis.** See PLEURISY.

**pleurobronchitis.** Pleurisy accompanied by bronchitis.

**pleurocele.** A hernia of the lung; an effusion of serum into the pleural cavity.

**pleurocentesis.** A surgical operation in which a needle is passed through the skin and into the pleural space to remove a sample of fluid for laboratory investigation of its content and germs. Sometimes done to remove part of a large pleural effusion which is disturbing breathing and heart function.

**pleurodynia.** 1. A severe pain caused by fibrositis of the muscles between the ribs. 2. There is also an epidemic form of pleurodynia that is characterized by the acute onset of a feverish condition, with pain in the chest, upper abdomen, and back; also called *Bornholm disease, devil's grip.*

**pleuropericarditis.** Pleurisy associated with pericarditis.

**pleuroperitoneal.** Relating both to the pleura and peritoneum.

**pleuropneumonia.** Inflammation of both pleura and lung.

**pleuropneumonolysis.** Surgical removal of some of the ribs on one side of the chest to bring about collapse of the lung. Also called *thoracoplasty.*

**pleuropulmonary.** Relating to the pleura and the lungs.

**pleurothotonos.** A muscular spasm which bends the body to one side. See also OPISTHOTONOS.

**pleurotomy.** A surgical incision into the pleura.

**plexiform.** Resembling a plexus or network.

**plexor.** The hammer used to elicit tendon reflexes. Also called *patellar hammer.*

**plexus.** A network of interlacing nerves or anastomosing blood vessels or lymphatics.

**plica.** A fold.

**plicate.** Folded.

**plicotomy.** Surgical division of the posterior fold of the eardrum.

**plumbism.** Lead poisoning.

**Plummer-Vinson syndrome.** Iron deficiency anemia accompanied by inability to swallow. Also called *Kelly-Paterson syndrome.*

**pluriglandular.** Relating to two or more glands or to their secretions.

**plurigravida.** See MULTIGRAVIDA.

**pluripara.** See MULTIPARA.

**pneumatic.** Relating to air or respiration.

**pneumatocele.** A sac or tumor containing gas, especially the scrotum, if filled with gas. Also called *pneumonocele, pneumocele.*

**pneumatogram.** A tracing showing the characteristics of the breathing movements.

**pneumatometer.** An instrument for measuring the pressure of respiratory

movements. Also called *pneumometer, pneumonometer.*

**pneumatosis.** The presence of air or gas in abnormal places in the body.

**pneumatothorax.** See PNEUMOTHORAX.

**pneumaturia.** The presence of gas or air in the urine.

**pneumectomy.** See PNEUMONECTOMY.

**pneumocele.** See PNEUMATOCELE.

**pneumococcaemia.** See PNEUMOCOCCEMIA.

**pneumococcemia.** A condition in which the germ pneumococcus is present in the blood.

**pneumococcal.** Relating to pneumococci.

**pneumococcus.** An alternative name for the germ more correctly called *Diplococcus pneumoniae*, which frequently causes pneumonia. Fifty-five varieties of the germ have been described and it can also cause arthritis, meningitis, otitis media and pericarditis.

**pneumoconiosis.** A chronic inflammation of the lungs caused by the inhalation of mineral dust; an occupational disease in certain trades.

*All recognized forms of pneumoconiosis are due to mineral dust; neither irritations of the air passages or lungs nor acute infections resulting from inhalation of other types of dust are classed as pneumoconiosis. The prominent reaction to the constant presence of the dust is a fibrosis which varies with each type of dust. The main forms of pneumoconiosis known to cause disability are silicosis, due to silica dust; and asbestosis, due to asbestos dust. Other forms are: anthracosis, due to carbon dust; siderosis, due to iron dust; calcinosis, due to marble dust; and baritosis, due to barium dust. Silicosis can often be complicated by tuberculosis of the lung, and asbestosis by cancer·of the lung. Although anthracosis and silicosis are both diseases occurring in coal miners, there is an essential difference between the two. In anthracosis there is an irritating bronchitis, with the coughing up of black spit, which is merely due to the inhalation of coal dust, whereas silicosis is a much more serious condition occurring after years of inhaling coal dust, in which the essential tissues of the lungs are altered and fibrosed, producing very serious, chronic, and permanent disabilities.*

**pneumoderma.** The presence of air or gas under the skin. Also called *subcutaneous emphysema.*

**pneumoenteritis.** Inflammation of both lungs and intestines.

**pneumogastric.** Relating to the lungs and the stomach; or relating to the vagus nerve, which is also called the pneumogastric nerve.

**pneumogram.** A tracing made by a pneumograph.

**pneumograph.** An instrument for recording the chest movements during breathing.

**pneumohaemopericardium.** See PNEUMOHEMOPERICARDIUM.

**pneumohaemothorax.** See PNEUMOHEMOTHORAX.

**pneumohemopericardium.** The presence of air and blood in the pericardium.

**pneumohemothorax.** The presence of gas or air, and blood, in the pleural cavity of the chest.

**pneumohydrometra.** The presence of air and fluid in the womb.

**pneumohydropericardium.** The presence of air and fluid in the pericardium.

**pneumohydrothorax.** The presence of air or gas and fluid in the pleural cavity of the chest.

**pneumokoniosis.** See PNEUMOCONIOSIS.

**pneumolith.** A stone in the lung.

**pneumolithiasis.** The presence of stones in the lungs.

**pneumomassage.** Massage of the eardrum by pneumatic pressure.

**pneumometer, pneumonometer.** See PNEUMATOMETER.

**pneumomycosis.** Any lung disease caused by a fungus.

**pneumomyelography.** X-ray examination of the spinal canal after the injection of either air or oxygen.

**pneumonectasia, pneumonectasis.** Emphysema of the lungs. See EMPHYSEMA: PULMONARY EMPHYSEMA.

**pneumonectomy.** Surgical removal of part of the lung.

**pneumonia.** Inflammation of the lungs. Also called *pneumonitis, pulmonitis.*

**aspiration pneumonia.** Pneumonia produced from inhaling fluid, food, or vomit during light coma or anesthesia.

**bronchial pneumonia.** Inflammation, often patchy, which has spread to the lung tissue from infected bronchi. Also called *broncho pneumonia.*

**double pneumonia.** Pneumonia affecting both lungs.

**hypostatic pneumonia.** Stagnation and congestion of the lowest parts of the lungs; usually seen in bedridden elderly patients who remain in one position for a long time.

**lipoid pneumonia.** Pneumonia produced by inhaling oil into the lungs, such as cod-liver oil, oily nose drops, and liquid paraffin.

**lobar pneumonia.** Pneumonia which involves one or more lobes of the lung.

**metastatic pneumonia.** Pneumonia produced by infected emboli entering the lungs.

**virus pneumonia.** Pneumonia caused by a virus as opposed to a bacillus infection.

**pneumonic.** Pertaining to the lungs or to pneumonia.

**pneumonitis.** See PNEUMONIA.

**pneumonocele.** A hernia of the lung.

**pneumonokoniosis.** See PNEUMOCONIOSIS.

**pneumonolysis.** A surgical operation to permit the lung to collapse by freeing it from adhesions to the chest wall.

**intrapleural pneumonolysis.** Surgical stripping apart of the two layers of pleura, the one lining the chest and the other covering the lungs.

**pneumonomelanosis.** Anthracosis of the lung. See PNEUMOCONIOSIS.

**pneumonometer.** An instrument for measuring the capacity of the lungs. Also called *spirometer.*

**pneumonopathy.** Any lung disease.

**pneumonorrhaphy.** Suturing of the lung.

**pneumonosepsis.** Inflammation or infection of the lung.

**pneumonosis.** Any lung disease.

**pneumonotomy.** Surgical incision into the lung. Also called *pneumotomy.*

**pneumopaludism.** A not very common term for malarial disease of the lungs.

**pneumopericardium.** The presence of air in the pericardium.

**pneumoperitoneum.** The presence of gas in the peritoneal cavity of the abdomen.

**pneumopyopericardium.** The presence of any gas and pus in the pericardium.

**pneumopyothorax.** The presence of air and pus in the cavity of the chest, especially in the pleural cavity.

**pneumorrhagia.** Bleeding into the air cells and tissues of the lungs. See also HEMOPTYSIS.

**pneumotherapy.** The use of air in treatment; the treatment of lung diseases.

**pneumothorax.** The presence of air or gas in the pleural cavity, causing complete or partial collapse of the lung. Incidence, causes, and symptoms are given under spontaneous pneumothorax.

**artificial pneumothorax.** The introduction into the pleural cavity of air or gas to produce collapse or immobility of the lung; once extensively used to treat pulmonary tuberculosis.

**extrapleural pneumothorax.** Collapse of the lung obtained by stripping the pleural membrane off the chest wall and introducing gas into the space thus formed. It was performed in cases in which artificial pneumothorax could not be used, but fell out of use because of the frequency of secondary infection and spread of the current disease to the extrapleural space.

However, since secondary infection can now be controlled with antibiotics there has been some revival in this operation.

**spontaneous pneumothorax.** Pneumothorax occurring from causes other than the deliberate introduction of air or gas into the pleural cavity from without; more common in men, the maximum incidence is between the ages of 20 and 40 years. It may be due to: air escaping from the lungs and bronchi, probably from rupture of a vesicle on the lung surface; rupture of a lung abscess; gangrene of the lung; rupture of an empyema into the lungs; accidental puncture of the lung during surgical tapping of the pleural cavity; perforation of a lung by a broken rib; penetrating wounds of the chest; an ulcerating growth in the gullet; rupture of a diseased bronchial gland; an ulcer of the stomach or duodenum perforating the diaphragm into the pleural cavity; or an accumulation of gas due to infection by a gas-producing organism—generally the result of wounds. A sudden spontaneous pneumothorax in an apparently healthy person is not very unusual and is known as simple benign pneumothorax. It is sudden in onset and the patient's condition may become quite alarming at once. On the other hand, the condition may develop quietly, with surprisingly little pain or dyspnea, and may only be discovered on routine x-ray examination of the chest. When acute in onset, the patient is seized with pain while coughing or engaged in extra exertion. There is often a feeling of "something giving way" in the chest and at once there is great shortness of breath, with signs of collapse, and often severe mental anguish. The skin may be blue, cold, and clammy, breathing is rapid and shallow, the temperature subnormal, with rapid heartbeat, and weak pulse. The patient is often restless, very alarmed, and unable, or afraid, to speak. In rare cases, death occurs within minutes, but as a general rule the acute symptoms subside within a few hours, though the temperature rises and the rapid breathing persists for a time. Course and prognosis are profoundly influenced by the originating cause, but in the majority of cases no treatment is required, other than a few days' rest in bed, with repeated x-rays to watch the progress of reexpansion of the lung. Where there is other complicating disease then, of course, the picture is altered and the pneumothorax is but a complication of the more general disorder. Also called *simple pneumothorax.*

**pneumotomy.** Surgical incision into the lung.

**pneumotympanum.** The presence of air in the tympanic cavity.

**pock.** A pustule seen in eruptive diseases, such as smallpox; the scar left by such a pustule.

**pockmarked.** Marked with the scars of smallpox.

**poculum.** A cup.

**podagra.** Gout.

**podalgia.** Any pain in the feet.

**podalic.** Relating to the feet.

**podalic version.** Manipulation of the unborn baby into a position in which the feet can be pulled down the birth canal to effect delivery feet first instead of the more normal head first.

**podedema.** Swelling of the foot.

**podelcoma.** Maduromycosis of the foot. Also called *Madura foot.* See MADUROMYCOSIS.

**podobromidrosis.** Offensive sweating of the feet.

**pododynia.** Pain in the foot, especially in the heel.

**podoedema.** See PODEDEMA.

**pogoniasis.** Excessive growth of beard, especially when it occurs in a woman.

**poikiloblast.** A large red blood cell of irregular shape, varying in size.

**poikilocyte.** A red blood cell which is irregular in shape.

**poikilocytosis.** A condition of the blood in which there are numerous irregularly shaped red blood cells; seen in such diseases as pernicious anemia.

**poikilodermia.** A vivid red skin eruption, showing fine veins in the skin, pigmentation, and eventually atrophy of the skin, which closely resembles damage due to excess x-ray radiation. Some cases progress to a certain point and then become stationary, while others continue to spread and end fatally. Also called *poikiloderma of Iacobi, poikiloderma atrophicans vasculare.*

**point.** 1. A small area or spot. 2. To approach the surface at a definite place, like the pus of a boil.

**poison.** Any substance, biological or chemical, noxious to the body.

**poker-back.** See SPONDYLITIS: SPONDYLITIS DEFORMANS.

**polioencephalitis.** Inflammation of the grey matter of the brain.

**polioencephalitis hemorrhagica superior.** A rare condition often associated with either pregnancy or chronic alcoholism, characterized by disease of the blood vessels in the brain, which become blocked and cut off the blood supply to certain parts of the brain, resulting in the death of these parts. The disease is characterized by paralysis of the eye muscles, nystagmus, incoordinate movements and tremors of the limbs, dysarthria, optic neuritis, disorders of consciousness, delirium, and hallucinations. Also called *Wernecke's disease.*

**poliomyelencephalitis.** A combination of polioencephalitis and poliomyelitis.

**poliomyelitis.** Inflammation of the grey matter of the spinal cord. There are several forms.

**acute anterior poliomyelitis.** An infectious disease, characterized, when fully developed, by muscular paralysis. Although no age is immune it was called infantile paralysis because early in this century its maximal incidence was among two- and three-year-old children. The young are still mostly attacked, but at present the biggest risk appears to be in the five- to ten-year-old group and the young adult. Infants under one year seem to be completely immune. There appear to be three degrees of poliomyelitis: abortive cases, called the "minor illness"; nonparalytic and preparalytic; and paralytic. While this classification is justifiable and useful on practical grounds there are no actual subdivisions in the disease, as the three degrees may shade off imperceptibly one into the other. *The "minor illnesses":* these cases occur sporadically, being particularly plentiful during epidemics. The symptoms are easily confused with those of influenza or the early stages of an infectious fever such as measles or glandular fever, and consist of a feeling of being unwell, with headache, mild fever, aching in the back and limbs, and sometimes a sore throat or mild gastrointestinal upset, but at this stage or in this condition there is no muscular paralysis. *Nonparalytic and preparalytic poliomyelitis:* the symptoms are essentially the same as the "minor illness" but tend to be more intense and prolonged. The onset is often abrupt and a high temperature is almost invariable, usually lasting from two to four days and then gradually subsiding, though there may be a secondary rise for a few days before paralysis appears. Back and limb pains are more severe and flexing the spine is painful. Vomiting and loss of appetite are common and there is often slight diarrhea. After a day or so the headache becomes intensified at the back of the head, and is associated with classical symptoms of brain irritation—irritability, neck stiffness, and photophobia. The back and limb muscles are often tender and may show tremors and loss of reflexes. Such a picture in a young adult or child in summer or early autumn is extremely suggestive of poliomyelitis. *Paralytic poliomyelitis:* in these cases muscle paralysis usually appears at the height of the general body disturbance and may be confined to muscles which receive their nerve supply from the spinal cord, the "spinal form" as it is called, or affect muscles which receive their nerve supply direct from the brain, the so-called "bulbar poliomyelitis." In spinal poliomyelitis, the paralysis occurs usually between the second and fifth days of the illness but may be delayed as long as the tenth day if the fever persists. It usually reaches its height within 24 hours, but in rare cases it may continue to progress for several days. In the gravest cases all four limbs become completely paralyzed very quickly and the patient is at once engaged in a life and death struggle in order to breathe. At the other end of the scale are cases so mild that the paralysis is not apparent until the patient tries to walk. Generally speaking, the legs and lower trunk muscles suffer more frequently and severely than the upper parts of the body, especially when diarrhea has been a feature of the early stages. Bulbar poliomyelitis commences with mental confusion and drowsiness, rapidity and irregularity of the pulse, irregularity of breathing, flushing, and congestion of the skin and eyes. There may be paralysis of the throat and gullet, making it difficult or impossible to swallow. The larynx, tongue, and palate may become paralyzed, causing nasal speech and regurgitation of fluids down the nose. Paralysis of one side of the face may occur, and occasionally the patient cannot keep the jaw shut. In this type of poliomyelitis the prognosis is always very grave, but if the patient survives the cranial nerve paralysis he usually makes a remarkably complete recovery. Now that protective inoculation against "polio" is available, it is an astonishing fact that those who seek it are but a small proportion of those who actually need it. The present practice is to give two inoculations at monthly intervals, followed by a third after some months and a fourth injection a year later. There is a move, however, to go over to oral vaccine (three doses at monthly intervals), and research is being made to find a vaccine to include diphtheria, whooping cough, and polio and so cut down the number of injections that have to be given to children. Also called *infantile paralysis, polio.*

**poliomyeloencephalitis.** Inflammation of the grey matter of the spinal cord and brain, such as occurs in acute anterior poliomyelitis.

**poliosis.** Premature greying of the hair.

**Politzer's bag.** An instrument used to produce a sudden increase of air pressure in the nose in order to inflate the Eustachian tube, which communicates with the middle ear, and to overcome an obstruction which may be due to catarrh or other causes. If the Eustachian tube becomes blocked, the atmospheric pressure drives in the eardrum, prevents it vibrating, and causes temporary deafness.

**Politzer's cone of light.** A light-reflecting triangle on the eardrum.

**politzerization.** The use of Politzer's bag.

**pollex.** The thumb.

**pollex pedis.** The big toe.

**pollinosis.** Hay fever.

**pollution.** 1. The act of rendering impure. 2. The production of a sexual orgasm by a stimulus other than sexual intercourse.

**nocturnal pollution.** A nocturnal involuntary discharge of semen. Also called *wet dream.*

**self-pollution.** Masturbation.

**Polya's operation.** An operation for ulcer of the duodenum or stomach, or of cancer of the stomach. Part of the stomach and the first part of the duodenum are removed, and a loop of jejunum is passed through an opening in the transverse mesocolon and connected to the back wall of the stomach to form a posterior gastroenterostomy.

**polyaemia.** See POLYEMIA.

**polyalgesia.** A curious condition in which the patient feels a single pinprick in several places at the same time.

**polyarteritis nodosa.** See PERIARTERITIS NODOSA.

**polyarthric.** Relating to several joints.

**polyarthritis.** Inflammation of many joints.

**polyarticular.** Affecting many joints. Also called *multi-articular.*

**polychromatic.** Showing many colors.

**polychromia.** Abnormal formation of pigment.

**polycyesia, polycyesis.** Multiple pregnancy.

**polycystic.** Composed of or containing many cysts.

**polycythaemia.** See *polycythemia.*

**polycythemia.** An increase in the number of red cells in the circulating blood. The upper limits of normality are 6.5 million red cells per cubic millimeter of blood, but in polycythemia this may reach 7–14 million per cubic millimeter. The condition is merely a symptom and may be caused by any dehydrating illness such as the diarrhea of cholera, which concentrates the blood; by a diminution in the available oxygen, such as is experienced at high altitudes; by certain heart diseases marked by cyanosis; by emphysema, asthma, and fibrosis or growths which interfere with normal ventilation of the lungs; by chronic poisoning with chemical agents such as arsenic, phosphorus, carbon monoxide, or aniline derivatives. Cirrhosis of the liver, tuberculosis of the spleen, and conditions associated with splenic enlargement are rare causes.

**polycythemia vera.** This is a disease in itself, as opposed to polycythemia, which is merely a symptom of another disorder. Characterized by a well-marked and persistent increase in the red cells in the blood due to an excessive production of blood cells by the bone marrow, it is a disease of the second half of life and more common in males than females. Symptoms include nervousness, headache, lack of concentration, vertigo, disturbance of vision, loss of speech, and even paralysis, which may recover completely in a few hours. Itching of the skin, particularly after a hot bath, is common. Other symptoms are loss of weight and strength, shortness of breath on exertion, angina, abdominal pain, and dyspepsia. There is cyanosis of the exposed surfaces, especially the cheeks, tip of the nose, and ears. The facial color varies with the temperature, being scarlet in a warm atmosphere and almost dark blue in cold weather. The eyeballs are often bloodshot and sometimes deep red. The risk to the patient is due to the increased volume, extra density, and sluggish flow of the blood, which may contain from 7 to 14 million red corpuscles per cubic millimeter, as opposed to the normal 4 to 5 million. There may be massive hemorrhages, especially from the stomach, nose, lungs, bowel, womb, bladder, or internally. Treatment is usually begun by removing a pint of blood twice weekly, and may be necessary to do this for five or six weeks to reduce the level to normal. This level may then be maintained by venesection at longer intervals, or by the use of various agents, such as radioactive phosphorus, which slow up the bone marrow production of red cells. X-ray treatment to the long bones, which contain the bone marrow, may also be used. Also called *erythremia, Osler-Vaquez disease, polyglobulism.*

**polydactylism.** The presence of more than the normal number of fingers or toes.

**polydipsia.** Abnormal thirst, such as occurs in those suffering with untreated diabetes.

**polydontia.** The presence of more than the normal number of teeth.

**polyemia.** An abnormal increase in the total volume of blood in the body.

**polygalactia.** An abnormally large secretion of milk.

**polygastria.** Abnormally increased secretion of gastric juices.

**polygenesis.** The production of many children.

**polyglobulism.** See POLYCYTHEMIA.

**polygraph.** An instrument for recording pulsations simultaneously, such as the radial and jugular pulses. In some machines the record is produced as a photograph and in others by means of an ink-writing arm; used as a so-called lie detector.

**polyhidrosis.** Excessive sweating.

**polyhydramnios.** The presence of abnormally large quantities of liquor amnii.

**polymastia, polymazia.** Having more than two breasts.

**polymenorrhea.** Too frequent menstrual periods.

**polymenorrhoea.** See *polymenorrhea.*

**polymorph.** A polymorphonuclear leukocyte (a white blood cell that attacks and ingests germs). Pus is a mass of these white cells and dead germs.

**polymorphic.** Having several forms.

**polymorphism.** The condition of being polymorphic.

**polymorphocyte.** See MYELOCYTE.

**polymorphonuclear.** Having nuclei of many forms.

**polymorphous.** Polymorphic.

**polymyalgia.** Pain in several muscles.

**polyneuritis.** Neuritis attacking several different nerves. See NEURITIS: MULTIPLE NEURITIS.

**polynuclear, polynucleate.** Having several nuclei.

**polyodontia.** See POLYDONTIA.

**polyonychia.** The presence of more than the normal number of nails.

**polyp, polypus.** A tumor that usually arises from a mucous membrane and is connected to it by a pedicle. Polyps may be found in the nose, urinary bladder, stomach, large intestine, or womb.

**polyphrasia.** Excessive talkativeness.

**polypiferous.** Having or producing polyps.

**polyplasmia.** An abnormal amount of plasma in the blood.

**polypnea.** Very rapid breathing, such as panting.

**polypoid.** Resembling a polyp.

**polyposis.** 1. An abnormal thirst; polydipsia. 2. Affected with polyps.

**polypotome.** A surgical instrument for removing polyps.

**polyserositis.** Inflammation of such membranes as the pleural membrane, pericardial membrane, and the peritoneal membrane. See also PICK'S DISEASE.

**polysinusitis.** Inflammation of several sinuses at once.

**polyspermia, polyspermism.** The excessive secretion of seminal fluid.

**polyspermy.** Fertilization of the ovum by more than one spermatozoan.

**polytendinitis.** Inflammation of several tendons at the same time.

**polythelia.** The presence of more than one nipple on a breast.

**polytocous.** Producing many young at a birth.

**polytrichia, polytrichosis.** The excessive growth of hair.

**polyuria.** The passing of an excessive amount of urine.

**pompholyx.** A skin disease characterized by the presence of tiny vesicles and bullae on the palms of the hands and soles of the feet. See also CHEIRO-POMPHOLYX.

**pomphus.** A wheal.

**pomum adami.** The Adam's apple, the prominence in the front of the throat which is the thryoid cartilage of the larynx.

**pons.** 1. Any bridge of tissue connecting two parts of an organ. 2. Part of the base of the brain which receives impulses from the brain cortex and sends them to the opposite side of the cerebellum.

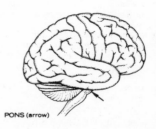

PONS (arrow)

**popliteal.** Related to or situated in the area at the back of the knee joint.

**porcupine disease.** See ICTHYOSIS.

**pore.** 1. A minute opening on a surface. 2. The opening of the duct of a sweat gland in the skin.

**porencephalia, porencephalus, porencephaly.** A congenital abnormality in which the brain cavities communicate with the surface.

**porencephalic, porencephalous.** Affected with porencephalia.

**porokeratosis.** A rare, hereditary, chronic, and progressive skin disease characterized by a ring of elevated thickened skin about an irregular patch of depressed atrophic skin.

**porosis.** 1. Rarefaction; increased translucency to x-rays. 2. Formation of pores; cavity formation.

**porosity.** The quality of being porous.

**porous.** Having pores.

**porphyria.** An inborn error of metabolism in which there is abnormal production of chemicals called porphyrins and in which large amounts of uroporphyrin appear in the urine. There are three separate types.

**porphyria acuta.** The commonest and most important of the three types of porphyria. Acute attacks usually occur between the ages of 20 and 30 years, and classically there is severe burning or colicky abdominal pain, vomiting, and constipation with involvement of the nervous system, giving rise to paralysis of limbs and trunk and later of cranial nerves. Psychological disturbances, rapidity of the heart, raised blood pressure, and signs of angina are not unusual. Remissions are sometimes dramatic but the ultimate prognosis is poor. The urine is reddish-brown or purple, either when passed or after it has been left standing for some hours. Certain barbiturate and sulphonamide drugs are reputed to precipitate the attacks.

**porphyria congenita.** A very rare hereditary disease appearing early in life. Porphyrins are found in bones, teeth, and urine, which are, in consequence, red or chocolate-brown in color. There is marked photosensitivity, with scarring of the skin, loss of fingers, and an overgrowth of hair.

**porphyria cutanea tarda.** This condition appears in early adult life. Photosensitivity of the skin may be accompanied by abdominal colic and jaundice. During the attacks porphyrins are diverted from the feces to the urine, due possibly to episodes of liver insufficiency.

**porphyrinaemia.** See *porphyrinemia.*

**porphyrinemia.** The presence of porphyrins in the blood.

**porphyrins.** Chemical pigments formed during the production of blood proteins such as hemoglobin.

**porphyrinuria.** The passing of porphyrins in the urine.

**porrigo.** Ringworm and other scalp diseases.

**porta.** That part of an organ through which the nerves and blood vessels pass. Also called *hilum.*

**portal.** Relating to the porta or hilum of an organ.

**portal vein.** The main vein to the liver.

**portio.** A term applied to various body structures; used without qualification, it usually refers to the portio vaginalis uteri, the portion of the womb situated within the vagina.

**port wine mark, port wine stain.** See NEVUS: NEVUS FLAMMEUS.

**porus.** A pore or opening.

**porus acusticus externus.** The opening of the external ear.

**porus acusticus internus.** The opening of the internal auditory canal into the cranial cavity.

**porus sudoriferus.** The opening of a sweat gland.

**position.** Place, location, attitude, posture.

**anatomical position.** The attitude of a person standing erect, with arms at the sides and the palms facing forward.

**apparent position.** A term used in ophthalmology to indicate the position in space to which the mind projects a visual image.

**bronchoscopic position.** The patient lies flat with the head hyperextended to bring the larynx and trachea in a straight line, so as to permit the introduction of the bronchoscope.

**dorsal position.** The attitude of a person when lying on his back.

**dorsosacral position.** The position of the patient when lying on the back, with the legs flexed on the thighs and the thighs flexed on the abdomen and widely separated at the knees.

**flipper position.** A position a patient adopts in cases of bleeding into the midbrain, following fractures of the bones of the middle or posterior compartments of the skull. The body is stiff, the arms extended and rotated inwards, with the wrists flexed, the legs rigid, and the feet pronated.

**Fowler's position.** The posture the patient assumes when the head of his bed is raised 18 to 20 inches from the level. A similar position is achieved by the use of a backrest; the position in which most "chest" cases are nursed.

**genupectoral position.** The position the patient adopts when resting on the knees and chest.

**high pelvic position.** See TRENDELENBURG'S POSITION.

**Jones' position.** Acute flexion of the forearm on the arm in the treatment of elbow fractures involving the condyles.

**knee-chest position.** See GENUPECTORAL POSITION, above.

**knee-elbow position.** The posture in which the patient lies upon the knees and elbows, the head resting upon the hands.

**latero-abdominal position.** See SIMS'S POSITION, below.

**left lateral position.** See SIMS'S POSITION, below.

**lithotomy position.** See DORSOSACRAL POSITION, above.

**mentoanterior position.** A midwifery term to indicate the baby's position in the uterus. The head is sharply

extended so that the back of the skull is in contact with its back and the face looks downwards towards the vagina. It is a position which makes delivery difficult or impossible and the doctor must alter it or use an alternative means of delivery.

**mentoposterior position.** A midwifery term to indicate that the baby within the uterus has its head sharply extended so that the back of the skull is in contact with the baby's back and the face looks downwards and backwards. This position makes delivery difficult or impossible and the doctor must either alter it or consider another means of delivery.

**occipitoanterior position.** A midwifery term to indicate the baby's position within the uterus, in which the back of the baby's skull is directed forwards towards the mother's abdomen. It is the normal and easiest position for delivery.

**occipitoposterior position.** A midwifery term to indicate that the baby's position within the uterus is with the back of the skull towards the rear with the face towards the mother's abdomen.

**position effect.** A term used in genetics, which expounds the view that the expression of a gene depends, in part, upon its relation to adjacent genes. Electronic microscope studies of genes within the chromosomes of the fertilized egg cell are slowly revealing the characteristics likely to be passed on to the new baby.

**Simon's position.** The dorsal posture with the legs and thighs flexed, the hips raised, and the thighs widely separated.

**Sims's position.** The posture of the patient when lying on the left side with the right knee and thigh drawn up, the left arm placed along the back and the chest inclined forward. Also called *semiprone, three-quarter-prone position.*

**Trendelenburg's position.** The posture of a patient lying on an operating table, which has been tilted upwards to about 40 to 50 degrees, with the legs and feet hanging over the upper end.

**Walcher's position.** The posture of a patient lying on his back, with the thighs and legs hanging over the edge of the bed or operating table; sometimes adopted in midwifery to facilitate difficult delivery.

**posological.** Relating to posology.

**posology.** The science of the dosage of medicines.

**postcentral.** Behind a center. Usually refers to the area behind the central fissure of the brain.

**postcerebellar.** Situated in the rear of the cerebellum.

**postcerebral.** Situated in the back of the cerebrum.

**postcibal.** After eating.

**postclavicular.** Behind the clavicle.

**postclimacteric.** Occurring after the menopause.

**postconcussional syndrome.** Headache, head noises, dizziness, insomnia, irritability, emotional excitement, and inability to withstand noise—a condition following concussion.

**postcondylar.** Situated behind a condyle.

**postconnubial.** Occurring after marriage.

**postconvulsive.** Occurring after a convulsion.

**postdiastolic.** Following a diastole.

**postdigestive.** Happening after digestion.

**postdiphtheritic.** Happening following diphtheria.

**postdural.** Situated behind the dura mater.

**postencephalitis.** The condition which sometimes remains after recovery from epidemic encephalitis. This period is sometimes marked by freakish, bizarre, and peculiar behavior.

**postepileptic.** Following an attack of epilepsy, such as postepileptic automatism. See also EPILEPSY; AUTOMATISM.

**posterior.** Behind or to the rear.

**postesophageal.** Behind the esophagus.

**postfebrile.** After the temperature has subsided.

**postganglionic.** Behind a ganglion.

**postglenoid.** Situated behind the glenoid cavity. The term is applied to a dislocation of the arm in which the head of the humerus is displaced backwards. It is then said to be in the postglenoid position.

**posthaemorrhage.** See *posthemorrhage.*

**posthaemorrhagic.** See *posthemorrhagic.*

**posthemiplegic.** Following hemiplegia.

**posthemorrhage.** When one hemorrhage succeeds another.

**posthemorrhagic.** Occurring after hemorrhage.

**posthepatic.** Behind the liver.

**posthetomy.** An infrequently used term for circumcision.

**posthitis.** An infrequently used term for inflammation of the prepuce.

**posthumous.** Occurring after death.

**posthumous child.** One born after the death of its father, or removed by cesarean operation from the dead body of its mother.

**posthypnotic.** Following hypnotism.

**posthypophysis.** The posterior part of the pituitary gland in the brain.

**postischial.** Situated posterior to the ischium bone of the pelvis.

**postmalarial.** Following malaria.

**postmastoid.** Behind the mastoid process.

**postmedian.** Posterior to the middle transverse line of the body.

**postmediastinal.** Behind the mediastinum.

**postmenopausal.** After or following the menopause.

**postmesenteric.** Behind the mesentery.

**post-mortem.** After death; an examination of a dead body. Also called *autopsy, necropsy.*

**post-mortem lividity.** Discoloration of the dependent parts of a corpse, caused by blood accumulating at the lowest points. See also HYPOSTASIS.

**postnasal.** Behind the nose.

**postnatal.** After birth or after delivery.

**postocular.** Behind the eye.

**postoesophageal.** See POSTESOPHAGEAL.

**postoperative.** Following a surgical operation.

**postparalytic.** Happening after an attack of paralysis.

**postpartum.** Happening after delivery of a baby.

**postprandial.** After a meal.

**postsacral.** Behind the sacrum.

**postscapular.** Behind the scapula.

**postscarlatinal.** Following scarlet fever.

**posttraumatic.** Following or in consequence of an injury.

**posttraumatic personality disorder.** A psychosis resulting from direct injury to the head or brain. The symptoms include headache, emotional instability, a tendency toward fatigue, and sometimes convulsions.

**postulate.** A proposition that is assumed without positive proof.

**Koch's postulate.** A medical law which states that to prove that a certain germ causes a certain disease the following conditions must obtain: (1) The germ must be present in all cases of the disease; (2) the germ must be cultivated in pure culture; (3) the culture must produce the disease when injected into susceptible animals; and (4) the germ must be obtained from such animals and again be cultivated in pure culture.

**postural.** Pertaining to position or posture; performed by means of adopting a special posture.

**posture.** Position, especially of the body. See POSITION.

**posture sense.** The power of perceiving, without actually seeing, the position in which a limb has been placed.

**postuterine.** Behind the uterus.

**postvaccinal.** Following vaccination.

**potable.** Fit to drink.

**potency.** Strength or power; in homeopathy, the extent of the dilution of a medicine.

**potentia coeundi.** Ability to perform the sexual act.

**potential.** 1. The inherent ability to perform. 2. In electricity, when bodies of different potentials are put in communication, a current passes between them. If they are of the same potential no current passes.

**potion.** A drink.

**potomania.** Delirium tremens. Also called *mania a potu.*

**Pott's curvature.** Kyphosis of the spine, resulting from tuberculosis of the spine.

**Pott's disease.** Tuberculosis of the spine. Also called *spondylitis tuberculosa.*

**Pott's fracture.** A fracture of the fibula bone of the leg, occurring about three inches above the ankle and sometimes accompanied by a splitting of the lower end of the tibia.

**Pott's gangrene.** Gangrene occurring in elderly people. Also called *senile gangrene.*

**Pott's paralysis.** The paralysis of both legs caused by tuberculous disease of the spine.

**Pott's puffy tumor.** Swelling produced by inflammation of the bone of the skull.

**potter's asthma, consumption, or rot.** See SILICOSIS.

**pouch.** A sac or hollow space.

**pouch of Douglas.** The space between the rectum and the womb.

**poultice.** A soft, semiliquid mass applied to the skin for the purpose of supplying heat. Although the use of poultices has been largely discontinued, the kaolin poultice is still useful in bringing comfort to arthritic joints. There are numerous methods of preparing it, but one of the easiest is to spread kaolin at least a quarter-inch thick on the smooth side of white lint and cover with a layer of gauze. Then place it on the upturned lid of a saucepan half full of boiling water and heat for 20-30 minutes. The area to be poulticed should be well greased with butter, lanolin, or petroleum jelly and the poultice applied, gauze side towards the skin. Cover with cotton wool to retain the heat, and bandage into position. This can be repeated every three or four hours.

*In the past, poultices consisted of many strange ingredients, from a mixture of dry mustard and flour in water to the pigeon-dung poultice applied to the feet of King Charles II to draw "bad blood" from his brain when he was lying in coma from a stroke.*

**pox.** Any disease producing vesicles or pustules; an obsolete slang term for syphilis.

**p.p. factor.** An abbreviation of pellagra preventing factor. See PELLAGRA.

**praecoid.** See PRECOID.

**praecox.** Occurring early, as in dementia praecox. See SCHIZOPHRENIA.

**praevia.** Coming before. See PLACENTA: PLACENTA PRAEVIA.

**pragmatism.** The doctrine that the whole meaning of an idea lies in its practical consequences.

**praxis.** The performance of an action or deed.

**preagonal.** Occurring immediately before the death agony.

**preanaesthesia.** See PREANESTHESIA.

**preanesthesia.** The giving of a drug to make the patient sleepy before administering a general anesthetic.

**preaortic.** Situated in front of the aorta.

**preataxic.** Before the onset of ataxia.

**prebrachial.** Situated on the front of the upper arm.

**precancerous.** A condition that may develop into a cancer. Also called *premalignant.*

**precardiac.** In front of the heart.

**precentral.** In front of the central fissure of the brain.

**precipitant.** An agent causing precipitation.

**precipitate.** 1. To cause a solid in a solution to settle down; the deposit that forms after precipitation. 2. To cause or initiate; headlong or hasty, as in precipitate labor.

**precipitation.** The act of precipitating solids in solution.

**precipitin.** An antibody to a soluble antigen. A precipitate is formed when the soluble antigen is mixed with the antibody.

**precipitinogen.** Any substance capable of producing a specific precipitin.

**precocious.** Developing at an age earlier than usual.

**precoid.** Like dementia praecox. See SCHIZOPHRENIA.

**preconscious.** A psychoanalytical term for mental processes of which the individual is unaware but which he can recall as opposed to unconscious processes, which he cannot recall. Also called *foreconscious.*

**preconvulsive.** Before a convulsion.

**precordia.** The area of the chest in front of the heart. Also called *precordium.*

**precordial.** Relating to the precordia.

**precordium.** Precordia.

**precostal.** In front of the ribs.

**precranial.** Situated in the front of the cranium.

**prediastole.** The time interval just before diastole.

**predigestion.** The partial digestion of food by artificial means before it is eaten.

**predisposing.** Rendering susceptible to disease.

**predisposition.** The condition of being susceptible to disease.

**preeclampsia.** A state of toxemia in the pregnant woman, associated with edema, headache, the presence of albumin in the urine, and increased blood pressure but not accompanied by convulsions.

**preepiglottic.** Situated in front of the epiglottis.

**preeruptive.** Anything which precedes the characteristic rash of a disease.

**prefrontal.** 1. Lying in the front part of the frontal lobe of the brain; 2. The middle part of the ethmoid bone in the skull.

**prefrontal leucotomy.** Surgical division of the conducting nerve paths in the front lobe of the brain. See also LEUCOTOMY.

**preganglionic.** In front of a ganglion.

**pregnancy.** The condition of the woman during the period between conception and the birth of a child. Normally this is about 280 days, ten lunar months, the expected date of birth being calculated from the first day of the last menstrual period. In practice, this method has proved to be remarkably accurate to within two or three days, but it is possible to be wrong by as much as four weeks, for the doctor can never be sure whether the mother became pregnant just after her last menstrual period or just before her next expected menstruation. Another basis of error is due to the fact that some women do menstruate during pregnancy, and while this may seem an anomaly, the explanation seems to be that the pregnancy does not fill the womb until after the third month and so it is possible for it to occupy the top half of the womb and for the lower half to still menstruate. While this theory may be true, in practice it is extremely rare.

**ectopic pregnancy.** A pregnancy occurring outside the uterus. It occasionally happens that, due to a kink or obstruction in the Fallopian tube, the fertilized egg, unable to pass the obstruction, continues to grow where it is. This can only continue for a short time before it ruptures the Fallopian tube, causing an internal hemorrhage and requiring urgent surgical operation. The symptoms are severe lower abdominal pain, mainly with the passage of some blood from the vagina, and vomiting and collapse in a woman who has missed one or two menstrual periods. The differential diagnosis is always between ectopic pregnancy and early abortion. In early abortion the bleeding is more severe and occurs before the pain; in ectopic pregnancy the pain is severe and comes on first, bleeding from the vagina is slight, and the patient very rapidly becomes surgically shocked and collapsed. Also called *extra-uterine pregnancy.*

**false pregnancy.** See PSEUDOCYESIS.

**tubal pregnancy.** Development of a fertilized egg in the oviduct.

**prehemiplegic.** Occurring before the onset of hemiplegia.

**prehensile.** Capable of grasping.

**prehension.** The act of grasping.

**prehyoid.** Situated in front of the hyoid bone in the neck.

**prehypophysis.** The anterior lobe of the pituitary gland in the brain.

**premalignant.** Precancerous.

**premaniacal.** Prior to insanity.

**premature.** Occurring before the proper time.

**premaxilla.** The intermaxillary bone.

**premaxillary.** Anterior to the maxilla.

**premedication.** The giving of a drug to induce a sleepy state prior to administering a general anesthetic.

**premenstrual.** Happening prior to the menstrual period.

**premolar.** One of the two teeth between the canine and the first molar, a bicuspid. Often incorrectly applied to a molar tooth of the first dentition. The premolars replace these so-called deciduous molars.

**premonitory.** Forewarning.

**premonitory symptoms.** Symptoms heralding the onset of a disease.

**prenatal.** Before birth.

**preneoplastic.** Occurring before the development of a definite tumor. See PRECANCEROUS.

**preoccipital.** Situated in front of the occipital region.

**preoperative.** Occurring prior to a surgical operation.

**preoral.** In front of the mouth.

**prepalatal.** In front of the palate.

**prepatellar.** Lying in front of the patella.

**prepatellar bursitis.** A swelling over the top of the knee cap due to the presence of fluid in the bursa situated in that position. Also called *housemaid's knee.* See also BURSITIS.

**prepuce.** The foreskin.

**preputial.** Relating to the prepuce.

**prepyloric.** In front of the pylorus.

**prerectal.** In front of the rectum.

**prerenal.** Lying in front of the kidney.

**preretinal.** Lying in front of the retina.

**presbyatrics.** The treatment of diseases occurring in old age. Also called *geriatrics.*

**presbycusis, presbykousis.** The loss of hearing occurring in old age.

**presbyope.** A person affected with presbyopia.

**presbyopia.** A condition of middle age in which the crystalline lens of the eye loses its elasticity and powers of accommodation, with the result that the individual requires reading glasses although his distance vision may remain unimpaired.

**presbysphacelus.** Senile gangrene.

**presenile, presenility.** Premature old age.

**present.** Said of the part of a baby that first appears at the mouth of the womb.

**presentation.** That part of the unborn baby first felt when an examination is made through the opening of the uterus at the beginning of labor. The relation of the part of the baby to the birth canal determines the type of presentation.

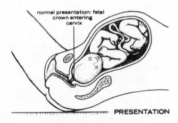

normal presentation: fetal crown entering cervix

PRESENTATION

**breech presentation.** Presentation in which the buttocks appear at the mouth of the womb.

**brow presentation.** Presentation in which the brow presents at the mouth of the womb.

**cephalic presentation.** Presentation in which any part of the head presents at the mouth of the womb.

**face presentation.** Presentation of the face with the chin leading at the mouth of the womb.

**footling presentation.** Presentation in which the baby is lying with the feet foremost.

**presentation of the cord.** A condition in which the umbilical cord drops down in front of the baby at the beginning of labor.

**transverse presentation.** Presentation in which the child lies with its long axis across the womb, so that the presenting part to the mouth of the womb may be the shoulder, back, or abdomen.

**vertex presentation.** The normal presentation with the back part of the skull presenting at the mouth of the womb.

**pressor.** Stimulating.

**pressor substance.** Any substance which increases blood pressure.

**pressure.** Force, weight, or tension.

**abdominal pressure.** The rise in pressure within the abdomen caused by the diaphragm contracting against a rigid abdominal wall, such as occurs in urination or defecation. Also called *abdominal strain, abdominal sqeeze, bearing down.*

**after pressure.** The sense of pressure that remains after a removal of an object from the body surface.

**arterial pressure.** The tension of the arterial wall due to the pressure of blood within it.

**atmospheric pressure.** The pressure exerted by the atmosphere on the earth's surface. It is about 15 pounds per square inch at sea level.

**back-pressure effect.** A damming back of blood in the venous system caused when the heart is unable to pump blood from the venous system to the arterial system as fast as it is received.

**bipolar pressure.** Pressure on both ends of a bone. It is sometimes used to differentiate a bone fracture from simple contusions, because springing the two ends of the bone with moderate force will produce a pain at the fracture site if one is present.

**blood pressure.** The pressure of the blood on the walls of the arteries. It is measured by a sphygmomanometer, which consists of a hollow rubber bag connected by a rubber tube to a column of mercury calibrated in millimeters and a small bellows. The bag is wound round the middle of the upper arm. The doctor listens through a stethoscope to the pulsation of the artery in front of the elbow. The rubber bag is then inflated until the arterial pulse sound can no longer be heard through the stethoscope, after which the pressure is released until the artery can be heard pumping again. The number of millimeters recorded on the mercury column at this point is referred to as the systolic pressure. Air pressure is further released slowly from the bag until the arterial pulse becomes quieter or even silent; the reading on the mercury column at this point is referred to as the diastolic pressure. Normal blood pressure in a healthy unemotional young adult is approximately 120 systolic and 80 diastolic. Nervous emotion and violent physical exercise cause temporary rises in blood pressure, but permanent rises may be due to heart and kidney diseases or to arteriosclerosis.

**critical pressure.** The pressure on a gas or vapor which will, at the critical temperature, convert it into a liquid.

**endocardial pressure.** The pressure of blood within the heart.

**hydrostatic pressure.** Pressure exerted in a fluid system as by the effect of gravity or by the energy of muscular contraction, such as the blood pressure created by the heartbeat.

**imbibition pressure.** Pressure due to the increase in volume of a gel by the absorption of liquid.

**intra-abdominal pressure.** See ABDOMINAL PRESSURE.

**intracranial pressure.** Pressure occurring within the skull.

**intraocular pressure.** Pressure arising within the globe of the eye.

**intrathoracic pressure.** Pressure within the chest cavity.

**negative pressure.** The force of suction or absence of pressure.

**oncotic pressure.** The osmotic pressure exerted by colloids in a solution; the pressure varies owing to the variation of colloidal molecules.

**osmotic pressure.** The pressure exerted by the passage of a solvent through a semipermeable membrane from a weak solution into a more concentrated one. See also OSMOSIS.

**pulse pressure.** The difference between systolic and diastolic pressures. See BLOOD PRESSURE.

**solution pressure.** The tendency of molecules to leave the surface of a solute and pass into the solvent.

**venous pressure.** The pressure of blood within the veins.

**pressure sore.** A bed sore.

**presystole.** The period of time before systole.

**presystolic.** Preceding the systole.

**pretarsal.** In front of the tarsus.

**prethyroid.** In front of the thyroid gland in the neck.

**pretibial.** In front of the tibia.

**pretracheal.** In front of the trachea.

**prevertebral.** Situated in front of the vertebrae.

**priapism.** Persistent painful erection of the penis due to disease and injuries of the spinal cord, stone in the bladder, or injury to the penis.

**prickly heat.** An acute skin eruption common among white people in the tropics, and characterized by papules and vesicles at the sweat gland openings. It is probably caused by profuse sweating, which leaves chemical salts that irritate and inflame the sweat gland openings. Mild forms can be controlled by frequent washing with soft water, especially shower baths, and changing into clean linen. In the severer forms, the openings of the sweat glands become blocked by horny plugs, and unless the condition is treated sweating is interfered with and the patient may suffer from tropical anhidrotic asthenia, a condition allied to heat exhaustion, which results in exhaustion, irritability, heat intolerance, vertigo, headache, dyspnea, and palpitations. Also called *heat rash, lichen tropicus, miliaria papillosa, miliaria rubra.*

**primary.** First in order or first in importance.

**primary lesion.** The original lesion from which subsequent disease develops.

**primary sore.** The initial ulcer of syphilis; chancre; hardsore.

**primigravida.** A woman in her first pregnancy.

**primipara.** A woman who has had her first child.

**primiparity.** The state of being a primipara.

**primiparous.** Bearing one child.

**privates.** A colloquial name for the genital organs.

**probang.** A flexible rod used to remove foreign bodies from the gullet.

**probe.** A slender, flexible rod used to explore channels, a wound, or a cavity.

**process.** 1. A course of action. 2. A group of phenomena, as an inflammatory process. 3. A prominence or outgrowth, such as the spinous process of a vertebra or the axis cylinder of a nerve. 4. In chemistry, a method of procedure, reaction, or test.

**prochoresis.** The movement of food through the pylorus or along the alimentary canal.

**procidentia.** The falling down of a part; a prolapse; usually refers to prolapse of the womb, which drags down with it the lining of the vagina, urinary bladder, and rectum.

**procreation.** The act of begetting offspring.

**proctalgia.** Pain in the anus or rectum.

**proctatresia.** A congenital condition in which there is no opening for the anus or rectum.

**proctectasia.** Dilation of the anus or rectum.

**proctectomy.** Surgical removal of the anus or rectum.

**proctencleisis.** Stricture of the rectum or anus.

**proctitis.** Inflammation of the anus or rectum.

**proctocele.** Prolapse of a part of the rectum.

**proctoclysis.** Slow injection of a liquid into the rectum.

**proctococcypexia, proctococcypexy.** Suturing of the rectum to the coccyx.

**proctodynia.** Pain in or about the anus or rectum.

**proctogenic.** Originating from the anus or rectum.

**proctology.** That branch of medical science dealing with the anatomy and diseases of the rectum.

**proctoparalysis.** Paralysis of the anal or rectal muscles.

**proctopexia, proctopexy.** Fixation of the rectum to another part by sutures.

**proctophobia.** A morbid dread or apprehension about diseases of the anus, common in persons suffering with disorders of the rectum and anus. In some neurotic personalities it may become obsessional.

**proctoplasty.** Plastic repair of the rectum or anus.

**proctoptoma, proctoptosis.** Prolapse of the rectum.

**proctorrhagia.** Bleeding from the anus.

**proctorrhaphy.** Plaiting of prolapsed rectal walls by suturing to reduce their circumference.

**proctorrhea.** The escape of mucus from the anus.

**proctorrhoea.** See PROCTORRHEA.

**proctoscope.** An instrument for examining the rectum.

**proctoscopy.** Inspection of the rectum with a proctoscope.

**proctosigmoidectomy.** A surgical operation in which the rectum and part of the sigmoid colon are removed and the stump of the sigmoid colon is joined to the stump of the rectum.

**proctosigmoiditis.** Inflammation involving the rectum and sigmoid colon.

**proctostenosis.** Stricture of the rectum or anus.

**proctostomy.** Surgical creation of a permanent artificial opening into the rectum. Also called *rectostomy.*

**proctotomy.** Surgical incision into the rectum or anus performed for stricture or for congenital inperforate anus. Also called *rectotomy.*

**prodromal.** Relating to a prodrome.

**prodromal period.** This is very commonly seen in children who are "off color" for a few days but have no signs of any specific disease, which follow later.

**prodrome.** An early manifestation of impending disease, before the specific symptoms begin.

**prodromous.** Prodromal.

**progeria.** Senile appearance at an early age, sometimes associated with pituitary dwarfism.

**progesterone.** The hormone of the corpus luteum of the ovary, which induces premenstrual changes of the uterus lining following ovulation and

probably inhibits contractions of the uterus during early pregnancy. It is used in the treatment of recurrent and threatened abortions and for disturbances of menstruation. Also called *progestin.*

**progestin.** See PROGESTERONE.

**prognathism.** Abnormal projection of the jaw.

**prognathous.** Having projecting jaws.

**prognosis.** The medical forecast of the outcome of a disease.

**prognostic.** Relating to prognosis.

**prognosticate.** To make a prognosis.

**progressive.** 1. Steadily advancing. 2. Going from bad to worse.

**progressive lenticular degeneration.** A disease characterized by loss of muscle tone, muscular weakness, poverty of movement, tremors, cirrhosis of the liver, and progressive deterioration of the mental faculties.

**progressive muscular atrophy.** Progressive muscular wasting, due to degeneration in certain cells of the spinal cord, resulting in degeneration of anterior nerve routes and wasting of the muscles supplied by them. Also called *chronic anterior poliomyelitis.*

**prolabium.** The red outer part of the lip.

**prolactin.** The milk-producing hormone of the anterior lobe of the pituitary gland.

**prolapse.** The falling forwards or downwards of a part, frequently used to indicate prolapse of the womb.

**prolapse of the cord.** Expulsion of the umbilical cord before the baby is born.

**prolapsus ani.** Prolapse of the anus.

**prolapsus uteri.** Prolapse of the uterus.

**prolepsis.** The return of an attack or paroxysm before the expected time or at progressively shorter intervals.

**proleptic.** Recurring sooner than expected.

**proliferate.** To multiply.

**proliferating, proliferous.** Multiplying; usually refers to the formation of new tissues or cells.

**proliferation.** The act of multiplying.

**prominence.** A projection.

**promontory.** A projection.

**pronation.** The condition of being prone; the act of placing in a prone position; the turning of the palm of the hand downwards.

**pronator.** A muscle which produces the movement of pronation.

**prone.** Lying face downwards; the position of the hand with palm turned downwards.

**propagation.** Reproduction.

**prophylactic.** Pertaining to prophylaxis; any agent which prevents disease.

**prophylaxis**

**prophylaxis.** The prevention of disease.

**proprioceptor.** A nerve ending located in a muscle, tendon, or joint, whose impulses, together with those of the labyrinth (organ of balance in the ear), supply the information by which we are informed of our position in space or the position of various parts of the body.

**proptosis.** 1. A falling downwards; prolapse. 2. Exophthalmus.

**propulsion.** 1. The act of propelling or pushing forwards; 2. A tendency to fall forwards in walking, such as is seen in paralysis agitans.

**prosopalgia.** See TIC: TIC DOULOUREUX.

**prosoponeuralgia.** Facial neuralgia.

**prosopoplegia.** Paralysis of the face.

**prosopospasm.** See RISUS SARDONICUS.

**prosopotocia.** A face presentation of the baby during labor.

**prospermia.** Uncontrollable precipitate ejaculation of seminal fluid. Also called *ejaculatio praecox.*

**prostatalgia.** Pain in the prostate gland.

**prostate gland.** The organ surrounding the neck of the bladder and beginning of the urethra in the male. It con-

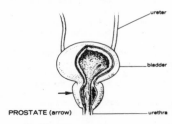

PROSTATE (arrow)

sists of two lateral lobes and a middle lobe and is composed of muscular and glandular tissue. Numerous ducts open from the prostate into the urethra, and it is probable that the gland secretes a fluid which mixes with the semen and acts both as a nutrient medium and as a lubricant to assist the semen on its long journey to fertilize the female egg.

*With advancing years the prostate tends to enlarge and interfere with the passage of urine. At first there is merely difficulty in maintaining a normal stream and this may go on for several years, gradually becoming worse until an acute obstruction sets in, which can only be relieved by the passage of a catheter or an operation. The usual conditions which precipitate such a crisis are either a long car drive, especially in cold weather, or following the consumption of alcohol and a journey*

*home in cold weather. In the early stages of difficulty it is imperative to empty the bladder at least every two hours, because once it overfills obstruction is likely to set in. This stage can be a sore trial to judges, clergymen, bus drivers, and others committed to being before the public for many hours, but their life can be transformed from one of acute and constant misery to one of complete comfort by the fitting of a portable, rubber urinal until such time as the gland has reached a size when only an operation will bring relief.*

**prostatectomy.** Surgical removal of the prostate gland. The operation usually results in male sterility but does not preclude sexual intercourse.

**prostatic.** Pertaining to the prostate gland.

**prostatitic.** Pertaining to prostatitis.

**prostatitis.** Inflammation of the prostate gland.

**prostatomy.** Surgical incision into a prostate gland.

**prostatorrhea.** A urethral discharge of catarrhal character from the prostate gland.

**prostatorrhoea.** See PROSTATORRHEA.

**prostatovesiculectomy.** Surgical excision of the prostate gland and the seminal vesicles.

**prostatovesiculitis.** Combined inflammation of the prostate gland and the seminal vesicles.

**prosthesis.** An artificial substitute for a part that has been removed surgically or is missing; for instance, a denture or artificial limb.

**prosthetics.** The branch of surgery which deals with prostheses.

**prostrate.** 1. Exhausted. 2. Lying at full length.

**prostration.** Great exhaustion of nervous or muscular energy.

**nervous prostration.** A form of neurasthenia.

**protal.** Congenital.

**protean.** 1. Any disease or eruption which takes on many forms or shapes. 2. An insoluble derivative of protein, being the first product due to the action of water or enzymes.

*Derived from Proteus, a Sea God who assumed different shapes when captured.*

**protein.** One of a group of complex nitrogenous substances of high molecular weight, which are found in various forms in animals and plants and are characteristic of living matter. On hydrolysis, they yield amino acids. The sources of protein in the human diet are numerous but largely derived from the flesh of mammals, birds, and fish. It is the constituent of the diet which largely replaces the wastage of body tissue in the human being. The other

ingredients derived from the diet are carbohydrates, fat, salts, chemicals, water, and vitamins.

**proteinaemia.** See PROTEINEMIA.

**proteinase.** A protein splitting enzyme.

**proteinemia.** An abnormal amount of protein in the blood.

**protein fever.** Artificial fever produced by the injection of foreign proteins.

**proteinic.** Pertaining to protein.

**proteinuria.** The presence of protein in the urine.

**proteoclastic.** The splitting up of proteins.

**proteolysis.** The conversion of proteins into simpler substances by the action of enzymes.

**proteolytic.** Pertaining to proteolysis.

**Proteus.** A genus of microorganisms belonging to the family *Enterobacteriaceae.* Members of this group have been associated with such diseases as pleurisy, peritonitis, cystitis, and abscesses, and one species has been isolated in cases of summer diarrhea in infants. See also PROTEAN.

**prothrombin.** A substance in blood plasma essential for the clotting of blood. In the presence of thromboplastin and calcium, prothrombin is converted to thrombin, which, in turn, converts fibrinogen into fibrin, which then contracts to form a clot.

**protodiastole.** The first part of the diastole of the ventricles of the heart, during which the pressure in the ventricles and aorta is falling rapidly.

**protopathic.** Descriptive of the cruder and more primitively developed sensations such as heavy pressure on the skin and pain. The finer sensations, such as light touch, are described as epicritic.

**protoplasm.** The viscid material contained within a living cell, upon which all the vital functions of life depend.

**protopsis.** Protrusion of the eyeball.

**Protozoa.** The lowest phylum of animal life, which consists of unicellular organisms that have neither a nervous system nor a circulatory system. Some are pathological to man and produce such diseases as amebic dysentery, Leishmaniasis, kala-azar, oriental sore, malaria, American trypanosomiasis, and East African sleeping sickness.

**proud flesh.** A colloquial term for the excessive production of granulation tissue in a wound.

**proximad.** Towards the proximal or nearest end.

**proximal, proximate.** Nearest.

**prurigo.** A group of itching, papular eruptions of the skin. Many experts consider the itching to be the primary

140

feature and the papules to be a reaction of the skin to scratching. Others believe the papules themselves are the essential feature and cause the itching. Prurigo, like other itching infections, is often complicated by secondary infection with germs and with the production of an eczematous condition produced by scratching.

**besnier's prurigo.** A condition characterized by intense, paroxysmal itching, often worse at night and showing seasonal variations and very resistant to treatment. There are often associated disorders, such as asthma, hay fever, migraine, or urticaria. There is a clear relationship between this condition and emotional states. The eruption particularly affects the folds of the knees and elbows, the face and the neck, with thickening, pigmentation, roughening of the skin, and papules. It usually begins in childhood. The subject is often highly strung and sensitive and may have a dry skin. It is probably an inherited defect. With careful management some improvement may be expected to occur and there is often a change for the better at puberty, but the tendency to relapse is apt to persist throughout life and the condition is prone to show itself under any emotional stress.

**common prurigo.** See LICHEN: LICHEN SIMPLEX.

**prurigo nodularis.** A rare chronic skin disease occurring chiefly in women and characterized by itching, the presence of nodules, and wartlike lesions in the skin. It is regarded as an atypical nodular form of lichen simplex.

**pruritus.** Itching.

**pruritus ani.** Extreme itching around the anus. Although popularly believed to be due to piles, it seldom is, the condition always being associated with anxiety and nervous and emotional instability. It frequently arises during periods of nervous tension. Treatment is not of the itchy area around the anus but of the anxiety state which it reflects.

**pruritus vulvae.** Intense itching about the vulva. It may also be associated with emotional stress and worry or be precipitated by vaginal discharges, such as leukorrhea.

**pseudaesthesia.** See PSEUDESTHESIA.

**pseudarthritis.** An hysterical disorder of a joint, simulating arthritis.

**pseudarthrosis.** A false joint.

**pseudesthesia.** An imaginary sensation for which there is no activating cause, for instance, pain felt in a limb that has been amputated.

**pseudoangina.** A condition arising in neurotic individuals, who complain of the symptoms associated with heart pain but have, in fact, no heart disease.

**pseudobulbar.** A term usually applied to a form of paralysis which appears to result from a lesion in the bulb of the brain but does not in fact do so.

**pseudocoxalgia.** See PERTHES' DISEASE.

**pseudocroup.** Also called *false croup.* See LARYNGISMUS: LARYNGISMUS STRIDULUS.

**pseudocyesis.** An hysterical manifestation in which a woman shows all the superficial signs and symptoms of pregnancy but is not, in fact, pregnant. Also called *false pregnancy.*

**pseudodiphtheria.** An inflammatory condition, producing a false membrane on the surface of the throat lining, but not caused by the germ of diphtheria and thus not producing the diphtheria toxin that has such a malignant effect on man. Also called *diphtheroid.*

**pseudoedema.** A condition resembling edema.

**pseudogeusia.** Hallucinations of taste.

**pseudohermaphroditism.** A condition in which secondary sexual characters, body appearance, and often emotional outlook are largely of one sexual type, while the essential sex organs are of the opposite sex.

**pseudohernia.** An inflamed hernial sac resembling a strangulated hernia.

**pseudohypertrophy.** Apparent increase in the size of an organ not due to enlargement of essential functional tissue. For instance, apparent enlargement of a muscle due to deposits of fat within it. Also called *false hypertrophy.*

**pseudo-icterus.** False jaundice.

**pseudoleukaemia.** See PSEUDOLEUKEMIA.

**pseudoleukemia.** A term formerly applied to blood disorders other than leukemia.

**pseudomelanosis.** The dark staining of the body tissues with blood pigments after death.

**pseudomembrane.** A false membrane.

**pseudomeningitis.** See MENINGISM.

**pseudomenstruation.** A bleeding from the womb which is not a true menstrual period.

**pseudomnesia.** A perversion of memory in which the patient seems to remember things that never occurred.

**pseudomucin.** A type of mucin seen in ovarian cysts.

**pseudomyxoma.** A skin tumor containing much mucus, but so interspersed with tissue that, superficially, it suggests a myxoma tumor.

**pseudomyxoma peritonei.** Widespread implantation, into the peritoneal membrane of the abdominal cavity, of growths that have spread from malignant disease of the ovary; the presence in the peritoneal cavity of mucus from a ruptured mucous cyst of the appendix.

**pseudoneoplasm.** A phantom tumor. See PHANTOM TUMOR.

**pseudoneuroma.** A false neuroma.

**pseudo-oedema.** See PSEUDOEDEMA.

**pseudoparalysis.** Apparent paralysis or loss of muscular power without true paralysis, marked by defective coordination of movements or repression of movements due to pain.

**pseudoparesis.** An hysterical or other condition simulating paresis.

**pseudophthisis.** A wasting disease arising from causes other than tuberculosis.

**pseudoplegia.** Hysterical paralysis.

**pseudopregnancy.** False pregnancy. See PSEUDOCYESIS.

**pseudoptosis.** Narrowing of the opening of the eyelids.

**pseudosclerosis.** A condition similar in symptoms to multiple sclerosis of the nervous system. A familial degenerative disease, poorly defined but characterized by the gradual onset of tremors, rigidity, and mental deterioration. A greenish ring at the outer edge of the cornea is considered diagnostic. It is closely allied to progressive lenticular degeneration.

**pseudosmallpox.** See ALASTRIM.

**pseudosmia.** Delusions of the sense of smell.

**pseudotumor.** A phantom tumor. See PHANTOM TUMOR.

**pseudotumour.** See PSEUDOTUMOR.

**psilosis.** 1. A falling out of the hair. 2. Sprue.

**psilosis pigmentosa.** See PELLAGRA.

**psittacosis.** A virus disease of birds, especially parrots, transmissible to man, in whom it runs a course resembling severe typhoid fever without abdominal symptoms, but with lung disturbances resembling pneumonia. Also called *ornithosis, parrot disease, parrot fever.*

**psoas abscess.** A cold abscess caused by tuberculous disease of the spine, which descends in the sheath of the psoas muscle in the lumbar region and erupts in the groin.

**psora.** 1. Scabies. 2. Psoriasis.

**psoriasis.** A chronic inflammatory skin disease of unknown cause, characterized by the development of reddish patches covered with silvery-white scales, affecting especially the extensor surfaces of the body and the scalp, though no region is excluded. It is not contagious or infectious. Existing attacks can be cleared by ultraviolet light treatment or by ointments and lotions, but there is no completely curative treatment. Women with psoriasis usually lose it completely during a pregnancy but, as a rule, it subsequently reappears. The main problem is a cosmetic one, especially in women, as the condition is unsightly and a great embarrassment.

**psoriatic.** Pertaining to psoriasis.

**psorous.** Affected with psora or the itch.

**psyche.** The mind.

**psychiatric.** Pertaining to psychiatry.

**psychiatric compensation.** A psychic phenomenon in which strong feelings of guilt or inferiority prompt an excessive defensive reaction. A typical example is the little man, extremely aware of his small stature, who shouts at the top of his voice as though fearful of not being recognized.

**psychiatrics.** Psychiatry.

**psychiatrist.** A physician skilled in psychiatry.

**psychiatry.** The science of diagnosis, treatment, and prevention of mental diseases and disorders.

**psychic, psychical.** Pertaining to the mind.

**psychoanalysis.** The method developed by Sigmund Freud for the exploration of patterns in emotional thinking and development used in the treatment of emotional disorders, particularly neuroses. It relies essentially upon inducing the patient to discover valuable information of which he was formerly unaware, and by bringing to the conscious state ideas and experiences from the unconscious part of the mind. The term also applies to the investigation by the psychoanalytical method which reveals the conflicts between infantile instincts and striving, and parental or social demands, and the manner in which this conflict affects emotional growth, character development, and the formation of mental and emotional disorders.

**psychoanalyst.** A specialist in the practice of psychoanalysis.

**psychoasthenia.** Feeble-mindedness.

**psychocortical.** Pertaining to the cortex of the brain as the seat of the mind.

**psychogenesis.** The development of mental characteristics.

**psychogenia.** Disease due to faulty psychic activity.

**psychogenic.** Psychic.

**psychognosis.** The study of the patient's mind while he is under hypnosis.

**psychology.** The study of mental processes, especially as they are shown in behavior.

**psychometer.** An apparatus used in psychometry.

**psychometry.** The measurement of the time taken to perform mental processes.

**psychomotor.** Pertaining to voluntary movement.

**psychoneuroses.** A large group of clinical disorders, all of a functional, nonorganic, basis, which result in only partial disorganization of the psyche. Psychoeuroses may be characterized by such symptoms as emotional states of anxiety and fear, lack of emotion, preoccupation, obsession, and psychosomatic tension in different body systems. The difference between psychoneurosis and psychosis is that in psychoneurosis the patient is aware of the symptoms as such and more or less capable of dealing with reality in a socially acceptable way, whereas in a psychosis he is not. See also PSYCHOSIS.

**psychoparesis.** Feeble-mindedness.

**psychopath.** One who suffers from a psychopathic illness.

**psychopathia.** See PSYCHOPATHY.

**psychopathic.** Pertaining to disease of the mind.

**psychopathology.** The pathology of psychoneuroses and psychoses.

**psychopathy.** Any mental disorder.

**psychoplegia.** Mental weakness of sudden onset.

**psychoplegic.** Pertaining to psychoplegia; any drug which lessens the excitability of the brain.

**psychosis.** A disease of the mind, especially one without organic disease. The term is generally applied to the more severe forms of mental derangement in which the patient is not aware of his condition as such and is incapable of dealing with reality in a socially acceptable way.

**affective psychosis.** A manic-depressive psychosis. There are two types: the manic type is characterized by increased motor activity, and the depressive type by melancholia.

**alcoholic psychosis.** A psychosis caused by alcoholism; chronic alcoholic delirium.

**arteriosclerotic psychosis.** A mental disturbance in which arteriosclerosis is the exciting cause.

**climacteric psychosis.** A mental disorder associated with the climacteric.

**degenerative psychosis.** A psychosis in which the patient becomes infantile in behavior.

**famine psychosis.** A psychosis seen in war-torn countries when starvation is severe and widespread.

**gestational psychosis.** A psychosis arising during pregnancy.

**involutional psychosis.** A psychosis due to senility.

**manic-depressive psychosis.** See AFFECTIVE PSYCHOSIS, above.

**menopausal psychosis.** See CLIMACTERIC PSYCHOSIS, above.

**organic psychosis.** A psychosis associated with definite disease, such as brain tumor, paralysis, pellagra, and brain injury.

**postinfection psychosis.** A mental disturbance following a severe acute disease such as pneumonia or typhoid fever.

**puerperal psychosis.** A psychosis following childbirth.

**reactive psychosis.** A psychosis precipitated by an environmental condition or intolerable situation.

**senile psychosis.** A psychosis occurring in old age.

**toxic psychosis.** A psychic disorder caused by poisons or poisonous agents, such as opium or alcohol.

**psychosomatic.** A body-mind relationship in which bodily symptoms are produced by an emotional, psychic, or mental reaction. An example is the shy person who gets an attack of nervous diarrhea which provides the excuse for not attending a social function.

**psychotherapeutic.** Relating to psychotherapy.

**psychotherapy.** The treatment of disease by suggestion; the treatment of mental diseases.

**psychotic.** Pertaining to psychosis.

**psychro-algia.** A painful feeling of cold.

**psychrotherapy.** Treatment of disease by the application of cold.

**ptarmic.** Pertaining to or inducing sneezing.

**ptarmus.** Spasmodic sneezing.

**pterion.** The junction of the frontal, parietal, temporal, and sphenoid bones of the skull.

**pterygium.** 1. Anything wing-shaped. 2. A triangular patch of mucous membrane growing on the conjunctiva, usually starting on the side nearest the nose with the apex towards the pupil.

**pterygium unguis.** The fold of skin which furnishes the base of the nail plate of the fingers and toes. It advances over the nail plate in varying degrees.

**pterygoid.** Wing-shaped.

**ptilosis.** Loss of the eyelashes.

**ptomaines.** Poisons produced by bacterial decomposition of proteins.

**ptosis.** Prolapse, abnormal depression, or the falling down of an organ, especially drooping of the upper eyelid due to paralysis of the levator palpebrae superioris muscle in the eyelid.

**ptyalogogue.** A medicine which produces an increased flow of saliva. Also called *sialogogue*.

**ptyalin.** A substance contained in saliva, which converts starch into maltose and dextrose.

**ptyalism.** Excessive salivation.

**ptyalocele.** A cyst containing saliva.

**ptyalorrhea.** Excessive flow of saliva.

**ptyalorrhoea.** See PTYALORRHEA.

**puberal.** Relating to puberty.

**pubertas praecox.** Puberty coming on at an earlier age than usual; precocious development.

**puberty.** The period at which the sex organs become functional. This is shown in the male by the voice breaking, the appearance of facial hair, and other changes, and in the female by the appearance of menstruation.

**pubes.** That region of the abdomen immediately above the external genitals; the hair covering the pubic region; the pubic bones.

**pubescence. 1.** The presence of fine, soft hair. **2.** Puberty; the coming on of puberty.

**pubic.** Relating to the pubes.

**pubic bone.** The os pubis, one of two bones forming the front of the pelvis.

**pubiotomy.** Surgical division of the pubic bone to allow enlargement of the birth canal during difficult labor. It is now seldom performed.

**pubis.** See PUBIC BONE.

**pubofemoral.** Relating to the pubic bone and the femur.

**pubovesical.** Relating to the pubic bone and the bladder.

**pudenda.** Plural of pudendum.

**pudendagra.** Pain in the sexual organs, especially of the female.

**pudendagra pruriens.** See PRURITUS VULVAE.

**pudendal.** Pertaining to the pudendum.

**pudendum.** The external sex organs, especially of the female.

**pudic.** Relating to the pudenda.

**puerile.** Relating to childhood.

**puerpera.** A woman recently delivered of a child.

**puerperal.** Pertaining to childbirth.

**puerperal eclampsia.** Convulsions or fits occurring in and related to pregnancy.

**puerperal fever.** An acute febrile disease of women caused by a germ infection during childbirth. The term milk fever arose because the onset of fever coincided with engorgement of the breasts with milk and the two conditions were associated. There is, in fact, no connection between breast engorgement and puerperal fever. Also called *childbed fever, milk fever.*

**puerperal insanity.** A form of mental derangement following childbirth. It usually occurs in either middle-aged women or those of an unstable disposition. Complete recovery is invariably the rule.

**puerperant.** A woman in the puerperium.

**puerperium.** The condition of being recently delivered of a child; the period of confinement after childbirth.

**puffiness.** Swelling of tissues.

**puking.** Vomiting. It commonly occurs in babies, who throw up some of their milk feed. As long as the child maintains a normal progressive increase in weight, it is of no significance and requires no treatment, apart from insuring that the child does not feed too quickly or swallow air to excess.

**pulex.** A flea.

**pulicide.** Any agent that destroys fleas.

**pulmo.** A lung.

**pulmoaortic.** Pertaining to the lungs and the aorta.

**pulmolith.** A stone in the lung, formed by the lung, and not one that has been inhaled.

**pulmometer.** An instrument for measuring the volume of the lungs. Also called *spirometer.*

**pulmometry.** Estimation of the volume of the lungs.

**pulmonary.** Pertaining to the lungs.

**pulmonectomy.** See PNEUMONECTOMY.

**pulmonic.** Pertaining to the lungs; pulmonary; relating to the pulmonary artery.

**pulmonitis.** An infrequently used term for pneumonia.

**pulp.** The soft interior of an organ.

**dental pulp.** The soft tissue filling the pulp chamber of a tooth and responsible for its vitality. It consists of connective tissue, blood vessels, and nerves.

**digital pulp.** The sensitive, elastic prominence on the end of the finger or toe.

**enamel pulp.** The jellylike cells between the outer and inner enamel layers of the enamel organ of a tooth.

**intervertebral pulp.** The soft substance in the center of the cartilaginous discs between each pair of spinal vertebrae.

**splenic pulp.** The proper substance of the spleen.

**pulpitis.** Inflammation of the dental pulp.

**pulpy.** Pulplike.

**pulsate.** To beat or throb.

**pulsatile.** Pulsating or throbbing.

**pulsation.** Pulsating, throbbing, or beating.

**pulse.** The throb in an artery due to an increase in the tension of its walls following a heartbeat. The pulse is usually counted on the thumb side of the wrist, but may be taken over any artery that can be felt. The normal pulse is regular, even, and occurs some 70 to 80 times a minute, but is increased during excitement, physical activity, and as a sequel to a rising temperature. It is unusually slow in some athletes, where physical activity is a normal phenomenon.

**alternating pulse.** A pulse in which there are alternations in volume of the pulse waves, so that large pulsations alternate with small ones in cycles of equal length; a sign of heart failure.

**anacrotic pulse.** A pulse with a notch in the ascending limb, which is both palpable and seen on sphygmograms, especially in aortic stenosis.

**anatricrotic pulse.** A pulse wave with three breaks on the ascending curve of a tracing of pulse beats.

**angry pulse.** A small, rapid, tense pulse, which feels like a cord; observed in cases of acute peritonitis.

**ardent pulse.** A pulse with a quick, full wave which seems to strike the finger at a single point.

**bigeminal pulse.** A pulse in which the beats occur in pairs so that the longer pause follows every two beats.

**capillary pulse.** A pulsation which can be seen in the skin capillaries under the fingernail or on the forehead. It is common in aortic regurgitation (backflow of blood into the heart).

**collapsing pulse.** The pulse observed in aortic regurgitation, characterized by a rigid rise and fall.

**contracted pulse.** A small pulse with high tension.

**Corrigan's pulse.** A collapsing pulse.

**decurtate pulse.** A progressively decreasing pulse.

**dicrotic pulse.** A pulse in which the recoil wave is exaggerated. It is seen when the arterial tension is low and gives to the finger the impression of a double beat.

**entoptic pulse.** A condition sometimes noticed after violent exercise in which, with every beat of the heart, the vision darkens. It is due to mechanical irritation of the retinal rods by the pulsating retinal arteries. The victim often describes this sensation as threatened blackouts.

**febrile pulse.** The pulse characteristic of fever. It is full, soft, and frequent, and exhibits a well-marked dicrotism.

**filiform pulse.** A small, thready, almost imperceptible pulse.

**formicant pulse.** A small, feeble pulse, likened to the movement of ants.

**frequent pulse.** A pulse recurring at short intervals.

**full pulse.** A pulse in which the artery contains a large volume of blood and feels distended.

**funic pulse.** The arterial pulse felt in the umbilical cord.

**goat-leap pulse.** A pulse marked by a weak pulsation followed by a strong one.

**guttural pulse.** A pulse felt in the throat.

**hard pulse.** A pulse characterized by high tension and rigidity.

**high-tension pulse.** The pulse felt in hardened arteries with consequent raised blood pressure. It is gradual in impulse, long in duration, and slow in subsiding, and the artery feels like a firm round cord between the beats.

**hyperdicrotic pulse.** A pulse in which the dicrotic wave is abnormally palpable.

**incisura pulse.** A pulse showing a sharp fall in pulse pressure.

**infrequent pulse.** A pulse with a slower than normal rate.

**intermittent pulse.** A pulse in which one or more beats are dropped or missing.

**intricate pulse.** An irregular, small, and infrequent pulse.

**irregular pulse.** A pulse in which the beats occur at irregular intervals or in which the force, or rhythm and force, varies.

**jerky pulse.** A pulse in which the artery is suddenly and markedly distended as occurs in aortic regurgitation.

**jugular pulse.** Pulsation of the jugular veins in the neck.

**low-tension pulse.** A pulse that is sudden in its onset, short, and quick to decline. It is easily obliterated by pressure.

**monocrotic pulse.** A pulse in which dicrotism is entirely absent.

**paradoxical pulse.** A pulse that is weaker during inspiration; a condition sometimes observed in cardiac compression.

**pistol-shot pulse.** The pulse produced by rapid distension and collapse of an artery, as occurs classically in aortic regurgitation. It produces a sound resembling a pistol shot when heard through a stethoscope.

**plateau pulse.** The prolonged pulse seen in aortic stenosis.

**quadrigeminal pulse.** A pulse in which there is a pause after every fourth beat.

**quick pulse.** A pulse that strikes the finger rapidly but leaves it just as rapidly.

**Quincke's pulse.** See CAPILLARY PULSE, above.

**respiratory pulse.** The modification in the pulse during respiration.

**running pulse.** A very weak, frequent pulse, with no tension in the arteries, one pulse wave running into the next with no apparent intervals.

**soft pulse.** A pulse that is readily compressed.

**supradicrotic pulse.** A pulse in which the preceding dicrotic wave falls on the ascending limb of the next pulse wave.

**thready pulse.** A scarcely perceptible pulse.

**tricotic pulse.** A pulse in which the three waves normally present are abnormally distinct.

**trigeminal pulse.** A pulse in which a pause occurs after every third beat.

**vagus pulse.** A slow pulse due to the inhibitory action of the vagus nerve on the heart.

**venous pulse.** A pulse observed in a vein.

**water-hammer pulse.** See COLLAPSING PULSE, above.

**wiry pulse.** A small, rapid, tense pulse which feels like a cord, sometimes observed in acute peritonitis.

**pulsimeter.** An instrument used for measuring the force or rate of the pulse.

**pulsus.** The pulse.

**pultaceous.** Pulpy or mushy.

**pulverulent.** Resembling powder.

**pulvis.** A powder.

**pump.** An apparatus for drawing up a liquid or gas.

**breast pump.** A pump used to remove milk from the breast.

**dental pump.** A pump used to remove saliva during dental procedures.

**stomach pump.** A pump for removing the contents of, or washing out, the stomach.

**punctate.** Having numerous dots or punctures.

**punctum.** A point or small aperture.

**P.U.O.** Abbreviation for "pyrexia of unknown origin." It indicates that the patient has a temperature from a cause not yet determined.

**pupil.** The opening in the iris of the eye to allow the passage of light. It generally opens or narrows according to the intensity of the light, but drugs, emotions, and other factors may affect the size of the opening.

**pupillary.** Relating to the pupil.

**purgation.** Bowel evacuation produced by the administration of purgatives.

**purgative.** A purge.

**purge.** To cause the evacuation of the bowels; an agent that produces an evacuation of the bowels.

**puriform.** Resembling pus.

**purpura.** A condition in which hemorrhages occur in the skin, mucous membranes, serous membranes, and elsewhere, either without definite cause, or due to slight injury, to a blood disorder or disease. The hemorrhages may be of pinpoint size or quite large patches and often the presenting symptom is the patient's complaint of bruising easily.

**hemorrhagic purpura.** See IDIOPATHIC THROMBOCYTOPENIC PURPURA, below.

**idiopathic thrombocytopenic purpura.** A systemic disease characterized by multiple hemorrhages into the skin or from mucous membranes. The blood has a reduced number of platelets, a prolonged bleeding time, but a normal coagulation time. The condition is controlled by blood transfusions and cortisone, and in some cases by removal of the spleen. Also called *essential thrombocytopenia, land scurvy, morbus maculosus hemorrhagicus of Werlhof, Werlhof's disease.*

**non-thrombocytopenic purpura.** A mixture of types of purpura, characterized by the presence of purpura, colic, vomiting, and diarrhea, and sometimes accompanied by urticaria, edema, and swollen joints. This group includes purpura simplex, rheumatic purpura, and Schonlein's purpura. The cause may be a germ poison or sensitization to foods, in which case the disease is cured by removing the offending item from the diet. Also called *Henoch-Schoenlein syndrome, Henoch's purpura, anaphylactoid purpura, hemorrhagic capillary toxicosis.*

**symptomatic purpura.** This type may accompany acute infectious of chronic diseases, such as malignant tumors, inflammation of the kidneys, and blood disorders, and may follow the administration of certain drugs. Also called *secondary purpura.*

**purpuric.** Pertaining to purpura.

**purulence, purulency.** The state of suppuration.

**purulent.** Pertaining to pus.

**puruloid.** Resembling pus.

**pus.** The liquid product of inflammation. It contains huge numbers of white blood cells which have ingested bacteria and died in the process.

*Pus formation is one of the body's protective mechanisms, and the first surgical principle is that when pus is present it must be drained from the body. Before there was any knowledge of antiseptics, of asepsis, or of germs, most wounds became infected and pus formation was looked upon with approval as an indication that the wound was following a normal course, and it was even referred to as "laudable pus."*

**pustula maligna.** Malignant pustules. See also ANTHRAX.

**pustular.** Characterized by the formation of pustules.

**pustulation.** A blisterlike swelling on the skin containing pus.

**pustule.** A small pus-containing elevation or blister on the skin.

**pustulent.** To produce pustules.

**pustulocrustaceous.** Marked by the formation of pustules and scabs.

**putrefaction.** Decomposition.

**putrefactive.** Pertaining to putrefaction.

**putrefy.** To decompose or become putrid.

**putrescence.** The condition of putrefaction.

**putrescent.** To rot or become putrid.

**putrid.** Rotten.

**putrid fever.** See TYPHUS FEVER.

**pyaemia.** See PYEMIA.

**pyarthrosis.** Suppuration within a joint.

**pycnocardia.** See PYKNOCARDIA.

**pycnolepsy.** See PYKNOLEPSY.

**pycnophrasis.** See PYKNOPHRASIS.

**pycnosis.** See PYKNOSIS.

**pycnotic.** See PYKNOTIC.

**pyelectasis.** Dilation of the pelvis of the kidney.

**pyelic.** Pertaining to the pelvis of the kidney.

**pyelitic.** Pertaining to pyelitis.

**pyelitis.** Inflammation of the pelvis of the kidney.

**pyelocystitis.** Inflammation of the pelvis of the kidney and of the urinary bladder.

**pyelography.** X-ray examination of the kidney and ureter after they have been filled with a substance opaque to x-rays.

**intravenous pyelography.** A method of pyelography in which the substance is injected into a vein and excreted by the kidney.

**retrograde pyelography.** A method of pyelography in which the opaque medium is introduced into the ureter via the urinary bladder. Also called *ascending pyelography.*

**pyelolithotomy.** Surgical removal of a stone from the kidney pelvis.

**pyelonephritis.** Inflammation of both the pelvis and the substance of the kidney.

**pyelonephrosis.** Any disease of the kidney and its pelvis.

**pyelopathy.** Any disease of the pelvis of the kidney.

**pyelotomy.** Surgical incision into the pelvis of the kidney.

**pyemia.** A disease due to the presence of pus-forming germs in the blood and the formation of abscesses wherever these organisms lodge.

**pyemic abscess.** An abscess caused by pus-producing organisms in the blood.

**pyesis.** Suppuration.

**pyknic.** Of short, stocky build.

**pyknocardia.** See TACHYCARDIA.

**pyknolepsy.** A very mild form of petit mal epilepsy. It appears as a fleeting mental blankness, associated with a momentary stare and a fleeting arrest of movement. There are no seizures or fits, no falls, and no convulsions nor loss of consciousness.

**pyknophrasia.** Thickness of speech.

**pyknosis.** 1. Thickness or inspissation.
2. A degenerative change in body cells, whereby the nuclei of the cells are condensed and shrink to dense, structureless masses.

**pyknotic.** Relating to pyknosis.

**pylephlebitis.** Inflammation of the portal vein. It is usually secondary to disease of the intestine, generally suppurative in character, and gives rise to the symptoms of pyemia.

**pylethrombophlebitis.** Inflammation and thrombosis of the portal vein.

**pylethrombosis.** Thrombosis of the portal vein.

**pylic.** Pertaining to the portal vein.

**pylorectomy.** Surgical removal of the pylorus.

**pyloric.** Pertaining to the pylorus.

**pyloric stenosis.** An obstruction of the pylorus occurring in babies. It causes profuse vomiting and unless relieved the child goes steadily downhill, since it can take neither fluid nor food. The condition is cured by Ramstedt's operation.

**pyloroplasty.** Plastic surgical repair of the pylorus.

**pyloroscopy.** Examination of the pylorus.

**pylorospasm.** Spasm of the pylorus.

**pylorostenosis.** Stricture of the pylorus.

**pylorostomy.** Formation of an opening through the abdominal wall into the pyloric end of the stomach.

**pylorotomy.** Surgical incision into the pylorus.

**pylorus.** The opening of the stomach into the duodenum. It is marked by a thickening of the circular muscular coat of the intestine in this region, forming a valve.

**pyocolpocele.** A pus-containing swelling of the vagina.

**pyocolpos.** The presence of pus in the vagina.

**pyocyst.** Any cyst containing pus.

**pyodermatitis.** Any inflammation of the skin which is accompanied with pus or pustule formation.

**pyodermatosis.** Any pus-producing skin affection.

**pyogenesis.** Pus formation.

**pyogenic.** Producing pus.

**pyogenic microorganism.** Any microorganism which produces pus.

**pyohaemia.** See PYOHEMIA.

**pyohaemothorax.** See PYOHEMOTHORAX.

**pyohemia.** See PYEMIA.

**pyohemothorax.** The presence of blood and pus in the chest cavity.

**pyoid.** Resembling pus.

**pyometra, pyometrium.** The presence of pus in the womb.

**pyonephritis.** Inflammation of the kidney accompanied by the formation of pus.

**pyonephrolithiasis.** The presence of pus and stones in the kidney.

**pyonephrosis.** A collection of pus in the pelvis of the kidney.

**pyonephrotic.** Characterized by pyonephrosis.

**pyo-ovarium.** An abscess in the ovary.

**pyopericarditis.** Inflammation of the pericardium accompanied by pus formation.

**pyopericardium.** An accumulation of pus in the pericardium.

**pyoperitoneum.** A collection of pus in the peritoneal cavity of the abdomen.

**pyophthalmia.** Suppuration and inflammation of the eye.

**pyopneumopericarditis.** Inflammation of the pericardium accompanied by pus and gas collection in the pericardium.

**pyopneumoperitoneum.** An accumulation of pus and air in the peritoneal cavity of the abdomen.

**pyopneumoperitonitis.** Peritonitis accompanied by pus and air in the peritoneal cavity of the abdomen.

**pyopneumothorax.** A collection of air and pus or gas and pus in the chest cavity.

**pyopoiesis.** Suppuration.

**pyorrhea.** A discharge of pus. Commonly applied to inflammation of the gums accompanied by necrosis of tooth sockets. It is progressive and frequently necessitates removal of all the teeth.

**pyorrheal.** Relating to pyorrhea.

**pyorrhoea.** See PYORRHEA.

**pyorrhoeal.** See PYORRHEAL.

**pyosalpingitis.** Inflammation and pus formation in the Fallopian tube.

**pyosalpinx.** The presence of pus in the Fallopian tube.

**pyosapraemia.** See PYOSAPREMIA.

**pyosapremia.** A suppurative infection of the blood.

**pyosclerosis.** Suppurative sclerosis.

**pyosepticaemia.** See PYOSEPTICEMIA.

**pyosepticemia.** The presence of both pyemia and septicemia.

**pyostatic.** Anything which prevents the formation of pus.

**pyothorax.** A collection of pus in the chest cavity.

**pyretic.** Relating to fever.

**pyretotyphrosis.** Fever delirium.

**pyretotyposis.** Fever of intermittent character.

**pyrexia.** The rise of the body temperature above the normal level of about 98.6° F. See FEVER.

**pyrexial.** Relating to pyrexia.

**pyriform.** Pear-shaped.

**pyrogen.** Any fever-producing agent.

**pyrogenic.** Producing fever.

**pyromania.** A mad, recurring impulse to set fire to objects and buildings.

**pyrometer.** An instrument for measuring intensities of heat beyond the range of an ordinary thermometer.

**pyrophobia.** A neurotic fear of fire.

**pyrosis.** Heartburn.

**pyuria.** The presence of pus in the urine.

# Q-R

**Q fever.** See QUEENSLAND FEVER.

**quadripara.** A women who has borne her fourth child or is in her fourth confinement. Also called *quartipara.*

**quadriparous.** Having had four children. Also called *quartiparous.*

**quadripartite.** Divided into four parts.

**quadriplegia.** Paralysis of all four limbs.

**quadroon.** The child of one white and one mulatto parent.

**quadruplet.** Any one of four children born of one pregnancy.

**quarantine.** The segregation of people or animals that have been exposed to communicable disease, for a time equal to the longest usual incubation period of the disease to which they have been exposed; the place where such persons or animals are detained; the act of detaining ships, travelers, or aircraft that have arrived from suspected or infected places; places authorized to carry out inspection or disinfection.

**quartan.** 1. Recurring on the fourth day. 2. Intermittent malaria in which the paroxysm occurs about every 72 hours.

**double quartan.** Intermittent malaria in which there are two concurrent cycles of fever, not synchronous with each other, ordinarily resulting in fever on two successive days.

**triple quartan.** Intermittent malaria in which there are three concurrent cycles of fever, not synchronous with each other, ordinarily resulting in fever every day.

**quarter evil.** See ANTHRAX.

**quartipara.** See QUADRIPARA.

**quartiparous.** See QUADRIPAROUS.

**Queensland fever.** An acute infection caused by the germ *Coxiella burnettii,* and characterized by pneumonia, high temperature, nausea, and vomiting. It is of short duration and there is, almost invariably, recovery. Also called *Q fever.*

**quick.** 1. A sensitive part. 2. The flesh beneath a nail. 3. Pregnant and able to detect fetal movements.

**quickening.** The first feeling by a pregnant woman of the baby's movements within the womb. It usually occurs about the twentieth week of pregnancy and may feel to the mother like a feather brushing across the abdomen, or there may be convulsive movements as the child moves its limbs.

**quinine.** An alkaloid obtained from cinchona bark, quinine kills malaria organisms and arrests the attacks. It is used in cold and influenza remedies for its ability to reduce body temperature, is employed as a tonic in convalescence, and taken in tablet form at night, is used to ward off muscle cramps in the legs. Quinine tablets have also been used to toughen the skin of people who sunburn easily, though it is not known why it has the ability when taken in tablets to increase the skin's resistance to ultraviolet light. By far its largest use today is in the making of so-called "tonic water," and though the drug is still used for malaria it has largely been replaced by synthetic substances. An historical note on quinine is given under CINCHONA.

**quinine fever.** A disease marked by high temperature and skin rashes, occurring in people exposed to quinine during its manufacture.

**quinsy.** An abscess behind the tonsil which pushes the swollen tonsil right across the midline of the throat and makes speaking and swallowing almost impossible until the abscess bursts.

**quintan.** A fever which recurs every five days.

**quintessence.** The highest concentrated extract which can be made of any substance.

**quintipara.** A woman who has had five children or is in labor for the fifth time.

**quintuplet.** Any one of five children born of a single pregnancy.

**quotidian.** 1. Recurring each day. 2. An intermittent fever which recurs each day.

**Q wave.** The electrocardiographic wave associated with the contraction of the ventricles of the heart.

**rabid.** Affected with rabies; pertaining to rabies.

**rabies.** A fatal disease in animals caused by a virus transmitted to other animals and man by the bite of an infected animal. All animals are subject to rabies, but it occurs most frequently in the wolf, the cat, and the dog. The incubation period is from one to six months, and the virus has a special affinity for the nervous system, being found in large numbers in the saliva and other secretions. In man there are usually three stages of the disease; the first or preliminary stage is marked by restlessness, apprehension, and obvious ill health; in the second or furious stage the patient is very active and has spasms of the muscles of swallowing and breathing; the third or paralytic stage begins with drooling of saliva due to poor muscular control, and terminates fatally with a general paralysis ascending the spinal column. It is during the second stage that the sight of water or anybody drinking promotes wild tetanic spasms termed *hydrophobia.* Humans contract rabies most often through the bite of a rabid dog. Also called *hydrophobia.*

**rachialgia.** Pain in the spine.

**rachianesthesia.** Spinal anesthesia.

**rachicentesis.** See LUMBAR PUNCTURE.

**rachidial, rachidian.** Pertaining to the spinal column.

**rachiocampsis.** Spinal curvature.

**rachiochysis.** An accumulation of fluid in the spinal canal.

**rachidynia.** Pain in the spinal column.

**rachiokyphosis.** Hunchback, kyphosis.

**rachiomyelitis.** Inflammation of the spinal cord.

**rachioparalysis.** Paralysis of the spine.

**rachiopathy.** Any spinal disease.

**rachioplegia.** Paralysis of the spine.

**rachiotome.** A surgical instrument for cutting the vertebrae.

**rachiotomy.** Surgical cutting into or through the vertebral column.

**rachis.** The spinal column.

**rachischisis.** A congenital cleft in the vertebral column.

**rachitic.** Produced by or resembling rachitis.

**rachitis.** See RICKETS.

**radial.** 1. Relating to the radius bone. 2. Radiating, spreading out like a fan or the rays of the sun. 3. Pertaining to the radius of a circle.

**radiant.** 1. Emitting rays. 2. Diverging from a common center.

**radiant energy.** Energy traveling in the form of electromagnetic rays.

**radiation.** 1. The act of radiating or diverging from a central point, as of light; having the appearance of rays. 2. In neurology, any group of nerve fibers diverging after leaving their place of origin. 3. The use of x-rays or radium in the treatment of disease. Deep x-rays are gradually being replaced in treatment by the cobalt-bomb machine, which has a more effective penetration; see also RADIUM.

**radiation sickness.** A condition sometimes caused by treatment with deep x-rays or radium; characterized by nausea, vomiting, headache, cramps, and diarrhea. The term is also applied to the effects of radiation produced by nuclear explosions, characterized by loss of hair and teeth, decreasing red and white blood cells, and hemorrhages in various parts of the body. In the severe cases there is no treatment, but for individuals who have only received a slight dose of radiation, treatment consists of absolute rest and blood transfusions.

**radical.** 1. Belonging to the root, going to the root, or attacking the cause of a disease; a form of treatment especially operative treatment, which aims at the total eradication of a disease and the diseased tissues. 2. The haptophore group of an antibody.

**radicle.** 1. A little root. 2. The smallest branches of a nerve or blood vessel.

**radicotomy.** Surgical division of nerve roots.

**radicula.** A radicle.

**radicular.** Pertaining to a radicle or spinal nerve root.

**radiculectomy.** Surgical removal or the cutting of nerve roots.

**radiculitis.** Inflammation of nerve roots, usually spinal nerve roots.

**radioactive.** Possessing the properties of radioactivity.

**radioactivity.** A property of certain substances of spontaneously emitting alpha, beta, or gamma rays from the nucleus of the atom. It is a natural phenomenon in such substances as radium; or it can be artificially induced by placing a substance inside a thermonuclear pile and bombarding it with high-velocity particles, thus producing radioactive isotopes. See also ISOTOPE; TRACER.

*Radioactivity exists in measurable quantities quite naturally in the earth and rocks and is emitted by luminous paint on watch dials and by television tubes, but collectively radiation from these sources is well below what is considered a dangerous level. However, frequent x-ray examinations are now avoided because these also contribute to the total irradiation of the body. Many countries now maintain testing stations which daily record the radioactivity in the atmosphere and food, lest fallout from nuclear explosions or nuclear power stations should reach a dangerous level. In sufficient quantity the gamma rays from radioactivity causes the condition known as radiation sickness.*

**radiocarbon.** A radioactive isotope of carbon used for chronological research, and in medicine for diagnosis and treatment. Also called *carbon-14.*

**radiocarpal.** Relating to the radius and the carpus.

**radiodermatitis.** The skin reaction produced by exposure to deep x-rays.

**radiodiagnosis.** Diagnosis by means of radiography.

**radiodigital.** Relating to the radius and the fingers.

**radioelement.** Any element possessing radioactive powers.

**radiogenic.** Produced by radioactive rays.

**radiograph.** An x-ray photograph; to take such photographs.

**radiographer.** One trained in taking x-ray photographs.

**radiography.** Photography with x-rays.

**radiohumeral.** Relating to the radius and the humerus.

**radioisotope.** An isotope which is radioactive and produced artificially from the element in question, as carbon-14.

**radiologist.** One trained in radiology.

**radiological.** Relating to radiology.

**radiology.** The study of x-ray photography; the treatment of disease with radiant substances; the science of radiant energy.

**radionecrosis.** The destruction of tissues caused by exposure to radium or x-rays.

**radiopaque.** Any substance which stops the passage of x-rays. See also CONTRAST MEDIA.

**radiophosphorus.** Phosphorus that has been made radioactive by being placed inside a cyclotron. It is used in the treatment of blood disorders.

**radioresistant.** A tissue or tumor which is not affected by being irradiated by x-rays or radium.

**radiostereoscopy.** Examination of the internal structure of the body by means of x-rays.

**radiosurgery.** Originally the term meant the surgical use of radium, but it is now also applied to many forms of irradiation.

**radiotherapeutic.** Pertaining to radiotherapy.

**radiotherapeutist.** One skilled in radiotherapy.

**radiotherapy.** The treatment of disease by x-rays, radium rays, and other radiant substances.

**radiothorium.** Radioactive thorium. It gives off thorium X, which is used in the treatment of some superficial skin disorders.

**radio-ulnar.** Relating to the radius and the ulna, the two bones in the forearm. The radius is on the outer, or thumb side, and the ulna on the inner, or little finger side.

**radium.** A highly radioactive metal element discovered in 1898 by Pierre and Marie Curie, who separated it from pitchblende. The chloride and bromide salts of radium are usually used in treatment. They continuously emit heat, light, and three distinct kinds of radiation: *gamma* rays, which are similar to x-rays, *alpha* rays, and *beta* rays. Radium is used either in platinum needles or platinum plaques (small, flat containers) which are placed either into or over a tumor to destroy it. Radium also gives off radon and has a half-life of 1600 years.

**radius.** 1. A ray. 2. The bone on the thumb side of the forearm.

**radix.** A root; any of the spinal nerve roots.

**radon.** A decay product of radium. It is a colorless, gaseous, radioactive element.

**radon seed.** A small glass capillary tube containing radon, which is placed inside a small gold or platinum tube for implantation into tissues or tumors in order to destroy them.

**ragweed fever.** See HAY FEVER.

**rale.** An abnormal respiratory sound heard through a stethoscope placed over the chest, and indicating some pathological condition. Rales are generally characterized by such self-explanatory terms as coarse, medium, and fine. The adjectives "moist" and "dry" are also widely used, but in a descriptive sense only. They are not intended to imply that the sound has originated in a moist or dry physical environment. Many doctors hold that all rales originate in the presence of abnormal moisture.

**consonating rale.** A moderately coarse rale which sounds unusually loud and close to the ear, as though it were being reinforced by transmission through an area of consolidated lung, with which it is usually associated.

**crepitant rale.** A fine, dry, crackling sound, like that of hairs being rubbed together; often heard transiently round the lower margins of normal lungs during the first few forced inspirations. It may be heard at the beginning or during the resolving stages of a congested lung, such as occurs in pneumonia, pulmonary collapse, and lung edema.

**posttussive rale.** A form of rale heard after the patient takes a deep breath and coughs.

**rhonchus rale.** An extremely coarse rale which originates in the larger air passages and sets up vibrations that, in addition to being heard quite clearly through a stethoscope, usually can even be felt with the hand when it is laid on the chest.

**sibilant rale.** A dry, high-pitched, hissing or whistling sound, heard usually in cases of bronchiolar spasm.

**sonorous rale.** A dry, low-pitched, resonant, snoring sound, heard most often in cases of bronchiolar spasm.

**vesicular rale.** See CREPITANT RALE, above.

**ramal.** Relating to a ramus; branching.

**rami.** The plural of ramus.

**ramification.** Branching of any organ or part.

**ramify.** To branch.

**ramisection.** Surgical division of some of the rami of the sympathetic nervous system.

**ramitis.** Inflammation of a nerve root.

**ramose.** Having many branches.

**Ramstedt's operation.** The operation employed to relieve pyloric stenosis in infants. An incision is made into the circular muscular coat of the pylorus to allow the lining of mucous membrane to push through and open up the inner canal.

**ramus.** 1. A branch, usually of a nerve or blood vessel. 2. A slim process projecting from a large bone, such as the ramus of the lower jaw.

**ranine.** 1. Pertaining to a frog. 2. Pertaining to a ranula.

**ranula.** A cystic tumor beneath the tongue, due to blockage of the duct of either the sublingual or submaxillary salivary gland.

**ranular.** Pertaining to a ranula.

**rape.** Sexual intercourse with a woman without her consent.

**raphe.** A seam or ridge, especially one indicating the line of junction of two symmetrical halves.

**rarefaction.** The condition of becoming or being less dense; a diminution of density and weight but not of volume. The term is used in radiography to describe the x-ray appearance of a bone which is less dense than normal.

**rasceta.** Transverse lines on the inner surface of the wrist, which show when the hand is flexed on the wrist.

**rash.** A skin eruption.

**raspberry mark.** A nevus.

**rat-bite fever.** A chronic type of relapsing fever transmitted by the bite of rats and characterized by inflammation of the glands, rigors, high temperature, and a rash. Also called *rat-bite disease, sodoku, sokoshio.*

**rational.** Based upon reason; reasonable. In medical therapeutics it indicates treatment based on reasoning as opposed to empirical treatment, which is based on experience.

**ratsbane.** The popular name for white arsenic (arsenic trioxide).

**rattle.** A rale.

**ray.** A beam of light or heat emanating from a common source; one of a number of lines diverging from a common center. Alpha, beta, and gamma rays are dealt with under radium.

**Raynaud's disease.** Intermittent attacks of pallor or congestion of the extremities, with the return of the skin to normal color in between the attacks. A common disease among young women, it is an excessive reaction to cold in otherwise normal blood vessels, which go into spasm and cut off the blood supply to the fingers or toes. The wearing of warm clothing and protection of the hands with gloves or mittens help to prevent the attacks, and there are also several drugs which relieve the blood-vessel spasms. If these measures fail and the condition is severe, a cure can be obtained by dividing the sympathetic nerves to the arm where they occur in the neck.

**reaction.** 1. The response to stimulation. 2. In chemistry, the interaction of two or more chemical substances. 3. In psychiatry, the mental response to a particular condition or event.

**abortin reaction.** See BRUCELLERGEN REACTION, below.

**addition reaction.** Direct union of two or more molecules to form a new molecule.

**affective reaction.** In psychiatry, moods of abnormal elation or depression, characteristic of psychotic states, such as involutional melancholia and manic-depressive psychosis.

**agglutination reaction.** The clumping of cellular antigens, bacteria for instance, upon mixture with immune serum.

**allergic reaction.** A reaction based on hypersensitivity to an antigen. It may be present in many forms, such as an outbreak of urticaria or edema of the face and throat after contact with a substance to which the individual is allergic.

**amphoteric reaction.** The reaction of a compound as an acid or base, depending upon the substance on which it acts.

**anaphylactic reaction.** The reaction occurring in anaphylactic shock. See also ANAPHYLAXIS.

**antigen-antibody reaction.** A combination of an antigen with its specific antibody.

**Aschheim-Zondek reaction.** A test for pregnancy performed by injecting the urine of a woman into immature female mice. If the woman is pregnant her urine will contain ovarian hormones which stimulate the mice sexually and this can be seen on post-mortem examination of the mice.

**Brucellergen reaction.** A skin reaction produced by the intradermal injection of antigens from bacteria of the genus *Brucella*, in the diagnosis of undulant fever.

**cholera red reaction.** A nonspecific test for cholera in which a pink color develops upon the addition of sulfuric acid to a growth of cholera germs.

**complement-fixation reaction.** An antigen-antibody combination with complement (a dissolving substance found in normal serum).

**conjunctival reaction.** Instillation of a suspected substance into the eye to test whether the patient is allergic to it. If positive, the white of the eye becomes pink and engorged.

**consensual reaction.** A reaction independent of the will.

**constitutional reaction.** Generalized reaction of the body to an allergen, other than the symptoms evoked at the site of injection.

**cross reaction.** Reaction between an antibody and an antigen which is closely related to, but not identical with, the specific antigen. The reaction in a hypersensitive skin to the presence of an antigen may be of swelling, edema, redness, or a rash.

**delayed reaction.** An allergic reaction occurring hours or days after contact with an allergen. The reaction may be localized at the site of contact or generalized and constitutional.

**diazo reaction.** A urine reaction which may be obtained in some febrile illnesses, such as typhoid fever, typhus, measles, and smallpox.

**distant reaction.** An allergic response to an allergen at a site remote from its introduction or application to the body.

**false-negative reaction.** An erroneous or deceptive negative reaction due to faulty technique or evaluation.

**false-positive reaction.** A deceptive positive reaction due to faulty technique or evaluation.

**focal reaction.** An exacerbation or recurrence at the site of an active, quiescent, or healed lesion distant from the place of introduction or point of origin of the exciting agent.

**immune reaction.** A reaction which demonstrates the presence of an antibody.

**inflammatory reaction.** A reaction exhibiting the characteristic signs of inflammation, such as the part becoming red, hot, swollen, or painful.

**Jarisch-Herxheimer reaction.** Increase of symptoms of syphilis following initial doses of arsenicals or penicillin. It lasts from 12 to 24 hours.

**local reaction.** The phenomena or lesions occurring at the site of application of an exciting agent.

**Mantoux reaction.** A skin test for tuberculosis.

**myasthenic reaction.** A reaction in which the normal contraction of a muscle, stimulated by direct electrical current, becomes less intense and of shorter duration with each successive stimulus and finally ceases as the muscle becomes exhausted.

**myotonic reaction.** An increase in muscle irritability seen in the diseases called myotonias.

**neutral reaction.** A reaction that indicates the absence of both acidity and alkalinity. It is expressed as pH 7.

**Rh reaction.** The result of Rh testing. See RHESUS FACTOR.

**specific reaction.** In allergy, phenomena produced by an agent identical with one that previously produced alteration in capacity to react.

**symptomatic reaction.** A reaction following therapeutic injection of an allergen and characterized by the reproduction of the original symptoms under investigation or treatment.

**transfusion reaction.** A reaction that occurs when incompatible blood is transfused. There is both clotting and dissolving of some of the blood cells.

**tuberculin reaction.** Localized inflammation of the skin following injection of a small quantity of tuberculin, indicating that the body has been sensitized by tubercle bacilli.

**van den Bergh reaction.** A blood test which detects impaired liver function.

**Widal reaction.** A blood test used in typhoid fever.

**reactivate.** To render active again.

**reactivation.** Rendering an inactive serum active again by the addition of complement.

**reagent.** Any substance involved in a chemical reaction, or used for the detection or determination of another substance by chemical or microscopical means.

**reagin.** An antibody.

**reamputation.** A second amputation performed on a limb to shorten it further.

**Réaumur's thermometer.** See THERMOMETER.

**rebound.** Sudden contraction of a muscle after it has relaxed and not been excited by a further stimulus.

**receptor.** 1. Peripheral nerve endings in the skin and special sense organs. 2. The atomic lateral chain or haptophore group, which exists in each tissue cell in addition to the nucleus. It combines with intermediary bodies, such as toxins, food molecules, and foreign substances, and is a part of the side-chain theory.

**recess, recessus.** A hole or cavelike recess. Also *fossa, ventricle, ampulla*.

**recession.** A drawing away.

**recession of the gums.** The shrinking away of the gums from the necks of the teeth, such as is seen in pyorrhea.

**recessive characteristic.** In biology, a characteristic which appears in the offspring only when both members of a pair of recessive genes are present. This may be contrasted with a dominant characteristic, which develops in the presence of only one gene for the trait. See also MENDELISM.

**recidivation.** 1. The relapsing of a disease. 2. In criminology, a relapsing into crime.

**recidivist.** 1. A patient who returns for treatment, especially an insane person who so returns. 2. In criminology, a criminal who, after punishment, returns to a life of crime.

**recipient.** The receiver of a blood transfusion.

**reconstitution.** The act of adding water to a powder to reconstitute it to its original form.

**recrement.** Any secretion, such as saliva, that is reabsorbed into the body after it has fulfilled its function.

**recrudescence.** The return of a disease after apparent recovery—the period being shorter than that referred to as a "relapse."

**rectal.** Pertaining to the rectum.

**rectalgia.** Pain in the rectum. Also called *proctalgia*.

**rectectomy.** Surgical removal of the rectum.

**rectification.** 1. A straightening, such as of a crooked limb. 2. Redistillation of liquids to obtain a product of higher purity or greater concentration.

**rectified.** Corrected or refined.

**rectified spirit.** Alcohol containing 94 percent of ethyl alcohol.

**rectitis.** Inflammation of the rectum.

**recto-abdominal.** Pertaining to the rectum and the abdomen.

**rectocele.** Prolapse of the rectum.

**rectococcygeal.** Pertaining to the rectum and the coccyx.

**rectococcypexy.** Suturing or tethering the rectum to the coccyx.

**rectopexy.** Surgical fixation of a prolapsed rectum.

**rectophobia.** A morbid foreboding, often encountered in patients with rectal diseases.

**rectoscope.** A surgical instrument for examining the rectum.

**rectosigmoid.** The region of the lower sigmoid colon and the upper part of the rectum.

**rectostenosis.** Stricture of the rectum.

**rectostomy.** See PROCTOSTOMY.

**rectotomy.** See PROCTOTOMY.

**rectourethral.** Pertaining to the rectum and urethra.

**rectouterine.** Pertaining to the rectum and uterus.

**rectovaginal.** Pertaining to the rectum and vagina.

**rectovesical.** Pertaining to the rectum and urinary bladder.

**rectum.** The last five inches of the large intestine, from the sigmoid colon to the anus.

**rectus.** Straight.

**recurrent.** Returning at intervals. In anatomy, a turning back of a structure to its source of origin.

**recurrent fever.** See FAMINE FEVER.

**red fever.** See DENGUE; ADEN FEVER.

**redintegration.** Full restoration of an injured part.

**red mite.** The red larva of the harvest mite or chigger. It lives in long grass and underbrush and attacks man, producing weals on the skin, which itch ferociously.

**redressement force.** Forcible correction of a deformity.

**reduce.** 1. To return a part to its normal position, such as a hernia or a fracture. 2. In chemistry, to bring back to metallic form by depriving of oxygen. 3. To lose weight by dieting.

**reducible.** Capable of reduction.

**reduction.** Restoration to normal.

**reduplicated.** Doubled.

**reduplication.** 1. The doubling of paroxysms in some forms of intermittent fever. 2. The doubling of the first or second sounds of the heartbeat.

**reflex.** Involuntary automatic response to a stimulus.

**abdominal reflex.** Contraction of the abdominal muscles, induced by tracing the fingernails across the corresponding side of the abdominal wall.

**accommodation reflex.** Adjustment by the eyes for near vision. The pupils constrict, the eyes converge, and the convexity of the lenses increases.

**Achilles tendon reflex.** Contraction of the calf muscles and plantar flexion of the foot caused by striking the Achilles tendon sharply.

**ankle clonus reflex.** Clonic contractions of the calf muscles in response to pressure against the sole of the foot.

**Babinski reflex.** Upward turning of the big toe on stimulating the sole of the foot. In adults, it indicates lesions of motor tracts in the brain or spinal cord.

**Brudzinski's reflex.** In meningitis, flexion of the patient's head also causes flexion of the ankle, knee, and hip. The test can also be performed by flexing one leg at the hip joint, which causes the other leg to flex automatically.

**conditioned reflex.** A reflex acquired as a result of repeated training. A famous example is the Pavlov dog, which salivated when offered food at the simultaneous ringing of a bell. Eventually the mere sound of the bell was sufficient to cause the dog to salivate.

**conjunctival reflex.** Automatic blinking of the eye when the white of it is touched.

**cough reflex.** A cough caused by irritation of the lining of the larynx. Also produced by syringing the ear.

**eyeball compression reflex.** Slowing of the heart caused by pressure on the eyeball.

**gastrocolic reflex.** Increased contraction of the colon induced by the entrance of food into the empty stomach. This is the reason why so many people have the urge to go to the toilet after eating.

**gastrosalivary reflex.** Salivation produced by the introduction of food into the mouth or stomach, especially if it contains meat or articles with a tart taste.

**grasp reflex.** A reflex seen in babies when the stimulation of the palm of the hand causes the finger to make a grasping movement.

**jaw jerk reflex.** Clonic contraction of the jaw muscles elicited by striking the relaxed and open jaw with a percussion hammer; seen in diseases of the nervous system.

**knee jerk reflex.** An involuntary jerk of the leg due to sudden contraction of the muscles when the tendon below the knee cap is quickly struck with a percussion hammer.

**light reflex.** 1. A cone of light seen on the healthy, normal eardrum. 2. The circular area of light reflected from the retina during examination of the eye 'with retinoscopic instruments; contraction of the pupil in response to light.

**palatal reflex.** Elevation of the soft palate or swallowing produced by touching the soft palate; both are absent in hysteria.

**patellar reflex.** See KNEE JERK REFLEX, above.

**plantar reflex.** See BABINSKI REFLEX, above.

**pupillary reflex.** See LIGHT REFLEX, above.

**rectal reflex.** The mechanism by which the feces are evacuated from the rectum, characterized by contraction of the rectal muscles and relaxation of the internal and external sphincter valves of the anus.

**red reflex.** A red glow of light seen to emerge from the eye when its interior is illuminated.

**stretch reflex.** Contraction of a muscle in response to sudden brisk stretching.

**tendo-Achillis reflex.** See ACHILLES TENDON REFLEX, above.

**triceps reflex.** Extension of the forearm in response to a brisk tap against the triceps tendon behind the elbow joint.

**urinary reflex.** The desire to pass urine in response to its accumulation within the bladder.

**vomiting reflex.** Vomiting induced by tickling the back of the throat.

**winking reflex.** Sudden closure of the eyelids in response to the unexpected appearance of an object within the field of vision.

**reflexophil.** Marked by reflex activity.

**reflux.** A return flow.

**refract.** 1. To cause deviation. 2. To estimate the extent of visual defect in an eye.

**refraction.** 1. The process of deviation. 2. The deviation of a ray of light passing through one transparent medium to another of different density. For instance, an object that is half in and half out of water and appears to be bent at the surface of the water. 3. The process of correcting errors of defective vision by providing spectacles.

**refractionist.** One who corrects defective vision by providing corrective spectacles.

**refractive.** Relating to refraction.

**refractory.** Resistant to treatment.

**refracture.** Rebreaking of a fractured bone in order to reset it into a better position.

**refrangibility.** Capacity of being refracted.

**refusion.** Injection of blood into the circulation after its prior removal from the same patient.

**regenerate.** To renew or reproduce.

**regeneration.** The repair of tissues damaged by disease or injury.

**regimen.** A systematic course or plan to maintain or improve the health. This may include diet, sanitary arrangements, hygiene, exercise, and drug medication.

**region.** Any division of the body with definite boundaries.

**abdominal region.** See ABDOMEN; ABDOMINAL AREAS.

**antecubital region.** The area in front of the elbow joint.

**axillary region.** The armpit.

**femoral region.** The thigh.

**gluteal region.** The buttocks.

**infraclavicular region.** The area below the clavicle.

**inframammary region.** The area below each breast.

**infrascapular region.** The area below the scapula.

**inguinal region.** The groin.

**ischiorectal region.** The area between rectum and ischium.

**olfactory region.** The interior of the nose.

**perineal region.** The area in front of the anus.

**popliteal region.** The area behind the knee.

**precordial region.** The area on the chest in front of the heart.

**scapular region.** The area of the back corresponding to the position of the scapula.

**sternal region.** The area overlying the sternum.

**sublingual region.** The floor of the mouth below the tongue.

**submaxillary region.** The area below the jaw.

**submental region.** The area below the chin.

**supraclavicular region.** The area above the clavicle.

**regression.** 1. A turning back. 2. The tendency for children to deviate less from the average of the population than did their parents. 3. In psychology, a mental state and mode of conduct when dealing with difficult or unpleasant situations, which although satisfying and appropriate at an earlier stage of development, no longer befits the age and social status of the individual. Childlike behavior in an adult. See also RETROGRESSION.

**regurgitant.** A flowing backwards.

**regurgitation.** 1. A backflow of blood through a defective heart valve. 2. Return of food from the stomach to the mouth soon after eating without the ordinary expulsive efforts of vomiting.

**rehabilitate.** To restore to good health; to restore working capacity.

**reimplantation.** Replacement of a tissue or organ into its original site or at a new site; in dentistry, replacement of an extracted tooth into its original socket.

**reinfection.** A second infection by the same type of germ.

**reinoculation.** A second inoculation with the same kind of germ.

**reinversion.** Correction of an inverted womb by applying pressure to the top of it.

**relapse.** The return of a disease after apparent recovery has begun.

**relapsing fever.** See FAMINE FEVER.

**relaxant.** An agent that reduces tension; a loosening.

**relaxation.** A diminution of tension in a part; a diminution in functional activity; popularly, "taking it easy."

**remedial.** Curative.

**remission.** The abating of symptoms during a disease; the period during which such abatement occurs.

**remittent.** Alternately subsiding and recurring.

**remittent fever.** A paroxysmal fever in which the daily differences in temperature vary by more than one degree.

**ren.** A kidney; an almost obsolete term though there are many derivations, such as *renal.*

**renal.** Pertaining to the kidneys.

**reniform.** Shaped like a kidney.

**renin.** A hormone released by damaged kidneys. It is thought to be responsible for one form of high blood pressure.

**renipuncture.** Surgical puncture of the kidney capsule.

**renitis.** Inflammation of the kidney.

**rennet.** An enzyme obtained from the walls of the fourth stomach of the calf which when added to milk causes curdling. Also called *rennin.*

**rennin.** Rennet.

**renogastric.** Pertaining to kidneys and intestine.

**repercolation.** Repeated percolation.

**repercussion.** 1. An aftereffect. 2. Ballottement.

**replication.** Refolding or duplication of a part.

**reposition.** Replacing back into its normal position.

**repression.** In psychopathology, a psychic mechanism by which threatening, painful, or shameful impulses or experiences are deliberately thrust back from a conscious into a subconscious level and become part of the unconscious.

**resect.** To surgically cut away.

**resection.** Surgical removal of part of an organ.

**reserpine.** An alkaloid obtained from the plant, *Rauwolfia serpentina,* and used as a tranquilizer.

**residual.** 1. A remainder. 2. Pertaining to that which cannot be evacuated or discharged, such as the residual air in the lungs or the residual urine left in the bladder in cases of enlargement of the prostrate gland.

**residue, residuum.** The balance or remainder.

**resilience.** Elasticity.

**resilient.** Elastic.

**resolution.** 1. The returning to normal. 2. In chemistry, the separation of a substance into its isomers. 3. The ability of the eye or a lens to register small detail; the resolution of the human eye being one minute of arc.

**resolvent.** Causing solution or dissipation of tissue; an agent causing resolution.

**resonance.** 1. The prolonged, nonmusical, composite sound which results from vibration of the normal chest. 2. The attribute of relatively long duration possessed by certain sounds.

**amphoric resonance.** A sound similar to that produced by blowing over the neck of an empty bottle.

**cracked-pot resonance.** A charac-teristic clinking sound which can be obtained occasionally when tapping over tuberculous cavities in the chest.

**vesicular resonance.** The sound obtained over a normal air-containing lung.

**vocal resonance.** The vibrations of the spoken voice transmitted through the lungs and chest wall and detected through the stethoscope. These vibrations are altered when the lungs are collapsed or solid, or if the chest cavity contains fluid.

**resonant.** Producing a vibrating sound or hollow sound on auscultation.

**resorption.** 1. The removal by absorption. 2. The process which causes the disappearance of the roots of the first set of teeth.

**respirable.** Capable of being breathed.

**respiration.** The act of breathing; the taking of air into and its expulsion from the lungs. The volume of air taken into the lungs and given out during an ordinary breath is the *tidal air* and is about 500 cubic centimeters; the volume that can be inspired in addition by a forcible intake of breath is *complemental air* and is about 1500 cubic centimeters; the amount of air that remains in the lungs after a normal expiration is the *reserve or supplemental air* and is about 1500 cubic centimeters; the amount remaining in the lungs after the most complete expiration is the *residual air,* and is about 1200 to 1600 cubic centimeters; and the volume of air that can be expelled after the most forcible inspiration is termed the *vital or respiratory capacity* and is equal to the tidal, complemental, and reserve air—about 3,500 cubic centimeters.

**abdominal respiration.** Breathing, in which there is more movement of the abdominal wall than of the chest wall.

**amphoric respiration.** A hollow blowing sound heard over cavities in the lungs due to the echo produced from the walls of the cavity.

**artificial respiration.** Breathing maintained either manually or mechanically. See ARTIFICIAL RESPIRATION; RESPIRATOR.

**bronchial respiration.** The sound of breathing as heard over the main air passages in health.

**cavernous respiration.** A blowing breath sound of low pitch, alternating with gurgling and emerging from a cavity in the lung.

**Cheyne-Stokes respiration.** Rhythmical breathing which starts with small breaths and each succeeding breath gets bigger up to a climax, after which each succeeding breath gets smaller till breathing practically stops—the cycle being repeated again and again. It occurs in grave disorders of the nervous system, heart, lungs, or in uremia, and is frequently a sign of impending death.

**cogwheel respiration.** Breathing in which either the intake or output of air is not a smooth, continuous process but is interrupted by jerks.

**costal respiration.** Breathing in which the chest movements predominate—the opposite of abdominal respiration.

**diaphragmatic respiration.** See ABDOMINAL RESPIRATION, above.

**dyspneic respiration.** Rapid breathing; shortness of breath.

**stertorous respiration.** The sound produced by heavy breathing through the nose and mouth at the same time, causing vibration of the soft palate between the two currents of air; seen in cases of cerebral compression and stroke.

**respirator.** An appliance which filters the air breathed through it, or which provides artificial respiration for paralyzed or unconscious patients.

**cabinet respirator.** A respirator in which the body is totally enclosed, with the exception of the head and neck. Also called *iron lung.*

**cuirass respirator.** A respirator which is attached only to the chest, and which alternately compresses the chest and relaxes it to induce breathing.

**respiratory.** Pertaining to respiration.

**respire.** To breathe.

**respirometer.** An instrument which determines the character of respiration.

**response.** The reaction of the body to a stimulus.

**responsibility.** 1. The accountability for professional acts. 2. The capacity to differentiate right from wrong. Legally, this turns upon the question of whether or not the person is of sound mind and capable of controlling his actions and thoughts.

**rest.** 1. Cessation of labor or action; repose. 2. Tissue cells which were misplaced during growth within the womb and which remain present in the adult body.

**restitution.** 1. A return to the normal condition. 2. Rotation of the baby's head immediately after its delivery.

**restocythemia.** The presence of broken-down red cells in the blood.

**resuscitation.** Restoring to life those apparently dead, by artificial respiration and external cardiac massage. See ARTIFICIAL RESPIRATION.

**resuscitator.** An apparatus for giving artificial respiration.

**retardation.** A slowing up.

**retch, retching.** An attempt at vomiting.

**rete.** Any network of fibers or blood vessels.

**retention.** Holding back or stopping.

**retial.** Pertaining to a rete.

**reticula.** A network.

**reticular.** Resembling or pertaining to a network.

**reticulate.** Possessing netlike meshes.

**reticulocyte.** A netlike red blood cell observed during the process of blood regeneration; an immature red blood cell.

**reticulocytosis.** An excess of reticulocytes in the blood.

**reticuloendothelial system.** A system of cells found in the spleen, lymph glands, liver, and bone marrow, which is involved in the formation of blood cells and bile, the metabolism of iron and blood pigments, and in the destruction of blood cells after they have served their purpose.

**reticulosarcoma.** A very malignant form of cancer which arises within lymph gland cells.

**reticulum.** A network.

**retiform.** Net-shaped.

**retina.** The light-sensitive membrane at the back of the eye, which registers visual images. It is formed by the expansion of the optic nerve and is composed of eight layers, seven of which are nervous and one pigmented. The central area is used for normal vision in bright light, and the outer area has special organs for use during periods of dim lighting. The peripheral distribution of these night-sensitive organs enables one to see more clearly out of the sides of the eye at night than when looking directly at a poorly illuminated object.

**retinaculum.** A band serving to keep an organ in its place.

**retinitis.** Inflammation of the retina.

**retinochoroiditis.** Inflammation of both retina and choroid.

**retinoscope.** An instrument used for measuring the refraction of the eye.

**retinoscopy.** The art of measuring the refraction of the eye.

**retractile.** Capable of being drawn back.

**retractility.** The power of drawing back.

**retractor.** An instrument used to draw back wound edges or an organ so that the surgeon has a clear operative field.

**retrad.** Toward the rear.

**retrahent.** Drawing back.

**retrenchment.** A plastic surgical operation in which superficial tissues are removed so as to obtain contraction of a scar.

**retrobronchial.** Situated behind the bronchi.

**retrobulbar.** Situated behind the eyeball.

**retrocaecal.** See RETROCECAL.

**retrocecal.** Situated behind the cecum.

**retrocardiac.** Situated behind the heart.

**retrocedent.** Disappearing from the surface.

**retrocession.** A going backward; displacement backward.

**retrocolic.** Situated behind the colon.

**retrocollic.** Pertaining to the back of the neck.

**retrocollis.** Also called *wryneck*. See TORTICOLLIS.

**retrodisplacement.** Displaced backwards.

**retrodural.** Behind the dura mater.

**retroesophageal.** Behind the esophagus.

**retroflexed.** Bent backwards.

**retrography.** A reversal of the normal order of writing. Also called *mirror writing*.

**retrogression.** 1. In biology, the passing from a more complex to a simpler type of structure in the development of an animal. 2. In medicine, a going backwards, degeneration, involution, atrophy, or the subsidence of a disease or its symptoms.

**retroinfection.** Infection of the mother by her unborn baby.

**retromammary.** Behind the mammary gland.

**retromandibular.** Behind the mandible.

**retromastoid.** Behind the mastoid process.

**retronasal.** Behind the nose.

**retro-ocular.** Behind the eyeball.

**retro-oesophageal.** See RETROESOPHAGEAL.

**retroperitoneal.** Behind the peritoneum.

**retroperitoneum.** The space between the peritoneum and the front of the spinal column. Also called *retroperitoneal space*.

**retroperitonitis.** Inflammation of the retroperitoneum.

**retropharyngeal.** Behind the pharynx.

**retropharyngitis.** Inflammation of the back of the pharynx.

**retropharynx.** The back of the pharynx.

**retroplacental.** Behind the placenta.

**retropulsion.** 1. A driving or turning backwards. 2. A running backwards sometimes seen in paralysis agitans.

**retrospection.** An exercise of the memory; going back into the past.

**retrosternal.** Behind the sternum.

**retrosymphyseal.** Behind the symphysis.

**retrotarsal.** Behind the tarsal plate (framework) of the upper eyelid.

**retro-uterine.** Behind the uterus.

**retrovaccination.** Vaccination with virus obtained from a cow that has previously been inoculated with smallpox virus obtained from a human subject.

**retroversion.** A turning backwards.

**retroversion of the uterus.** A tilting backwards of the uterus without curvature of its axis.

**reversion.** 1. A returning to a previous condition. 2. The reappearance of characteristics that existed in distant ancestors.

**revulsion.** The drawing of blood from a distant part of the body to another part.

**revulsive.** An agent producing revulsion; causing revulsion.

**Rh factor.** See RHESUS FACTOR.

**rhabdoid.** Rod-shaped.

**rhabdomyolysis.** Dissolution of body muscles producing the red urine of myoglobinuria.

**rhabdomyoma.** A tumor composed of striated muscle fibers.

**rhabdomyosarcoma.** A malignant tumor arising in striated muscle.

**rhachialgia.** See RACHIALGIA.

**rhachianaesthesia.** See RACHIANESTHESIA.

**rhachicentesis.** See RACHICENTESIS.

**rhachidial, rhachidian.** See RACHIDIAL, RACHIDIAN.

**rhachiocampsis.** See RACHIOCAMPSIS.

**rhachiochysis.** See RACHIOCHYSIS.

**rhachiodynia.** See RACHIODYNIA.

**rhachiokyphosis.** See RACHIOKYPHOSIS.

**rhachiomyelitis.** See RACHIOMYELITIS.

**rhachioparalysis.** See RACHIOPARALYSIS.

**rhachiopathy.** See RACHIOPATHY.

**rhachioplegia.** See RACHIOPLEGIA.

**rhachiotome.** See RACHIOTOME.

**rhachiotomy.** See RACHIOTOMY.

**rhachis.** See RACHIS.

**rhachischisis.** See RACHISCHISIS.

**rhachitic.** See RACHITIC.

**rhachitis.** See RACHITIS.

**rhacoma.** 1. Excoriation or chapping. 2. A pendulous scrotum.

**rhacous.** Lacerated, excoriated.

**rhagades.** Cracks or fissures in skin that has lost its elasticity through infiltration and thickening; seen in syphilis, intertrigo, keratoderma, and other affections. Also called *rimae*.

**Rhesus factor.** A substance discovered in 1940 to be present in the blood of 85 percent of human beings; so named because it was first found in the blood of Rhesus monkeys. The terms Rhesus positive and Rhesus negative are applied, respectively, to blood that possesses or lacks this factor, and Rhesus is commonly abbreviated to Rh. The presence of the Rh factor in the blood of an unborn child of an Rh-negative mother and an Rh-positive father irritates the mother's blood to produce antibodies against the Rh factor in the baby's blood. The antibodies then cross the placental barrier and immediately being to dissolve the red blood cells of the fetus. This may result in the baby being born with a blood disorder known as hemolytic disease of the newborn with jaundice. Unless this blood is drained off and replaced by other blood within 48 hours of birth, there is a risk of brain damage resulting in mental retardation. This does not always occur, for the first and usually the second baby of such parents are not affected—it is in the third and fourth pregnancies that trouble arises. Approximately 17 women in every 100 are Rh negative and of these 17, three have Rh-negative husbands. Of the 14 with Rh-positive husbands only about seven will have a Rh-positive baby, so that in every 100 pregnancies there are, on the average, only ten in which the mother is Rh-negative and the baby Rh-positive. Only a few of these babies will have hemolytic disease of the newborn. Routine prenatal care involves determining the mother's Rh classification. If it is Rh-negative the father's blood is also tested, and if this is also Rh-negative there is no problem. If, however, the father's blood is Rh-positive, the mother's blood is tested at intervals during pregnancy to check whether she is manufacturing Rh antibodies. Should this occur, towards the end of pregnancy, arrangements are made to change the baby's blood at birth. However, it does not automatically follow that because the mother's blood contains Rh antibodies her baby will necessarily suffer from hemolytic jaundice. Also called *Rh factor.*

**rheum.** An obsolete term for any watery or catarrhal discharge.

**rheumarthrosis, rheumarthritis.** Acute rheumatism of the joints.

**rheumatalgia.** Pain due to rheumatism.

**rheumatic fever.** A feverish disease characterized by painful arthritis and a predilection for heart damage, leading to chronic valvular disease of the heart. The cause is not definitely known but it is related to streptococcal infections of the throat and possibly to an hereditary susceptibility. It is essentially a disease of childhood, girls being more frequently affected than boys, and multiple attacks are common. The heart complications are the important feature of this disease; permanent damage to the joints seldom occurs and they may not even be involved.

**rheumatism.** A much misused term, popularly applied to any pain affecting muscles, tendons, joints, bones, or nerves, which produces discomfort or disability in such widely varied disorders as rheumatoid arthritis, degenerative joint disease, spondylitis, bursitis, fibrositis, myositis, neuritis, lumbago, sciatica, and gout.

**rheumatoid.** Resembling or pertaining to rheumatism.

**rheumatoid arthritis.** Contrary to popular belief, this is really a disease of the whole body, which attacks the joints as a complication, so that the patient may feel ill, depressed, lose his appetite, and become anemic as well as having swollen and painful joints. The origin of the disease is unknown, and apart from causing inflammation of tissues in and around joints, several of which are usually attacked at the same time, it may affect nearly all the body systems. Although it may occur at any age, the majority of patients are between 25 and 40 years, and women are affected about three times as often as men. The small joints of the hands and feet are usually affected first. Not every attack is severe; many are quite mild and end in quick recovery, but even in severe cases the ailment eventually burns itself out, leaving behind damaged joints. In the acute stage of a well-established attack, physical and mental rest are highly important and heroic attempts to keep going and "work it off" only make matters worse. The diet should be a full, mixed one with plenty of meat, fish, eggs, milk, cheese, and a variety of vegetables. There is no special item to take or avoid, and since the disease is not due to acid there is no reason to restrict acid food and fruit, however tart their flavor. Treatment consists in first trying to induce the disease to burn itself out quickly and then in preventing the affected joints from becoming deformed. This latter is done by applying splints and by exercising the muscles to strengthen them, often by making them work against resistance, such as lifting weights. There must be close cooperation between patient and doctor, for only the patient can strengthen his own muscles by special exercises.

**rheumic.** Pertaining to rheum.

**rhexis.** Rupture of an organ or vessel.

**rhinal.** Pertaining to the nose.

**rhinalgia.** Pain in the nose. Also called *rhinodynia.*

**rhinitis.** Inflammation of the lining of the nose. It may be due to an infection such as acute coryza, or to an allergy, when it is called allergic rhinitis (hay fever).

**rhinocleisis.** Obstruction to the nose.

**rhinodynia.** Pain in the nose. Also called *rhinalgia.*

**rhinolalia.** A nasal tone of voice such as is heard when the nose is obstructed in the course of a head cold.

**rhinolaryngitis.** Inflammation of the interior of the nose and larynx.

**rhinolaryngology.** The science which deals with the diseases and the structure of the nose and larynx.

**rhinolith.** A stone which forms in the nose.

**rhinolithiasis.** The formation of rhinoliths.

**rhinologist.** An expert in rhinology.

**rhinology.** The science dealing with the diseases and structure of the nose.

**rhinomeiosis.** See RHINOMIOSIS.

**rhinomiosis.** Operative reduction of the size of the nose.

**rhinommectomy.** Surgical removal of the inner canthus of the eye.

**rhinomycosis.** Any fungus infection of the lining of the nose.

**rhinonecrosis.** Necrosis of the nose bones.

**rhinopathy.** Any disease of the nose.

**rhinopharyngeal.** Pertaining to the nose and pharynx.

**rhinopharyngitis.** Inflammation of the nose and pharynx.

**rhinopharynx.** The nasopharynx.

**rhinophonia.** A nasal voice.

**rhinophore.** A nasal cannula to aid in breathing.

**rhinophyma.** A disfiguring condition of the nose in which it enlarges in all its tissues, producing a lobulated and usually a highly colored appearance. Although it is also called toper's nose and whisky nose, the condition may not be due to alcohol, but is more likely a manifestation of acne rosacea, a skin disease. The basic cause is an instability of skin, blood vessels, and nerves, and is shown by the patient's reaction to mental, physical, and physiological stimuli, largely influenced by emotional upsets. There may also be associated gastrointestinal disorders, and there is a tendency for it to occur in families.

**rhinoplasty.** Surgical repair of the nose.

**rhinopolyp, rhinopolypus.** Polyp of the nose. An innocent tumor arising from the lining of the nose and resulting in obstruction to the nasal passage.

**rhinorrhagia.** A nosebleed. Also called *epistaxis.*

**rhinorrhea.** The discharge of mucus from the nose.

**rhinorrhoea.** See RHINORRHEA.

**rhinosalpingitis.** Inflammation of the lining of the nose and the Eustachian tube.

**rhinoscleroma.** A growth of almost stony hardness commencing in the skin of the nose about the nostrils. The lesions consist of flat, isolated patches or nodules, which coalesce; the growth is painful when pressed.

**rhinoscope.** An instrument used to examine the inside of the nose.

**rhinoscopy.** Examination of the interior of the nose by means of a rhinoscope.

**rhinostenosis.** Nasal obstruction.

**rhinotomy.** Surgical incision into the nose.

**rhizomelic.** Pertaining to the roots of the limbs; that is, the hip or shoulder joints.

**rhizoneure.** A cell forming a nerve root.

**rhizotomy.** Surgical division of the spinal nerve roots.

**rhodogenesis.** The regeneration of rhodopsin which has been bleached by light. See also RHODOPSIN.

**rhodophylaxis.** The power of the retina of the eye to produce rhodogenesis.

**rhodopsin.** A light-sensitive, purple-red pigment contained in the rods of the retina of the eye. It is bleached by yellow light and is part of the mechanism by which the retina interprets vision. Also called *visual purple.*

**rhombocoele.** A small dilation of the lower end of the spinal cord.

**rhonchal, rhonchial.** Pertaining to a rhonchus.

**rhonchus.** A rattling sound in the throat or bronchial tubes. See also RALE.

**rhotacism.** Overuse of the R sound in speech.

**rhubarb.** The rhizome of a plant belonging to the genus *Rheum* which is dried and powdered and included in medicine as a stomachic and as a laxative.

**rhypophobia.** A neurotic fear of dirt. Also called *rupophobia.*

**rhythm.** Something which recurs at regular intervals.

**rhytidectomy.** A cosmetic operation for the removal of wrinkles.

**rhytidosis.** A wrinkling, especially of the cornea; one of the indications of approaching death.

**rib.** One of the 24 long, flat, curved bones forming the wall of the chest. See also BONE.

**abdominal ribs.** The floating ribs.

**cervical rib.** Excessive enlargement of the transverse process of the seventh cervical vertebra which sticks out. The bone resembles a rib and causes pressure on nerves and blood vessels, producing attacks of "pins and needles" in the arms and hands.

**false ribs.** The five lower ribs on each side, which are not attached directly to the sternum. This makes them somewhat weaker than the other ribs and

more liable to damage when compressed.

**floating ribs.** The last two ribs on each side which have their front ends free and not attached to the sternum.

**slipping rib.** Excessive mobility of a lower intercostal joint.

**sternal ribs.** See TRUE RIBS, below.

**true ribs.** The seven upper ribs on each side that are attached in front to the sternum.

**riboflavin.** Vitamin B$_2$; present in milk, eggs, muscle and organ meats, green leafy vegetables, malted barley, and yeast.

**rice-water stools.** A descriptive term for the bowel discharges in cholera.

**rickets.** A deficiency disease of infancy due to lack of vitamin D, which alters calcium and phosphorous metabolism. There is slight fever and sweating. The softened bones become deformed due to the muscles pulling upon them. Closure of the fontanelles is often delayed and so is the appearance of the teeth. Nervous symptoms, such as laryngismus stridulus may occur. Also called *rachitis.*

**fetal rickets.** See ACHONDROPLASIA.

**renal rickets.** A form of rickets resulting from failure of the kidneys to maintain a normal ratio of calcium to phosphate in the blood. Also called *renal osteodystrophy.*

**Rickettsia.** A class of bacterialike microorganisms responsible for typhus and other types of fever.

**rickety.** Affected with rickets.

**Rideal-Walker coefficient.** A number which expresses the disinfecting value of a substance. A dilute solution of carbolic acid is used as a standard and the disinfecting action of the same dilution of the substance being tested is compared with it.

**rider's bone.** An infiltration of bone into the adductor longus muscle on the inner side of the thigh. It is caused by prolonged pressure between the muscle and the saddle in riding horseback.

**ridgel, ridgling.** Any male animal with one testicle.

**Rift Valley fever.** A mild disease caused by a virus that produces inflammation of the liver.

**rigor.** Rigidity; a shivering fit which, in the adult, sometimes arises with the onset of an infectious fever and a rising termperature.

**rigor mortis.** Stiffening and rigidity after death due to coagulation in the muscles. The time of onset depends upon the air temperature and upon the age and physical condition of the person before death. It normally begins in 5 to 6 hours, though it can start in 15 minutes or be delayed for 12 or 15 hours. Rigor mortis usually com-

mences in the neck and lower jaw, spreading downwards over the body. Since the flexor muscles are more powerful than the extensors, the arms and legs become flexed. It usually disappears within 36 hours. Also called *post-mortem rigidity.* See also SPASM: CADAVERIC SPASM.

**rima.** A chink or cleft.

**rimose, rimous.** Marked by cracks or fissures.

**rimula.** A small cleft.

**ring.** A circular opening or organ.

**inguinal ring.** The hole in the abdominal muscles through which the testicles pass from the region near the kidney to the scrotum. The ring is normally closed at birth but occasionally closure is incomplete and portions of the abdominal contents, such as intestine, protrude to form an inguinal hernia.

**ring pessary.** A rubber appliance inserted into the vagina to correct the position of the womb or to prevent it from prolapsing.

**Ringer's solution.** See SOLUTION: RINGER'S SOLUTION.

**ringworm.** A skin disease caused by a fungus type of organism and characterized by pigmented areas of skin. See also TINEA.

**Rinne's test.** A test of hearing performed with a tuning fork to detect whether air or bone conduction of sound is the better of the two.

**risus sardonicus.** The sardonic grin. A distortion of the face caused by muscle spasm, and seen in some cases of tetanus.

*The term originated from a legend about a plant (sardonia) found on Sardinia, which, if eaten, caused people to laugh so violently that they died.*

**roborant.** Any tonic remedy.

**Rochelle salt.** A mixture of potassium and sodium tartrate first discovered at La Rochelle in France.

**roentgen rays.** See X-RAYS.

**roentgenism.** 1. Therapeutic application of roentgen rays. 2. The bad effects produced by overdosage of roentgen rays.

**roentgenography.** Photography by means of roentgen rays. Also called *radiography, skiagraphy.*

**roentgen therapy.** Treatment of disease by roentgen rays.

**Romberg's sign.** Swaying of the body when the eyes are covered and the feet placed together. It is a sign of incoordination and is a test used in the early stages of locomotor ataxia and in drunkenness.

**rongeur forceps.** A surgical instrument used for cutting bone.

**röntgen rays.** An alternative spelling for roentgen rays.

**roof of mouth.** The palate.

**root.** That part of an organ, such as a tooth or hair, embedded in the tissues.

**anterior root.** A bundle of nerve fibers emerging from the front portion of the spinal cord to form a spinal nerve. Also called *motor root.*

**dorsal root.** See POSTERIOR ROOT, below.

**motor root.** See ANTERIOR ROOT, above.

**nerve root.** The beginning of nerve fibers which emerge from the central nervous system and join to form a nerve trunk.

**posterior root.** A bundle of nerve fibers arising from a spinal ganglion and passing to the central nervous system. They carry sensory impuses from the body to the brain. Also called *sensory roots.*

**root of the lung.** That area of the lung which contains the pulmonary blood vessels, lymphatics, and nerves connecting the lung with the heart and trachea.

**root of the mesentery.** That portion of the abdominal peritoneum extending from the junction of the duodenùm and jejunum to the ileocecal junction.

**root of the nail.** That portion of the finger- or toenail that just emerges from underneath the skin.

**root of the nose.** That part of the forehead between the eyes from which the nose commences.

**sensory root.** See POSTERIOR ROOT, above.

**ventral root.** See ANTERIOR ROOT, above.

**rosacea.** A chronic skin disease of the face, characterized by redness and the formation of pustules. It ultimately leads to a coarsening of the skin. See ACNE ROSACEA; RHINOPHYMA.

**Rosenbach's disease.** An erysipelas-like skin disorder which occurs on the hands of people who deal with fish.

**roseola.** 1. Any rose-colored rash or eruption. 2. An obsolete name for rubella.

**rose spots.** Rose-colored spots appearing on the abdomen and loins in typhoid fever. Also called *typhoid roseola, typhoid spots, taches rosées lenticulaires.*

**rotenone.** A poisonous chemical obtained from derris root and used as a horticultural insecticide.

**rotheln.** The German name for rubella. See GERMAN MEASLES.

**roughage.** The cellulose or fibrous, and indigestable, part of the diet.

**rouleau.** A roll of red blood corpuscles, like a pile of coins.

**roundworm.** A common worm, *Ascaris lumbricoides,* found in the small intestines, often causing diarrhea and pain, and especially common in children. Also called *ascaris.*

**Rous's sarcoma.** A cancerlike growth found in some fowls, and from which can be obtained a virus, which on inoculation into other fowls reproduces a similar cancerlike growth. When first discovered, it aroused great medical interest as the possible answer to all forms of cancer.

**rubedo.** Blushing.

**rubefacient.** Anything which, when applied, produces reddening of the skin.

**rubella.** See GERMAN MEASLES.

**rubeola.** 1. Measles. 2. Rubella.

**rubescent.** Blushing; becoming reddened.

**rubor.** The redness of inflammation.

**ructus.** The burping of gas from the stomach.

**rudimentary.** Vestigial; incompletely developed; abortive.

**ruga.** A ridge, wrinkle, or fold.

**rugitus.** Intestinal rumbling. Also called *borborygmus.*

**rugose.** Characterized by folds.

**rugosity.** A wrinkle.

**rumination.** 1. Chewing the cud. 2. A persistent habit in unhappy babies, who regurgitate their food and retaste it with intense satisfaction. 3. In psychiatry, an obsessional concentration on an idea which cannot be dislodged from the mind; seen in anxiety states.

**rupia.** A skin disease usually seen in the third stage of syphilis and characterized by the formation of large blisters and scabs.

**rupophobia.** See RHYPOPHOBIA.

**rupture.** 1. Forcible tearing of a part. 2. A hernia.

**Ryle's tube.** A rubber tube, slightly weighted, which is passed down the mouth and gullet into the stomach, in order to remove samples of its contents or to give a fractional test meal.

# S

**sabulous.** Gritty or sandy.

**saburra.** Dirt or filth, particularly the brown crusts that collect around the lips and teeth in patients suffering with fevers. See SORDES.

**saburral.** Relating to saburra.

**sac.** A cyst, pouch, or baglike structure.

**saccate, sacchated.** Sac-shaped; contained within a sac.

**saccharated.** Containing sugar.

**saccharephidrosis.** Excessive sweating with the discharge of sugar in the sweat.

**sacchariferous.** Yielding or containing sugar.

**saccharification.** Conversion into sugar.

**saccharimeter.** An instrument for measuring the sugar content of a solution. Also called *saccharometer.*

**saccharin.** A chemical 280 times sweeter than ordinary sugar, used as a sugar substitute in reducing diets and diabetes mellitus.

**saccharine.** Pertaining to or characteristic of sugar.

**saccharogalactorrhea.** The secretion of milk containing an excess of sugar.

**saccharogalactorrhoea.** See SACCHAROGALACTORRHEA.

**saccharolytic.** A substance capable of chemically splitting up sugar.

**saccharometer.** A saccharimeter.

**Saccharomyces.** A genus of fungi which includes the yeasts.

**saccharomycosis.** Any disease produced by the yeast fungus.

**saccharorrhea.** The presence of sugar in the urine. See GLYCOSURIA.

**saccharorrhoea.** See SACCHARORRHEA.

**saccharose.** Cane sugar. Also called *sucrose.*

**saccharosuria.** The presence of saccharose in the urine.

**sacciform, saccular.** Like a sac.

**sacculated.** Composed of saccules.

**saccule.** A small sac.

**sacculus.** A saccule or pouch.

**saccus.** A sac or bursa.

**sacrad.** Towards the sacrum.

**sacralgia.** Pain in the sacrum.

**sacrectomy.** Surgical removal of the sacrum.

**sacred bark.** A popular name for the purgative cascara sagràda.

**sacrificial operation.** An operation in which some part or organ is completely removed and sacrificed because there is no alternative if the patient is to be helped.

**sacro-anterior.** 1. A midwifery term descriptive of the position of an unborn baby whose back faces the front of the mother—one of the positiqns in breech presentation. 2. A position of the sacrum in which it is directed forward.

**sacrococcygeal.** Pertaining to the sacrum and the coccyx.

**sacrocoxitis.** Inflammation of the sacro-iliac joint.

**sacrodynia.** Pain in and around the sacrum.

**sacro-iliac.** Relating to the sacrum and the ilium.

**sacrolumbar.** Relating to the sacrum and the loins.

**sacroperineal.** Pertaining to the sacrum and the perineum.

**sacroposterior.** A midwifery term descriptive of the position of an unborn baby whose back faces the mother's spine.

**sacrosciatic.** Pertaining to the sacrum and the ischium.

**sacrospinal.** Relating to the sacrum and the spine.

**sacrotomy.** Surgical removal of part of the sacrum.

**sacro-uterine.** Pertaining to the sacrum and the uterus.

**sacrovertebral.** Pertaining to sacrum and the vertebrae.

**sacrum.** A curved, triangular bone composed of five united vertebrae, situated between the last lumbar vertebra above, the coccyx below, and the innominate bones on each side, and forming the rear wall of the pelvis. The ancient Romans called it the *os sacrum*, the sacred bone.

**saddlenose.** A nose with a depressed bridge, sometimes seen in congenital syphilis.

**sadism.** 1. A sexual perversion in which sexual pleasure is obtained from the infliction of cruelty upon another. 2. In a broader sense, the infliction of anxiety or discomfort on another for no apparent reason. The term is derived from the Marquis de Sade (1740-1814), who wrote about this perversion.

**sadist.** One who practices sadism.

**sadistic.** Pertaining to sadism.

**sagittal.** 1. Arrow-shaped. 2. The middle longitudinal plane of the body from front to back.

**sal.** Latin for salt.

**sal volatile.** Ammonium carbonate.

**salacious.** Lustful.

**salacity.** Lustful desires.

**salicylate.** Any salt of salicylic acid.

**salicylic acid.** A compound used in ointments to soften hard skin.

**saline.** Salty; a salt of an alkali.

**saline solution.** Normal, more correctly physiological, saline solution contains 0.9 percent of sodium chloride and is in balance with the salinity of body tissues so that no osmotic pressure is exerted in either direction when it is used as a bland irrigating solution. For first aid, so-called "normal" saline can be prepared by dissolving a level teaspoonful of ordinary salt in a pint of boiled water.

**saliva.** A clear, tasteless and weakly alkaline fluid secreted by the salivary glands. It contains digestive enzymes such as ptyalin, and its functions are to moisten the food, to commence the digestion of starches, to facilitate tasting, and to enable dry foods to be swallowed. Between two and three pints of saliva are secreted in 24 hours. Also called *spittle*.

**salivant.** Any agent that promotes the flow of saliva.

**salivary.** Pertaining to saliva.

**salivary calculus.** A stone in a duct of a salivary gland.

**salivary fistula.** An opening between a salivary gland or its duct with the surface of the skin.

**salivary glands.** Glands in the mouth region that secrete saliva by way of ducts into the mouth cavity. The important ones are the three pairs called sublingual, submaxillary, and parotid. See also MUMPS.

**salivate.** To produce an excessive quantity of saliva.

**salivation.** Excessive flow of saliva. It may be produced by mercury poisoning, pilocarpine (a drug), and by emotional disturbances. In severe mercurial poisoning, ulceration of the gums and loosening of the teeth occurs. Also called *ptyalism, ptyalorrhea, sialism, sialismus.*

**salivator.** An agent producing salivation.

**salivatory.** Producing salivation.

**Salmonella.** A genus of microorganisms which cause acute infective enteritis (food poisoning) and closely resemble the germs which cause paratyphoid fever. They are named after the bacteriologist who discovered them, not because they are contained in tinned salmon. The germ may be spread by an immune carrier or animals such as cattle and pigs, milk from infected cows, sausages, poultry, and eggs, especially duck eggs. Commercial "rat viruses" sold as rat poison consist of cultures of germs of *Salmonella.* Although it is claimed the virus used is harmless to man, this is open to question.

**salmonellosis.** A form of food poisoning brought about by infection with certain species of *Salmonella.*

**salpingectomy.** Surgical removal of a Fallopian tube.

**salpingemphraxis.** Closure of a Fallopian tube or a eustachian tube.

**salpingian.** Relating to a Fallopian tube or eustachian tube.

**salpingitis.** Inflammation of a Fallopian tube or of a eustachian tube.

**salpingocatheterism.** Passing a catheter into a eustachian tube.

**salpingocyesis.** A pregnancy occurring in a Fallopian tube. Also called *tubal pregnancy.*

**salpingo-oophorectomy.** Surgical excision of a Fallopian tube and its adjacent ovary.

**salpingopharyngeal.** Pertaining to the eustachian tube and the pharynx.

**salpingoplasty.** Surgical repair of a Fallopian tube.

**salpingorrhaphy.** Suture of a Fallopian tube.

**salpingostaphyline.** Pertaining to the eustachian tube and the uvula.

**salpingostomy.** Surgical creation of an opening into a Fallopian tube.

**salpingotomy.** Surgical incision into a Fallopian tube.

**salpinx.** A tube, particularly a Fallopian tube or a eustachian tube.

**salt.** A compound produced by the combination of a base, commonly a metallic oxide, with an acid.

**saltation.** 1. The dancing, skipping and jumping sometimes seen in chorea. 2. In genetics, an abrupt change of sequence or variation of a species; a mutation.

**saltatory.** Pertaining to leaping.

**saltpeter.** Potassium nitrate.

**saltpetre.** See SALTPETER.

**salubrious.** Healthy.

**salutary.** Beneficial to health.

**salve.** An ointment.

**sanative, sanatory.** Promoting health.

**sandfly fever.** See PAPPATACI FEVER.

**sanguicolous.** Living in the blood.

**sanguifacient.** Forming blood.

**sanguine.** 1. Resembling blood, bloody. 2. Hopeful, optimistic.

**sanguineous.** Pertaining to or containing blood.

**sanguinolent.** Tinged with blood.

**sanguinopoietic.** Blood forming.

**sanguis.** The Latin word for blood.

**sanguisuga.** A leech.

**sanies.** A thin, purulent discharge from an ulcer, wound, or fistula.

**sanious.** Pertaining to sanies.

**sanity.** The state of being of sound mind; normal mentality.

**santonin.** A chemical used to kill intestinal worms.

**saphena.** One of two large veins in the leg.

**saphenous.** 1. Manifest or superficial. 2. Pertaining to the two large veins in the legs and the nerves which accompany them.

**saphenous nerves.** Two nerves, the inner and the outer, which follow the course of the saphenous veins.

**saphenous veins.** The *internal, or great, saphenous vein* arises beneath the skin in the arch of the foot and runs up the inner side of the leg, just below the skin, to the groin. It is the longest individual vein in the body. The *external, or small, saphenous vein* also arises in the foot but runs up the outside of the leg and ends behind the knee. Both veins have a tendency to become varicose.

**sapid.** Having an agreeable taste.

**sapo.** Latin for soap.

**saponaceous.** Of a soapy nature.

**saponification.** The process of converting into soap.

**sapphism.** Sexual practices occurring between two females.

**sapraemia.** See SAPREMIA.

**sapraemic.** See SAPREMIC.

**sapremia.** Poisoning caused by the absorption into the blood of the products of putrefaction.

**sapremic.** Relating to sapremia.

**saprodontia.** An infrequently used term for caries of the teeth.

**saprogenic, saprogenous.** Producing or caused by putrefaction.

**saprophilous.** Living upon putrefying matter. The term is mainly applied to certain types of bacteria.

**saprophyte.** A plant that lives on decaying organic matter.

**saprophytic.** Pertaining to a saprophyte.

**sapropyra.** See TYPHUS FEVER.

**saprotyphus.** Malignant typhus fever. See also TYPHUS FEVER.

**saprozoite.** Any animal which lives upon decaying organic matter.

**sarcitis.** Inflammation of the flesh, particularly muscle.

**sarcoadenoma.** A malignant growth arising in gland tissue. Also called *adenosarcoma*.

**sarcocarcinoma.** A malignant growth composed of both sarcoma and carcinoma cells.

**sarcocele.** A swelling of the testicle resembling muscle.

**sarcocyst.** A cyst growing in muscle caused by a parasite of the genus *Sarcocystis*.

**sarcoenchondroma.** A growth composed of both sarcoma cells and cartilage cells.

**sarcogenic.** Strictly, this term means flesh-forming, but it is frequently used to indicate a growth productive of malignant sarcoma.

**sarcoid.** 1. Resembling flesh. 2. The characteristic lesion in sarcoidosis. 3. Resembling a sarcoma.

**sarcoidosis.** The cause of this disease is uncertain, and while some consider it to be a reaction to the poison of the tuberculosis germ, others regard it as an allergy disease. It is characterized by granulomatous lesions, principally affecting lymph glands, skin, lungs, and bones, especially in the distal parts of the extremities, but they may arise in any tissue of the body. Sarcoidosis may occur in relationship with leprosy and syphilis, or with the entrance into the body of foreign substances such as silica particles or beryllium. Most patients are middle-aged adults, women being affected more frequently than men. When the lungs are affected they exhibit on the x-ray photograph a diffuse, mottled appearance. An appearance similar to this is also seen in the lungs of some hairdressers who have inhaled shellac hair sprays over a long period. This last aspect of the disease has been subject to an investigation by the British Medical Research Council who found only one case out of 506 hairdressers investigated and recommended further research. In the United States, 14 cases were discovered and given the name of thesaurosis. It was believed the cause was breathing air heavily impregnated with insoluble hair spray. The lesions may heal spontaneously or steadily progress and cause increasing disability. Occasionally tuberculosis develops and the sarcoid lesions disappear, while in other cases the patient becomes dangerously ill due to the destruction of the bone marrow by sarcoid infiltration. Also called *Boeck's sarcoid, Besnier-Boeck disease, Besnier-Boeck-Schaumann disease, lupus pernio of Besnier, lymphogranulomatosis of Schaumann, benign lymphogranulomatosis.*

**sarcolemma.** The delicate sheath which surrounds every striated muscle fiber.

**sarcology.** The study of the anatomy of soft tissues.

**sarcoma.** A highly malignant growth arising from connective tissue cells. There are several types, each named after the type of tissue from which the growth arises. Chondrosarcomas arise in cartilage, fibrosarcomas in fibrous tissue, liposarcomas in fat, melanosarcomas in mucous tissue, and osteosarcomas in bone.

**sarcomatosis.** The presence of sarcomas in various parts of the body at the same time.

**sarcomatous.** Of the nature of sarcoma.

**sarcomelanin.** The black pigment present in melanotic sarcoma.

**sarcosis.** The state of having sarcomatosis.

**sarcostosis.** The formation of bone in muscle tissues. Habitual horseback riders can develop bone formation in the muscles of the inner side of the thigh where it rubs against the saddle.

**sarcostyle.** A bundle of muscle fibers.

**sarcotic.** Pertaining to the growth of flesh.

**sarcous.** Relating to flesh.

**sardonic grin.** See RISUS SARDONICUS.

**sartian.** An epidemic skin disease of central Asia, characterized by the appearance of nodules in the skin of the face which becomes ulcerated.

**saturnine.** 1. Pertaining to lead. 2. Of a gloomy disposition.

**saturnism.** Lead poisoning.

**satyriasis.** Excessive sexual desire in the male. Also called *satyromania.*

**sauriderma.** See ICHTHYOSIS.

**sauroid.** Lizardlike.

**sausage poisoning.** A disease with symptoms of gastroenteritis caused by eating incompletely cooked infected sausages or improperly canned food. See also BOTULISM.

**scab.** Dried exudate covering a wound or ulcer. A crust.

**scabies.** A contagious skin disease produced by a parasite, the itch mite, which burrows into the skin and lays its eggs. The eggs eventually liberate young itch mites and it is their movement across the skin that produces the intense irritation, which is most intense when in bed and warm at night. The disease is often present in several members of a family and can usually be controlled by two thorough applications of benzyl benzoate lotion on all the skin from the chin downwards, followed by a further application a few days later, and the disinfestation of clothing. Also called *the itch.*

**scabious.** Scabby or scaly.

**scabrities.** Roughness or scabbiness of the skin.

**scabrities unguium.** Rough and thickened toenails or fingernails.

**scald.** A burn caused by hot fluids or vapors. If more than 30 percent of the body surface is involved, severe surgical shock is produced and the patient must be taken to the hospital.

**scalenotomy.** A surgical operation in which the scalenus anterior muscle is divided to remove pressure on the nerves to relieve the symptoms of cervical rib. See RIB: CERVICAL RIB.

**scalenus anterior syndrome.** Pain, numbness, and weakness of the arm due to compression of the brachial plexus (a network of nerves in the neck) by the edge of the scalenus anterior muscle.

**scall.** Any disease of the skin, such as psoriasis or impetigo, characterized by scabs or scales.

**scalp.** The hair-bearing skin on the upper part of the head.

**scanning speech.** A peculiar, slow, and measured form of speech observed in various diseases of the nervous system such as multiple sclerosis.

**scaphocephalic.** Possessing a boat-shaped head.

**scaphocephalus.** A boat-shaped appearance of the cranium.

**scaphoid.** Boat-shaped.

**scaphoid bone.** A boat-shaped bone on the thumb side of the wrist and the inner side of the instep of the foot. Also called *navicular bone.*

**scaphoiditis.** Inflammation of a scaphoid bone.

**scapula.** The shoulder blade.

**scapulalgia.** Pain in the area of the scapula.

**scapular.** Pertaining to the scapula.

**scapulectomy.** Surgical removal of part or the whole of the scapula.

**scapuloclavicular.** Pertaining to the scapula and the clavicle.

**scapulodynia.** Pain in the region of the shoulder.

**scapulohumeral.** Pertaining to the scapula and the humerus.

**scapulopexy.** Surgical fixation of the scapula to the ribs.

**scapulothoracic.** Pertaining to the scapula and the thorax.

**scapulovertebral.** Pertaining to the scapula and the vertebrae.

**scar.** The mark resulting from the healing of a wound or disease process in a tissue, especially the skin. Also called *cicatrix*. See also KELOID.

**scarfskin.** The epidermis or cuticle, especially that of the nail.

**scarification.** The making of multiple pricks or incisions into the skin, such as is done in one method of smallpox vaccination.

**scarificator.** A surgical instrument composed of numerous pinpoints, used to produce scarification.

**scarify.** To make many small incisions.

**scarlatina.** Mild scarlet fever.

*In the past scarlatina was popularly considered to be a disease different from scarlet fever, probably because the term was less horrifying to use than scarlet fever, which was considered a very serious complaint. The presence of scarlet fever in a house usually so frightened the neighbors that the occupants were shunned for as long as six or eight weeks.*

**scarlatinal.** Pertaining to scarlet fever.

**scarlatinoid.** Resembling scarlet fever.

**scarlet fever.** An acute febrile contagious illness caused by the hemolytic streptococcus, with sore throat, headache, high temperature, and a scarlet rash. The characteristic features are a pale area around the mouth, in spite of the rest of the face being pink, and a two-stage change in the appearance of the tongue; the first stage is called white strawberry tongue, and as the coating disappears the tongue takes on a red, raw appearance called red strawberry tongue. The disease is promptly cured by antibiotics, though in the past it frequently produced acute inflammation of the kidneys. Also called *scarlatina.*

**Schaefer's method.** A method of artificial respiration in which the patient is placed face downwards on a firm surface and intermittent pressure is made on the lower part of the chest.

**Schaumann's disease.** See SARCOIDOSIS.

**Scheuermann's disease.** Osteochondritis of the growing points of the vertebrae.

**Schick's test.** A test to measure immunity to diphtheria by injecting the germ toxin of diphtheria into the thickness of the skin.

**Schilder's disease.** A progressive disease of the nerve cells of the brain producing increasing failure of cerebral function. Often the disease starts with blindness not due to eye disease, followed by deafness, incoordination of muscles, spastic paralysis and finally complete mental deficiency. The actual cause of the disease is unknown and there is no treatment that has any influence on its course.

**schindylesis.** A type of joint in which a thin plate of one bone is received into the fissure in another.

**schistasis.** A splitting; usually refers to a congenital defect in the form of a split in some part of the body.

**schistocoelia.** A congenital split in the abdomen.

**schistocormia.** A congenital split in the torso.

**schistocystis.** A congenital cleft in the bladder.

**schistocyte.** A fragmented red blood cell.

**schistocytosis.** The presence of many schistocytes in the blood.

**schistoglossia.** A fissure in the tongue.

**schistomelia.** A congenital fissure of a limb.

**schistoprosopia.** A congenital cleft of the face.

**schistorrhachis.** See SPINA BIFIDA.

**schistosis.** See SILICOSIS.

**Schistosoma.** A genus of blood flukes which can attack man.

**schistosomiasis.** Infestation with blood flukes of the genus *Schistosoma*, which are parasitic on snails in tropical and subtropical lakes. These parasitic worms enter the human body through the skin of those who swim or wade in water infested with them and then pass into the blood. There are many types of fluke belonging to this group, and each causes a different form of disease. Within two to eight weeks of the flukes entering the body, the patient has an outbreak of urticaria and this may be followed by rigors, abdominal pain, enlargment of the liver and spleen, shortness of breath, bronchitis, loss of appetite, diarrhea, and fever, which lasts from a few days to several weeks—severer cases often simulating typhoid fever. If the flukes settle in the urinary system, they cause congestion, inflammation, and pain, and the patient passes bloody urine. Many drugs are used to treat this group of diseases, including tartar emetic, Stibophen, and emetine. The disease was common among troops in the Middle East during the Second World War. Also called *bilharziasis, bilharziosis, "Bill Harris" disease.*

**schistothorax.** A congenital cleft of the chest.

**schizogenesis.** Reproduction by the splitting of a cell into two.

**schizogony.** See SCHIZOGENESIS.

**schizoid.** Resembling schizophrenia.

**schizomycetes.** A class of fungi.

**schizomycosis.** Any disease caused by schizomycetes.

**schizont.** 1. A stage in the asexual life of the malarial parasite. 2. The mother cell in coccidia, which produces swarms of crescent-shaped spores.

**schizonychia.** Fissuring of the nails.

**schizophrenia.** A chronic mental disorder, usually of young people or young adults, characterized by one or more of the following patterns of behavior: (1) *Introversion.* The patient is reticent, a poor mixer, sensitive, and passively stubborn, shows little interest in what goes on around him and lives in a world of fantasy. (2) *Mental disintegration.* Although he may well be intelligent, the patient lacks the capacity to apply himself to his studies, his work, or to well directed logical thought. Instead, he may behave hysterically or be childish and silly. His conduct becomes meaningless, unexpected, and inconsistent. (3) *Paranoid trends.* He becomes suspicious and thinks everybody and the world in general are against him. He hears imaginary voices, and, as his condition worsens, he suffers from hallucinations and delusions. Also called *dementia praecox.*

**schizophrenic.** Pertaining to schizophrenia; one suffering with schizophrenia.

**Schlatter's disease.** A form of osteochondritis of the tuberosity of the tibia just below the knee cap. It is a common disorder of the early teens, males being affected more frequently than females. The symptoms are pain, and swelling, worse after exercise, occurring below the knee cap, with tenderness over the upper tibia and sometimes a feeling of heat. Passive movements are painless, but active extension of the area causes pain. The disease runs a course lasting from a few months to a couple of years, complete recovery takes place without treatment, and in many cases there is no need even to restrict physical activity. The probable cause is the great strain placed on the immature bone by the patellar ligament, which pulls at the bone during periods of great physical activity, such as playing football. Also called *Osgood-Schlatter's disease.*

**Schönlein's disease.** See PURPURA: NON-THROMBOCYTOPENIC PURPURA.

**Schüller's disease.** A disease caused by the production of granulomas that contain "foam cells," so-called because of the characteristic appearance given by the deposition of cholesterol esters within them. The lesions occur most often in the skull, and frequently at the base, where they may interfere with the pituitary gland, causing symptoms of pituitary disorder such as diabetes insipidus, and infantilism. Any bone can be affected and deposits may be found in the liver, kidneys, brain, and other organs. Also called *Christian-Schüller syndrome, Hand-Schüller-Christian disease, lipoid granulomatosis, lipoidosis, Schüller-Christian disease, xanthogranulomatosis.*

**Schultz-Charlton reaction.** A reaction occurring when scarlet fever antitoxin is injected into an area of skin showing the bright red rash of scarlet fever, and a blanching of the skin occurs at the site of the injection.

**Schwann's sheath.** The membrane covering a nerve fiber.

**schwannoma.** A tumor arising from a nerve sheath.

**Schwartze's operation.** A surgical operation on the mastoid, in which the external auditory meatus (ear opening) is preserved.

**sciage.** A to-and-fro sawing movement performed in massage.

**sciatic.** Pertaining to the sciatic nerve or to the ischium.

**sciatica.** Originally defined as inflammation of the sciatic nerve, by common usage the term now refers to any condition producing pain in the course of this nerve. Sciatica is commonly caused by a prolapsed vertebral disc pressing on the sciatic nerve roots as they emerge from the spinal cord and spine.

**scirrhoid.** Like a scirrhus.

**scirrhoma.** A scirrhus.

**scirrhosis.** The formation of scirrhus cancer.

**scirrhous.** Hard.

**scirrhus.** A hard cancer, especially of the breast and sometimes of the intestine.

**scission.** Fission.

**scissor-leg.** A deformity in which the legs are crossed over in walking, due to disease of both hip joints.

**scissura.** A splitting.

**Sclavo's serum.** Serum used in the treatment of anthrax.

**sclera.** The tough, fibrous, white outer membrane of the eyeball. Also called *sclerotic coat.*

**scleral.** Pertaining to the sclera.

**sclerectasia.** Localized bulging of the sclera.

**sclerecto-iridectomy.** Surgical removal of a portion of the sclera and of the iris in the treatment of glaucoma.

**sclerectomy.** 1. Surgical excision of the sclera. 2. Surgical removal of diseased ossicles.

**sclerema.** Sclerosis or hardening of tissue, particularly of the skin.

**sclerema neonatorum.** A disease of the newborn characterized by a hardening of the subcutaneous tissues, especially of the legs and feet, due to the presence of an abnormally dense deposit of fat.

**sclerencephalia.** Hardening of the brain tissues.

**scleritic.** Sclerous.

**scleritis.** Inflammation of the sclera.

**sclerochoroiditis.** Inflammation of both the sclera and the choroid.

**scleroconjunctivitis.** Inflammation both of the sclera and the conjunctiva.

**sclerocornea.** The sclera and the cornea.

**sclerodactylia, sclerodactyly.** An ailment of the fingers and toes resembling scleroderma.

**scleroderma.** A disease characterized by induration and thickening of the skin either in localized patches or diffuse areas and associated with pigmentation. The skin becomes firmly adherent to the underlying tissues, sometimes causing joints to become fixed and immovable. Ulceration may also occur. Also called *scleriasis, dermatosclerosis, chorionitis, morphoea, white spot disease, sclerodermia, sclerodactylia, acrosclerosis, systemic sclerosis.*

**sclerodermatitis.** Inflammation and hardening of the skin.

**sclerodesmia.** Hardening of the ligaments.

**sclerogenous.** Producing hard tissues.

**scleroid.** Tough or hard.

**sclero-iritis.** Inflammation of both the sclera and the iris.

**sclerokeratitis.** Inflammation of the sclera and the cornea.

**scleroma.** Any hardening, thickening, or induration of a tissue.

**scleromalacia.** Softening of the sclera.

**scleromeninx.** The dura mater.

**sclerometer.** An instrument designed to measure the hardness of a substance.

**scleronychia.** Hardness and dryness of the nails.

**scleronyxis.** Perforation of the sclera.

**sclero-oophoritis.** Thickening, induration and inflammation of an ovary.

**sclerosarcoma.** A hard tumor of fleshy tissue.

**sclerose.** To harden.

**sclerosed.** Affected with sclerosis.

**sclerosing.** Causing or undergoing sclerosis.

**sclerosis.** Hardening of a part by the overgrowth of fibrous tissue. The term is applied particularly to hardening of

the nervous system from atrophy or degeneration of the nerve elements, and to a thickening of the coats of arteries by the excessive production of fibrous connective tissue.

**amyotrophic lateral sclerosis.** A degenerative disease of the pyramidal tract (the course of the motor nerves from the brain to the spinal cord) and lower motor neurones, characterized by weakness and spasm of the limb muscles associated with wasting and twitching of muscles and increasing helplessness.

**arterial sclerosis.** See ARTERIOSCLEROSIS.

**atrophic sclerosis.** Sclerosis accompanied by wasting.

**cerebrospinal sclerosis.** See MULTIPLE SCLEROSIS, below.

**combined sclerosis.** Simultaneous sclerosis of the posterior and lateral columns of the spinal cord.

**diffuse sclerosis.** Sclerosis extending through a large part of the brain and spinal cord.

**disseminated sclerosis.** See MULTIPLE SCLEROSIS, below.

**focal sclerosis.** Sclerosis confined to a particular region of the brain or spinal cord.

**generalized arteriolar sclerosis.** Sclerosis affecting the small arteries of the kidney, liver, brain, intestinal tract, muscles, and other organs. More frequently found in those suffering with severe high blood pressure.

**hereditary cerebellar sclerosis.** A disease of the cerebellum. Some forms of the disease occur in early infancy, and others do not manifest themselves until later in life, when they are called delayed cerebellar sclerosis. The disease affects both sexes and causes a slowly developing ataxia, producing a reeling movement when the patient attempts to walk. Also called *Marie's ataxia, Marie's delayed cortical cerebellar atrophy.*

**hereditary spinal sclerosis.** A progressive disease starting in childhood and characterized by ataxia, paralysis, and contractures due to lesions in the spinal cord. Also called *Friedreich's ataxia.*

**insular sclerosis.** See MULTIPLE SCLEROSIS, below.

**lateral sclerosis.** See AMYOTROPHIC LATERAL SCLEROSIS, above; PRIMARY LATERAL SCLEROSIS, below.

**lobal sclerosis.** Atrophy of a lobe of the brain, resulting in dementia. Also called *convolutional atrophy of the brain, circumscribed atrophy of the brain.*

**miliary sclerosis.** Small areas of sclerosis which occur in the spinal cord of some cases of pernicious anemia, accompanied by subacute combined degeneration of the spinal cord.

**multilocular sclerosis, multiple cerebral sclerosis, multiple cerebrospinal sclerosis.** See MULTIPLE SCLEROSIS, below.

**multiple sclerosis.** Patches of sclerosis which appear in different parts of the nervous system. The principal symptoms are scanning speech, nystagmus, muscular weakness, and tremors of the arms and legs on trying to perform some voluntary movements.

**neural sclerosis.** Sclerosis accompanied by neuritis.

**posterior spinal sclerosis.** A form of sclerosis seen in tabes dorsalis.

**posterolateral sclerosis.** Degeneration of the spinal cord affecting the posterior column and pyramidal tract (the course of the motor nerves from brain to spinal cord) and characterized by a mixture of pins and needles sensations in the limbs, spasticity of muscles, and with signs of pernicious anemia. Also called *subacute combined degeneration of the cord.*

**presenile sclerosis.** Degeneration of the brain cells due to disease of the brain arteries and producing so-called "softening of the brain." The patient becomes irritable, egotistic, moody, easily tired; his conversation is slow, he is depressed or paranoidal; he may complain of headache, giddiness, noises in the ear, faintness, and insomnia; there may be disturbance of speech and writing; the memory deteriorates. The most important feature is that the patient continues to look normal and sensible when already mildly demented. Emotional control falls off so that he weeps and storms when he would rather be calm, and he may make extravagant allegations such as that his bowels have not been opened for six months, or he has not slept for three weeks. Any sudden change, such as moving from home or a transfer to hospital, may be too much for the outward appearance of normality and the patient goes to pieces. Also called *Alzheimer's disease.*

**primary lateral sclerosis.** A form affecting the pyramidal tracts of the spinal cord, characterized by paralysis of the limbs, with rigidity, exaggerated tendon reflexes, and absence of sensory disorders. A peculiarly characteristic jerking gait is produced.

**progressive muscular sclerosis.** Pseudohypertrophic muscular paralysis.

**renal sclerosis.** Involvement of the kidney in high blood pressure vascular disorders, causing disturbances in kidney function, and a clinical picture identical to that of chronic nephritis. Also called *nephrosclerosis.*

**sclerosis dermatis.** An obsolete term for scleroderma.

**tuberous sclerosis.** A condition characterized by multiple tumors on the skin of the cheeks and face, mental deficiency, and epileptic fits. Also called *adenoma sebaceum, epiloia.*

**vascular sclerosis.** See ARTERIOSCLEROSIS.

**sclerostenosis.** Hardening with contracture of a part.

**sclerotic. 1.** Hard or indurated; affected with sclerosis. **2.** Pertaining to the sclera. **3.** Connected with or obtained from ergot; see SCLEROTIS.

**sclerotica.** Sclera.

**scleroticectomy.** Surgical excision of part of the sclera.

**scleroticotomy.** Surgical incision into the sclera.

**sclerotis.** Ergot of rye. See ERGOTISM.

**sclerotitis.** See SCLERITIS.

**sclerotomy.** Surgical cutting into the sclera.

**anterior sclerotomy.** Incision into the anterior chamber of the eye.

**posterior sclerotomy.** Incision into the vitreous chamber of the eye.

**sclerous.** Hard.

**scolecology.** The study of the infestation of man by worms. Also called *helminthology.*

**scolex.** The head of a tapeworm.

**scolioma.** See SCOLIOSIS.

**scoliometer.** An instrument used to measure spinal curvatures.

**scoliopathexis.** Malingering.

**scoliorhachitic.** Pertaining to scoliosis and rickets.

**scoliosiometry.** The measurement of spinal curvatures.

**scoliosis.** Abnormal curvature of the spine, especially in a lateral direction. If a lateral curve to the spine occurs in one direction there is usually a compensatory curve which brings the general direction of the spine back to the upright position.

**congenital scoliosis.** A spinal curvature due to a congenital defect in the development of the spine.

**functional scoliosis.** A bending of the spine to one side due to persistent faulty posture. At first this is mobile and can be voluntarily straightened, but if the faulty posture is continued for a long period it may become permanent and form a structural scoliosis.

**organic scoliosis.** Spinal curvature due to a disease process, such as rickets or inflammation; paralysis of the spinal muscles; deformities of the chest; or disease of the hips or legs.

**structural scoliosis.** A condition in which a series of vertebrae remain constantly out of position and accompanied by some degree of rotation. Organic and congenital forms of scoliosis are structural and the functional type may become so.

**scoliotic.** Relating to scoliosis.

**scoop.** A spoonlike surgical instrument used for clearing out cavities.

**scopolamine.** An alkaloid used with morphine to produce so-called "twilight sleep." It is also one of the so-called "truth drugs" because under its influence a person becomes sleepy and easily encouraged to reveal most things in his mind. Therefore, when asked a question he tells the truth, or so it is alleged. Also called *hyoscine.*

**scopophobia.** Neurotic fear of being seen.

**scoracratia.** The involuntary release of feces; more commonly referred to as incontinence of feces.

**scorbutic.** Relating to or affected with scurvy.

**scorbutus.** See SCURVY.

**scotodinia.** Attacks of giddiness, associated with the appearance of black spots before the eyes.

**scotograph, scotogram.** An impression made on a photographic plate by radioactive substances, without the intervention of an opaque object.

**scotography.** See SKIAGRAPHY.

**scotoma.** A blind spot in the visual field.

**scotomatous.** Pertaining to scotoma.

**scotometer.** An instrument used for detecting and measuring scotomas.

**scotophobia.** A neurotic fear of darkness.

**scotopia.** The ability to see in the dark; dark adaptation.

**Scott's dressing.** Compound ointment of mercury applied as a counterirritant.

**screen. 1.** That which cuts off or protects. **2.** Loosely applied to an x-ray examination in which the patient stands behind a fluorescent screen while the radiologist studies a continuous x-ray picture on the front of the screen.

**screwworm.** The larva of a fly found in tropical America, where it may cause serious disease in man by burrowing into the lining of the nose or mouth.

**scrobiculate.** Pitted.

**scrobiculus.** Any small hollow or cavity.

**scrofula.** An old term for tuberculous glands in the neck. See KING'S EVIL.

**scrofulide.** See SCROFULODERMA.

**scrofuloderma.** A tuberculous disease of the skin.

**scrofulophyma.** A skin growth of tuberculous origin.

**scrofulosis.** A tendency to develop scrofula.

scrofulous. Pertaining to scrofula.

scrofulous abscess. A tuberculous abscess.

scrotal. Pertaining to the scrotum.

scrotitis. Inflammation of the scrotum.

scrotocele. Hernia of the scrotum.

scrotum. The bag or sac containing the testicles.

scruple. An apothecaries' weight of 20 grains.

scrupulosity. Overprecision or overconscientiousness.

scurf. See DANDRUFF.

scurvy. A disease caused by gross deficiency of vitamin C. It is characterized by extreme weakness, spongy gums, and a tendency for hemorrhages to occur under the skin, membranes, and periosteum. Until fresh fruit, such as limes, was carried on board ship, as practiced by Nelson, no ship returned from a long voyage without having lost from one-third to one-half of its crew from scurvy. It was this practice that earned British seamen the nickname "limey" in America.

scutiform. Shaped like a shield.

scutulum. 1. Any one of the thin, round, yellow crusts seen as the eruption of favus. 2. The scapula.

scutum. 1. Any shield-shaped bone. 2. The thyroid cartilage. 3. The patella.

scybalous. Having the nature of a scybalum.

scybalum. A collection of abnormally hard feces in the intestines.

scyphoid. Cup-shaped.

scytitis. Dermatitis.

seasickness. One of a group of disorders called motion sickness.

sebaceous. Relating to sebum.

sebaceous cyst. A swelling formed beneath the skin by blockage of the duct of a sebaceous gland. It can occur wherever sebaceous glands are located but is peculiarly common on the scalp.

sebaceous glands. Small glands situated in the skin of the body which secrete sebum, an oily substance, that keeps the skin soft and supple and acts as a protective covering.

sebastomania. Religious insanity.

sebiparous. Producing sebum.

sebolith. A stone formed within a sebaceous gland.

seborrhabia. See SEBORRHEA.

seborrhea. An excessive production of sebum from the sebaceous glands producing a greasy skin. It is an inherited characteristic and produces the condition favorable for the existence of acne and seborrheic dermatitis.

seborrheal. Pertaining to seborrhea.

seborrheic. Affected with seborrhea.

seborrheic dermatitis. This term covers a group of skin disorders all of which have the same constitutional pattern, namely the seborrheic state. Acne rosacea, acne vulgaris, pityriasis capitis, pityriasis corporis, and pityriasis rosea are included in this group, and are dealt with under those headings. Seborrheic dermatitis is associated with a scurfy scalp and may vary from an acute disorder to a long, drawn-out, chronic one. The eruption may be widespread on the trunk and limbs, consisting of round and oval scaling red areas, which are irritable and tend to form small blisters or plaques of thickened skin. The acute stage is treated with bland preparations, such as calamine liniment, or creams or pastes, some of which contain tar; and the chronic stage with preparations containing sulphur and salicylic acid. Attention has also to be paid to the general health, diet, psychological influences, climate, and the nature of the employment. Humidity, heat, and dust may have an effect on the skin, so that work underground in coal mines or residence in tropical and subtropical climates are contraindicated. Many patients have anxiety states which need treatment by mild sedatives and psychotherapy. Disturbances of the endocrine glands occur, therefore thyroid extract and estrogen hormone have a place in the treatment of seborrheic skin disorders. A diet rich in protein and vitamins with restricted starches, sugars, and fats should be adopted. Dental hygiene is important, and so is the treatment of nose and throat infections.

seborrhoea. See SEBORRHEA.

seborrhoeal. See SEBORRHEAL.

seborrhoeic. See SEBORRHEIC.

sebum. The oily secretion from the sebaceous glands of the skin.

secernent, secerning. Secreting; usually the secreting of a gland.

second intention. A term applied to the healing of a wound obtained either by suturing it for a second time or by suturing it a long time after it was inflicted, healing by first intention having failed. Healing by first intention takes place when the wound edges unite spontaneously or are sutured together soon after the wound is inflicted. Secondary suture is necessary either because the original sutures have broken or because they have been removed in order to drain the wound.

secondaries. Deposits of malignant growths which have spread throughout the body from the primary growth.

secreta. Secretions.

secretagogue. Any agent that stimulates secretion of glands.

secrete. To separate; particularly to separate from blood or to make out of materials furnished by the blood, a secretion.

secretin. A hormone produced in the cells of the duodenum. It is absorbed into the blood and conveyed to the pancreas, which it excites into activity.

secretion. The act of forming, by means of a gland, a substance which is either eliminated from the body as an excretion or carried by the blood to perform a special function elsewhere in the body; the substance produced by secretion.

secretory. Performing a secretion, or pertaining to a secretion.

section. 1. The act of cutting or dividing; a cut surface. 2. A division.

abdominal section. Surgical incision in the abdomen in order to open it.

cesarian section. Surgical cutting open of the abdomen and womb to remove the baby.

frozen section. A thin slice cut from frozen tissue for staining and examination under a microscope.

sector. 1. The area between the radii and the arc of a circle. 2. Medically it refers to an area of the body.

secundigravida. A woman pregnant for the second time.

secundines. The placenta and membranes expelled from the uterus after childbirth. See AFTERBIRTH.

secundipara. A woman who has had two pregnancies resulting in two viable offspring.

secundum artem. According to the approved method.

sedation. Calming.

sedative. An agent that produces calming.

sedentary. Not physically active; pertaining to sitting.

segment. 1. A part bounded by a natural or imaginary line; a natural division, resulting from segmentation. 2. The part of a limb between two consecutive joints; a subdivision, ring, lobe, somite, or metamere of any cleft or articulated body.

segmental. Pertaining to or composed of segments.

segmentation. Cleavage into a number of small sections.

segregation. 1. The placing apart or isolation of contacts (victims) of a serious infectious disease. 2. In genetics, the reappearance of contrasted inherited characteristics in the young; the separation of the paired maternal and paternal genes when the gametes are produced.

Seidelin's bodies. Small objects discovered in the red blood cells in cases of yellow fever, and believed to be the parasites which cause the disease.

Seidlitz powder. An effervescent powder supplied in two papers. The blue paper contains tartarated soda and sodium bicarbonate and the white, tartaric acid. The putting of the contents of both papers into water produces a fizzy alkaline drink. They are used as aperients.

**seismotherapy.** The therapeutic use of mechanical vibration.

**seizure. 1.** A sudden attack or recurrence of a disease. **2.** An epileptic fit, heart attack, or stroke.

**self-abuse.** An outmoded term for MASTURBATION.

**seltzer water.** A sparkling mineral water like that obtained from Seltzers in Prussia.

**semantic.** Pertaining to the meaning of words.

**semeiography.** A description of disease symptoms and signs.

**semeiology.** See SYMPTOMATOLOGY.

**semeiotic.** Pertaining to symptoms.

**semeiotics.** See SYMPTOMATOLOGY.

**semelincident.** Occurring only once for the same person.

**semen.** The thick, whitish fluid secreted chiefly by the testicles. It is composed of spermatozoa and secretions from the prostate gland, seminal vesicles, and other glands. See also SPERMATOZOAN.

**semenuria.** The presence of semen in the urine. Also called *seminuria.*

**semicartilaginous.** Partly composed of cartilage.

**semicircular canals.** The three minute, semicircular canals in the labyrinth of the ear which occupy three planes in space and form the organ of balance for posture. Each canal contains a fluid which, when the head is moved in a particular direction, runs around the canal and by stimulating minute nerve fibers sends impulses to the brain. The signals are interpreted as movement, so that even a blind person is able to tell whether he is in correct equilibrium. See also EAR.

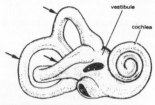

SEMICIRCULAR CANALS (arrows)

**semilunar.** Crescent-shaped or half-moon-shaped.

**seminal.** Pertaining to the semen.

**seminal vesicles.** Two small saccular glands attached to the posterior part of the urinary bladder. The ducts from

these join the ducts which carry semen from the testicles.

**semination.** The introduction of semen into the female. Also called *insemination. See also* A.I.; A.I.D.

**seminiferous.** Producing or carrying semen.

**seminormal.** Half normal.

**seminuria.** The presence of semen in the urine. Also called *semenuria.*

**semipermeable.** Allowing for the passage of certain molecules and hindering others, as in cell membranes.

**semis.** Half.

**senescence.** The process of growing old.

**senescent.** Growing old.

**senile.** Pertaining to old age.

**senilism.** Premature old age.

**senility.** Old age; the enfeebled mental and bodily state characteristic of old age.

**sense.** Any of the faculties by which we see, hear, touch, smell, and taste.

**sensitive.** Capable of responding to stimuli; sometimes used to refer to cases of extreme or abnormal responses to stimuli.

**sensitized.** Rendered sensitive, particularly to bacteria or proteins which produce an allergy. This is becoming a bugbear to doctors because the application of surface agents containing such drugs as antibiotics to treat skin disorders sometimes sensitizes the patient to that drug. The result is, that if the same drug is then given at a subsequent date for the treatment of an internal disease the patient immediately exhibits a violent reaction, such as skin rashes, compelling the doctor to stop treatment. It is becoming increasingly realized that no drug should be used for surface treatment which may have to be subsequently used for internal treatment, lest the patient should become sensitized to it, thus making its use in treatment impracticable or even dangerous.

**sensitizer.** Any agent which produces sensitization.

**sensorium.** A sensory nerve center in the brain.

**sensory.** Pertaining to sensation.

**sensory aphasia.** A condition characterized by difficulty in understanding speech or written words, and assumed to be due to a lesion of an area below the middle part of the first temporal convolution of the brain.

**sensualism.** The state of being controlled by primitive passions, instincts, or emotions.

**sentient.** Sensitive.

**sepsis.** The general bodily reaction, usually febrile, resulting from the action of germ poisons, usually from pathogenic bacteria.

**septaemia.** See SEPTEMIA.

**septemia.** Blood poisoning. Also called *septicemia.*

**septal.** Relating to a septum.

**septan.** Recurring every seventh day.

**septate.** Separated by a septum.

**septecomy.** Surgical removal of part of the nasal septum.

**septic.** Pertaining to sepsis.

**septic sore.** A veldt sore.

**septicaemia.** See SEPTICEMIA.

**septicaemic.** See SEPTICEMIC.

**septicemia.** Blood poisoning; the presence of harmful bacteria in the blood. Also called *septemia.*

**septicemic.** Pertaining to septicemia.

**septicopyaemia.** See SEPTICOPYEMIA.

**septicopyemia.** The state of having both bacteria and pus in the blood.

**septimetritis.** Inflammation of the walls of the womb caused by sepsis.

**septonasal.** Pertaining to the nasal septum.

**septotome.** A surgical instrument used in operations on the nasal septum.

**septotomy.** Surgical incision into the nasal septum.

**septum.** A partition or dividing wall.

**septuplet.** One of seven children produced during a single pregnancy.

**sequel, sequela.** (plural, sequelae). An abnormal condition following and caused by a previous disease.

**sequestral.** Pertaining to a sequestrum.

**sequestration. 1.** The production of a sequestrum. **2.** Isolation.

**sequestrectomy.** Surgical removal of a sequestrum.

**sequestrotomy.** The surgical cutting away and removal of diseased bone.

**sequestrum.** (plural, sequestra). A dead piece of bone that has separated from a normal healthy bone, usually the result of infection.

**seriflux.** A watery discharge.

**sero-albuminuria.** The presence in the urine of albumin derived from the blood serum.

**serobacterins.** Emulsions of killed bacteria that have been treated with a special serum to increase their effectiveness in producing immunity against a disease.

**serocolitis.** Inflammation of the serous coat of the colon.

**seroculture.** The culturing of bacteria on blood serum.

**serodermatosis.** A skin disease characterized by serous effusion into the skin.

**serodiagnosis.** Diagnosis founded on the blood-serum reactions of patients.

**sero-enteritis.** Inflammation of the serous coat of the intestine.

**sero-enzyme.** An enzyme derived from the blood serum.

**serofibrinous.** Consisting of both fibrin and serum.

**serofluid.** A fluid of serous character.

**serogastria.** The presence of blood serum in the stomach.

**seroglobulin.** The globulin of blood serum.

**serohepatitis.** Inflammation of the peritoneum covering the liver.

**sero-immunity.** The immunity produced by the injection of antiserum.

**serology.** The study of serums, especially of antigen–antibody reactions in the test tube.

**serolysin.** A substance in blood serum which has the ability to kill bacteria.

**seromembranous.** Composed of serous membrane.

**seromucous.** Composed of both serum and mucus.

**seronegative.** Negative to serological tests.

**seropneumothorax.** Serous effusion into the pleural cavity, associated with pneumothorax.

**seropositive.** Positive to a serological test.

**seropurulent.** Consisting of serum and pus.

**seropus.** A mixture of serum and pus.

**serosa.** Any serous membrane.

**serosanguineous.** A mixture of serum and blood.

**seroserous.** Pertaining to several serous surfaces.

**serositis.** Inflammation of a serous membrane.

**serosynovial.** Consisting of both serous and synovial membranes.

**serosynovitis.** Synovitis with a serous effusion. A typical example is "housemaid's knee." See also SYNOVITIS.

**serotherapy.** The treatment of disease by injecting human or animal blood serum containing antibodies.

**serous.** Pertaining to or resembling serum; producing serum; containing serum, as in a serous cyst.

**serpens.** Sinuous, winding, serpentlike.

**serpiginous.** Creeping; having the shape of a serpent.

**serpigo.** Any creeping eruption or rash.

**serra.** A sawlike structure.

**serratus, serrated.** The term is applied to muscles that are attached to bone by a series of processes like the teeth of a saw, such as the serratus anterior muscle of the shoulder.

**serrulate.** Minutely serrated.

**serum.** 1. The straw-colored fluid in which the blood cells float. 2. A serum obtained from humans or animals and containing protective properties against disease and used as treatment.

**serum gonadotrophin.** A sex hormone derived from pregnant mare's serum.

**serum sickness.** An allergic reaction characterized by urticaria and edema, resulting from the injection of serum.

**serum therapy.** The treatment of disease by the injection of serum obtained from immune animals or human beings, containing antibodies against the disease.

**serumuria.** See ALBUMINURIA.

**sesamoid.** Oval-shaped, like a sesame seed, as the small short bones in hands and feet, which are embedded in tendons.

**sessile.** 1. Without a stalk. 2. Applied to tumors that are not attached by a stalk but a broad base. (Tumors attached by a stalk are called penile, pedicled, or pedunculated.)

**setaceous.** Stiff and bristlelike.

**seven-day fever.** A fever related to dengue and usually affecting Europeans living in India.

**seventh nerve.** The seventh cranial nerve (the facial nerve).

**sex-.** A prefix indicating the numeral six.

**sex.** The state of being male or female.

**sex change.** See HERMAPHRODISM.

**sex chromosome.** The X and Y chromosomes, which determine the sex of the individual. See SEX DETERMINATION, below.

**sex determination.** The male sex cells or sperms are of two types: one type that carries among its 23 chromosomes the X sex chromosome, and the other type that carries the Y sex chromosome. When the female sex cell or egg is fertilized by a sperm carrying the X chromosome, the offspring is a female; when fertilized by a sperm carrying the Y chromosome, the offspring is a male. Thus the male determines the sex of an offspring.

**sex-limited.** Appearing in or affecting one sex only.

**sex-linked.** A type of inheritance that is applied to genes carried on the X chromosome only. In red-green color blindness and hemophilia, recessive genes are responsible for the traits; thus the conditions occur more frequently in males because the Y chromosomes are lacking the corresponding genes or allelomorphs, which if present would mask the effects of the recessive genes carried on the X chromosomes. See GENE; ALLELOMORPH; CHROMOSOME.

**sextigravida.** A woman pregnant for the sixth time.

**sextipara.** A woman who has produced six children.

**sextuplet.** One of six young born of the same pregnancy.

**sexual.** Relating to sex.

**sexual diseases.** A delicate expression for venereal diseases.

**sexual intercourse.** Coitus, copulation.

**sexuality.** The primary characteristics which differentiate a male from a female.

**sexual organs.** The genitalia.

**shaft.** The long slender part of a long bone. Also called *diaphysis*.

**shakes.** Rigors.

**shaking palsy.** See PARALYSIS; PARALYSIS AGITANS.

**shank.** The leg from the knee to ankle; the tibia.

**sharebone.** The pubic bone.

**sheath.** A sac; an envelope; a covering.

**Sheehan-Simmonds' disease.** See SIMMONDS' DISEASE.

**shell shock.** A term used during the First World War to describe a nervous breakdown alleged to be due to the noise of shell fire. A more modern conception is that shell shock was either due to battle fatigue in individuals subjected to strain beyond endurance; or, alternatively, to lack of moral fiber, in which the individual broke down as a means of escaping from unpleasant and intolerable conditions.

**Shigella.** A bacterium of the genus *Shigella*, some species of which cause dysentery.

**shin.** The sharp front edge of the tibia.

**shingles.** See HERPES ZOSTER.

**shivering.** An uncontrolled trembling or quivering of the body due to contraction of muscles, and being a physiological measure of heat production in man and other mammals.

**shock.** A term with two entirely different meanings, depending upon whether the cause is emotional or physical. The word is, however, popularly used in the emotional sense, with resultant confusion.

**anaphylactic shock.** Sudden profound collapse following the injection of a foreign protein. See ANAPHYLAXIS.

**emotional shock.** An emotional disturbance due to an unpleasant experience. The individual becomes agitated, anxious, depressed, or even hysterical.

**surgical shock.** A very serious condition of complete collapse of bodily functions, resulting from severe bleeding, extensive burns or scalds, or severe crush injuries.

**shock therapy.** The treatment of mental or psychiatric patients, by inducing coma, with or without convulsions, by means of drugs or by passing an electric current through the brain.

**shoddy fever.** A febrile illness associated with coughing and shortness of breath occurring in workers manufacturing shoddy.

**shoemaker's spasm.** A neurosis similar to writer's cramp, affecting shoemakers. See NEUROSIS: OCCUPATIONAL NEUROSIS.

**short circuit.** A surgical operation which by-passes a diseased area of intestine by joining together two other parts of the intestines.

**short-sightedness.** Myopia.

**short-windedness.** Dyspnea.

**shoulder blade.** The scapula.

**show.** The appearance of a small amount of blood prior to the onset of labor or to the onset of menstruation.

**sialaden.** A salivary gland.

**sialadenitis.** Inflammation of a salivary gland.

**sialadenoncus.** A tumor of a salivary gland.

**sialagogue.** An agent which stimulates the production of saliva.

**sialaporia.** Deficiency of saliva.

**sialic, sialine.** Pertaining to saliva.

**sialism, sialismus.** Excessive flow of saliva. Also called *ptyalism, ptyalorrhea, salivation.*

**sialoadenectomy.** Surgical removal of a salivary gland.

**sialoadenotomy.** Surgical incision into a salivary gland.

**sialoaerophagy.** Swallowing of saliva and air into the stomach.

**sialoangiectasis.** Dilatation of the salivary ducts.

**sialoangiitis.** Inflammation of the salivary ducts.

**sialocele.** A cyst of the salivary ducts or glands.

**sialogenous.** Producing a flow of saliva.

**sialogogue.** Any drug exciting the flow of saliva.

**sialoid.** Pertaining to the nature of saliva.

**sialolith.** A stone in a salivary duct or gland.

**sialolithiasis.** The formation of stones in the salivary ducts or glands.

**sialolithotomy.** Surgical incision into a salivary duct or gland to remove a stone.

**sialoncus.** A tumor beneath the tongue, commonly caused by the presence of a stone in the salivary duct producing obstruction.

**sialorrhea.** A flow of saliva.

**sialorrhoea.** See SIALORRHEA.

**sialoschesis.** Suppression of saliva.

**sib.** Related; a blood relation; a sibling.

**sibilant.** Hissing.

**sibilus.** A hissing noise in the chest.

**sibling.** One of the children of the same parents; a brother or sister.

**sick.** In poor health; affected with nausea.

**sick headache.** Headache accompanied by nausea and vomiting; migraine.

**sickle cell.** A sickle-shaped red blood cell.

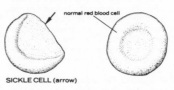

SICKLE CELL (arrow)

**sickle cell anemia.** An hereditary blood disorder, usually found only in Negroes, in which the red blood cells take on a sickle shape.

**sickness.** Any disease; the condition of being unwell.

**siderodromophobia.** Fear of trains.

**siderogenous.** Iron-forming.

**sideropenia.** Iron deficiency.

**siderophilous.** A term applied to cells, such as red blood cells, which have an affinity for iron.

**sideroscope.** An instrument for detecting small foreign bodies of iron or steel in the eye.

**siderosis.** Chronic inflammation of the lungs due to prolonged inhalation of dust containing iron, occurring in such workers as iron miners and arc welders. X-ray films of the chest show a characteristic nodular shadowing. The term is also applied to other conditions associated with iron, such as an excess of iron in the blood, pigmentation due to deposits of iron in the tissues, and degenerative changes in the eye due to the presence of a foreign body containing iron. Also called *arc-welder's disease, arc-welder's nodulation.*

**siderous.** Containing iron.

**sigh.** A long indrawn breath, followed by a short breathing out or a short intake of breath followed by a long, drawn-out expiratory effort. This sometimes occurs as a result of holding the breath when concentrating deeply, but as a rule it is of nervous origin.

**sigmatism.** Excessive use of the S sound in speech.

**sigmoid.** Shaped like a letter S.

**sigmoid colon.** The S-shaped bend in the colon above the rectum. Also called *sigmoid flexure.*

**sigmoid colostomy.** See SIGMOIDOSTOMY.

**sigmoidectomy.** Surgical removal of part or all of the sigmoid colon.

**sigmoiditis.** Inflammation of the sigmoid colon.

**sigmoidopexy.** Surgical fixation of the sigmoid colon, performed to cure a prolapse of the colon or rectum.

**sigmoidoproctostomy.** Surgical removal of a diseased portion of the sigmoid colon and the rectum and rejoin-ing of the cut ends; now rarely performed.

**sigmoidoscope.** An illuminated surgical instrument which is passed into the anus for the visual examination of the lower part of the bowel, up to a distance of about 14 inches.

**sigmoidoscopy.** Examination of the sigmoid colon with a sigmoidoscope.

**sigmoidostomy.** Surgical creation of an artificial anus by bringing the sigmoid colon to the surface of the abdomen. Also called *sigmoid colostomy.*

**sign.** Any objective evidence which the doctor is able to see, hear, or feel, as an indication or positive evidence of disease.

**signature.** That part of a doctor's prescription, usually placed on the container label, which directs the patient as to how the medicine is to be taken.

**doctrine of signatures.** An ancient and obsolete theory that the medicinal uses of a plant can be determined from its fancied physical resemblance to normal or diseased organs. Such plants include the liverwort, the lungwort, and the mandrake.

**silicosis.** The deposit of particles of silica in the tissues, especially the lungs. It is a variety of pneumoconiosis, and is caused by the inhalation of silica particles in trades in which silica, sandstone, sand, and the like are a feature. Also called *chalicosis, lithosis, schistosis, miner's phthisis, miner's asthma, grinder's asthma, grinder's rot, potter's asthma, potter's rot, potter's consumption.*

**silkworm gut.** A suture material made from silkworms. The silkworm is immersed in a fluid, broken in the middle, pulled apart into lengths, and dried.

**Silvester's method.** See ARTIFICIAL RESPIRATION: SILVESTER'S METHOD.

**Simmonds' disease.** A disorder due to destruction or atrophy of the pituitary gland and manifested by extreme wasting, absence of menstrual periods, and loss of appetite. In both sexes the pubic, axillary, and facial hair is lost, that on the scalp becomes thin and lusterless and the eyebrows disappear. Men also become impotent. Some characteristics resemble those of premature senility, and the disease occurs more often in women, since the commonest cause is atrophy of the pituitary gland following severe hemorrhages at childbirth. Other important causes are cysts or growths of the pituitary gland. Also called *hypopituitarism, panhypopituitarism, pituitary cachexia, Sheehan-Simmonds' disease.*

**Simon's posture.** See POSITION: LITHOTOMY POSITION.

**simples.** Herbal remedies.

**Sims's position.** See POSITION: SIMS'S POSITION.

**simul.** At once, at the same time; used on prescriptions.

**simulation. 1.** The feigning or counterfeiting of disease, as in malingering. **2.** The imitation of one disease by another.

**sinapism.** A mustard plaster.

**sincipital.** Pertaining to the sinciput.

**sinciput.** The front part of the head, as opposed to the occiput.

**sinew.** A tendon.

**singer's nodules or nodes.** Fibrotic nodules which appear on the vocal cords of singers.

**singultus.** A hiccup.

**sinister.** Left.

**sinistrad.** Towards the left.

**sinistral.** Pertaining to the left side or to a left-handed person.

**sinistrality.** Being left-handed.

**sinistraural.** Having better hearing in the left ear than the right.

**sinistrocardia.** Displacement of the heart to the left side of the chest.

**sinistrocerebral.** Pertaining to the left cerebral hemisphere.

**sinistrocular.** The ability to see better with the left eye than the right.

**sinistromanual.** Left-handed.

**sinistropedal.** Left-footed; as occurs in football players, who may be able to kick better with the left foot than the right.

**sinistrous.** Clumsy or unskilled.

**sinuous.** Wavy, undulating, or curving.

**sinus. 1.** A hollow, cavity, recess, or pocket. **2.** A large channel containing blood, usually venous blood. **3.** A suppurating tract. **4.** A cavity within a bone.

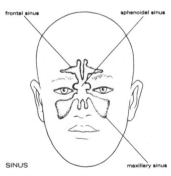

frontal sinus     sphenoidal sinus

SINUS     maxillary sinus

**nasal sinuses.** The air cavities, lined by mucous membrane, which communicate with the nose. The two maxillary sinuses are situated within the cheekbones, the two frontal sinuses within the bone on each side of the root of the nose, and the ethmoid sinuses communicate with the back of the nasal air passages. See also SINUSITIS.

**sinusal.** Pertaining to a sinus.

**sinusitis.** Inflammation of a sinus, especially a nasal sinus.

*Whenever the lining of the nose becomes thickened and engorged with catarrh or acute inflammation, the opening of the sinuses may become blocked. The resultant lack of drainage causes chronic infection in the sinus and pain.*

**sinusoid.** Resembling a sinus; one of the large spaces which constitute the venous circulatory system in the liver and other organs.

**sinusoidal. 1.** Pertaining to a sinusoid. **2.** Varying in proportion to the sine of an angle or of a time function. Thus, in sinusoidal alternating currents, the wave of current rises from zero to its maximum and then gradually falls back to near zero. Zero is never reached because a second rise to maximum begins and sends the wave upwards again.

**Sippy diet.** A treatment for peptic ulcer recommended by Dr. B. W. Sippy, an American physician (1866-1924). The diet consists of milk only for the first three or four days, after which small quantities of cereals and eggs are added. Amounts of food are gradually increased and purees added, until by the 24th day the patient is back to a normal diet.

**sitiergia.** An hysterical refusal of food. Probably closely allied to anorexia nervosa, a disorder in which there is a refusal to take food and for which there is always an underlying psychological disturbance.

**sitiology.** The science of dietetics. Also called *sitology*.

**sitiophobia.** See SITOPHOBIA.

**sitology.** See SITIOLOGY.

**sitomania.** A neurotic craving for food.

**sitophobia.** A morbid aversion to food.

**sitotherapy.** Medical treatment by dieting.

**sitz bath.** A hip bath or any bath taken sitting.

**sixth disease.** An acute infectious disease affecting small children, characterized by the sudden onset of a temperature with signs of malaise. The temperature falls abruptly and is immediately followed by a measleslike rash, which spreads from back and shoulders to abdomen and lastly to face and limbs. The rash fades after about two days. The whole complaint is over in a few days. Also called *three-day fever*.

**sixth nerve.** One of the cranial nerves which supplies the external rectus muscle of the eyeball. Also called *abducent nerve*.

**skatole.** A chemical product found in the feces due to decomposition of protein material, and causing the characteristic odor of feces.

**skatophagy.** The eating of feces, a behavior disorder of children. Also called *coprophagy*. See also PICA.

**skeletal.** Pertaining to the skeleton.

**skeletal traction.** Traction exerted directly upon the long bones by transfixing them with pins, wire, tongs, and other mechanical devices to which wires and weights are attached in order to straighten fractured bones and keep them in position until the fracture is united.

**skeletogenous.** Producing bony structures.

**skeletology.** The branch of anatomy which deals with the skeleton.

**skeleton.** The bony framework of the body.

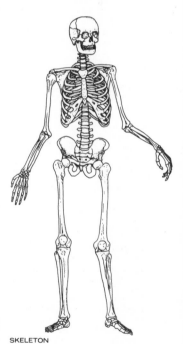

SKELETON

**skiagram.** A print of an x-ray photograph. The term is frequently loosely applied to an x-ray plate. Also called *skiagraph, scotograph*.

**skiagraph.** See SKIAGRAM.

**skiagraphy.** X-ray photography. Also called *radiography, scotography*.

**skiametry.** Measurement of the accommodation of the eye by skiascopy.

**skiascope.** An instrument used to examine the retina.

**skiascopy.** 1. Testing the vision of the eye with a skiascope. 2. Examination of the body by x-rays. Also called *fluoroscopy.*

**skin.** The outer integument, or covering, of the body. It consists of two layers: an outer layer called the epidermis, cuticle, or scarf skin; and an inner layer called the dermis, corium, cutis vera, or true skin. The skin contains sweat glands, grease glands, hair follicles, and the sense organs of touch, heat, cold, pressure, and pain, and its ability to sweat is an important part of the body's heat-control mechanism. The skin is just as much a live and vital organ as the brain, the liver, or the kidneys, and takes its part in the varying conditions of health and nervous stability of the body. It flushes with anger and pales with fear; it becomes irritable when the individual is nervous, and many of the skin rashes occurring in a tense and nervous individual are caused by scratching. The application of so-called cosmetic skin foods is sheer nonsense, for the skin is nourished by its blood supply, and all that external applications, such as soap, lanolin, or petroleum jelly, can

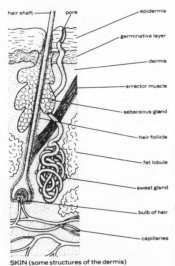

SKIN (some structures of the dermis)

do is to clean or grease the skin. Astringent preparations, such as petroleum products or witch hazel, just tighten the skin, and applications containing vitamins, hormones, lemon juice, and other cosmetically inspiring agents are also a complete waste of time, for they are neither absorbed nor do they have the slightest beneficial effect as beauty treatment. The bland ones apart, most other cosmetic skin preparations have the disadvantage that they may not only sensitize the skin but also cause skin rashes.

**anserine skin.** Goose flesh.

**atrophic skin.** A wasting change in the skin. Also called *dermatrophia.*

**bronzed skin.** Pigmentation of the skin seen in certain disorders of the adrenal gland.

**congestive skin.** Engorgement of the blood vessels in the skin. Also called *dermathemia.*

**edematous skin.** Effusion of serum into the skin. Also called *dermatoclysis.*

**farmer's skin.** See SAILOR'S SKIN, below.

**fish skin.** Dry, hard, scaly skin.

**glossy skin.** A peculiarly shiny skin seen when the nerve supply to the skin has been damaged.

**gold beater's skin.** A thin tenacious sheet from the gut of cattle, occasionally used as a surgical dressing.

**parchment skin.** An atrophic state of the skin.

**piebald skin.** See LEUKODERMA.

**pigmentation of the skin.** Coloration of the skin by natural body pigments or by the deposition of foreign substances. A common example is the yellow color of skin in jaundice due to the presence of bile pigments. Other natural pigments which can stain the skin are melanin, hemosiderin, and carotene. Foreign pigments include Atabrine and silver salts.

**sailor's skin.** A skin condition seen in exposed areas such as the face and forearms in elderly people. There is pigmentation and senile thickening, roughening, and drying of the skin.

**scarf skin.** The outer layer of skin. Also called *epidermis, cuticle.*

**toad skin.** A dry, roughened skin associated with deficiency of vitamin A in the diet.

**true skin.** The inner layer of the skin. Also called *dermis, corium, cutis vera.*

**skin grafting.** The application of portions of skin, either the outer layers or the full thickness, to a raw surface to promote healing or to replace a defect.

**skleriasis.** See SCLERODERMA.

**skotograph.** See SCOTOGRAPH.

**skull.** The entire bony framework of the head, consisting of the cranium and the face. The cranial bones are the occipital, frontal, sphenoid, ethmoid, two parietal, and two temporal bones. The face is composed of two nasal bones, two lacrimal, two zygomatic, two palate, two inferior turbinate bones, two maxillae, the vomer, and the mandible.

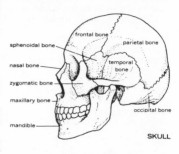

SKULL

**slaver.** To dribble saliva, especially if it is discharged involuntarily.

**sleep.** The period in which the bodily functions are partially suspended accompanied by a state of relative unconsciousness; a natural regular suspension during which body restoration takes place.

*This condition is still not clearly understood, but the importance of adequate sleep cannot be overemphasized. All that happens to the human body during waking hours are called external stimuli, and they include all that one sees, hears, feels, and thinks. The sum total of these stimuli is truly enormous, and it is small wonder that without sleep, during which most external stimuli are blocked, the body would collapse under the strain and the individual have a nervous breakdown. This was well illustrated during the Second World War, when attempts were made to abolish sleep by means of brain-stimulating drugs, and though this could successfully be endured for two and sometimes three nights, after that the individual had to sleep or collapse. So great is the recuperative power of sleep that it is employed medically to treat cases of anxiety and emotional disturbance, the patient being put to sleep for as long as two weeks by means of drugs and only wakened for food and general nursing and toilet attention. See also INSOMNIA.*

**sleeping sickness.** A disease marked by increasing sleepiness. There are several forms. Also called *African lethargy, encephalitis lethargica, trypanosomiasis.* See also BARBIERO FEVER.

**slipped disc.** The rupture of a disc or cartilage pad between the vertebrae.

**slit lamp.** An apparatus used by an eye specialist to study optical sections of the front portion of the eye.

**slough.** A mass of dead tissue in or separating from living tissue, as in a wound or ulcer.

**smallpox.** A highly contagious, infectious disease ushered in with severe febrile symptoms and followed in two or three days by a skin eruption appearing over all parts of the body. The eruption passes through various stages, beginning with small red spots that become vesicles, which then fill with pus and later dry up to form crusts which fall off leaving small pits, or pockmarks, in the skin. The spots appear about the third day, the pustules about the sixth day, and crusting around the twelfth day. The period of incubation is 12 to 21 days. There is no known specific treatment for the disease except prevention by vaccination. Also called *variola*.

*The differentiation between chickenpox and smallpox is important. Chickenpox is usually a mild disease of children and sometimes of adults while smallpox chiefly affects adults. Chickenpox presents the following distinctive characteristics: (1) The rash of chickenpox first appears on the trunk and is thickest on the trunk, face, perhaps the scalp, upper arms and thighs. It tends to avoid the extremities of the limbs. The presence of many spots on the palms and soles is heavily in favor of smallpox. (2) The eruption of chickenpox comes out in distinct crops for three to five days or more. (3) The vesicles of chickenpox come out within 24 hours, and at this early stage are not seen in smallpox. (4) In smallpox there is a very high temperature and complete bodily prostration, which is not usually seen in chickenpox.*

**smegma.** A thick, cheesy secretion found under the foreskin, and around the lips of the vagina.

**smegmatic.** Pertaining to smegma.

**smelling salts.** Preparations of ammonium carbonate scented with aromatic substances.

**Smith's disease.** Mucous colitis.

**Smith's dislocation.** Upward and backward dislocation of the metatarsal bones and the internal cuneiform bone of the foot.

**Smith's fracture.** The same as a Colles' fracture of the wrist with the displacement occurring in the reverse direction. Also called *reverse Colles' fracture.*

**Smith's operation.** 1. Crushing of hemorrhoids with clamps and the subsequent application of an electric cautery. 2. Extraction from the eye of a cataract with an intact capsule.

**Smith-Petersen nail.** A triflanged nail which is driven into the upper end of the femur in order to fix the head of

the femur in cases of fractures of the neck of the femur.

**smoker's patch.** An area of chronic inflammation on the tongue, seen in pipe smokers.

**smoker's sore throat.** A chronic catarrhal condition of the throat, common in heavy smokers.

**snare.** A wire loop used for removing polyps.

**Snellen's test types.** Lines of letters constructed from small squares, used to ascertain the visual acuity.

**snore.** The sound made during sleep, when breathing causes the soft palate to vibrate. Many cases are due merely to the mouth dropping open during sleep, and when this is so the snoring can be stopped by getting the individual to tie up his lower jaw by some form of sling, such as a lady's stocking tied under the jaw and fastened on top of the head. When the mouth breathing is due to nasal obstruction, then treatment by an ear, nose, and throat surgeon is required.

**snow, carbon dioxide.** Solid carbon-dioxide snow has a very low temperature and is used in the treatment of warts and skin moles. An application lasting from a few seconds to a minute causes the blood vessels of the wart to coagulate, after which the wart dies and drops off.

**snow blindness.** Irritation of the eyes caused by continuous exposure to the reflection of light from vast expanses of snow.

**snuffles.** A common condition of nasal catarrh in babies, causing them to make the characteristic snuffling sound. In some cases it is due to congenital syphilis.

**soap.** A salt of one or more of the fatty acids with an alkali or metal. Soap is used chiefly as a detergent and, in solution, as a vehicle for liniments. In constipation a solution of soap is used as an enema. In skin conditions soap is useful, not only for its detergent action in removing grease and dirt, but also because it has a softening action on the horny layer of the skin and possibly has a germicidal power as well.

*The effectiveness of soap is in direct proportion to its ability to loosen grease by altering the surface tension, and it can only act as a detergent if it itself is free from grease. Therefore it is almost a comical contradiction for soap manufacturers to claim that their product contains either cold cream or lanolin, because if either were present in anything but infinitesimal amounts the soap would neither lather nor act as a detergent. A good soap degreases and cleans, and that is all that can be expected from it. To add anything else*

*apart from a perfume and claim it as a skin food or skin treatment is largely an advertising gimmick. Medicated soaps have largely gone out of use in medical practice though sulphur soap is still, on occasions, ordered by doctors.*

**sobee.** Soya bean and barley flour mixed with olive oil, salt, and calcium; used as a milk substitute to feed infants who have an idiosyncrasy to cow's milk.

**soda.** A vague term which usually means sodium carbonate.

**baking soda.** Sodium bicarbonate.

**caustic soda.** Sodium hydroxide.

**chlorinated soda solution.** Bleaching powder solution (sodium hypochloride).

**soda ash.** Commercial sodium carbonate.

**soda lime.** A mixture of calcium hydroxide with sodium hydroxide, potassium hydroxide, or both; used to absorb carbon dioxide in rebreathing anesthesia machines.

**soda lye.** Sodium hydroxide.

**soda mint.** Solution of soda and mint.

**soda nitre.** Sodium nitrate.

**soda water.** Water charged with carbon dioxide gas.

**washing soda.** Sodium carbonate.

**sodium.** A metallic element belonging to the alkaline metals. It is a silver-white color and lustrous when freshly cut, but it rapidly oxydizes when exposed to air, becoming dull and grey. Sodium violently decomposes water, forming sodium hydroxide and hydrogen. It is usually stored, covered by kerosene, in tightly stoppered containers. Sodium metal and its salts are widely used in industry and in medicine. The sodium ion is the least toxic of all metallic ions and is therefore the base of choice when it is desired to obtain the effects of various acid ions.

**sodium amytal.** A sedative and sleeping tablet.

**sodium bicarbonate.** Baking powder, used as an antacid.

**sodium carbonate.** Washing soda.

**sodium chloride.** Common table salt.

**sodium citrate.** A compound administered to render the urine alkaline, and used as an anticoagulant in blood for transfusion.

**sodium iodide.** A compound used in the treatment of syphilis.

**sodium salicylate.** A compound used in the treatment of rheumatism.

**sodium sulphate.** Glauber's salts, used as a mild purgative, one or two teaspoonfuls being added to a full tumbler of tepid water.

**sodomist, sodomite.** One who practices sodomy; named after the ancient town of Sodom.

**sodomy.** Sexual contact between humans and animals, or anal contact between humans.

**sodoqu.** Japanese for rat-bite fever.

**soft sore.** See CHANCROID.

**sokoshio.** See RAT-BITE FEVER.

**solanoid.** Resembling a raw potato.

**solanoma.** A cancerous growth with the texture of a raw potato.

**solar.** Pertaining to the sun.

**solar plexus.** A popular term for the celiac plexus, a collection of nerves from the sympathetic nervous system, situated on the front of the spine and level with the upper part of the abdomen. A heavy blow in this region may cause such a severe impulse to this plexus as to stop the heart.

**solarization.** Exposure to sunlight.

**sole.** The bottom surface of the foot.

**solenoid.** A coil of wire wound round an inert core, such as a tube of plastic. When a current flows through the wire a magnetic field is set up in the vicinity.

**solution.** The process of dissolving; a homogeneous mixture of a solid, liquid, or gaseous substance in a liquid, from which the dissolved substance can be recovered by crystallization. The formation of a solution is not accompanied by permanent chemical change and is thus commonly considered a physical phenomenon.

**alkaline solution.** A solution containing potassium bicarbonate, sodium borate, thymol, eucalyptus, and methyl salicylate, used as a nasal douche, mouthwash, or gargle.

**Benedict's solution.** A solution containing an easily reduced copper salt, used for determining the presence of glucose in the urine.

**buffer solution.** A solution prepared from a weak acid, or a weak base and a salt of the weak base. The solution resists any appreciable change in the p H (acid-alkali balance) on the addition of small amounts of acid or alkali or by dilution with water.

**chlorinated soda solution.** A solution of sodium hypochlorite used as a disinfectant and antiseptic; made into a cream, it was employed as an antidote for mustard gas burns.

**colloidal solution.** A homogeneous system consisting of either single, large molecules, such as proteins, or aggregations of smaller molecules suspended in a liquid, solid, or gas. Colloidal dispersions in which a solid is the dispersed phase and a liquid is the dispersing phase are called sols.

**Dakin's solution.** A solution of bleaching powder (sodium hypochlorite).

**Fehling's solution.** A solution containing an easily reduced copper salt, used for determining the presence of sugar in the urine.

**hypertonic solution.** A solution which has an osmotic pressure greater than that of blood serum.

**hypotonic solution.** A solution having an osmotic pressure less than that of blood serum.

**isosmotic solution.** A solution having an osmotic pressure equivalent to that of blood serum. See also NORMAL SALINE SOLUTION, below.

**isotonic solution.** See ISOSMOTIC SOLUTION, above.

**normal saline solution.** A solution prepared by adding approximately one level teaspoonful of common table salt to a pint of water. Much purer and more accurate solutions are employed in surgery. Also called *isotonic solution, normal salt solution.*

**normal salt solution.** Normal saline solution.

**physiological salt solution.** An aqueous solution of sodium chloride with a few other components, and having an isosmotic pressure equal to that of blood serum.

**Ringer's solution.** Sodium chloride, potassium chloride, and calcium chloride, dissolved in distilled water. It is used in cases where these chemicals and body fluids have been lost through vomiting or diarrhea or both.

**saturated solution.** One that normally contains the maximum amount of substance able to be dissolved.

**soma.** 1. The body as distinguished from the mind. 2. The whole body, excluding the germ cells. 3. The main part of the body without the limbs.

**somaesthetic.** See SOMESTHETIC.

**somasthenia.** An obsolete term for bodily deterioration and exhaustion.

**somatic.** Pertaining to the body cells exclusive of the germ cells.

**somatomegaly.** Gigantism.

**somatometry.** Measurement of the human body with the soft parts intact.

**somatopathic.** Pertaining to somatopathy.

**somatopathy.** Any bodily disease, as distinguished from a mental disease.

**somatophrenia.** A mental disease in which bodily disorders are imagined or exaggerated.

**somatopsychic.** Pertaining to both body and mind.

**somesthetic.** Pertaining to the general sensory structures of the body.

**somite.** A primitive segment found in the developing embryo and from which various organs are derived.

**somitic.** Pertaining to a somite.

**somnambulism.** 1. Sleepwalking. 2. A hypnotic condition in which the patient is possessed of all his senses and appears to be awake, but his mind is under the control of the hypnotist.

**somnambulist.** A sleepwalker.

**somnifacient.** Any agent or drug that causes sleep.

**somniferous.** Inducing sleep.

**somniloquence, somniloquism, somniloquy.** Talking out loud while asleep.

**somnolence.** Drowsiness, sleepiness.

**somnolent.** Sleepy, drowsy.

**somnolentia.** To be drunk with sleep, a condition of incomplete sleep in which some of the faculties are excitable while the others are in repose; somnolence.

**sonde coudé.** A catheter having a beaklike bend near the end.

**Sonne dysentery.** A form of enteritis caused by the Sonne strain of the germ *Shigella dysenteriae.* The disease is characterized by the sudden onset of colic followed by urgent diarrhea, malaise, vomiting, headache, muscular pains, and a high temperature. The stools are at first watery and full of mucus, but later contain blood and mucopus. The disease is spread by pollution of the water supply from feces, contamination of food by flies which have had access to infected feces, or by food handlers who are carriers of the disease. Uncooked vegetables and salads which have been grown on soil manured with human excrement are also often a source of infection. Also called *bacillary dysentery.*

**sonorous.** Resonant.

**soot cancer.** A form of cancer of the scrotum occurring in chimney sweeps. The constant presence of soot in that region acts as a surface irritant and starts skin cancer between the legs.

**sopor.** Deep sleep.

**soporiferous.** An agent that induces profound sleep.

**soporific.** Causing deep sleep; any agent or drug which induces sleep.

**soporose, soporous.** Pertaining to or affected with sound sleep.

**sorbefacient.** Promoting absorption; a medicine or agent which induces absorption.

**sorbite.** See SORBITOL.

**sorbitol.** A chemical allied to mannitol. It is used largely by diabetics as a substitute for sugar.

**sordes.** The Latin for filth or dirt. The term is applied especially to the brown crusts which accumulate on the teeth and lips of patients suffering with continued fevers. Also called *saburra.*

*The condition can be avoided by ensuring that the patient's mouth, lips, and teeth are cleaned two or three times a day during the illness. Giving the patient fresh pineapple to suck not only keeps the mouth clean, because of the presence of an enzyme in fresh pine-*

*apple juice, but has a most refreshing effect on the palate.*

**sore.** Painful or tender; an ulcer or wound.

**soroche.** Mountain sickness of the Andes; so-called because it was incorrectly believed to be due to contact with the antimony (*soroche* in Spanish), which is mined in these mountains.

**souffle.** A soft, blowing murmur heard through the stethoscope.

**cardiac souffle.** A heart murmur.

**foetal souffle.** A murmur heard through the stethoscope, coming from the womb during pregnancy.

**funic souffle.** A hissing sound heard over the abdomen of a pregnant woman and supposed to be produced by blood flowing through the umbilical cord of the baby.

**placental souffle.** A sound thought to be produced by blood vessels in the placenta.

**splenic souffle.** A sound heard over the spleen in cases of malaria and leukemia.

**uterine souffle.** A soft, blowing sound, synchronous with the mother's heartbeat, heard over the abdomen at the sides of the womb and due to the circulation of blood in the enlarged uterine arteries.

**sound.** 1. The sensation produced by stimulation of the organ of hearing. 2. An instrument for insertion into a cavity to detect a foreign body or structure. 3. A noise, normal or abnormal, heard within the body.

**bandbox sound.** The resonant percussion sound elicited in cases of emphysema.

**bell sound.** A bell-like or ringing sound that is heard through the stethoscope after striking a coin placed over a chest that has a pneumothorax.

**bellows sound.** A heart murmur which sounds like a bellows.

**blowing sound.** A blowing heart murmur.

**bottle sound.** A sound, similar to that produced by blowing over the neck of a bottle, which is heard when the stethoscope is placed over a cavity in the lung.

**breath sound.** The sound heard over the chest by the stethoscope during respiration.

**bronchial sound.** The harsh sound produced by air passing through the bronchial tubes.

**cardiac sounds.** The heart sounds.

**coin sound.** See BELL SOUND, above.

**cracked-pot sound.** A resonant noise heard through a stethoscope and indicating the presence of a cavity in the lung.

**foetal heart sounds.** The sounds of the unborn baby's heart heard through the mother's abdomen.

**friction sound.** A sound like two pieces of rough leather being rubbed together, which is heard in cases of dry pleurisy or pericarditis before an effusion has taken place.

**heart sounds.** Sounds heard over the cardiac area. The first, dull and prolonged, is said to sound like "lubb" and is due to contraction of the ventricles, the second sound, sharp and short, is said to sound like "dup" and is caused by the closure of the heart valves. Also called *cardiac sounds*.

**humming-top sound.** Venous hum. A humming sound heard over the right jugular vein in anemia and sometimes in health.

**kettle-singing sound.** A chest sound sometimes heard in early pulmonary tuberculosis; said to resemble the sound of water boiling in a kettle.

**pulmonary sound.** See RESPIRATORY SOUND, below.

**respiratory sound.** Any sound heard through the stethoscope placed over any portion of the respiratory tract.

**sawing sound.** A to-and-fro heart murmur.

**to-and-fro sound.** The friction sound heard in cases of dry pericarditis and dry pleurisy.

**tubular sound.** The sound of air passing down the trachea.

**Southey's tubes.** Small metal tubes for insertion into the tissues to drain them of fluid in cases of edema. They have largely fallen out of use with the introduction of diuretic drugs.

**soya bean.** The bean of a plant originally grown in China but now extensively harvested in the United States. High in certain forms of protein, it yields an oil used in the making of margarine, a flour which is used to make a milklike food for children allergic to cow's milk, a fertilizer, cattle cake, and is the source of numerous chemicals, one of which is similar to female sex hormones in its effect upon the body.

**space.** An enclosed or partly circumscribed area in or about the body. There are about 70 such areas of the body and each has a special name, for example the axillary space or armpit.

**Spanish fly.** A fly which when dried is used as a blistering agent and as an aphrodisiac. See also CANTHARIDES.

**spanogyny.** A decline in the number of females being born.

**spanopnea.** Infrequency of respiration.

**spanopnoea.** See SPANOPNEA.

**spargosis.** Expansion or distension of a part, especially of the breasts with milk.

**spasm.** A sudden muscular contraction.

**Bell's spasm.** A facial tic; a habit spasm.

**bronchial spasm.** Asthma.

**cadaveric spasm.** A condition resembling rigor mortis. If sudden death occurs associated with damage to the nervous system or after great nervous strain or exhaustion, some muscles may go rigid in permanent spasm. This is seen in suicides who die clutching a gun which can only be removed from the hand with difficulty. The condition is of great medico-legal importance.

**carpopedal spasm.** A spasm of the hands and feet associated with tetany.

**clonic spasm.** An intermittent spasm.

**fatigue spasms.** See OCCUPATIONAL SPASMS, below.

**habit spasm.** A nervous tic.

**night spasm.** Painful contracture of the calf muscles just after getting into bed at night. If not caused by general bodily disease, many night spasms or night cramps of the legs can be cured by a nightly dose of quinine.

**nodding spasm.** One characterized by nodding of the head.

**occupational spasms.** A group of affections characterized by spasm of muscles, brought about by attempting to use those muscles, the exciting cause being limited to an action associated with the individual's trade or occupation, writer's cramp for example. Also called *business spasms, coordinated business neuroses, functional spasms, handicraft spasms, movement spasms, occupation spasms, professional spasms.* See also NEUROSIS, OCCUPATIONAL NEUROSIS.

**spasmodism.** A spasmodic condition produced by an excitable state of the brain.

**spasmophilia.** A morbid tendency to convulsions and tonic spasms, such as those observed in tetany.

**spasmophilic.** Characterized by a tendency to spasms.

**spasmotoxin.** The poison of tetanus.

**spasmous.** Of the nature of a spasm.

**spasmus.** A spasm.

**spastic.** Relating to or characterized by spasm. The term is also applied to one who suffers from congenital spastic paralysis.

**spasticity.** The condition of being spastic.

**spastic paralysis.** Paralysis in which the muscles affected have an increased tone. See also DIPLEGIA.

**spatial.** Pertaining to space.

**spay.** To surgically remove the ovaries.

**specific. 1.** Produced by a single type of microorganism. **2.** A medicine specially indicated for a particular disease.

**spectral.** Pertaining to a spectrum.

**spectrograph.** A spectroscope for photographing a spectrum.

**spectrometer.** An instrument for measuring the deviation of light rays and the wavelengths of spectral lines.

**spectrometry.** The science of using a spectrometer.

**spectroscope.** An instrument in which rays of light are split up through a prism into colored bands. By inserting chemicals in the light path, black lines or absorption bands are revealed in the resulting spectrum. In this way the presence of certain chemicals can be rapidly identified. In pathological laboratories these instruments are frequently used to identify the composition of solutions which are placed in the light path. The absorption bands are then studied. A similar method is used to identify the chemical composition of stars.

**spectrum.** The colors produced (red, orange, yellow, green, blue, indigo, and violet) when white light is refracted by means of a prism.

**speculum.** A surgical instrument, sometimes fitted with reflectors, and sometimes with electric lights, used for examining the interior of body cavities.

**sperm.** A spermatozoon.

**spermacetti.** A waxy substance obtained from the head of a sperm whale, used chiefly to add firmness to ointments; an ingredient of many cosmetic creams such as rose-water ointment or skin food.

**spermacrasia.** Deficiency of spermatozoa.

**spermatemphraxis.** An obstruction to the discharge of semen.

**spermatic.** Relating to semen.

**spermatic cord.** The tube which, surrounded by its various membranes, blood vessels, and nerves, carries the semen from the testicles.

**spermatism.** An emission of semen.

**spermatocele.** A cystic swelling arising in or around the testicle.

**spermatoclemma.** An involuntary discharge of semen, such as happens during the night in boys reaching puberty. Also called *wet dream.*

**spermatocyst.** A seminal vesicle.

**spermatocystitis.** Inflammation of the seminal vesicles.

**spermatocyte.** The germ cell in the testicle from which the spermatozoon develops.

**spermatogenesis.** The production of spermatozoa.

**spermatogenic.** Producing spermatozoa.

**spermatoid.** Like semen.

**spermatolysis.** Destruction of spermatozoa.

**spermatopathy.** Any disorder of the sperm cells.

**spermatophobia.** Neurotic dread of the emission of semen.

**spermatopoietic.** Pertaining to the production of semen.

**spermatorrhea.** The involuntary discharge of semen without sexual intercourse.

**spermatorrhoea.** See SPERMATORRHEA.

**spermatoschesis.** Suppression of semen.

**spermatovum.** A fertilized ovum.

**spermatozoa.** The male reproductive cells. The plural of spermatozoon.

**spermatozoan.** Pertaining to spermatozoa.

**spermatozoid.** A spermatozoon; in botany, a motile male reproductive cell found in certain algae, mosses, and ferns.

**spermatozoon.** The male germ cell manufactured in the testicles. It has an oval-shaped head and a long tail, which it uses to propel its way over the moist internal surface of the uterus to gain entry into the Fallopian tube, where it meets the ovum. The head

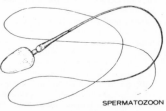

SPERMATOZOON

passes into the ovum and the tail drops off, and the moment this occurs the ovum produces a thickening of its capsule to prevent further spermatozoa entering. About three million spermatozoa are liberated with each male ejaculation, and only one is necessary to produce pregnancy. They are capable of living for some days in the female genital tract. Also called *sperm.*

**spermaturia.** The presence of semen in the urine.

**spermectomy.** Surgical removal of part of the spermatic cord.

**spermolith.** A stone in the spermatic duct.

**spermolysis.** The destruction of spermatozoa.

**spermoneuralgia.** Neuralgic pain in the spermatic cord.

**sphenoethmoid.** Relating to the sphenoid and ethmoid bones of the skull.

**sphenofrontal.** Relating to the sphenoid and frontal bones of the skull.

**sphenoid. 1.** Shaped like a wedge. **2.** The wedge-shaped bone at the base of the skull.

**sphenoidal.** Pertaining to the sphenoid bone of the skull.

**sphenoiditis.** Inflammation of the sphenoid sinus.

**sphenomalar.** Relating to the sphenoid and malar bones of the skull.

**sphenomaxillary.** Relating to the sphenoid and maxillary bones of the skull.

**spheno-occipital.** Relating to the sphenoid and occipital bones of the skull.

**sphenopalatine.** Relating to the sphenoid bone of the skull and to the palate.

**sphenoparietal.** Relating to the sphenoid and parietal bones of the skull.

**sphenotemporal.** Relating to the sphenoid and temporal bones of the skull.

**spherocyte.** A red blood cell which is nearly spherical and more fragile than normal.

**sphincter.** A muscular valve surrounding and closing an orifice. Such sphincters control the emergence of urine from the bladder and feces from the anus; there are many others in various parts of the body.

**sphincteral.** Pertaining to a sphincter.

**sphincteralgia.** Pain in and around the anal sphincter.

**sphincterectomy.** Surgical excision of a sphincter, especially of the pyloric sphincter.

**sphygmic.** Relating to the pulse.

**sphygmocardiogram.** The record made by a sphygmocardiograph.

**sphygmocardiograph.** An instrument which registers the pulse and the heartbeat.

**sphygmochronograph.** A self-registering sphygmograph.

**sphygmogram.** The tracing produced by the sphygmograph.

**sphygmograph.** An instrument used to make recordings of the pulse.

**sphygmography.** The recording of pulse tracings.

**sphygmoid.** Resembling a pulse.

**sphygmomanometer.** An instrument for measuring arterial blood pressure. See also PRESSURE: BLOOD PRESSURE.

**sphygmophone.** An instrument for rendering audible the pulse vibrations.

**sphygmoscope.** An instrument which indicates visually the pulsations of an artery.

**sphygmoscopy.** Examination of the pulse.

**sphygmotonometer.** An apparatus for determining the elasticity of the arterial walls.

**sphygmous.** Pertaining to the pulse.

**sphyra.** The malleus.

**sphyrectomy.** Surgical removal of the malleus.

**sphyrotomy.** Surgical removal of part of the malleus.

**spica.** A bandage applied in the form of a figure eight.

**spicule.** A needlelike projection.

**spiloma.** A nevus.

**spiloplania.** A skin condition characterized by transient spots.

**spiloplaxia.** Spots on the skin symptomatic of pellagra; a red spot seen on the skin in leprosy.

**spilus.** A nevus.

**spina.** Any spinous process.

**spina bifida.** A congential deformity in which there is a fissure in the lower part of the spine, allowing the spine membranes to protrude. Also called *schistorachis*.

**spina dorsalis.** The spinal column.

**spinal.** Relating to a spine, the spinal cord, or spinal column.

**spinal analgesia.** The injection into the spinal canal of local anesthetics, which paralyze the body below the level of injection.

**spinal column.** The vertebral column, consisting of the vertebrae, the intervertebral discs, and associated ligaments. See also VERTEBRA.

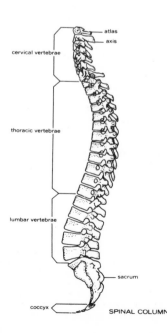

cervical vertebrae

atlas
axis

thoracic vertebrae

lumbar vertebrae

sacrum

coccyx

SPINAL COLUMN

**spinal cord.** The nerve structures and nerve pathways within the spinal column, extending from the skull opening to the level of the first or second lumbar vertebra.

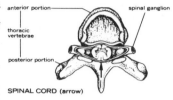

anterior portion

thoracic vertebrae

posterior portion

spinal ganglion

SPINAL CORD (arrow)

**spinate.** Shaped like a thorn.

**spina ventosa.** Enlargement and thinning of a bone due to destruction or malignant growth.

**spine.** 1. A slender, thornlike process of bone. 2. The spinal column.

**spinobulbar.** Pertaining to the spinal cord and the medulla.

**spinocerebellar.** Relating to the spinal cord and the cerebellum.

**spinoneural.** Pertaining to the spinal cord and the nerves.

**spinous.** Relating to the spine.

**spinous process.** A bony backward projection from a spinal vertebra. These projections can be felt as firm knobs under the skin if the fingers are run up the spinal column.

**spirillaemia.** See SPIRILLEMIA.

**spirillemia.** The presence of spirilla in the blood.

**spirillosis.** Any disorder caused by a microorganism of the genus *Spirillum*. This germ may produce a cattle disease commonly found in the Transvaal and a fatal disease of poultry and some other birds. One species produces rat-bite fever.

**spirillum, pl. spirilla.** A bacterium of the genus *Spirillum*, which is spiral-shaped; the species, *S. minus*, is pathogenic.

**spirobacteria.** The spinal bacteria, a group which includes the spirillum, the spirochete, and the vibrio.

**spirochaetaemia.** See SPIROCHETEMIA.

**spirochaete.** See SPIROCHETE.

**spirochaetosis.** See SPIROCHETOSIS.

**spirochaeturia.** See SPIROCHETURIA.

**spirochete.** A bacterium distinguished by slender spiral filaments and of the genus *Spirochaeta*. A general term for any bacterium of the order *Spirochaetales*, which includes the species responsible for syphilis.

**spirochetemia.** The condition in which spirochetes are found in the blood.

**spirochetosis.** A generalized infection with spirochetes.

**spirocheturia.** The presence of spirochetes in the urine.

**spirograph.** An instrument used for recording respiration.

**spiroid.** Resembling a spiral.

**spirometer.** An instrument used for measuring the capacity of the lungs. Also called *pneumonometer*.

**spirometry.** The measurement of respiration.

**spirophore.** An apparatus for performing artificial respiration.

**spissated.** Thickened; inspissated.

**spissitude.** The condition of being inspissated.

**splanchna.** The intestines or viscera.

**splanchnectopia.** Abnormal position or location of an organ.

**splanchnemphraxis.** Intestinal obstruction.

**splanchnic.** Pertaining to the viscera.

**splanchnicectomy.** Surgical excision of a part of a splanchnic nerve.

**splanchnicotomy.** Surgical division of a splanchnic nerve.

**splanchnocele.** Hernial protrusion of any abdominal organ.

**splanchnodynia.** Abdominal pain.

**splanchnolith.** An intestinal stone or concretion.

**splanchnolithiasis.** The presence of stones in the intestines.

**splanchnology.** The branch of medicine which deals with the viscera.

**splanchnomegaly.** Abnormal increase in the size of the viscera.

**splanchnomicria.** Unusual smallness in the viscera.

**splanchnopathy.** Any disease of the viscera.

**splanchnoptosis.** Prolapse of the viscera.

**splanchnosclerosis.** Hardening of the viscera.

**splanchnoscopy.** Visual inspection of the viscera.

**splanchnoskeleton.** The part of the skeleton relating to the viscera.

**splanchnotomy.** Dissection of the viscera.

**splanchnotribe.** A surgical instrument for crushing the intestines.

**splash fremitus.** A noise heard sometimes in cases of pleural effusion.

**splash in the stomach.** A sound symptomatic of lack of tone in the stomach.

**splayfoot.** Flatfoot. Also called *pes planus*.

**spleen.** A ductless, glandlike organ lying just below the diaphragm on the left side of the upper abdomen. It is purple colored, is shaped like a flattened oblong about five inches long, and weighs about six ounces. The spleen breaks down the red blood cells and has other important functions, not all of which are fully understood, but, while important, it is not essential to life. Certain diseases, such as leukemia and malaria, cause the spleen to become grossly enlarged. Animal spleens sold as pet food are called "melts."

**splenaemia.** See SPLENEMIA.

**splenalgia.** Pain arising from the spleen.

**splenatrophy.** Atrophy of the spleen. Also called *splenophthisis.*

**splenauxe.** Enlargement of the spleen. Also called *splenectasis, splenomegaly.*

**splenectasis.** Enlargement of the spleen. Also called *splenauxe, splenomegaly.*

**splenectomy.** Surgical removal of the spleen.

**splenelcosis.** Ulceration of the spleen.

**splenemia.** Splenic leukemia.

**splenemphraxis.** Congestion of the spleen.

**splenetic.** 1. Pertaining to the spleen. 2. Ill-tempered.

**splenotopia.** Displacement of the spleen. Also called *floating spleen.*

**splenic.** Pertaining to the spleen.

**spleniculus.** An accessory spleen. Also called *splenulus.*

**splenitis.** Inflammation of the spleen.

**splenization.** The alteration of a tissue or organ by congestion, so that its appearance resembles that of a spleen; usually refers to the congested state of a lung.

**splenocele.** Hernia of the spleen.

**splenocolic.** Pertaining to both the spleen and the colon.

**splenocyte.** A phagocyte found in the spleen.

**splenodynia.** Pain in the spleen.

**splenohemia.** Hyperemia of the spleen.

**splenoid.** Resembling the spleen.

**splenokeratosis.** Hardening of the spleen.

**splenoma.** A tumor of the spleen. Also called *splenoncus.*

**splenomalacia.** Softening of the spleen.

**splenomegaly.** Enlargement of the spleen. Also called *splenauxe, splenectasis, splenomegalia.*

**splenoncus.** A splenoma.

**splenopathy.** Any disease of the spleen.

**splenopexia, splenopexis, splenopexy.** Surgical fixation of a prolapsed spleen by suturing it to the abdominal wall.

**splenophrenic.** Pertaining to the spleen and the diaphragm.

**splenophthisis.** Atrophy of the spleen. Also called *splenatrophy.*

**splenopneumonia.** Pneumonia marked by alteration of the lung tissue, which takes on the appearance of spleen tissue.

**splenoptosis, splenoptosia.** Prolapse of the spleen.

**splenorrhagia.** Hemorrhage from the spleen.

**splenorrhaphy.** Suture of wounds of the spleen.

**splenotomy.** Surgical incision of the spleen.

**splenulus.** An accessory spleen; a small spleen. Also called *spleniculus.*

**spondylalgia.** Pain in a vertebra.

**spondylarthritis.** Inflammation of a vertebral joint.

**spondylarthrocace.** Tuberculosis of a vertebra.

**spondyle.** A vertebra.

**spondylexarthrosis.** Dislocation of a vertebra.

**spondylitis.** Inflammation of a vertebra.

**spondylitis ankylosans.** See SPONDYLITIS DEFORMANS, below.

**spondylitis deformans.** Spondylitis, alleged to be caused by a rheumatic affection of the joints of the spine, which become fixed, causing forward spinal deformity. The patient may be so bent forward that he has to look through his eyebrows to see where he is going. Two varieties are recognized: *Strumpell-Marie type.* This type starts in the hip joint and travels upwards fixing joints as it goes, even progressing as far as the shoulder joints. *Bechterew's type.* A rare form in which the spinal discs change into bone, the whole spine becoming one long continuous length of bone. Also called *ankylosing spondylitis.*

**spondylitis tuberculosa.** Tuberculosis of the vertebral column. Also called *Pott's disease.*

**spondylodynia.** Pain arising in the vertebrae.

**spondylolisthesis.** Deformity of the spinal column produced by the sliding forwards of a lumbar vertebra on the sacrum, thus obstructing the inlet of the pelvis.

**spondylopathy.** Any disease of the vertebrae.

**spondylopyosis.** Any suppurative disease of the vertebrae.

**spondyloschisis.** A congenital cleft in the arch of one or more vertebrae.

**spondylosis.** A painful disease complex affecting the spinal column. Degenerative changes similar to those occurring in osteoarthritis affect not only the vertebral joints but also the spinal discs and the surrounding tissues, so that pain is produced either by pressure on the nerve roots or by changes in the joints themselves.

**spondylosyndesis.** A surgical operation in which vertebrae are joined.

**spontaneous.** Voluntary, automatic; occurring without external influence.

**spontaneous fractures.** Fractures due to defects in the bone and not to violence. The bone may be thinned by a growth or be inherently weak, as in such diseases as fragilitas ossium. In these cases, the bone eventually fractures from some quite ordinary movement such as turning over in bed or even shaking hands.

**spore.** A reproductive cell from a germ or plant. This type of cell usually has a thick wall which enables it to lie inert and to survive in adverse conditions for many years. When conditions change and favor its growth, the spore loses its protective coating and commences to grow again even after such a long interval.

**sporicidal.** Destructive of spores.

**sporiferous.** Bearing spores.

**sporiparous.** Spore-producing.

**sporogenesis.** Reproduction by means of spores.

**sporogenic.** Producing spores.

**sporotrichosis.** Infection by a fungus of the genus *Sporotrichum.* It is a subacute and chronic disease usually affecting the skin, producing abscesses which are slow to heal. The condition occurs among farmers, florists, and others working with soil.

**sport.** Any animal or plant deviating from the normal.

**sporulation.** Spore formation.

**sporule.** A minute spore.

**spot.** A macula.

**sprain.** The wrenching of a joint. Not even a doctor can tell by superficial examination whether a sprain has also a fracture present, so all sprains should be treated as fractures until the part has been x-rayed. First-aid treatment consists in cold compresses and immobilization of the part.

**sprew.** See SPRUE.

**sprue.** A nonfebrile, chronic disease common in Caucasians in Sri Lanka, southeastern Asia, the East Indies, and the West Indies. It is due to an inability of the intestines to adequately absorb fat, glucose, calcium, and certain vitamins, and is characterized by the passage of large, soft, frothy stools, weakness, wasting, changes in the tongue, and anemia. Also called *tropical sprue, Ceylon sore mouth, Cochin-China diarrhea, psilosis of the intestines.*

**nontropical sprue.** This disease occurs in people who have never lived in the tropics, and although resembling sprue in many respects it is really the adult variety of celiac disease. The underlying disturbance is interference with the function of the small intestine and is related to an intolerance to glutin, which interferes with the absorption of fat. The main features of the condition are steatorrhea with or without diarrhea, and sometimes dilatation of the colon, tetany, osteomalacia, anemia of various types, skin eruptions, and frequently failure of development. With certain rare exceptions, the condition arises in childhood, although it may remain unrecognized until adult life. It is more common in females than males, and sometimes runs in families. Also called *adult celiac disease, Gee-Herter disease, Gee-Thaysen disease, Herter-Heubner disease.*

**spud.** A surgical instrument. One type is used to detach foreign substances from the cornea and another to strip off mucous membrane in operations necessitating the removal of bone.

**spur.** A sharp projection or point, usually of bone.

**spurious.** Not genuine.

**sputum.** The material ejected from the mouth. It is saliva mixed with mucus and other substances from the respiratory tract.

**squama.** A scale or scalelike substance.

**squamate.** Scaly.

**squamous.** Shaped like a scale; scaly.

**squarrious, squarrose, squarrous.** Scurfy.

**squint.** See STRABISMUS.

**convergent squint.** One in which the eye is turned inwards.

**divergent squint.** One in which the eye is turned outwards.

**stable.** Unlikely to break down or dissolve; likely to retain its composition under the application of physical or chemical forces.

**staff.** An instrument for passing through the urethra into the bladder and used as a guide in operations on the bladder or for operating on strictures.

**stage.** The definite period of a disease characterized by certain symptoms.

**staggers.** A term applied to various diseases which are characterized by lack of coordination in movement and a staggering gait, such as gid of sheep, encephalomyelitis of horses, botulism, loco poisoning, grass tetany, and some brain diseases, such as Parkinson's disease and tabes dorsalis.

**stagnation.** 1. A cessation of motion. 2. In pathology, a cessation of motion in any fluid; stasis. 3. In dentistry, the accumulation of debris on a tooth because its antagonist in the other jaw has been removed.

**staircase sign or phenomenon.** A difficulty in walking downstairs, an early symptom of locomotor ataxia.

**stammering.** Hesitant or interrupted speech. This is a frequent speech de-

fect in emotional children and persists only when the child loses confidence in his ability to speak and when his difficulty becomes an obsession. Encouragement is the best cure—teasing makes the difficulty worse. See also STUTTERING.

**stanch.** To restrain or stop a flow, particularly of blood.

**stapedectomy.** Surgical removal of the stapes.

**stapedial.** Pertaining to or shaped like the stapes.

**stapediovestibular.** Pertaining to both the stapes and the vestibule.

**stapes.** The innermost of the three ossicles of the ear. It is shaped like a stirrup.

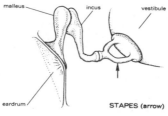

STAPES (arrow)

**staph.** An abbreviation for staphylococcus.

**staphyle.** The uvula.

**staphylectomy.** Surgical removal of the uvula.

**staphyline.** Pertaining to the uvula.

**staphylitis.** Inflammation of the uvula.

**staphyloangina.** An inflammation of the throat, producing a pseudomembrane, caused by staphylococci.

**staphylococcaemia.** See STAPHYLOCOCCEMIA.

**staphylococcemia.** The presence of staphylococci in the blood. Also called *staphylohemia.*

**staphylococcal.** Pertaining to staphylococci.

**staphylococcic.** Pertaining to staphylococci.

**Staphylococcus.** A genus of bacteria, so called because when cultured on nutrient media they form into clusters resembling a bunch of grapes. There are many different types of staphylococci, only a few of which are harmful to man.

**Staphylococcus albus.** A species of bacteria which grows in white colonies. It may cause boils but is only weakly poisonous to man.

**Staphylococcus aureus.** A species of bacteria which grows in yellow colonies and the most virulent of the group. It is found in boils and carbuncles.

**Staphylococcus citreus.** A species of bacteria which grows in lemon-yellow colonies and is not very poisonous to man.

**staphylodermatitis.** Inflammation or disease of the skin caused by staphylococci.

**staphyledema.** Edema of the uvula.

**staphyloedema.** See STAPHYLEDEMA.

**staphylohaemia.** See STAPHYLOHEMIA.

**staphylohemia.** The presence of staphylococci in the blood. Also called *staphylococcemia.*

**staphyloma.** A bulging of the cornea or sclera.

**staphylomatous.** Pertaining to the staphyloma.

**staphyloncus.** A tumor or swelling of the uvula.

**staphyloplasty.** Surgical repair of the uvula.

**staphyloptosis.** Elongation of the uvula.

**staphylorrhaphy.** The suturing of a cleft soft palate.

**staphyloschisis.** A cleft of the uvula.

**staphylotome.** A surgical knife used in operations on the uvula.

**staphylotomy.** 1. Incising or detaching a part of the uvula. 2. Incision into a staphyloma.

**stasimorphy.** The deformity caused by arrested development.

**stasis.** Cessation of flow of any body fluid, particularly the blood.

**intestinal stasis.** Constipation.

**venous stasis.** Venous congestion or insufficiency.

**state.** A condition.

**anxiety state.** A psychoneurosis marked by almost continuous anxiety and apprehension, with attacks of fear and panic, and characterized by palpitations, shortness of breath, nausea, and other physical effects of nervous irritability of the organs.

**cataleptic state.** The retention of limbs in positions into which they are placed, such as occurs in hypnosis.

**cataleptoid state.** A condition due to neuromuscular excitability and differing from true catalepsy in that the limbs must be held in fixed attitudes for a few seconds before they may retain that position.

**depressive state.** Mental disorders characterized by extreme depression.

**resting state.** In biology, a state of suspended activity—the condition of perennial plants, spores, and seeds during their period of dormancy.

**typhoid state.** A condition in which the patient is slumped in bed in stupor, with dry, brown tongue, sordes on the teeth, rapid feeble pulse, incontinence of feces and urine, and rapid wasting; seen in typhoid and other continued fevers.

**statoliths.** Minute stones or concretions found in the labyrinth of the ear.

**status.** A state or condition, often a severe or intractable condition.

**status asthmaticus.** Rapidly recurring attacks of asthma; or a prolonged asthmatic attack which refuses to respond to treatment and in which the patient's general condition is deteriorating.

**status epilepticus.** A condition in which one epileptic fit follows another in rapid succession without periods of consciousness between them.

**status lymphaticus.** A condition in which the lymphoid tissues are very prominent in the body, especially the thymus gland and spleen. It is alleged to cause sudden death, especially if the patient has to undergo anesthesia. Many authorities dispute the existence of this condition.

**statuvolence.** A voluntary, self-induced state of hypnotism.

**stauroplegia.** Crossed hemiplegia, which is paralysis affecting a part on one side of the body and another part on the other side.

**steapsin.** Lipase, an enzyme of the pancreatic juice.

**steariform.** Resembling fat.

**stearodermia.** A disease of the sebaceous glands of the skin.

**stearorrhea.** See SEBORRHEA.

**stearorrhoea.** See SEBORRHEA.

**steatitis.** Inflammation of fatty tissues.

**steatocele.** A fatty swelling occurring within the scrotum.

**steatogenous.** Producing fat.

**steatolysis.** The chemical process through which fats pass prior to their absorption into the system.

**steatolytic.** Pertaining to steatolysis.

**steatoma.** A fatty tumor; a sebaceous cyst.

**steatomatosis.** The formation of a large number of sebaceous cysts.

**steatopathy.** Any disease of the sebaceous glands.

**steatopygia.** Excess accumulation of fat in the buttocks.

**steatorrhea.** An increased flow of the secretion of the sebaceous glands in the skin; fatty stools.

**steatorrhoea.** See STEATORRHEA.

**steatosis.** An obsolete term for fatty degeneration or disease of sebaceous glands; also applied to abnormal fat deposits.

**stegnosis.** The closing of a passage. Also called *stenosis*.

**stellate.** Star-shaped.

**stellectomy.** Surgical removal of the stellate nerve ganglion (a spinal nerve network in the neck).

**stenocardia.** See ANGINA PECTORIS.

**stenocephalia, stenocephaly.** Abnormal narrowness of the head.

**stenocephalous.** Possessing a narrow head.

**stenochoria.** Partial obstruction, narrowing, particularly narrowing of a lacrimal duct.

**stenocoriasis.** Narrowing of the pupil of the eye.

**stenokoriasis.** See STENOCORIASIS.

**stenopaeic.** See STENOPEIC.

**stenopeic.** Having a narrow slit.

**stenosed.** Constricted.

**stenosis.** Contriction or narrowing, especially of a channel or aperture.

**aortic stenosis.** Narrowing of the aorta. It may particularly refer to a narrowing of the aortic valve area in the heart.

**cicatricial stenosis.** Contracture or narrowing produced by a scar.

**granulation stenosis.** Narrowing caused by the encroachment or contraction of granulation tissues.

**mitral stenosis.** Narrowing of the mitral valve of the heart, causing obstruction to the flow of blood through the left atrioventricular opening. It is a sequel to rheumatic fever.

**pyloric stenosis.** A congential obstruction of the pyloric opening of the stomach, resulting in intractable, forcible vomiting in babies. The usual cure is an operation to split the pyloric muscular valve. See RAMSTEDT'S OPERATION.

**stenostomia.** Narrowing of the mouth, usually the result of scarring.

**stenothermal.** Capable of resisting only a small range of temperature.

**stenothorax.** Unusual narrowing of the chest.

**stenotic.** Marked or caused by stenosis.

**Stensen's duct.** The tube carrying the saliva from the parotid gland into the mouth and opening on the inside of the cheek.

**stepping gait.** The peculiar high-stepping gait seen in tabes dorsalis and some forms of multiple neuritis.

**stercobilin.** The chief constituent of the brown coloring found in feces; derived from bilirubin, which originates in the gall bladder, and reduced by the action of bacteria in the intestine. When there is complete obstruction to the entry of bile into the intestinal tract, there is an absence of stercobilin in the stools. Also called *hydrobilirubin, urobilin.*

**stercolith.** A calcified, fecal concretion.

**stercoraceous, stercoral, stercorous.** Fecal.

**stercus.** Dung; feces.

**stereoagnosis.** Failure to recognize an object by touching. Also called *astereognosis.*

**stereognosis.** The faculty of recognizing the nature of an object by touch.

**stereognostic.** Relating to sterognosis.

**stereogram, stereography.** A stereoscopic x-ray picture.

**Stereo-orthopter.** A proprietary mirror-reflecting instrument for treating squints by orthoptics.

**stereoscope.** An instrument by which two pictures can be viewed simultaneously, thereby giving a three-dimensional effect.

**stereoscopic.** Pertaining to stereoscopy.

**stereoscopy.** The combination of two pictures by means of a stereoscope.

**stereoskiagraphy.** Stereographic photography by means of x-rays.

**sterile.** 1. Barren, infertile. 2. Free from germs, aseptic.

**sterile abscess.** An abscess in which bacteria or other causal agents have ceased to exist, the inflammation has subsided, and the pus remains a cyst.

**sterility.** 1. The condition of being incapable of producing young. 2. Freedom from germs.

**sterilization.** 1. The removal or destruction of all forms of life, especially microorganisms. 2. Any procedure, such as a surgical operation, which renders an individual incapable of reproduction.

*Substances may be sterilized by physical or chemical methods, heat being the most important. Moist heat at temperatures above the boiling point of water will kill the most resistant spores formed by germs, within a short time, and germs may be destroyed by putting the article to be sterilized in an autoclave (a high-pressure steam apparatus). A tablespoonful of methylated spirit thrown into the bottom of a bucket and then carefully lit will sterilize the walls of the bucket. Heating dressings between two enamel pie dishes in an oven will dry-sterilize the dressings, and metal objects can be sterilized by boiling them in water for ten minutes. Chemical agents, such as disinfectants, will sterilize objects if the objects are immersed for a given length of time. Irradiation by rays will sterilize without contaminating the objects and is used for sterilizing both hypodermic syringes and food. Drains can be sterilized by strong disinfectants such as the cresol derivatives.*

**sterilize.** To make sterile.

**sterilizer.** An apparatus for destroying germs by heat.

**sternad.** Towards the sternal aspect of the body.

**sternal.** Relating to the sternum.

**sternalgia.** Pain in the sternum.

**sternoclavicular.** Pertaining to the sternum and the clavicle.

**sternocostal.** Pertaining to the sternum and the ribs.

**sternoid.** Like the sternum.

**sternomastoid.** Pertaining to the sternum and the mastoid process (a projection of the temporal bone behind the ear).

**sternothyroid.** Pertaining to the sternum and the thyroid cartilage.

**sternotracheal.** Pertaining to the sternum and the trachea.

**sternum.** The breastbone. It is composed of three parts: the top part is called the manubrium, and articulates with the clavicles, the center portion is called the gladiolus; and the lower end is known as the ensiform, or xiphoid, cartilage. The first seven ribs on each side are attached to the sternum by cartilaginous joints.

**sternutation.** An obsolete term for sneezing.

**sternutator.** An agent capable of inducing sneezing, as certain war gases.

**sternutatory.** Producing or causing sneezing.

**steroid.** A group name for compounds which resemble cholesterol chemically. The group includes sex hormones, bile acids, sterols, and some cancer-stimulating hydrocarbons.

**stertor.** Snoring.

**stertorous.** Marked by stertor.

**stethograph.** An instrument for registering the respiratory movements of the chest.

**stethokyrtograph.** An instrument for measuring the curves of the chest.

**stethoscope.** An instrument for the detection and study of sounds arising from within the body.

**binaural stethoscope.** This is the familiar type of stethoscope in common use. It consists of a bell or cup-shaped endpiece of metal or hard rubber connected to two rubber tubes which conduct the sound to both ears of the doctor.

**electronic stethoscope.** A type of stethoscope consisting of a minute microphone attached to an amplifier, from which the sounds are boosted either directly to the doctor's ears or to a loudspeaker. It is of great advantage not only for studying very faint and distant sounds arising from within the body but also to doctors who are hard of hearing.

**obstetric stethoscope.** A type of stethoscope used for listening to the unborn baby's heart through the mother's abdomen. It resembles the original stethoscope and consists of a slender metal or plastic tube with a small flange at one end and a wide trumpetlike opening at the other.

*Invented by the French physician Laennec in 1816, the early stethoscope consisted of a slender wooden tube with a flange at each end. One end was applied to the patient's chest or abdomen and the other to the doctor's ear.*

*When Dr. Laennec first used his stethoscope his patients regarded it with suspicion and accused him of impudently prying into God's secrets. They labeled the instrument "The Devil's Trumpet," and so great was their superstition that they claimed the stethoscope left "round, red, witch marks on their skins, dried up their lights, made them spit blood, and threw them into sweats." Thus did these early patients, suffering with symptoms of tuberculosis, blame the doctor for their disease.*

**stethoscopic.** Relating to a stethoscope.

**stethoscopy.** Examination by means of a stethoscope.

**Stevens-Johnson syndrome.** A severe variety of erythema multiforme characterized by skin rashes involving the mouth and by lesions on the cornea and conjunctiva, which may lead to blindness. See also ERYTHEMA: ERYTHEMA MULTIFORME.

**sthenia.** Normal health and strength.

**sthenic.** Strong and active.

**stibialism.** Poisoning with antimony.

**stictacne.** Acne in which the pustules are tiny and surround the blackhead.

**stigma.** 1. A small spot or mark, especially a hemorrhagic spot in the palm or sole, sometimes found in hysterical people; any mark or sign characteristic of a disease or condition. 2. An opening between cells; a stoma.

**baker's stigmas.** Corns on the backs of the fingers from kneading dough.

**hereditary stigmas.** Psychic stigmas resembling those of an ancestor and supposed to be inherited.

**hysterical stigmas.** The peculiar symptoms characteristic of hysteria, such as anesthesia (loss of sensitivity), hyperesthesia (increase of sensitivity), reversal of the visual color field, loss of vision when excited, and impairment of hearing, taste, and muscular sense.

**psychic stigmas.** Certain mental states characterized by susceptibility to particular suggestions.

**stigmata.** The plural of stigma; stigmas.

**stigmata nigra.** The black spots caused by grains of gunpowder in the skin. In legal medicine, proof that a gunshot wound must have been made at close range.

**stigmatic.** Relating to a stigma.

**stigmatism.** 1. The condition of having stigmata. 2. The property of a lens system in which rays of light from a single point converge on a single focal point.

**stigmatization.** The formation of stigmata.

**stilbestrol.** A chemical with all the properties of the female sex hormone. It is used in small doses to control the symptoms of the menopause. In large doses, it will suppress breast milk in the nursing mother and control some forms of cancer in the male.

**stilboestrol.** See STILBESTROL.

**stilet, stilette.** A probe.

**stillbirth.** The birth of a dead child after the 28th week of pregnancy. Prior to the 28th week of pregnancy it would be called a miscarriage or abortion.

**stillborn.** Born dead.

**Still's disease.** Chronic polyarthritis which affects children and is marked by enlargement of lymph glands and spleen and by irregular fever.

**sting.** A sharp prick with an acute burning sensation. It can be caused when the fine hairs on the stinging nettle—the stinging organ located in the tail of the wasp and bee, the head of gnats, or the claws of centipedes—inject poison into the skin. The skin reaction is usually of a local, temporary, reversible inflammatory type, but if the sting apparatus carries pollen this may cause a violent constitutional reaction in hypersensitive people. Some people can become so sensitized by a sting that on receiving a subsequent sting of the same type, they develop an anaphylactic reaction, which has, on occasions, killed the victim. If the insect's sting apparatus is still embedded in the skin, it should be gently eased out with the point of a sterile needle rather than squeezed, for squeezing merely empties more of the poison into the wound. Since the insect may have carried germs to the spot on its feet, first aid consists of applying an antiseptic and then either a soothing cream made up of bicarbonate of soda or calamine lotion. Doctors sometimes prescibe the application of an antihistamine cream, and, in severe cases, the taking of an antihistamine tablet internally.

**stirrup.** See STAPES.

**stitch.** 1. A sudden sharp pain occurring in a muscle, usually the diaphragm, after unaccustomed exercise. 2. To sew with thread, catgut, etc. through tissue, as treatment in fixing an organ or aligning edges of a wound. 3. A suture.

**stitch abscess.** An abscess occurring around the knot of a surgical stitch.

**Stokes-Adams disease.** Also called *Stokes-Adams syndrome.* See ADAMS-STOKES DISEASE.

**stoma.** 1. A minute opening or pore in a surface of a plant or animal. 2. A small opening providing communication between neighbouring lymph cells. 3. An opening created on the surface of the abdominal wall by operations such as colostomy.

**stomacace.** Ulceration of the mouth. Also called *stomatocace.* See also STOMATITIS; ULCERATIVE STOMATITIS.

**stomach.** The oval-shaped digestive pouch situated below the diaphragm in the upper part of the abdomen. The upper, or cardiac, end connects with the esophagus and the lower, or pyloric, end with the duodenum. The stomach is made up of four coats: an outer peritoneal, or serous, coat; a muscular coat made up of longitudinal, oblique, and circular fibers; a submucous coat; and a mucous coat. The mucous coat contains glands that secrete the gastric juice, which contains mucus and hydrochloric acid.

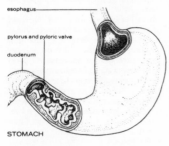

esophagus

pylorus and pyloric valve

duodenum

STOMACH

**stomachalgia.** Pain in the stomach.
**stomachic.** Pertaining to the stomach; any substance which stimulates the secretory activity of the stomach and thus enhances appetite.
**stomatalgia.** Pain in the mouth.
**stomatitis.** Inflammation of the mouth.
  **aphthous stomatitis.** A form characterized by the presence of small, white vesicles on the lining membrane of the mouth, whether on tongue, lips, or cheek. These minute blisters break down and leave a raw, sensitive ulcer which makes eating painful. Great relief can be obtained by painting each ulcer with either carbolic or chromic acid. The exact cause of this condition has not yet been determined.
  **arsenical stomatitis.** Necrotic stomatitis due to arsenical poisoning.
  **catarrhal stomatitis.** A simple form of stomatitis characterized by swelling.
  **epidemic stomatitis.** An acute infectious condition of the mouth occurring in epidemics.
  **epizootic stomatitis.** See FOOT AND MOUTH DISEASE.
  **gangrenous stomatitis.** Inflammation of the mouth accompanied by necrosis. Also called *cancrum oris, noma, stomatonecrosis.*
  **herpetic stomatitis.** A form of stomatitis characterized by the presence of blisters or cold sores.

  **membranous stomatitis.** Inflammation of the mouth accompanied by the presence of an adventitious membrane.
  **mercurial stomatitis.** Stomatitis due to the excessive absorption of mercury.
  **mycotic stomatitis.** See THRUSH.
  **parasitic stomatitis.** See THRUSH.
  **ulcerative stomatitis.** A type of stomatitis characterized by shallow ulcers on tongue, cheeks, and lips. Also called *stomacace, stomatocace.*
  **Vincent's stomatitis.** A gangrenous, membranous form of stomatitis associated with the presence of Vincent's spirillum. Also called *trench mouth.*
**stomatocace.** Ulcerative stomatitis. Also called *stomacace.*
**stomatology.** The study of diseases of the mouth.
**stomatomycosis.** Any fungous disease of the mouth.
**stomatonecrosis.** Also called *cancrum oris.* See NOMA.
**stomatonoma.** Gangrene of the mouth.
**stomatopathy.** Any disease of the mouth.
**stomatoplasty.** Surgical repair of the mouth.
**stomatorrhagia.** Bleeding from the mouth.
**stomatoschisis.** See HARELIP.
**stone.** A concretion or calculus.
**stool.** The feces; the matter evacuated from the bowels.
  **acholic stools.** Light grey or clay-colored stools having the consistency of putty, which follow the obstruction of the flow of bile into the duodenum. They contain an abnormal amount of undigested fat, and are usually associated with jaundice, and with bile in the urine. Stools of similar color may occur in disorders of the pancreas, when they contain an excessive amount of fat but there is no associated obstruction to the flow of bile.
  **caddy stools.** Stools resembling fine, dark, sandy mud and seen in yellow fever.
  **fatty stools.** Stools in which fat is present due either to pancreatic disease, sprue, or celiac disease.
  **green stools.** Stools seen in babies when the contents of the intestine are rushed through before the bile has been digested, so that they emerge as green instead of the normal yellow-brown. If the baby is symptom free and gaining weight regularly and adequately it is of no significance.
  **lead-pencil stools.** Stools of small caliber, usually due to intestinal spasm, stricture, or to stenosis of the sigmoid colon or rectum. Also called *ribbon stools.*

  **meconium stools.** The pasty, greenish mass, consisting of mucous tissue cells, bile, lanugo hairs, and vernix caseosa that collects in the intestines and forms the first fecal discharge of the newborn three or four days after birth. It is a normal phenomenon.
  **mucous stools.** Stools which contain a lot of mucus; an indication of intestinal inflammation.
  **pea-soup stools.** Descriptive of the stools passed in typhoid fever.
  **putty stools.** See ACHOLIC STOOLS, above.
  **rice-water stools.** The watery stools occurring during attacks of cholera.
  **sheep-dung stools.** Small, round, fecal masses, similar to the dung of sheep, which may occur in cases of starvation or hunger or those on a severely restricted, nonresidual diet.
  **tarry stools.** Black stools which consist of digested blood due to bleeding occurring inside the intestinal tract. These have to be differentiated from the grey stools produced by taking bismuth medicines and the greyblack stools seen following the taking of iron medicines.
**strabismal, strabismic.** Relating to strabismus.
**strabismus.** A squint in the eye. In the early months of life transient squints are commonplace and do not signify anything untoward. In early infancy, pronounced and permanent squints usually indicate a disorder of the eyeball muscles. Variable and fleeting squints are sometimes seen during the course of a disease, such as meningitis. The commonest age to observe squints is from two to six years, and the most important causes are errors of refraction, general weakness, and nervous instability. In many cases, however, once the refractive error is corrected by spectacles the squint disappears. In the older child, squints can be treated by orthoptic methods, that is, by exercises designed to develop and train the eye muscles to become coordinated. If a squint remains uncorrected, the brain will eventually suppress, sometimes permanently, the vision in the affected eye. It is for this reason that a squinting eye is often completely covered for several months until the squint has been corrected, and why all children with squints should be seen by eye specialists to determine the best means of preserving the sight and correcting the squint. See also SQUINT.
**strabometer.** An apparatus for measuring the optical deviation in a squint.
**Strachan's disease.** See PELLAGRA.
**strain.** **1.** Excessive stretching or overuse of a part; the condition produced by wrong use or overuse, such as eye strain; to overexert, make violent

efforts. **2.** A group of organisms or plants closely related to each other. **3.** In pharmacy, to filter.

**strangle. 1.** To choke or throttle by compression of the trachea. **2.** The closing of any opening by constriction.

**strangulated.** Strangled; constricted in such a way as to stop the circulation, as for instance a strangulated hernia.

**strangulation.** The act of choking; occlusion caused by the arrest of circulation to a part.

**stranguria, strangury.** The passing of urine drop by drop accompanied by pain.

**stratified.** Arranged in layers.

**stratiform.** Formed in layers.

**stratum.** A layer.

**strawberry mark.** A nevus, a red mark visible on the skin of a baby shortly after birth.

**strawberry tongue.** The description of the tongue in cases of scarlet fever.

**strephosymbolia. 1.** A disorder in which objects seem reversed as in a mirror. **2.** The difficulty experienced by some children in learning to read through inability to distinguish between similar letters such as *p* and *q* or *n* and *u*. It is occasionally an expression of the fight between the left and right halves of the brain to determine which half is to be dominant, and many children with this difficulty eventually show themselves to be left-handed.

**streptobacillus.** A type of bacillus forming twisted chains.

**streptobacteria.** Short, rod-shaped bacteria grouped together in the form of twisted chains; a bacterium of the genus *Streptobacillus.*

**streptococcaemia.** See STREPTOCOC-CEMIA.

**streptococcemia.** The presence of streptococci in the blood.

**streptococcal.** Relating to a streptococcus.

**streptococcus.** Circular or oval-shaped bacteria which form chains and belong to the genus *Streptococcus.* There are many types; included in this classification is *Streptococcus pyogenes,* the germ that causes scarlet fever, erysipelas, and many other infections; also called *hemolytic streptococcus.*

**streptomycin.** An antibiotic drug.

**streptomycosis.** A disease condition caused by a fungus of the genus *Streptomyces.*

**streptosepticaemia.** See STREPTOSEP-TICEMIA.

**streptosepticemia.** The presence of streptococci in the blood, causing a form of septicemia.

**streptothricosis.** An infection caused by a fungus of the genus *Streptothrix.* Also called *streptotrichosis.*

**Streptothrix.** A genus of fungi.

**stria.** A streak or line.

**striae.** Plural of stria; streaks or lines.

**striae atrophicae.** Whitish wrinkles or lines on the skin of the abdomen or breasts following stretching by obesity, pregnancy, or other cause.

**striae gravidarum.** The white lines seen on the skin of the abdomen in women who have borne children or who have been pregnant.

**striate, striated.** Striped or streaked.

**striation.** The condition of being striped or streaked; any striated structure.

**stricture.** Abnormal narrowing of a canal or hollow organ being the result of inflammatory or other changes in the wall of the organ. Stricture occasionally occurs through external pressure.

**stridor.** A harsh, vibrating sound produced during expiration in certain conditions. See also LARYNGISMUS.

**stridulous.** Affected with stridor.

**strobiloid.** Having the appearance of tapeworm segments.

**stroke. 1.** A sudden severe attack, as in paralysis or sunstroke; a brain catastrophe in which a blood vessel bursts and bleeding occurs into the skull. **2.** To pass the hands gently over the body.

**apoplectic stroke.** A stroke due to the bursting of a blood vessel within the brain. The patient suddenly becomes unconscious, with a red face and stertorous breathing. If the patient survives, he may be left with one side of his body paralyzed.

**paralytic stroke.** Sudden loss of muscular power from some disease of the brain or spinal cord.

**stroke volume.** The quantity of blood ejected by the left ventricle during a single heartbeat.

**stroma.** The supporting framework of an organ.

**stromal.** Pertaining to a stroma.

**stromatolysis.** Destruction of a stroma.

**strongyloides.** A species of intestinal roundworms.

**strongyloidosis.** To be infested with strongyloides.

**strophulus.** A popular name for a skin condition of infants and young children, probably caused by a mild gastrointestinal disturbance. The skin eruption consists of shotty papules which may be pale or pink and are usually more numerous on the limbs, but which may occur on the loins and about the waist. Occasionally the rash may resemble urticaria. Itching may be a prominent feature of the eruption. Also called *lichen urticatus, papular urticaria, gum rash.*

**struma. 1.** Scrofula. **2.** A goiter.

**strumiprivous.** Caused by surgical excision of the thyroid gland.

**strumitis.** Inflammation of a thyroid gland already affected with goiter.

**strumoderma.** A skin disorder due to tuberculosis of the skin. Also called *scrofuloderma.*

**strumous.** Pertaining to scrofula or to goiter.

**strychnine.** A poisonous alkaloid obtained from the seeds of the tree *Strychnos nux vomica.* It is a powerful stimulant to the central nervous system, has a very bitter taste, and is used in medicines to stimulate the appetite and improve the digestion. In poisonous doses the drug causes violent contraction of muscles to a point when the body may be arched, resting on the heels and the back of the skull, and the violence may be such as to rupture the abdominal muscles. The violent muscular spasm also gives rise to a contorted grin called risus sardonicus.

**strychninism.** Poisoning by strychnine.

**strychninomania.** Delirium caused by strychnine poisoning.

**Strychnos.** A genus of tropical trees from the seeds of which strychnine is obtained.

**stupe.** A cloth used for applying heat or counterirritation, especially a cloth wrung out of hot water and sprinkled with a counterirritant, such as turpentine, eucalyptus, or eau de Cologne.

**stupefacient.** A narcotic.

**stupor.** Being only partly conscious.

**stuporous.** Affected with stupor; sleepy.

**stuttering.** A type of hesitating speech characterized by repeated attempts to pronounce a syllable or word. See also STAMMERING.

**sty, stye.** A tiny abscess formed in an eyelash follicle.

**stylet.** A small probe; a wire passed into a hollow, such as a hypodermic needle, in order to keep the channel clear. Also called *stilette.*

**styloid.** Shaped like a stylus.

**styloiditis.** Inflammation of the structures around the styloid process (a projection of the temporal bone).

**stylomastoid.** Pertaining to the styloid and the mastoid processes (projections of the temporal bone).

**stylomaxillary.** Relating to the styloid process (a projection of the temporal bone) and the maxilla.

**stylus, stylet.** A pointed instrument for making applications.

**stymatosis.** An obsolete term for a violent erection of the penis accompanied by hemorrhage.

**stype.** A plug of wool or sponge. Also called *tampon, pledget.*

**styptic.** An agent, such as alum or tannic acid, that checks bleeding by causing contraction of the blood vessels.

**subabdominal.** Below the abdomen.

**subacetabular.** Below the acetabulum.

**subacromial.** Beneath the acromion.

**subacute.** A stage between acute and chronic illness.

**subaponeurotic.** Beneath an aponeurosis.

**subarachnoid.** Located beneath the arachnoid.

**subarachnoid hemorrhage.** Bleeding into the subarachnoid space, that is, between the two innermost of the three membranes covering the brain. *This hemorrhage may be caused by head injuries or by disease. When caused by disease it is usually due to rupture of a small aneurysm of an artery on the brain surface. It may occur in a young adult without warning, causing a sudden blinding, intense headache, rapidly followed by loss of consciousness and accompanied by profuse sweating of the body. Sometimes the skull has to be opened in order to relieve the pressure on the brain, remove the blood clot, and tie the artery.*

**subarachnoiditis.** Inflammation of the undersurface of the arachnoid; a form of meningitis.

**subarcuate.** Slightly arched.

**subareolar.** Beneath the areolar space or pigmented tissue such as that surrounding the nipples.

**subastragalar, subastragaloid.** Beneath the astragalus (one of the bones forming the ankle joint).

**subastringent.** Slightly astringent.

**subaural.** Beneath the ear.

**subaxillary.** Below the axilla.

**subcartilaginous.** Beneath a cartilage.

**subcerebellar.** Beneath the cerebellum.

**subcerebral.** Beneath the cerebrum.

**subchondral.** Beneath a cartilage.

**subchordal.** Beneath or below the vocal cords.

**subclavian, subclavicular.** Beneath the clavicle.

**subclinical.** Appplied to a disease in which signs and symptoms are so slight as to be unnoticeable and even not demonstrable. A condition which is inferred rather than diagnosed.

**subconjunctival.** Lying beneath the conjunctiva.

**subconscious, subconsciousness.** State of being partly conscious.

**subcoracoid.** Beneath the coracoid process.

**subcortical.** Lying beneath the cortex of an organ.

**subcostal.** Beneath a rib.

**subcranial.** Beneath the cranium.

**subcrepitant.** Only slightly crepitant.

**subculture.** A secondary bacterial culture made from a primary culture.

**subcutaneous.** Beneath the skin.

**subcuticular.** Beneath the epidermis.

**subdelirium.** Mild delirium.

**subdiaphragmatic.** Beheath the diaphragm.

**subdiaphragmatic abscess.** See SUBPHRENIC ABSCESS.

**subdorsal.** Beneath the dorsal area.

**subdural.** Beneath the dura.

**subendocardial.** Beneath the endocardium.

**subendothelial.** Beneath the endothelial structure.

**subepidermal, subepidermic.** Beneath the epidermis.

**subepiglottic.** Below the epiglottis.

**subepithelial.** Beneath an epithelial surface.

**subepithelium.** A structure beneath an epithelial surface.

**subfascial.** Beneath a fascia.

**subfebrile.** A moderate rise in temperature.

**subfrontal.** Beneath a frontal lobe of the brain.

**subgingival.** Beneath the gums.

**subglenoid.** Beneath the glenoid cavity.

**subglossal.** Beneath the tongue; sublingual.

**subglottic.** Below the glottis.

**subhepatic.** Beneath the liver.

**subhyoid.** Beneath the hyoid.

**subicteric.** Slightly jaundiced.

**subiliac.** Below the ilium.

**subilium.** The lowest part of the ilium.

**subinfection.** A slight infection; a chronic poisoning of the system by small doses of germ toxin.

**subinflammation.** A slight degree of inflammation.

**subintrant.** Literally means to enter by stealth, and is applied to malaria and other fevers in which a fresh attack starts before the first one has ended.

**subinvolution.** Imperfect return to normal size of an organ after it has been enlarged; usually refers to incomplete contraction of the womb following childbirth.

**subjective.** Relating only to the individual concerned; a term used to indicate that the symptoms of which the patient complains are probably imaginary and for which there is no supporting evidence. On some occasions it is a polite way of indicating that the patient is malingering.

**sublatio.** Removal.

**sublatio retinae.** Detachment of the retina.

**sublimation.** 1. The act of vaporizing and condensing a solid. 2. In psychiatry, an unconscious psychic device whereby undesirable primitive cravings gain outward expression by converting their energies into socially acceptable activities. Freud used the term to indicate the deviation of sexual feelings to aims and objects of a nonsexual character.

**subliminal.** Below the threshold of consciousness or awareness.

**sublingual.** Beneath the tongue. Also called *subglossal.*

**sublobular.** Beneath a lobule.

**sublumbar.** Beneath the lumbar area.

**subluxation.** An incomplete dislocation of a joint.

**submammary.** Beneath the breast.

**submandibular.** Situated below the mandible.

**submarginal.** Beneath a marginal area.

**submaxilla.** The lower jaw. Also called *mandible.*

**submaxillary.** Beneath the lower jaw; relating to the submaxillary salivary glands.

**submedial.** Beneath the middle.

**submembranous.** Partly membranous.

**submeningeal.** Beneath the meninges.

**submental.** Beneath the chin. See also MENTAL

**submicron.** A particle so small that it is only visible with the aid of an electronic microscope.

**submicroscopical.** Too minute to be seen with a microscope.

**submorphous.** Partly crystalline and partly amorphous in nature.

**submucosa.** The space or area beneath a mucous membrane.

**submucous.** Beneath a mucous membrane.

**subneural.** Beneath a nerve.

**subnutrition.** Defective nutrition.

**suboccipital.** Beneath the occiput.

**suborbital.** Beneath the orbit of the eye.

**subordination.** 1. The condition of being under subjection. 2. The condition of organs that depend upon or are controlled by other organs.

**subparietal.** Beneath the parietal bone, situated on the side of the skull.

**subpatellar.** Beneath the patella.

**subpectoral.** Beneath the chest or beneath the pectoral muscle of the chest.

**subpeduncular.** Beneath a peduncle.

**subpericardial.** Beneath the pericardium.

**subperiosteal.** Beneath the periostium.

**subperitoneal.** Beneath the peritoneum.

**subpharyngeal.** Beneath the pharynx.

**subphrenic.** Beneath the diaphragm. Also called *subdiaphragmatic.*

**subphrenic abscess.** An abscess situated below the diaphragm. Also called *subdiaphragmatic abscess.*

**subpituitarism.** The state of having a poorly functioning pituitary gland.

**subplacenta.** The decidua basalis.

**subplacental.** Beneath the placenta; pertaining to the decidua basalis.

**subpleural.** Lying beneath the pleura.

**subplexal.** Beneath a plexus.

**subpreputial.** Beneath the prepuce.

**subprostatic.** Beneath the prostate gland.

**subpubic.** Beneath the pubic arch or symphysis of the pelvis.

**subpulmonary.** Beneath the lungs.

**subrectal.** Below the rectum.

**subretinal.** Beneath the retina.

**subscapular.** Beneath the scapula; relating to the subscapularis muscle.

**subscleral.** Beneath the sclera.

**subserous.** Beneath a serous membrane, such as those lining the joints.

**subsidence.** The gradual abatement of the signs and symptoms of a disease.

**subspinous.** Beneath a spine; beneath a spinal column.

**substantia alba.** The white matter of the brain and nerves.

**substantia cinerea.** The grey matter of the brain and spinal cord.

**substantia propria.** The essential tissue of a structure or organ; the framework of an organ.

**substernal.** Beneath the sternum.

**substitution.** 1. The replacement of one thing by another. 2. In chemistry, the replacing of one or more elements or radicals in a compound by other elements or radicals.

**substitution therapy.** Providing the patient with a substance which his body should normally be able to manufacture for itself; for instance, the provision of insulin in cases of diabetes and treatment by cortisone and hormones.

**subsultory.** Affected with twitching.

**subsultus tendinum.** Involuntary twitching of the muscles, especially the hands and feet, seen in some fevers.

**subtarsal.** Beneath the tarsus.

**subtertian fever.** A variety of malarial fever.

**subthalamic.** Beneath the thalamus, an area deep within the brain through which sensory information passes.

**subthalamus.** The motor portion of the thalamus. Also called *hypothalamus.* See SUBTHALAMIC.

**subtrochanteric.** Below a trochanter.

**subtrochlear.** Lying beneath a trochlea.

**subtympanic.** Below the tympanum.

**subtypical.** Not quite typical.

**sububeres.** Sucklings; babies at the breast.

**subumbilical.** Below or beneath the umbilicus.

**subungual.** Beneath a nail.

**suburethral.** Beneath the urethra.

**subvaginal.** 1. Below the vagina. 2. Situated beneath a sheath, as of a tendon or nerve.

**subvertebral.** Beneath a vertebra.

**subzygomatic.** Below the zygoma.

**succagogue.** An agent that stimulates the flow of gastric juice or other secretion.

**succedaneous.** Resembling a succedaneum.

**succedaneum.** A medicine which may be substituted for another of similar properties.

**succinous.** Relating to amber.

**succinum.** Amber.

**succorrhea.** Excessive flow of a secretion.

**succorrhoea.** See SUCCORRHEA.

**succus.** Latin for juice. It can refer to any animal or plant secretion.

**succus citri.** Lime juice.

**succus entericus.** Intestinal juice.

**succus gastricus.** Gastric juice.

**succus pancreaticus.** Juice of the pancreas.

**succus prostaticus.** Secretion of the prostate gland.

**sucrase.** An enzyme capable of converting cane sugar into glucose and fructose. It is found in the intestinal juices and in yeast. Also called *invertase.*

**sucrosaemia.** See SUCROSEMIA.

**sucrosemia.** The presence of sugar in the blood.

**sucrose.** Sugar obtained from sugar cane and sugar beet. Also called *saccharose.*

**sucrosoria.** The presence of sugar in the urine.

**sudamina.** Prickly heat.

**sudaminal.** Pertaining to sudamina.

**sudation.** Sweating or excessive sweating.

**sudatoria.** Excessive sweating. Also called *ephidrosis, hyperhidrosis, hyperidrosis.*

**sudatorium.** A hot air bath or chamber.

**sudorkeratosis.** Thickening around the orifices of the sweat glands.

**sudor.** Sweat.

**sudoral.** Pertaining to or characterized by sweating.

**sudoriferous.** Producing sweat.

**sudorific.** An agent that promotes sweating. Also called *diaphoretic.*

**sudoriparous.** Sweating.

**sudorous.** Sweaty.

**sudorrhea.** Excessive production of sweat.

**sudorrhoea.** See SUDORRHEA.

**suffocation.** The stoppage of breathing.

**suffumigation.** Fumigation.

**suffusion.** The spreading of any body fluid, blood for instance, into the surrouding tissues.

**sugar.** A carbohydrate having a sweet taste.

**acorn sugar.** Quercite.

**beet sugar.** Sucrose.

**blood sugar.** Glucose.

**brain sugar.** Cerebose, galactose.

**brown sugar.** Partially refined cane sugar.

**cane sugar.** Sucrose.

**corn sugar.** Glucose.

**fruit sugar.** Levulose, fructose.

**grape sugar.** Glucose.

**gum sugar.** Arabinose.

**honey sugar.** Glucose.

**invert sugar.** Equal parts of glucose and levulose, obtained by hydrolysis of sucrose.

**liver sugar.** Glycogen.

**malt sugar.** Maltose.

**maple sugar.** Chiefly sucrose; obtained from the sap of the sugar maple.

**meat sugar.** Inositol.

**milk sugar.** Lactose.

**mucin sugar.** Levulose.

**muscle sugar.** Inositol.

**pectin sugar.** Arabinose.

**refined sugar.** Purified cane sugar or beet sugar which contains sucrose.

**wood sugar.** Xylose.

**suggestion.** The artificial production of a psychic state in which the individual experiences sensations suggested to him, or ceases to experience those which he is instructed not to feel; the thing suggested.

**suggillatio, suggillation.** A bruise. Also called *ecchymosis.*

**suicidal.** An intention to commit self-destruction.

**suicide.** Intentional taking of one's own life; one who intentionally takes his own life.

**sulcate.** Furrowed.

**sulcus.** A furrow, particularly the fissures in the brain.

**sulfa drugs.** A group of chemicals which are bacteriostatic. This means they prevent germs from multiplying and have a stimulating effect on the blood's white cells, which then engulf more bacteria than they would normally do. They are effective against a large number of bacteria. The commonest of these preparations in use are sulfanilamide, sulfathiazole, sulfadiazine, sulfacetamide, and sulfadimidine. Also called *sulfonamides.*

**sulfonamides.** The sulfa drugs

**sulfur.** A nonmetallic element found in volcanic areas in combination with a number of metals, especially iron and copper, in the form of sulfides. Due to sulfur's local irritant action upon the lining of the intestines, it exerts a laxative effect, and because it liberates hydrogen sulfide, it acts as a poison to intestinal parasites such as worms. It is used on the skin in ointment and soap as a treatment for scabies, though it has now been largely replaced for this purpose by benzyl benzoate lotion. Sulfur dioxide, a product of sulfur and the main chemical ingredient of smog, is the cause of ulcerative bronchitis and other chest troubles. See also AIR POLLUTION.

*Sulfur is the only active ingredient of the old-fashioned brimstone and treacle (sulfur and molasses) much favored by grandmother as a spring tonic and restorative—a remedy which originated in a rather curious way. Mithridates, King of Pontus in the second century B.C., like so many royal personages of that time, considered himself something of a physician, and he noted that when vipers fought although they bit each other, they did not die of poison. He thus concluded that viper flesh was immune to viper venom, and as snake poisoning and other forms of poisoning were then so rife, and there were no antidotes, he made a preparation of dried, powdered viper flesh to use as an antidote to all forms of poisoning and called it Mithridaticum. The name became changed over the centuries to theriac, and this evil-looking, oily preparation contained some 63 ingredients, all of them worthless, the two main ones being sulfur and dried viper flesh. During the Renaissance the preparation of theriac became an elaborate affair supervised by city officials to prevent adulteration, and there were severe punishments, including death, for those who made unofficial preparations and sold them on the black market. Later, theriac was called treacle, which term was also applied to molasses, the crude unrefined product derived from sugar cane. Molasses was then added to the treacle and this preparation, consisting largely of sulfur and molasses, was eventually called brimstone and treacle. Thus a remedy which originated hundreds of years ago for snakebite ended up as one for threadworms.*

**summation.** The accumulation of effects, whether muscular, sensory, or nervous stimuli.

**summer diarrhea.** A form of infectious gastroenteritis of children, seen usually during summer and often initiated by food contamination from flies.

**summer diarrhoea.** See SUMMER DIARRHEA.

**sunburn.** An inflammation of the skin caused by excessive exposure to the sun's rays.

*The skin protects itself against the sun by producing melanin, a pigment which tans the skin. Excessive exposure to the sun's rays, particularly by those sensitive to ultraviolet light and especially redheads and blondes, will cause the skin to become fiery-red, blister, and ulcerate. Small children allowed to run around almost naked in the blazing sun are especially liable to this painful condition, and can even become dangerously ill. Therefore, those with pale skin should only expose it to the sun for a short period, after which it should be covered and reexposed later, thus allowing the skin time to provide its own protection against sunburn. Sunburned skin should be first covered to prevent further damage and, if it has not already ulcerated, the pain can be relieved by applying wet compresses of saturated Epsom salts. These compresses are made by adding to a quantity of water as much Epsom salts as will dissolve and then soaking pieces of linen or gauze in the solution. Calamine lotion or liniment are other soothing preparations which can be applied. People suffering from severe exposure to the sun can also have their night adaptation vision affected and they should remember this if they have to drive home at night after a long day sunning.*

**sunstroke.** See HEAT STROKE; HEAT EXHAUSTION.

**superciliary.** Relating to the eyebrow.

**supercilium.** The eyebrow.

**superdistension.** A marked degree of distension.

**superdural.** Situated above the dura mater.

**superego.** The mental processes which exert an influence over the ego.

**superexcitation.** Extreme excitement.

**superfecundation.** The fertilization of two or more egg cells, ovulated more or less at the same time, by two or more successive acts of sexual intercourse, not necessarily involving the same male.

**superficial.** Related to a surface. In referring to several layers, the top one may be called superficial as opposed to the lowest one, which is called deep; the superficial fascia and deep fascia beneath the skin, for instance.

**superficialis.** At or near the surface. A term applied to arteries, muscles, and nerves.

**superficies.** Any external surface.

**superfetation.** The production or development of a second baby while one is already present in the womb; conception by a pregnant woman.

**superfoetation.** See SUPERFETATION.

**superfunction.** Overactivity of an organ.

**superimpregnation.** See SUPERFECUNDATION, SUPERFETATION.

**superinduce.** To add a new factor or complication to a condition already existing.

**superinfection.** A second or subsequent infection caused by the same germ, as seen in tuberculosis for instance.

**superinvolution.** Shrinkage of an organ to smaller than normal, especially after enlargement. Also called *hyperinvolution.*

**superlactation.** Excessive or overprolonged secretion of milk from the breasts.

**supernatant.** The fluid which remains after the removal of suspended matter.

**supernormal.** Above the normal.

**supernumerary.** In excess of the usual number.

**supersaturate.** To saturate to excess; to add more of a substance than a liquid can normally and permanently dissolve. For instance, heating a liquid will sometimes enable more of a solid to be dissolved in it than if it was at room temperature.

**supersecretion.** Excessive secretion.

**supertension.** Excessive tension.

**supervirulent.** Extremely virulent.

**supination.** 1. Rotating the forearm so that the palm of the hand is uppermost. 2. Lying on the back.

**supine.** 1. Lying on the back. 2. Turning the palm upwards.

**suppository.** Medicinal substances incorporated into a gelatin or greasy base and intended for introduction into the rectum. See also PESSARY.

**suppression.** 1. A sudden cessation of secretion such as the urine or menstruation during pregnancy. 2. In psychiatry, a mode of adjustment to urges and desires considered to be unacceptable or unworthy, by attempting to control or prevent their occurrence or expression in consciousness; a form of repression.

**suppurant.** Inducing suppuration; an agent that induces suppuration.

**suppuration.** The formation of pus. See also PUS.

**suppurative.** Forming pus, or an agent favorable to suppuration.

**supra-acromial.** Above the acromion.

**supra-auricular.** Above the ear.

**suprachoroid.** Above the choroid.

**suprachoroidea.** The outer layer of the choroid.

**supraclavicular.** Above the clavicle.

**supracondylar, supracondyloid.** Located above a bony condyle.

**supracostal.** Above the ribs.

**supradiaphragmatic.** Above the diaphragm.

**supradural.** Above the dura mater.

**supraglenoid.** Above the glenoid cavity of the shoulder joint.

**suprahepatic.** Above the liver.

**suprahyoid.** Above the hyoid.

**supra-inguinal.** Above the groin.

**supraliminal.** Within the field of consciousness.

**supralumbar.** Above the loin.

**supramalleolar.** Above the malleolus.

**supramammary.** Above the breast.

**supramarginal.** Above an edge or margin.

**supramastoid.** Above the mastoid process.

**supramaxilla.** The upper jaw.

**supramaxillary.** Relating to the upper jaw.

**supraoccipital.** Above the occipital bone at the back of the head; in the upper part of the occipital bone.

**supraorbital.** Above the orbit (eye socket).

**suprapelvic.** Above the pelvis.

**suprapubic.** Above the pubic arch of the pelvis.

**suprarenal.** 1. Above the kidney. 2. The dried, partially defatted and powdered suprarenal gland of cattle, sheep, or swine, from which chemists have isolated over 20 derivatives closely related to the hormones derived from the reproductive system. Among the more potent is desoxycorticosterone and corticosterone. Also called *adrenal gland, suprarenal gland.* See also ADRENALINE.

**suprascapular.** Above the scapula.

**suprascleral.** On the outer surface of the sclera.

**supraseptal.** Above a septum.

**supraspinal.** Above a spine.

**supraspinous.** Above a spinous process.

**suprasternal.** Above the sternum.

**supratonsillar.** Above a tonsil.

**supratrochlear.** Above the trochlea.

**supravaginal.** 1. Above the vagina. 2. Above a muscle or nerve sheath or on its outer surface.

**supravergence.** Upward rotation of an eye, the other eye remaining stationary.

**sura.** The calf of the leg.

**sural.** Pertaining to the calf of the leg.

**suralimentation.** Forced feeding; excessive feeding.

**surditas.** Latin for deafness.

**surdity.** Deafness.

**surdomute.** A deaf-mute.

**surface.** The outer surface of the body; a term frequently used in anatomy to describe bones.

**buccal surface.** That part of the crown of a tooth next to the cheek.

**contact surface.** The surface of a tooth facing an adjoining tooth.

**distal surface.** The surface of the crown of a tooth away from the middle line.

**extensor surface.** The portion of the surface of a limb situated over the muscles which extend the limb.

**flexor surface.** The portion of the surface of a limb situated over the muscles which flex the limb.

**labial surface.** The surface of the crown of a tooth facing towards the lips.

**lingual surface.** The surface of the crown of a tooth next to the tongue.

**surface markings.** In anatomy, lines drawn on the skin to show the size and location of structures lying deep in the skin.

**mesial surface.** The surface of the crown of a tooth facing towards the middle line.

**occlusal surface.** The part of the crown of a tooth facing towards its antagonist.

**respiratory surface.** The entire surface of the lungs in contact with the respired air.

**surgery.** That branch of medicine which treats disease by manual or operative procedures.

**abdominal surgery.** Surgery performed on the abdominal organs.

**antiseptic surgery.** Surgery performed with antiseptic principles.

**aseptic surgery.** Operations at which all instruments, towels, rubber gloves, and the like, including the patient's skin, are first sterilized to produce germfree conditions.

**aural surgery.** Surgery performed on the ear.

**battle surgery.** Surgery performed in frontline areas in war time.

**brain surgery.** Surgery performed within the skull. Also called *neurosurgery.*

**clinical surgery.** The practice of surgical teaching.

**conservative surgery.** Surgery performed to save rather than remove a part.

**cosmetic surgery.** A branch of plastic surgery devoted to improving the appearance of a person, such as reshaping the nose, reducing the size of the breasts, face lifting, and the like.

**dental surgery.** Surgery performed on the teeth and jaws.

**general surgery.** Operations other than those of a specialist nature. Since chest and brain surgery are specialties the term usually infers surgery to the abdomen or limbs.

**major surgery.** Surgery which carries a risk to life.

**minor surgery.** Operations of a slight nature which can be performed under local anesthesia and carry no risk to life. It includes sewing up cuts, incision into and removal of superficial structures, bandaging, and the application of splints or plaster casts.

**neurosurgery.** Surgery performed on the nerves, including the brain.

**oral surgery.** Surgery performed within the mouth on teeth, jaws, and adjacent tissues.

**orthodontic surgery.** Correction of irregularities of the teeth.

**orthopedic surgery.** The correction of bone, ligament and joint disorders, and deformities by operation or manipulation.

**pelvic surgery.** Surgery performed chiefly on the female sex organs.

**plastic surgery.** The repair of defects sometimes involving the transplantation of tissue, bone, or skin from one part of the body to another. See also COSMETIC SURGERY, above.

**rectal surgery.** Surgical treatment of diseases of the rectum.

**repair surgery.** See PLASTIC SURGERY, above.

**thoracic surgery.** Surgery performed within the chest.

**veterinary surgery.** Surgery performed on animals.

**surgical.** Pertaining to surgery.

**surgical shock.** See COMA, SHOCK.

**surrogate.** Any medicine used as a substitute for a more expensive kind or for one to which there is a special objection in any particular case.

**sursumduction.** The ability to elevate the axis of either eye above that of the other; the degree to which such elevation can be made.

**sursumvergence.** The turning of the eyes upwards. Also called *supravergence.*

**susceptible.** To be sensitive to an influence; the liability to be infected by a disease.

**suspension.** 1. Temporary cessation in the function of an organ. 2. Hanging or fixing in a higher position, a method of treatment such as suspension of the womb. 3. The dispersion of solid particles throughout the body of a liquid.

**suspensory.** Serving to suspend; a muscle, ligament or contrivance such as a bandage or sling for suspending a part.

**suspiration.** A sigh.

**sustentacular.** Sustaining.

**sustentaculum.** A support, such as a ligament or bone.

**susurrus.** A murmur heard over cases of aneurysm of a blood vessel.

**sutura.** A suture.

**sutural.** Pertaining to a suture.

**suture.** 1. In anatomy, a line of junction or closure between bones, such as those in the cranium. 2. To close a wound by sewing. **3.** Fine cordlike structures, such as gut, silk, wire, or nylon, used to sew up a wound. **4.** The method of using a suture, such as interrupted sutures, mattress sutures, continuous sutures, purse-string sutures, or tension sutures. See also LIGATURE.

**swab.** Absorbent material used to make applications or to soak up blood during surgical operations.

**sweat.** The secretion of the sweat glands of the skin, perspiration. It is a transparent, colorless, watery fluid, holding in solution neutral fats, volatile fatty acids, traces of albumin and urea, free lactic acid, sodium lactate, sodium chloride, potassium chloride, and traces of alkaline phosphates, sugar, ascorbic acid; and its function is to help regulate the temperature of the body.

*Despite dreadful advertisements which imply that an individual's career or sex life is liable to be affected by the odor of sweat, it is comforting to know that sweat of itself is in fact odorless. However, if normal sweat is allowed to remain on the skin for several days it is attacked by bacteria resulting in the production of hydroxybutyric acid, which has an odor and is also an unpleasant ingredient of rancid butter. The obvious cure for a sweaty body odor, therefore, is regular and frequent bathing. The danger of succumbing to the blandishments of advertisers of deodorants is that these preparations may dry up and split the skin and cause either dermatitis or outbreaks of boils.*

**sweating.** The process of perspiring.

**sweating sickness.** A term applied to a variety of illnesses, such as malaria and pulmonary tuberculosis, in which sweating is a prominent feature.

**sweetbread.** The name given by butchers to the pancreas and thymus gland.

**swine plague.** A disease of pigs characterized by pneumonia and septicemia. This disease sometimes decimates pig herds, and for this reason many pig farmers routinely feed antibiotics to their piglets from birth. This practice is a danger to humans, for in eating pig flesh a person may also take in quantities of the antibiotic and become sensitized to it, with devastating results should he subsequently receive the same drug in the course of treatment. Also called *hog cholera.*

**swoon.** A fainting attack.

**sycoma.** A wart.

**sycosiform.** See SYCOSIS.

**sycosis.** An inflammatory disease affecting the hair follicles of the skin, particularly of the beard area (when it is called sycosis barbae or barber's rash), and characterized by papules and pustules together with crusting of the skin surface.

**Sydenham's chorea.** St. Vitus's dance. See CHOREA.

**syllable stammering.** Difficulty in pronouncing a whole word but able to pronounce its component syllables.

**symbion, symbiont.** Either of two organisms existing in close association.

**symbiosis.** A more or less close association or union between organisms of different species. In *mutualism* the organisms are mutually benefited and sometimes so dependent on each other that existence apart is impossible. Other forms of symbiosis include *commensalism*, in which neither organism is injured and one derives benefit from the association; and *parasitism*, in which the relationship of the two organisms is detrimental to one of them, the host, and beneficial to the other, the parasite.

*In the human body there appears to be an association between bacteria and fungi in which the bacteria control the fungi. This is a serious disadvantage when using antibiotics, for these drugs destroy all the bacteria present with the result that the fungi are no longer kept in check and they cause infections of the interior of the body, for which there is little treatment at present.*

**symbiotic.** Pertaining to symbiosis.

**symblepharon.** An adhesion of the eyelids to the eyeball.

**symblepharosis.** Adhesion of the eyelids to the eyeball or to each other.

**symbolism. 1.** A mental condition in which the patient interprets events or objects as a symbol of his own thoughts. **2.** The investment of a thing or an event with a significance other than its literal meaning.

**symbrachydactylia.** A congenital condition characterized by the presence of unusually short and adherent fingers; webbed fingers or toes.

**symparalysis.** Conjugate paralysis of the eye.

**sympathectomy.** Surgical removal of a portion of the sympathetic nervous system. It is performed in the hope of dilating blood vessels to increase the blood supply to a part.

**sympathetic. 1.** Pertaining to sympathy. **2.** Pertaining to the sympathetic nervous system.

**sympathetic nervous system.** Those parts of the central and peripheral nervous systems which supply motor innervation to smooth muscles, glands, and the heart; a part of the autonomic nervous system and which is thus not under the control of the will.

**sympatheticoparalytic.** Caused by paralysis of sympathetic nerves.

**sympatheticotonic.** Overaction of the sympathetic nervous system, producing, among other things, goose flesh of the skin, increased blood pressure, and spasm of blood vessels.

**sympathic.** Sympathetic.

**sympathomimetic.** Imitating the action of the sympathetic nervous system.

**sympathy.** The mutual relationship between two parts more or less distant, whereby a change in one has an effect upon the other.

**symphyseal.** Pertaining to a symphysis.

**symphysiectomy.** Surgical excision of the symphysis pubis.

**symphysion.** The most forward point of the lower jaw.

**symphysiorrhaphy.** The plastic repair of a cleft symphysis.

**symphysiotomy.** Surgical division of the symphysis pubis in order to increase the diameter of the pelvis and thus facilitate delivery in a difficult labor. It is fast becoming an obsolete operation, since most surgeons faced with a difficult labor would prefer to do a cesarian section.

**symphysis.** The junction line of two meeting bones.

**symphysis pubis.** The joint between the two pubic bones at the front lower part of the pelvis.

**symptom.** The complaint described by the patient as indicating some disease or disorder; opposed to a sign, which is what the doctor observes for himself.

**symptomatic.** Pertaining to a symptom.

**symptomatology.** The study of symptoms; all the symptoms of a disease considered as a whole.

**symptosis.** Wasting, collapse, emaciation.

**synaesthesia.** See SYNESTHESIA.

**synalgia.** Pain felt in one part but produced by damage to another.

**synalgic.** Pertaining to synalgia.

**synanastomosis.** The union of several blood vessels.

**synanthema.** A cluster of papules on the skin.

**synapse.** The region of communication between two nerve cells; the point at which a nerve impulse passes from one nerve cell to another.

**synapsis.** The conjugation of homologous chromosomes in meiosis.

**synaptic.** Pertaining to a synapsis.

**synarthrodia.** Synarthrosis.

**synarthrodial.** Pertaining to synarthrosis.

**synarthrosis.** A form of joint in which the bones are immovably bound together without any intervening lining joint membrane. There are three forms: *sutures or sutura*, in which bony processes are interlocked; *schindylesis*, in which a thin plate of one bone is inserted into a groove of another; and *gomphosis* in which a conical bony process is held by a socket in the other bone.

**syncheilia, synchilia.** Congenital fusion of the lips, leaving no mouth opening.

**synchondrosis.** A joint in which the surfaces are connected by a growth of cartilage.

**synchondrotomy.** Surgical division of the cartilage uniting two bones, especially that of the symphysis pubis.

**synchronism, synchronous.** Occurring at the same time, simultaneous.

**synchysis, scintillans.** Bright particles in the vitreous humor.

**synclitism.** A condition marked by similarity of inclination, as when the pelvic plane and the fetal head are parallel.

**synclonus.** 1. Tremor, or clonic spasm of several muscles simultaneously. 2. A disease characterized by tremor or spasm, such as St. Vitus's dance.

**syncopal.** Relating to syncope.

**syncope.** Swooning or fainting; temporary loss of consciousness from anemia of the brain.

**anginosa syncope.** An infrequently used term for angina pectoris.

**carotid sinus syncope.** Sudden attacks of unconsciousness and convulsions caused by overactivity of the nerves of the carotid sinus.

**laryngeal syncope.** Spasm of the larynx, associated with giddy attacks and loss of consciousness.

**local syncope.** Sudden pallor and insensibility of a part.

**vasovagal syncope.** The fainting attack seen in persons with unstable vasomotor systems. Emotional strain or pressure on the vagus nerve causes a lowering of blood pressure and slowing of the pulse, both of which combine to create a state of anemia of the brain.

**syncytial.** Pertaining to a syncytium.

**syncytioma.** A tumor arising within the womb consisting of syncytoid tissues. Also called *chorioma*.

**syncytium.** 1. A mass of cytoplasm with numerous nuclei. 2. The exterior covering of the chorionic villi, associated with the fetal membrane within the womb.

**syncytoid.** Like a syncytium.

**syndactylia, syndactylism, syndactyly.** Webbed fingers or toes, being congenital abnormalities.

**syndactylus.** A person affected with syndactylia.

**syndectomy.** Surgical removal of a piece of conjunctiva.

**syndesis.** Being fastened together.

**syndesmectomy.** Surgical removal of a ligament.

**syndesmitis.** 1. Inflammation of a ligament. 2. Conjunctivitis.

**syndesmoma.** A tumor composed of connective tissue.

**syndesmopexy.** Surgical fixation of a dislocation by using the ligaments of the dislocated joint.

**syndesmorrhaphy.** Suture or surgical repair of a ligament.

**syndesmosis.** A form of joint in which the bones are connected by ligaments. Also called *synneurosis*.

**syndesmotomy.** Surgical division of a ligament.

**syndesmus.** A ligament.

**syndrome.** A group of symptoms and signs which together characterize a disease.

**syndromic.** Pertaining to a syndrome.

**synechia.** Adhesion of parts, especially adhesion of the iris to the lens capsule or cornea.

**synechotomy.** Surgical cutting of a synechia.

**synechtenterotomy.** Surgical cutting of intestinal adhesions.

**syneresis.** 1. The contraction of a clot. 2. In colloid chemistry, the exudation of the liquid constituent of gels.

**synergetic.** Working together.

**synergist.** An agent which acts jointly with another agent, each enhancing the effect of the other.

**synergy.** The cooperative action of two or more agents or organisms or drugs.

**synesthesia.** A secondary sensation provoked by an actual perception, as for instance, sensations of color or sound aroused by the perception of taste.

**syngamy.** Sexual reproduction.

**syngenesis.** Sexual reproduction.

**synizesis.** Closure, blocking, or occlusion. Also called *synezesis*.

**synkinesia, synkinesis.** An involuntary movement occurring in the body simultaneously with a voluntary movement in another part of the body.

**synneurosis.** See SYNDESMOSIS.

**synocha, synochus.** A continued fever.

**synophthalmus.** An hereditary abnormality in which there is almost complete fusion of two eyes into one; a cyclops.

**synopsia.** Congenital fusion of both eyes.

**synoscheos.** Adherence between the skin of the penis and that of the scrotum.

**synosteology.** The study of joints, and their articulations.

**synosteosis, synostosis.** A union of normally separate bones by osseous material.

**synosteotomy.** The dissection of joints.

**synovectomy.** Surgical stripping of the lining membrane of joints.

**synovia.** The clear fluid contained in a joint cavity.

**synovial.** Pertaining to synovia.

**synovial membrane.** The membrane covering the articular surfaces of bones and the inner surfaces of ligaments forming a joint.

**synovin.** A variety of mucin present in synovia.

**synoviparous.** Secreting synovia.

**synovitis.** Inflammation of a synovial membrane. It usually leads to a vast output of fluid, causing the joint to swell.

**synovium.** A synovial membrane.

**synpneumonic.** Occurring at the same time as pneumonia.

**syntaxis.** An articulation or joint.

**synthesis.** 1. In chemistry, the operations necessary to build up a compound. 2. The formation of a complex concept by the combination of separate ideas. 3. In psychiatry, the process in which the ego accepts unconscious ideas and feelings and fuses them within itself more or less consciously.

**synthesize.** To produce anything by synthesis.

**synthetic.** Pertaining to synthesis; artificial.

**syntripsis.** A comminuted fracture.

**syntrophus.** Any congenital disease.

**syntropic.** Alike and turned in the same direction.

**synulosis.** Scarring.

**synulotic.** Leading to scarring; an agent that causes scarring.

**syphilelcosis.** Syphilitic ulceration; the condition of having a syphilitic chancre.

**syphilelcus.** A syphilitic ulcer.

**syphilid, syphilide.** Any skin disease caused by syphilis.

**syphilionthus.** Any copper-colored, scaly, syphilitic skin eruption.

**syphiliphobia.** A morbid dread of syphilis. Also called *syphilomania, syphilophobia*.

**syphilis.** A highly contagious venereal disease, caused by a spirochete, *Treponema pallidum*, and characterized by a variety of lesions, the chancre, the mucous patch, and the gumma being the most distinctive. The disease is usually acquired by sexual intercourse with an infected person, hence its earliest manifestations generally appear on the genital organs, but any abraded surface of the body, if brought into contact with the germ, may give entrance to the infection. The clinical course of syphilis is generally divided into three stages. The *primary stage* is characterized by the chancre, or primary sore, a painless ulcer which produces a slight watery or purulent discharge, and appears after a variable period of between ten days and three weeks. Shortly after the primary sore appears, the nearest lymph glands become enlarged and hard. The *secondary stage* is characterized by skin eruption, sore throat, general enlargement of the glands, and a generalized toxemia. The *tertiary stage* is characterized by gumma, a soft rounded nodule containing a gelatinous gummy material and varying in size from a pea to that of a small apple. It may be sited over flat bones, the meninges, the liver, spleen, and testicles. There is usually an interval of about six weeks between the appearance of the primary sore and the secondary stage, the tertiary stage following the secondary stage after a quiescent period of variable length. The disease may attack any organ of the body, and the late stages of untreated syphilis may produce meningitis, tabes dorsalis, paralysis, and other lesions. Also called *lues*. See also CONGENITAL SYPHILIS.

**syphilitic.** Pertaining to syphilis.

**syphilization.** Infected with syphilis.

**syphiloderm, syphiloderma.** Any skin disease caused by the germ of syphilis.

**syphilogenesis, syphilogeny.** The development of syphilis.

**syphiloid.** With the appearance of syphilis; like syphilis.

**syphilologist.** A specialist in the treatment of syphilis.

**syphilology.** The study of the origin and nature of syphilis.

**syphiloma.** A gumma.

**syphilomania.** Syphiliphobia.

**syphilopathy.** Any disease of a syphilitic nature.

**syphilophobia.** Syphiliphobia.

**syrigmophonia.** A whistling sound in the voice.

**syrigmus.** A ringing sound in the ears.

**syringectomy.** Surgical removal of the walls of a fistula.

**syringitis.** Inflammation of the eustachian tube.

**syringocoele.** An obsolete term for the central canal of the spinal cord.

**syringocystadenoma.** An enlargement of an inflammatory tumor arising in the sweat glands of the skin.

**syringocystoma.** A rare disease of the skin thought to begin in embryonic sweat glands. The lesions are pale, rose-colored, oval nodules, the size of a split pea and nearly level with the skin.

**syringomyelia.** A chronic disease characterized by the formation of long cavities in the spinal cord and brain stem. Due to compression and destruction of the spinal nerve pathway, the patient is unable to recognize pain and heat, and may, for instance, smoke a cigarette right down to the fingers and be unaware that he is burning his skin until he suddenly smells it being burnt.

**syringomyelitis.** Inflammation associated with syringomyelia.

**syringomyelocele.** A defect of the spine with protrusion of a sac containing a portion of the spinal cord, whose central canal is greatly distended with cerebrospinal fluid.

**syringotome.** A special kind of surgical knife.

**syringotomy.** Surgical incision of a fistula.

**syrinx.** A fistula.

**syspasia.** Spasmodic inability to speak.

**syssarcosis.** The uniting of bones by means of muscular tissue.

**systaltic.** Having a pulse; alternately contracting and expanding; having a systole.

**system.** 1. A methodical arrangement. 2. A combination of parts into a whole, such as the digestive, nervous, circulatory, and respiratory systems; the body as a whole.

**systemic.** 1. Relating to a system. 2. Relating to the entire organism or the body as a whole.

**systole.** The period of the heart's contraction; the contraction itself.

**systolic.** Relating to systole.

**systremma.** A cramp in the calf muscles of the leg.

# T

**T.A.B.** A vaccine which provides protection against typhoid, paratyphoid A, and paratyphoid B.

**tabagism.** The tobacco habit.

**tabatiere anatomique.** The anatomical snuff box, a hollow on the back of the hand at the base of the thumb and most obvious when the thumb is forced backwards. The scaphoid bone is beneath this hollow and in fractures of this bone pressure in the hollow causes pain.

**tabefaction.** Wasting away; emaciation.

**tabella.** A tablet.

**tabes.** 1. Any progressive wasting of the body or part of it. 2. The short term for tabes dorsalis.

**tabes dorsalis.** A disease of the nervous system due to untreated syphilis. The symptoms are lightning pains, unsteadiness, incoordination of voluntary movements, disorders of vision, and pain crises in the stomach, throat, and rectum. Also called *locomotor ataxia*.

**tabetic.** Relating to or affected with tabes or tabes dorsalis.

**tabetiform.** Resembling tabes.

**tabic.** Tabetic.

**tabification.** See TABEFACTION.

**table.** A flat layer of bone.

**taboparalysis.** See TABOPARESIS.

**taboparesis.** Muscular paralysis associated with tabes dorsalis.

**tabular.** Like a table.

**tache.** A spot; a blemish.

**tachetic.** Marked by spots.

**tachycardia.** Excessively rapid heartbeat. See also PAROXYSMAL: PAROXYSMAL AURICULAR TACHYCARDIA.

**tachycardiac.** Pertaining to tachycardia.

**tachylalia.** Abnormal rapidity of speech.

**tachyphrasia.** Abnormal volubility; sometimes a sign of mental disorder.

**tachyphrenia.** Abnormal activity of the mental processes.

**tachypnea.** Rapid breathing.

**tachynoea.** See TACHYPNEA.

**tactile.** Pertaining to the sense of touch.

**tactual.** Tactile.

**tactus.** Touch.

**taedium vitae.** A morbid weariness of life, a form of depression which sometimes leads to suicide.

**taenia.** Tapeworms belonging to the genus *Taenia*, being ribbonlike parasitic flatworms of the class *Cestoda*. The two commonest species in man are: *Taenia saginata*, acquired by eating undercooked infested beef; and *Taenia solium*, acquired by eating undercooked infested pork or pork products.

**taenia.** See TENIA.

**taeniacide.** See TENIACIDE.

**taeniafuge.** See TENIAFUGE.

**talalgia.** Pain in the heel or ankle.

**taliped.** A clubfooted person.

**talipes.** Clubfoot, a congenital deformity probably produced by the baby adopting an abnormal position in the womb. These deformities do not usually occur alone but in combination, the most common being talipes equinovarus, which accounts for about three-quarters of all the cases. Treatment is usually commenced on the day after birth, for unless it is started early a normal foot can seldom be obtained. See also PES.

**talipes calcaneus.** Club foot in which both ankle and foot are bent upwards.

**talipes equinovarus.** Clubfoot in which the heel is elevated and turned outward.

**talipes equinus.** Clubfoot in which the foot is bent downwards.

**talipes valgus.** Clubfoot in which the foot is both rotated and turned outwards.

**talipes varus.** Clubfoot in which the foot is both turned and rotated inwards.

**talipomanus.** Clubhand, a deformity similar to clubfoot.

**talocalcanean.** Pertaining to the talus and the calcaneum.

**talocrural.** Pertaining both to the talus and the leg bones.

**talofibular.** Pertaining both to the talus and the fibula.

**talotibial.** Pertaining both to the talus and the tibia.

**talpa.** A mole.

**talus.** The astragalus or anklebone; the ankle.

**tampon.** A plug of soft material inserted into a cavity; to plug a cavity with a tampon.

**tamponade.** The act of plugging with a tampon.

**cardiac tamponade.** Symptoms of back pressure on the heart due to disease in the chest causing obstruction to the flow of blood.

**tantalum.** A rare silver-white metal element which is very hard and resistant to corrosion and yet is malleable. It is used in surgery to bridge gaps in the skull caused by injury.

**tapeinocephaly.** Flattening of the skull. Also called *tapinocephaly.*

**tapeworm.** See TAENIA.

**tapinocephaly.** Tapeinocephaly.

**taphophobia.** A morbid fear of being buried alive.

**tapotement.** Tapping movements used in massage.

**tarantism.** Dancing mania, once popularly believed to be caused by the bite of the tarantula spider and cured by dancing. See CHOREA.

**tarantula.** A type of spider with a poisonous bite, named after the town of Taranto in Southern Italy.

**tarry stools.** See MELENA.

**tarsadenitis.** Inflammation of both the tarsal plate of the eyelid and of the meibomian glands.

**tarsal.** 1. Relating to the tarsus of the foot. 2. Relating to the tarsal plate of the upper eyelid.

**tarsalgia.** Pain in the foot.

**tarsectomy.** Surgical removal of part of the tarsus of the foot or of the tarsal plate in the upper eyelid.

**tarsectopia.** Dislocation of the tarsus of the foot.

**tarsitis.** Inflammation of the tarsal plate of the upper eyelid.

**tarsomalacia.** Abnormal softening of the tarsal plate of an eyelid.

**tarsomegaly.** Strictly, enlargement of the tarsus of the foot, but more commonly applied to enlargement of the heel bone.

**tarsometatarsal.** Relating to the tarsus and the metatarsus of the foot.

**tarso-orbital.** Relating to the tarsal plate in the upper eyelid.

**tarsophalangeal.** Pertaining to the tarsus and the phalanges (toe bones).

**tarsophyoma.** Any tumor of the tarsus.

**tarsoplasty.** Surgical repair of an eyelid. Also called *blepharoplasty.*

**tarsoptosis.** Flatfooted.

**tarsorrhaphy.** Sewing of the eyelids together to protect the eyeball from exposure in such conditions as corneal ulcer.

**tarsotibial.** Pertaining to the tarsus of the foot and the tibia.

**tarsotomy.** Surgical incision into either the tarsus of the foot or an eyelid.

**tarsus.** 1. The bones forming the instep of the foot. 2. The tissues forming the framework of an eyelid.

**tartar.** 1. The chalky substance deposited on teeth. 2. Acid potassium tartrate, the chemical found deposited on the inside of wine casks; also called *cream of tartar.*

**tartaric acid.** A chemical prepared from the argol and lees formed as a deposit after the fermentation of grape juice in winemaking. It is used in the preparation of effervescent powders, is a constituent of baking powder, and is used to make sherbert and fizzy drinks.

**tasikinesia.** An abnormal desire to walk.

**taste.** A sensation produced by stimulation of the taste buds in the tongue. Only three primary tastes are recognized—sweet, sour, and salty—all others being a combination of the primary sensations.

**taste blindness.** Inability to taste certain substances.

**tattooing.** The introduction of plant and mineral substances into the skin in order to color it. Many practicing this trade are less than careful with their antisepsis, and apart from adding their design, which most young men live to regret, there is a risk of introducing infections into the skin. Tattoos can only be removed by surgery.

**taxis.** 1. Manipulation of a misplaced organ into its normal position, as, for instance, the reduction of a rupture, or the replacing of a misplaced uterus. 2.

The involuntary response of an organism involving change of place, either towards (positive taxis) or away from (negative taxis) a stimulus.

**Tay's disease.** Inflammation of the choroid, occurring in old age and probably due to hardening of the arteries. Also called *Tay's choroiditis.*

**Tay-Sachs disease.** A family disease occurring chiefly among Jews and affecting children during the first year of life. The child appears to be quite healthy at birth, but later there appear progressive mental impairment ending in absolute idiocy, and progressive paralysis of the whole body together with progressive loss of vision, leading to blindness. A cherry-red spot on the retina is diagnostic of this disease, and almost invariably these children die before the age of two years. Nothing is known of the cause and there is no effective treatment. Also called *amaurotic family idiocy, Warren-Tay-Sachs disease.*

**tease.** To shred a tissue.

**technetium.** The first artificially produced chemical element not found in nature. It was prepared in 1937 by neutron bombardment of molybdenum. Formerly called *masurium.*

**technocausis.** Mechanical cauterization, such as with an electric current, as opposed to cauterization by chemicals.

**tecnotomia.** A little-used term for infanticide.

**tectiform.** Like a roof.

**tectocephaly.** Having a roof-shaped head.

**tectorial.** Acting as a roof.

**tectorium.** A covering.

**tectum.** Any rooflike structure.

**teeth.** Small bonelike structures set in the jaws for masticating food. See also TOOTH.

*The human child develops two sets of teeth: the 20 deciduous milk or temporary teeth appear first and fall out with the eruption of the 32 permanent teeth. It is not uncommon for a baby to be born with one or two central incisor teeth erupted; this may make it necessary to bottle feed the baby to avoid damage to the mother's nipple. The deciduous teeth begin to erupt about the end of the sixth month and all have appeared by about the end of the second year. They usually appear in three groups with intervals of six to twelve weeks between each; first come the eight incisors, then the four canines, followed by the four premolars and finally the four molars. There is no apparent eruption from the third to the seventh years of life, after which the deciduous teeth begin to fall out, starting with the incisors and ending about the twelfth year with the molars. The permanent dentition (consisting of eight incisors, four canines, eight premolars and twelve molars), with the exception of the wisdom teeth, is completed with the appearance of the second molars about the twelfth to the sixteenth year. The third molars, or wisdom teeth, appear between the sixteenth and twentieth years if they erupt at all. In many cases there is no room for the wisdom teeth to erupt and they are only seen when the jaw is x-rayed. If they partially erupt they may cause considerable discomfort and need to be removed.*

**teething.** The cutting of the teeth; dentition. During periods of tooth eruption, some apparently quite healthy infants become irritable, probably due to niggling discomfort in the gums.

**tegmen.** A roof or cover. Also called *tegumen.*

**tegmental.** Pertaining to the tegmentum.

**tegmentum.** A covering, the skin for example, but especially a portion of the midbrain.

**tegumen.** See TEGMEN.

**tegument.** The skin covering the body.

**tegumental.** Pertaining to the skin.

**teichopsia.** Attacks of temporary blindness accompanied by subjective visual images, flashes of light, or colored rings, experienced by those suffering with migraine headaches.

**teinodynia.** See TENODYNIA.

**tela.** Any weblike tissue.

**telaesthesia.** See TELESTHESIA.

**telalgia.** Referred pain, that is, pain occurring at a site distant from the disease process or lesion causing it. For instance, a disease causing pressure on spinal nerve roots in the small of the back may produce pain in the leg or foot.

**telangiectasia, telangiectasis.** Dilation of small blood vessels in the skin. One form is the weblike network of veins seen on the skin of the legs of middle-aged women.

**telangiitis.** Inflammation of the capillaries.

**telangiosis.** Any disease of the capillaries or small blood vessels.

**teledactyl.** A device used to pick up objects for those unable to stoop.

**telegrapher's cramp.** A neurosis seen in manual telegraph operators. See NEUROSIS: OCCUPATIONAL NEUROSIS.

**telencephalon.** The anterior portion of the brain. Also called *endbrain.*

**teleneuron.** Any nerve ending.

**teleologic.** Relating to the final causes.

**teleology.** The doctrine that explanations of phenomena are to be found in terms of the final causes, purpose, or design in nature.

**telepathist.** A thought reader.

**telepathy.** Thought reading. Also called *extrasensory perception.*

**telesthesia.** Perception at a distance; telepathy.

**telesystolic.** Pertaining to the end of the systole.

**teletactile.** Pertaining to the teletactor.

**teletactor.** An apparatus which enables the deaf to hear by means of a vibrating plate.

**temperament.** The combination of ideas and urges that make a person what he is.

**temperature.** The degree of intensity of heat, especially as measured by a thermometer.

**absolute temperature.** A temperature expressed in a number reckoned from absolute zero (-273.15°C. or -459.67°F.).

**basal body temperature.** The temperature of the body under conditions of absolute rest.

**body temperature.** The temperature of the body. Temperatures may be classified as: normal, 98°-99°F.; subnormal, below 98°F.; collapse, below 96°F.; febrile, above 99°F.; and hyperpyrexia, above 107°F. Pyrexia is a state of having a continuously high temperature coupled with thirst, headache, and a rapid pulse. The three principal types of fever accompanied by temperature are: *continued fever* or *continued temperature,* when the fever does not fluctuate more than about 1½°F. during 24 hours and at no time touches the normal; *remittent fever* or *remittent temperature,* when the daily fluctuations exceed 2°; and *intermittent fever* or *intermittent temperature,* when the fever is only present for several hours during the day. In many cases the temperature may be up in the morning and normal at night, or vice versa. Thus it is important to take the patient's temperature morning, afternoon, and evening before one can be certain that it has come down to normal properly. No patient should be allowed out of bed until the temperature has been normal or below normal morning, afternoon, and evening of one day and is still normal or below normal the following morning.

**critical temperature.** The temperature at which a gas can, by pressure, be reduced to a liquid.

**normal temperature.** The temperature of the body in health. It may vary between 98°-99°F., averaging 98.6°F.

**optimum temperature.** The temperature most favorable for a particular process, such as the cultivation of microbes or germs.

**temple.** The flat portion of the head behind the eye and above the ear.

**tempora.** The temples.

**temporal.** 1. Relating to the temple. 2. Relating to time.

**temporo-auricular.** Pertaining to the temporal and auricular areas.

**temporofacial.** Pertaining to the temples and the face.

**temporomandibular.** Pertaining to the temporal bone and the mandible.

**temporomaxillary.** Pertaining to the temporal bone and the maxilla.

**temporo-occipital.** Pertaining to the temporal and occipital regions.

**temporosphenoid.** Pertaining to the temporal and sphenoid bones of the skull.

**temulence.** Drunkenness.

**tenacious.** Adhesive, tough, sticky.

**tenaculum.** A hook-shaped implement for seizing or holding parts.

**tenalgia.** A pain in a tendon.

**tendinitis.** Inflammation of a tendon.

**tendinosuture.** The suturing of a tendon.

**tendinous.** Pertaining to a tendon.

**tendo.** A tendon.

**tendo Achillis.** The powerful tendon which joins the calf muscles to the back of the heel.

**tendon.** A tough, fibrous tissue forming the termination of a muscle and with which the muscle is attached to a bone.

**tendoplasty.** Surgical repair of a tendon. Also called *tendinoplasty.*

**tendovaginal.** Relating to both a tendon and its sheath.

**tendovaginitis.** Inflammation of a tendon and its sheath. See TENOSYNOVITIS.

**tenesmic.** Relating to a tenesmus.

**tenesmus.** A painful straining, particularly a painful straining effort to empty the bladder, or bowel, usually without success.

**tenia.** A flat band or strip of soft tissue. Also called *taenia.*

**teniacide.** An agent that destroys tapeworms.

**teniafuge.** An agent that expels tapeworms.

**tennis elbow.** A name commonly applied to almost every disorder in which there is pain at the side of the elbow caused by energetic use of the arm. Only in very few patients is the playing of tennis the original cause, for any occupation requiring a tight grip and rotary movements of the forearm may be responsible. The pain is due either to a stretching of the extensor muscles of the forearm or to a nipping of the membrane lining the joint between the articular surfaces of the radius and the humerus. Each case has to be treated on its merits and in some the arm is rested on a splint, while others respond to injections of local anesthetic or hydrocortisone. In yet others relief can be obtained by early manipulation, which does not require an anesthetic, unless the condition is of long standing and adhesions have formed.

**tenodesis.** Fixation of a joint by shortening the tendons passing about it.

**tenodynia.** Pain in a tendon.

**tenonectomy.** Surgical shortening of a tendon.

**tenonitis.** 1. Inflammation of a tendon; also called *tenontitis.* 2. Inflammation of Tenon's capsule (a fluid-containing sac on the back of the eyeball).

**tenontagra.** Pain in a tendon due to gout.

**tenophyte.** A growth of bone in a tendon.

**tenoplasty.** Surgical repair of a tendon.

**tenorrhaphy.** Suturing of a tendon. Also called TENOSUTURE.

**tenostosis.** Bony changes in a tendon.

**tenosuture.** See TENORRHAPHY.

**tenosynovitis.** Inflammation of a tendon and its sheath. Probably the most common example is that affecting the forearm. Normally, tendons are lubricated within their sheaths and are silent and painless when moved. In tenosynovitis the lubricant temporarily disappears so that one can almost hear, and certainly feel, the tendon rubbing against its dry sheath, causing pain when the part is used. Treatment consists of absolute rest, after which recovery is usually complete. Also called *tendosynovitis.*

**tenotome.** An instrument for cutting a tendon.

**tenotomy.** Surgical cutting of a tendon.

**tenovaginitis.** Inflammation of a tendon sheath. See also TENOSYNOVITIS.

**tensiometer.** An instrument for determining the surface tension of liquids.

**tension.** The act of stretching; the condition of being stretched.

**arterial tension.** The strain on the arterial walls at the height of the pulse wave on the contraction of the heart; equivalent to the systolic blood pressure.

**elastic tension.** Stretching by means of any elastic material.

**gaseous tension.** The tendency of a gas to expand; the pressure that this expansion causes.

**intraocular tension.** The pressure produced by the fluid within the eyeball. It may be estimated by a tonometer, or by palpation with the fingers. Increased intraocular tension causes glaucoma.

**intravenous tension.** The strain to which the wall of a vein is subjected by the pressure of the blood within it.

**muscular tension.** The state of muscular contraction which occurs when muscles are passively stretched.

**premenstrual tension.** Symptoms of headache, nausea, and fainting attacks occurring a few days before the onset of menstruation, the woman often being depressed and emotional. The cause is obscure, though many factors have been blamed, from fluid retention in the tissues to hormone imbalance and psychological causes. Each case has to be treated on its merits, with drugs, diet, or with psychological analysis.

**surface tension.** The force operating at surfaces, such as between a liquid and a gas, two liquids, or a liquid and a solid, due to the unequal molecular attraction on either side of the surface; the contractile force in the surface of a liquid, by which the surface tries to assume the smallest area possible. The surface tension of water against air at 20°C. (68°F.) is 72.5 dynes per centimeter.

**tensor.** Any muscle stretching a part.

**tent.** 1. A roll of absorbent material that increases in volume by the absorption of water; used to stretch a body canal or keep a wound open. 2. A fabric covering arranged as a tent over a patient in bed, and used for therapeutic purposes, such as the administering of oxygen in an oxygen tent.

**tentative.** Experimental.

**tenth nerve.** The tenth cranial nerve. Also called *vagus.*

**tentiginous.** Lecherous.

**tentigo.** Lecherousness.

**tentigo venerea.** Nymphomania.

**tentorium.** Part of the dura mater.

**tentum.** The penis.

**tenuis.** Slight, thin.

**tenuity.** The state of being thin.

**tenuous.** 1. Slight or thin in form. 2. Thin in consistency.

**tephromalacia.** Morbid softening of the grey matter of the brain or spinal cord.

**tephromyelitis.** Inflammation of the grey matter of the spinal cord.

**tephrosis.** Cremation.

**tepid.** At blood heat.

**teras.** A fetal monster.

**teratic.** Monstrous.

**teratism.** Any malformation, whether congenital or acquired.

**teratoblastoma.** See TERATOMA.

**teratogenesis.** The production of physical defects in offspring developing in the uterus.

**teratoid.** Like a monster.

**teratology.** The study of birth monstrosities.

**teratoma.** A tumor containing teeth, hair, or other material not found in the part wherein it grows; resulting from the misplacement of tissue during the growth of the fetus.

**teratophobia.** The morbid dread of giving birth to a monster.

**teratosis.** See TERATISM.

**terebinth, terebinthina.** Turpentine.

**terebinthinate.** Containing turpentine.

**terebinthism.** Turpentine poisoning.

**terebrant, terebrating.** Boring or piercing; usually refers to a piercing pain.

**terebration.** Surgical trephining of the skull.

**teres.** Round and smooth; applied to ligaments or muscles.

**terminad.** Towards a terminal or end point.

**terminal.** Pertaining to the end; being at the end; forming the end.

**terminology.** Nomenclature.

**terpene.** A modified form of turpentine.

**terra.** Earth.

**terra alba.** White clay.

**terra foliata.** Sulfur.

**terra japonica.** Catechu.

**tertian.** Occurring every third day.

**tertian fever.** A form of malaria.

**tertiary.** Third in order.

**tertiary syphilis.** The third stage of syphilis.

**tertigravida.** A woman in her third pregnancy.

**tertipara.** A woman who has had three pregnancies, each resulting in a viable offspring.

**tessellated.** Checkered.

**testa.** A shell.

**testaceous.** Pertaining to a shell.

**testectomy.** Castration; the surgical removal of a testicle or testicles.

**testes.** The testicles.

**testicle.** See TESTIS.

**testicond.** Undescended testicles.

**testicular.** Pertaining to the testicles.

**testicular fluid.** The semen.

**testis.** A testicle, one of the two male sex glands which manufacture semen.

**testopathy.** Any disease of the testicles.

**testosterone.** The male sex hormone. It is manufactured in the testicles and is responsible for the production of the secondary sex characteristics, such as the growth of the beard. It is also synthesized in the chemical laboratory without recourse to animal extracts.

**tetania.** Tetany.

**tetanic.** Pertaining to or causing tetanus.

**tetaniform.** Similar to tetanus.

**tetanilla.** A form of tetany.

**tetanization.** The inducing of tetanic spasms.

**tetanoid.** Like tetanus.

**tetanus.** An infectious disease, characterized by violent spasm of the muscles and convulsions. It is due to the poison produced by the tetanus bacillus, *Clostridium tetani,* which enters through a wound. Since this germ can grow only in the absence of oxygen, the character of the wound is important—the most dangerous being puncture, penetration, and crushing injuries. The germ normally inhabits the intestines of horses, therefore any wound contaminated with manure or manured soil bears an increased risk of developing tetanus. Since severe attacks may prove fatal, and once the disease is established treatment is often unsatisfactory, it has been suggested that children receiving diphtheria and whooping cough inoculations should also be inoculated against tetanus, thus giving them a lifelong protection. Also called *lockjaw*.

**tetany.** A disease characterized by intermittent, painful spasms of the muscles.

**tetartanopsia.** Defect of vision in the corresponding area of the visual field of each eye.

**tetrachromic.** Able to perceive four colors only.

**tetrad.** 1. A group of four bodies. 2. A chemical element able to combine with four other elements.

**tetraethyl lead.** An extremely poisonous organic compound of lead.

**tetralogy of Fallot.** A form of congenital heart disease described by L. A. Fallot, a French physician (1850-1911), and characterized by (1) narrowing of the pulmonary artery; (2) a hole in the septum between the ventricles; (3) dextroposition of the aorta; and (4) enlargement of the right ventricle.

**tetraplegia.** Paralysis of both arms and both legs.

**texis.** Childbearing.

**textural.** Relating to a tissue.

**texture.** The structure of a tissue.

**thalamic.** Pertaining to the thalamus, a region of the brain through which sensory information passes.

**thalamic syndrome.** Destruction by thrombosis of the optic thalamus resulting in hemiparesis with spontaneous involuntary movements on the side of the body opposite to the side of the brain damage. In addition there is hemianesthesia and a hypersensitivity to painful or thermal stimuli, such as tickling and rubbing, which may produce agonizing distress. Also called *Dejerine-Roussy syndrome*.

**thalamocoele.** The third ventricle of the brain.

**thalamocortical.** Pertaining to the thalamus and the cortex of the brain.

**thalamolenticular.** Pertaining to the thalamus and the lenticular nucleus of the brain.

**thalamus.** A mass of grey matter at the base of the brain, developed from and forming part of the wall of the third ventricle (a brain cavity). Practically all the sensory nerve impulses must pass through this area to reach the

sensory area in the cortex of the brain, and the primary centers for vision are situated in the rear portion of it.

**thalassanaemia.** See THALASSANEMIA.

**thalassanemia.** A disease occurring in the Mediterranean region, characterized by enlargement of the spleen, anemia, and changes in the bones, with pigmentation of the skin. Also called *Coolie's anemia*.

**thalassophobia.** A neurotic dread of the sea.

**thalassotherapy.** Treatment by means of sea bathing, sea voyages, sea air, and seaside holidays.

**thanatognomonic.** Indicating the approach of death.

**thanatoid.** Resembling death.

**thanatomania.** Suicidal mania.

**thanatophobia.** A neurotic fear of death.

**thanatopsy.** A post-mortem examination; necropsy.

**thanatosis.** Gangrene.

**thaumatropy.** The transformation of one structure into another.

**thaumaturgic.** Miraculous.

**theca.** A sheath or enclosing membrane, especially of a tendon or nerve.

**thecal.** Pertaining to a sheath.

**thecal abscess.** An abscess in a tendon sheath.

**thecate.** Sheathed or having a sheath.

**thecitis.** Inflammation of a tendon sheath.

**theic.** One addicted to tea.

**theine.** The active principle of tea; similar to caffeine, the active principle of coffee.

**theism.** The morbid condition resulting from excessive tea drinking, characterized by headache, palpitations, tremor, sleeplessness, and wasting of the body.

**thelalgia.** Pain in the nipple.

**theleplasty.** A surgical operation on the nipple. Also called *thelyplasty*.

**thelitis.** Inflammation of the nipple.

**thelium.** A nipple; a papilla.

**thelorrhagia.** Bleeding from the nipple.

**thelothism.** Jutting out of the nipple.

**thelygenic.** Producing only female children.

**thelyplasty.** See THELEPLASTY.

**thenad.** Towards the thenar eminence of the thumb.

**thenal.** Pertaining to the palm or to the thenar eminence of the thumb.

**thenar.** 1. The palm of the hand or sole of the foot, but especially the palm of the hand. 2. The fleshy mound of muscle at the base of the thumb; also called *thenar eminence*.

**theobromine.** A purine chemical closely related to caffeine and contained in cocoa.

**theomania.** Religious mania.

**theomanic.** One suffering with religious mania.

**theophobia.** Morbid fear of God.

**therapeutic.** Relating to therapeutics.

**therapeutics.** The application of remedies in the treatment of disease.

**therapeutist.** One skilled in therapeutics. Also called *therapist*.

**therapy.** See THERAPEUTICS.

**theriaca.** Treacle. See SULFUR.

**theriacal.** An agent useful as an antidote for snakebite.

**therm.** A unit of heat.

**thermaesthesia.** See THERMESTHESIA.

**thermaesthesiometer.** See THERMESTHESIOMETER.

**thermal.** Pertaining to heat.

**thermalgesia.** The condition in which heat causes pain.

**thermangesthesia.** See THERMO-ANESTHESIA.

**thermanesthesia.** See THERMO-ANESTHESIA.

**thermesthesia.** The power of perceiving heat.

**thermesthesiometer.** An instrument used to measure the sensitivity of heat.

**thermic.** Pertaining to heat.

**thermo-anaesthesia.** See THERMO-ANESTHESIA.

**thermo-analgesia.** Insensibility to heat, due to disease of the brain.

**thermo-anesthesia.** Loss of the normal powers of detecting heat. See SYRINGOMYELIA.

**thermocauterectomy.** Surgical removal by means of an electric cautery.

**thermocautery.** An instrument consisting of a loop of platinum, which is usually heated by an electric current to a dull red. It is used for cutting through tissues and by its burning action seals off bleeding points. There are other forms of cautery heated by different means, but the electric cautery is the one in common use.

**Thermogene wool.** A proprietary brand of pink-colored wool used as a counterirritant for painful joints. See also CAPSICUM.

**thermogenesis.** The production of heat, especially within the body.

**thermogenetic, thermogenic.** Pertaining to thermogenesis.

**thermograph.** An instrument for recording temperature variations.

**thermohyperaesthesia.** See THERMOHYPERESTHESIA.

**thermohyperalgesia.** The condition in which the application of even moderate heat causes excessive pain.

**thermohyperesthesia.** Abnormal sensitivity to the application of heat.

**thermoinhibitory.** Preventing the production of heat.

**thermolabile.** Detroyed or changed by heat.

**thermolysis.** The dissipation of body heat; chemical decomposition produced by heat.

**thermolytic.** Relating to thermolysis.

**thermometer.** An instrument for measuring temperatures.

**alcohol thermometer.** A thermometer in which the expansive substance is alcohol.

**celsius thermometer.** The centigrade thermometer.

**centigrade thermometer.** A thermometer in which the freezing point of water is 0° and the boiling point of water is at 100°, the interval between these two points being divided into 100 parts. Also called *Celsius thermometer*.

**clinical thermometer.** A thermometer used to ascertain the body temperature; constructed so that the point to which the mercury rises remains stationary after removal of the thermometer from the patient. The body temperature can be taken in the mouth, under the arm, in the groin, or in the rectum. When taken under the arms or in the groins the skin should first be wiped free of perspiration. Before the thermometer is used the mercury must be shaken to the bottom of the column. For those who find this difficult to do, there is a special thermometer case fitted with handles so that the mercury can be shaken down by centrifugal spinning of the case. For children, the armpit or the groin is most often used, while the rectum is often used to take the temperature of babies. The rectal temperature is often a degree higher than that taken under the armpit.

**Fahrenheit thermometer.** A thermometer in which the interval between the freezing point and the boiling point of water is divided into 180°, freezing point being 32° and the boiling point 212°.

**maximum and minimum thermometer.** A thermometer with two joining tubes, each containing a marker and which register the maximum and minimum temperatures to which it has been exposed.

**Reamur thermometer.** A thermometer in which the freezing point of water is 0° and the boiling point of water is 80°.

**wet and dry bulb thermometer.** A device for determining the relative humidity of the atmosphere. It consists of two thermometers, the bulb of one of which is kept saturated with water, the evaporation of the water having a cooling effect which depresses the temperature. The temperature difference of the two thermometers depends on the relative humidity.

**thermometry.** The use of the thermometer.

**thermoneurosis.** A rise of temperature due to nervous instability.

**thermophobia.** The neurotic dread of heat.

**thermophore.** 1. Any device for holding heat, such as a hot-water bottle. 2. A vessel containing chemicals which absorb a considerable amount of heat and give it off by degrees during the process of crystallization.

**thermoplegia.** Heatstroke.

**thermopolypnea.** Rapid breathing due to high temperature.

**thermopolypnoea.** See THERMOPOLYP-NEA.

**thermostable.** Not affected by heat.

**thermotactic.** Relating to thermotaxis.

**thermotaxis.** 1. The regulation or adjustment of body temperature. 2. Thermotropism.

**thermotherapy.** The treatment of disease by heat.

**thermotropism.** The property possessed by some cells and organisms of moving or growing towards, or away from, heat.

**thiamine.** See ANEURIN.

**Thiersch's graft.** A form of skin grafting which consists of slicing away thin strips of the top layer for transfer to a raw wound or ulcer.

**thigh.** That portion of the lower limb situated between the pelvis and the knee.

**thighbone.** The femur.

**thigh joint.** The hip joint.

**thigmaesthesia.** See THIGMESTHESIA.

**thigmesthesia.** Sensitivity to touch.

**thiouracil.** A drug used to treat overactivity of the thyroid gland.

**third cranial nerve.** The oculomotor nerve. It innervates most of the muscles that move the eyeball.

**Thomas' splint.** A splint consisting of a leather-padded ring which surrounds the top of the thigh and from which metal bars extend on either side of the limb. Slings are tied to the metal bars and the limb lies on these slings. It is used primarily as a first-aid treatment for fractures of the femur.

**Thomsen's disease.** See MYOTONIA CONGENITA.

**thoracal.** Pertaining to the chest.

**thoracentesis.** Tapping the chest with a hollow needle to remove fluid.

**thoracic.** Pertaining to the chest.

**thoracico-abdominal.** Pertaining to both the chest and the abdomen.

**thoracocyllosis.** Malformation of the chest.

**thoracocyrtosis.** Abnormal prominence of the chest.

**thoracodynia.** Any pain in the chest.

**thoracoplasty.** Surgical removal of parts of all the ribs on one side to allow both the chest wall and the underlying lung to collapse and close cavities in the lung. Also called *pleuropneumolysis*.

**thoracoscopy.** Examination of the chest with a thorascope.

**thoracostenosis.** Compression of the chest walls.

**thoracostomy.** Surgical creation of an opening in the chest wall to allow drainage of fluid contents.

**thoracotomy.** Surgical incision into the chest wall.

**thorascope.** A surgical instrument equipped with a light, which is inserted into the chest so that the surgeon may visually examine the inside of the chest cavity. Also called THORACOSCOPE.

**thorax.** The chest, that part of the body between neck and abdomen.

**thorium.** A radioactive metal named after Thor, the Norse god of thunder. It is used to produce thorium X, a substance used in the treatment of some skin diseases.

**threadworm.** Tiny inch-long worms which inhabit the intestine. Also called *oxyuris vermicularis*.

**three-day fever.** See DENGUE.

**threpsis.** Nutrition.

**threpsology.** The study of nutrition.

**threshold.** 1. The lower limit of stimulus capable of producing an impression upon consciousness or evoking a response. 2. The entrance of a canal.

**thrill.** A vibration felt by placing the hand over an underlying aneurysm, over a heart with valvular disease, or over hydatid cysts.

**thrix.** Hair.

**thrix annulata.** Ringed hair, a condition in which the hair appears banded with light and dark segments.

**throat.** The pharynx; the fauces; the front part of the neck.

**throb.** A pulsation or beat.

**throbbing.** A rhythmic pulsation.

**throe.** A paroxysm of severe pain.

**thrombectomy.** Surgical removal of a thrombus, usually from a vein.

**thrombin.** The enzyme that causes clotting of shed blood.

**thrombinogen.** A substance which is the precursor of thrombin. Also called *prothrombin, thrombogen, proserozyme*.

**thromboangiitis.** Thrombosis accompanied by inflammation of the lining of a blood vessel.

**thromboangiitis obliterans.** See BUERGER'S DISEASE.

**thromboarteritis.** Clotting accompanied by inflammation of an artery.

**thromboclasis.** The breaking up or destruction of a thrombus. Also called *thrombolysis*.

**thrombocystis.** The sac which sometimes encloses a thrombus.

thrombocyte

**thrombocyte.** A blood platelet. See PLATELET.

**thrombogen.** See THROMBINOGEN.

**thrombogenesis.** Clot formation.

**thrombogenic.** The formation or forming of a clot.

**thromboid.** Resembling the character of a thrombus or clot.

**thrombokinase.** A substance capable of transforming thrombinogen to thrombin, part of the mechanism of the formation of a clot.

**thrombokinesis.** The clotting of blood.

**thrombolymphangitis.** Lymphangitis accompanied by clot formation.

**thrombolysis.** The dispersal or breaking up of a clot or thrombus. Also called *thromboclasis.*

**thrombophlebitis.** Inflammation of a vein accompanied by clot formation.

**thrombophthisis.** Destruction of blood platelets caused by a disorder of bone-marrow function.

**thromboplastid.** A blood platelet. See PLATELET.

**thromboplastin.** A substance which causes coagulation of shed blood.

**thrombosed.** Clotted.

**thrombosis.** The formation of a thrombus or clot. See also PHLEBITIS.

**cavernous sinus thrombosis.** Septic phlebitis arising from infection in the area of the face being carried into one of the large blood sinuses in the skull.

**thrombotic.** Pertaining to a thrombosis.

**thrombus.** A clot of blood formed within the heart or blood vessels, usually due to a slowing of the circulation or to alteration of the blood or walls of the blood vessels.

**throwback.** The appearance of a characteristic which existed in ancestors.

**thrush.** An infection due to the fungus *Candida albicans.* It occurs usually in children and is characterized by small, whitish spots on the tip and sides of the tongue and the lining membrane of the mouth. It is rapidly amenable to applications of gentian violet. Also called *mycotic stomatitis, parasitic stomatitis.*

**thrypsis.** A comminuted fracture.

**thylacitis.** Inflammation of the sebaceous glands of the skin.

**thymectomy.** Surgical removal of the thymus gland.

**thymelcosis.** Ulceration of the thymus gland.

**thymion.** A wart.

**thymiosis.** A condition in which wart-like growths appear. See YAWS.

**thymitis.** Inflammation of the thymus gland.

**thymolysis.** The destruction of thymus tissue.

**thymopathy.** 1. Any disorder of the thymus gland. 2. Any mental disease.

**thymus.** A gland situated in the front upper region of the chest. It grows until about the second year, remains unaffected until the fourteenth year, when it passes through fatty changes and wastes away. It has no known function.

**thyremphraxis.** Obstruction of the thyroid gland.

**thyroadenitis.** Inflammation of the thyroid gland.

**thyrocele.** Any tumor of the thyroid gland; a goiter.

**thyrochondrotomy.** Surgical incision into the thyroid cartilage.

**thyroepiglottic.** Pertaining both to the thyroid and the epiglottis of the throat.

**thyroglossal.** Pertaining to the thyroid gland and the tongue.

**thyrohyoid.** Pertaining to the thyroid gland or cartilage and the hyoid bone in the throat.

**thyroid.** Shaped like a shield; relating to the thyroid gland or thyroid cartilage; the thyroid gland.

**thyroid gland.** One of the chief ductless glands of the body, it is situated in the front of the throat and is called the "master gland" of the body because it controls other ductless glands and hormones. Overactivity of the gland is called hyperthyroidism or Graves's disease and is characterized by loss of weight, tremors of the hands, lips and tongue, prominent, staring eyeballs, and disordered action of the heart. Poor activity of the thyroid gland results in a disease called myxedema, characterized by coarsening of the hair and skin, mental sluggishness, and other symptoms. Growths of the thyroid gland are called goiters or Derbyshire neck, and result from the inadequate intake of iodine in the diet. See also GOITER, HYPERTHYROIDISM, MYXEDEMA.

**thyroidectomy.** Surgical removal of part or the whole of the thyroid gland.

**thyroidism.** The condition resulting from overuse of thyroid gland preparations; the disturbances due to overactivity of the thyroid gland; the aftereffects caused by surgical removal of part or the whole of the thyroid gland.

**thyroiditis.** Inflammation of the thyroid gland.

**thyroidotomy.** Surgical incision into the thyroid gland.

**thyrolaryngeal.** Pertaining to the thyroid cartilage and arytenoid cartilage of the larynx.

**thyroncus.** An old term for a goiter or thyrocele.

**thyrophyma.** A tumor of the thyroid gland.

**thyroprival.** The result of inactivity of the thyroid gland.

**thyroprivus.** 1. Lacking a thyroid gland. 2. The symptoms of disease due to the loss of the thyroid gland.

**thyroptosis.** Displacement of a goitrous thyroid gland so that it is partially or completely concealed in the chest. Also called *plunging goiter.*

**thyrosis.** Any disease due to disordered thyroid action.

**thyrotome.** A surgical instrument for incising the thyroid cartilage.

**thyrotomy.** Surgical division of the thyroid cartilage; surgical incision of the thyroid gland.

**thyrotoxicosis.** Overactivity of the thyroid gland. Also called *hyperthyroidism.*

**thyrotrope.** One afflicted with a thyroid gland disorder.

**thyrotropism.** The state of having a constitution in which the influence of the thyroid gland predominates.

**thyroxine.** The active hormone of the thyroid gland. It can now be prepared by synthesis, and is used to treat underactivity of the thyroid gland.

**tibia.** The inner of the two large bones of the leg below the knee. Also called *shinbone.*

**tibial.** Pertaining to the tibia.

**tibialgia.** Pain in the tibia.

**tibiocalcanean.** Pertaining to the tibia and the calcaneus.

**tibiofemoral.** Pertaining to the tibia and the femur.

**tibiofibular.** Pertaining to the tibia and the fibula.

**tibiotarsal.** Pertaining to the tibia and the tarsus.

**tic.** A spasmodic twitching, especially of the facial muscles; a habit spasm.

**tic convulsive.** A muscular spasm occurring in the face, in the area supplied by the seventh cranial nerve.

**tic douloureux.** A form of intense neuralgia, occurring in the area at the side of the face supplied by the fifth cranial nerve. The pain is very severe and can be precipitated by a casual movement such as brushing the hair. Also called *prosopalgia, trigeminal neuralgia.*

**tick.** The popular name for a number of blood-sucking parasites.

**tick fever.** Any infectious disease transmitted by the bite of a tick, such as African relapsing fever, Rocky Mountain spotted fever, or Texas fever.

**tilmus.** The delirious picking at bedclothes seen in serious diseases associated with high fever.

**time.** The duration of an event or phenomenon.

**bleeding time.** The time it takes for a needle prick, usually in the ear lobe, to stop bleeding. In normal persons it is usually one to three minutes, but in those suffering from hemophilia the time may be indefinite.

**clot retraction time.** The time it takes for a sample of blood to form a contracted clot, usually about one hour.

**clotting time.** The time it takes a blood specimen to form a normal clot, usually five to eight minutes.

**prothrombin time.** The time required for oxylated plasma to clot after adding thromboplastin. The time is measured in seconds and is inversely proportional to the quantity of prothrombin present.

**reaction time.** The interval between the application of a stimulus and the beginning of a response, or, alternatively, the time it takes between seeing a situation and making some muscular movement, such as applying the brakes of a car when sighting an obstruction. In a normal, healthy young adult this is approximately one-fifth of a second.

**tincture.** An alcoholic extract of a drug.

**tinea.** Ringworm; a fungus infection of the skin.

**tinea barbae.** Ringworm of the beard area. Also called *barber's itch, barber's rash, tinea sycosis.* See also SYCOSIS.

**tinea capitis.** Ringworm of the scalp. In its earliest stage, it appears as a small scaly spot, with a few broken hairs present on the patch. It may occur in epidemic form among children through wearing each other's caps.

**tinea circinata.** See TINEA CORPORIS, below.

**tinea corporis.** Ringworm occurring anywhere on the skin and characterized by a patch tending to heal in the center with a well-defined advancing edge, red in color, scaly, and sometimes with small vesicles or pustules. Also called *tinea circinata, tinea glabrosa.*

**tinea cruris.** Ringworm involving the skin of the groin and the areas around the anus and vagina. This form appears to be highly contagious and is eradicated with difficulty when it appears in residential institutions. It is often associated with ringworm of the feet, and is rarely seen in women, except in hot climates. Infection may also come from shower-bath floors, duckboards, bath mats and possibly lavatory seats, towels, and borrowed clothing. Also called *gym itch, jockey itch, dhobie itch.*

**tinea favosa.** A chronic fungus infection often limited to the scalp, the characteristic lesions being sulfur-yellow cups, about one-eighth inch in diameter, which produce a peculiar mouselike odor.

**tinea imbricata.** A form of ringworm

normally found in the tropics and consisting of patches or concentric scaly rings on the skin, which spread out and produce an appearance like watered silk. The scales are thin flakes, like tissue paper, firmly attached towards the margin of the ring and free towards the center. Also called *gogo, scaly ringworm, Tokelau ringworm, tropical tinea circinata.*

**tinea pedis.** Ringworm of the feet. Also called *athlete's foot, epidermophytosis.*

**tinea unguium.** A chronic fungus infection involving the nails of the hands and feet. The affected nails become discolored, opaque, and brittle and a scaly mass forms under the free margin of the nail, above which the nail plate breaks away unevenly, leaving a spiked, upturned edge.

**tinea versicolor.** A chronic condition in which the lesions are fawn-colored, pale pink, or café-au-lait tinted; well-defined patches usually spread over the skin of the trunk. The factors which maintain this infection are excessive sweating, infrequent washing with soap and water, and wearing underclothes that are not boiled in the wash. Also called *pityriasis versicolor.*

**tinnitus.** A singing, rushing, or roaring sound in the ears. It may be high-pitched, like the hissing of steam, or low-pitched, like the roaring of an underground train. In some cases it is due to hardening of the minute artery of the eardrum, in which case the patient is listening to his own circulation. Tinnitus, when accompanied by deafness and giddy attacks, is called Ménière's disease. It may also result from taking excessive quantities of drugs such as aspirin and quinine.

**tiqueur.** One affected with the spasmodic movements called tics.

**tisane.** An infusion prepared by pouring boiling water over an herb such as mint. Depending on the herb used, these decoctions are alleged to have health-promoting or restorative properties.

**tissue.** An aggregate of cells usually of similar structure which perform the same or related functions, as muscle tissue.

**titillation.** Tickling.

**titre.** A standard of strength or purity.

**titurbation.** A reeling gait observed in diseases of the cerebellum.

**tobacco.** A plant, the dried leaves of which contain the poisonous alkaloid nicotine. Unquestionably tobacco plays a large part in producing in smoker's chronic bronchitis, heart disease, and cancer of the lung. The stalks of the tobacco leaves are

crushed into a powder and mixed with menthol and other aromatics and used as snuff. Regular snuff takers are liable to develop cancer of certain parts of the nose.

**tobacco amblyopia.** Loss of vision caused by smoking excessive quantities of heavy shag.

**tobacco heart.** An irritable condition of the heart caused by excessive use of tobacco.

**tocology.** The science of midwifery.

**tocophobia.** Excessive fear of childbirth.

**tokus.** An obsolete term for childbirth.

**tolerance.** The capacity to endure the influence of a drug, particularly when it is being administered for a long time.

**tolerant.** Withstanding the effects of a drug without coming to any harm.

**tomograph.** A special form of x-ray apparatus which takes a picture of different sections or layers of the body.

**tomomania.** An excessive desire to undergo or to perform surgical operations.

**tonaphasia.** Loss of the ability to sing due to disease of the brain.

**tone.** 1. The normal state of tension of a part. 2. A particular quality of sound or of the voice.

**tongue.** The movable muscular organ attached to the floor of the mouth and concerned with tasting, masticating, swallowing, and speaking. It is covered by a mucous membrane, from which project numerous papillae containing the organs of taste. When the tongue is extruded from the mouth, as in examining the back of the throat, a number of large papillae come into view. These, to the uninitiated, look abnormal and many patients fear they have some form of growth, but in fact, these papillae are quite harmless and a normal configuration of the back part of the tongue. The tongue's movements are limited by a fold of tissue, called the *frenum linguae,* connecting the undersurface of the tongue with the floor of the mouth. In some individuals the frenum linguae is too short, thus limiting the movement of the tongue. Such a condition is called being tongue-tied.

**geographic tongue.** See LINGUA GEO-GRAPHICA.

**tonic.** 1. Pertaining to tone, causing normal tone; marked by tension, contraction, or spasm; an agent imparting normal tone to a part or to a whole organism. 2. A form of medicine to which is ascribed potent powers of stimulating the body to a better state of health. In point of fact, so-called tonics are either bitter or stimulating and have nowhere near the pharmacological action ascribed to them by the patient. Many doctors are convinced that there is no such thing as a tonic.

**tonicity.** The state of normal tone of the body.

**tonitrophobia.** Morbid fear of thunder.

**tonometer.** An instrument for measuring tension, especially that within the eyeball, to test for glaucoma.

**tonsil.** 1. One of the two small, oval-shaped, fleshy bodies, situated on each side of the back of the throat. They are probably part of the system which produces antibodies in the presence of germs and serve a real purpose in early life. 2. A small lobe of the cerebellar hemisphere.

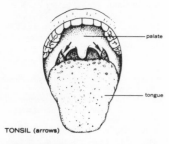

TONSIL (arrows)

**tonsilla.** A tonsil.

**tonsillar.** Pertaining to a tonsil; acting upon a tonsil.

**tonsillar crypt.** The small holes in the tonsil that sometimes become filled with a cheeselike material which shows as whitish areas when the tonsil is examined. This cheesy substance is largely composed of waste products, bacteria, and bits of food.

**tonsillectome.** A surgical instrument used to remove a tonsil.

**tonsillectomy.** Surgical removal of a tonsil. This operation is performed much less frequently today than it was in the past, for it is now realized that many of the indications for removing tonsils in children are no longer valid. In most cases it is only the adenoids behind the nose that need removing in order to promote drainage of the eustachian tube. Many parents have an exaggerated idea of the advantages of having the tonsils removed and expect that once this has been done they will see a tremendous improvement in their child's health. Such expectations are largely illusory. The tonsils are removed only because they are septic and will cause further trouble if left, not because their removal will suddenly release a flood of good health into a child. The one classical and compulsory indication for removing the tonsils is a history of quinsy. Once the quinsy has burst and recovered, it leaves an infected space behind the tonsil which forms a breeding ground for germs, and the only way to eradicate this space is to remove the tonsil over it.

**tonsillitis.** Inflammation of a tonsil.

**tonsillolith.** A stone formed in a tonsil.

**tonsillotome.** A surgical instrument used in removing a tonsil.

**tonsillotomy.** Surgical cutting away of the whole or part of a tonsil.

**tooth.** One of the calcified structures which grow from the jaws and which serve to masticate food, aid speech, and influence facial contours. Each tooth consists of (1) a mass of dentin surrounding a cavity which contains the dental pulp, the nerve, and blood vessels; (2) a crown covered by enamel; (3) a root, which may be single, double, or treble, covered by cementum; and (4) a neck which is the junction between the crown and the root. See also TEETH.

**artificial tooth.** A tooth made by a dentist; part of a denture.

**bicuspid tooth.** See PREMOLAR TOOTH, below.

**buck tooth.** A protruding tooth.

**canine tooth.** A tooth with a conical crown, situated between the lateral incisor and the first premolar.

**cheek tooth.** One of the molar teeth which act as grinders of food.

**cuspid tooth.** See CANINE TOOTH, above.

**deciduous tooth.** One of the twenty temporary or milk teeth which are replaced about the age of seven years by the permanent teeth.

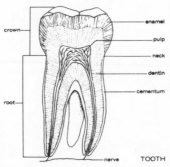

TOOTH

**eye tooth.** The upper canine tooth.

**incisor tooth.** One of the two cutting teeth nearest the midline.

**milk tooth.** See DECIDUOUS TOOTH, above.

**molar tooth.** One of the back teeth which act as grinders of food. In the human jaw there are three molars in each quadrant, behind the premolars.

**multicuspid tooth.** See MOLAR TOOTH, above.

**notched tooth.** A tooth with an irregular cutting edge due to maldevelopment.

**permanent tooth.** One of the 32 teeth in the second dentition in the human being, consisting of eight incisors, four canines, eight premolars, and twelve molars.

**pivot tooth.** An artificial crown pegged onto a natural tooth.

**premolar tooth.** One of the two teeth with two cusps, situated between the canine and the first molar tooth in each quadrant of the permanent dentition.

**stomach tooth.** The lower canine tooth.

**supernumerary tooth.** A tooth additional to the normal complement of teeth.

**temporary tooth.** 1. A tooth of the first dentition; also called *milk tooth, deciduous tooth.* 2. A provisional set of artificial teeth inserted immediately following dental extractions and used only until the gums have shrunk.

**wisdom tooth.** The third molar tooth. This normally erupts at about the age of 20 or 21 years but in many cases does not erupt at all. In many cases there is no room for the wisdom tooth, so that when it does try to erupt it frequently causes trouble and has to be extracted.

**toothpaste.** See DENTIFRICE.

**Tooth's atrophy.** The peroneal type (starting in the muscles on the outer side of the lower leg) of progressive muscular atrophy. Also called *Tooth's. type.*

**topaesthesia.** See TOPESTHESIA.

**topagnosis.** Loss of sensitiveness to touch localization.

**topalgia.** See TOPOALGIA.

**toper's nose.** See RHINOPHYMA.

**topesthesia.** Local sensitivity to touch.

**tophaceous.** Gritty.

**tophus.** A mineral concretion in the body, especially about the joints; deposits of sodium urate in the skin about a joint, in the ear, or in a bone; a characteristic of gout. The term is also occasionally applied to dental tartar or a syphilitic node.

**topical.** Local; referring to a particular spot.

**topoalgia.** Local pain, common in cases of neurasthenia and hysteria, and often appears suddenly after an emotional disturbance or crisis. Also called *topalgia.*

**topography.** Study of the areas of the body and its parts.

**toponeurosis.** Any localized neurosis.

**toponymy.** The names pertaining to the position of organs.

**topophobia.** The neurotic dread of certain places.

**toric.** Relating to a torus.

**tormina.** Gripping pain in the intestines.

**torminal, torminous.** Pertaining to or affected with griping pains in the intestines.

**torpent.** 1. Any agent that allays irritation. 2. Inactive, incapable of normal function.

**torpid.** Sluggish or inactive.

**torpidity.** Sluggishness.

**torpor.** Sluggishness; lack of reaction to normal stimuli.

**torrefaction.** Drying up by the application of strong heat, roasting.

**torrefy.** To dry up by the application of strong heat; to parch; to roast.

**torsion.** 1. A twisting. 2. The rotation of the eye about its visual axis; the tilting of the vertical meridian of the eye.

*Medically, torsion has often an ominous significance, because the twisting of an organ may cut off its blood supply and produce death of the organ or gangrene requiring an emergency surgical operation, as for instance in torsion of a freely hanging fibroid tumor of the womb.*

**torso.** The trunk of the body.

**torticollis.** A contraction of the neck muscles causing the head to be carried in an abnormal posture. Also called *wryneck*.

**torulus.** A small prominence or elevation.

**torus.** A swelling or bulging projection.

**touch.** The sense by which contact of some part of the body, especially the fingers, to an object gives evidence of the object's qualities; tactile sense.

**tourniquet.** Any apparatus for controlling bleeding from any part of the body where direct pressure can be brought upon the blood vessels by means of straps, cords, rubber tubes, or pads. See also HEMORRHAGE.

*Tourniquets are made in a multiplicity of forms, from the simplest emergency adaptation of a handkerchief or a piece of clothing wound round a limb and tightened with a stick, to elaborate instruments which apply pressure by screws acting upon metal pads or by a rubber hose encircling the limb and distended with air by means of a pump. Tourniquets have largely fallen into disuse as a first-aid means of controlling bleeding because of the risks involved in using them, such as damage to nerves and blood vessels. The safest method of arresting bleeding is by a firmly applied pad and bandage or, if this proves ineffective, by a rubber constrictive bandage.*

**toxaemia.** See TOXEMIA.

**toxanaemia.** See TOXANEMIA.

**toxanemia.** Anemia caused by poison.

**toxemia.** A general infection or blood poisoning in which the blood contains germ poisons but not the actual germs. It may also be caused by poisonous products of body cells. Also called *toxicohemia, toxinemia*.

**toxic.** Poisonous, relating to a toxin.

**toxicity.** Poisonous.

**toxicoderma.** Skin disease caused by poison.

**toxicodermatitis.** Inflammatory skin disease caused by poison.

**toxicogenic.** Producing a poison.

**toxicohaemia.** See TOXICOHEMIA.

**toxicohemia.** See TOXEMIA.

**toxicoid.** Resembling a poison.

**toxicologist.** One skilled in the study of poisons, their detection, and treatment.

**toxicology.** The study of poisons.

**toxicomania.** A neurotic desire for poisonous substances.

**toxicopathy.** Any disease produced by poison.

**toxicopexis.** Neutralization of poisons.

**toxicophobia.** Neurotic dread of being poisoned.

**toxicosis.** A condition of being poisoned.

**toxidermitis.** A skin condition produced by poison.

**toxiferous.** Producing or transmitting poison.

**toxigenous.** Producing poisons.

**toxin.** A poisonous product of animal or plant cells which, on injection to animals or man, causes the formation of antibodies called antitoxins. The most important toxins are those produced by higher plants, some animals, and pathogenic bacteria.

**phytotoxins.** Toxins produced by plants.

**zootoxins.** Those toxins produced by animals. They include snake venom and the poisons of spiders.

**toxinaemia.** See TOXINEMIA.

**toxin–antitoxin.** A mixture in which the toxin present is almost neutralized by the presence of the appropriate antitoxin. See also TOXIN.

**toxinemia.** See TOXEMIA.

**toxinfection.** Infection caused through a germ toxin.

**toxinic.** Pertaining to a toxin.

**toxinicide.** Any agent capable of destroying toxins.

**toxinosis.** Any disease caused by a poison.

**toxiphobia.** The neurotic dread of being poisoned.

**toxoid.** A nonpoisonous product similar to a toxin but with the ability to provoke the body into producing antibodies after it has been injected.

**toxoid–antitoxoid.** A mixture of toxoid and antitoxin serum.

**toxolysin.** A substance capable of neutralizing a specific germ poison. Also called *antitoxin*.

**toxophile.** Having an affinity for poisons.

**toxophore.** The poisonous element of a toxin.

**toxophorous.** Pertaining to a toxophore.

**toxoplasmosis.** A disease caused by a small banana-shaped protozoon, many of which collect together in body cells, like herrings in a barrel, and form cysts, which may remain dormant for years. The source of infection may be dogs, cats, mice, hens, or ducks. The disease appears in various guises resembling chorioretinitis, hemolytic disease of the newborn, or neonatal purpura, or it may resemble typhus fever or glandular fever. Sometimes there occurs myocarditis, pericarditis, or encephalitis.

**trabecula.** Any of the septa (connective tissue partitions) passing from a capsule into the interior of an organ.

**trabecular.** Pertaining to a trabecula.

**trabeculate.** Pertaining to a trabecula.

**tracer.** A radioactive isotope which, because of its unique physical properties, can be detected in extremely minute quantities, and hence is used to trace the chemical behavior of the natural element. Such use of isotopes is referred to as a tracer study. The isotope itself is the tracer. See also ISOTOPE.

**trachea.** The cartilaginous tube extending from the larynx to the bronchi and serving as the passage for conveying air to and from the lungs. Also called *windpipe*.

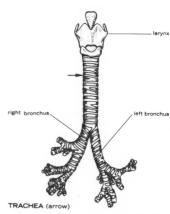

TRACHEA (arrow)

**tracheaectasy.** Dilation of the trachea.

**tracheal.** Pertaining to the trachea.

**trachealgia.** Any pain in the trachea.

**tracheitis.** Inflammation of the trachea. This is the "raw chest" experienced during a cold or early attack of bronchitis. Also called *trachitis.*

**trachelagra.** Gout in the neck.

**trachelectomopexy.** A surgical operation in which part of the womb is removed and the neck of the womb is surgically fixed.

**trachelismus.** Spasmodic contraction of the neck muscles; a bending backward of the neck, sometimes seen in epileptic attacks.

**trachelitis.** Inflammation of the neck of the womb. Also called *cervicitis.*

**trachelomyitis.** Inflammation of the neck muscles.

**trachelopexia, trachelopexy.** Fixation of the neck of the womb.

**tracheloplasty.** Surgical repair of the neck of the womb.

**trachelorrhaphy.** The sewing up of a laceration of the neck of the womb.

**trachelotomy.** Surgical incision into the neck of the womb.

**tracheobronchial.** Pertaining to the trachea and the bronchi.

**tracheobronchitis.** An inflammation involving both the trachea and the bronchi.

**tracheo-esophageal.** Pertaining to the trachea and the esophagus.

**tracheolaryngeal.** Pertaining to the trachea and the larynx.

**tracheolaryngotomy.** Combined laryngotomy and tracheotomy, an operation to open both the larynx and the trachea.

**tracheomalacia.** Morbid softening of the cartilages of the trachea.

**tracheo-oesophageal.** See TRACHEO-ESOPHAGEAL.

**tracheopathia, tracheopathy.** Any disease of the trachea.

**tracheopharyngeal.** Pertaining to the trachea and the pharynx.

**tracheoscopy.** Examination of the interior of the trachea by means of an instrument fitted with an electric light and a mirror.

**tracheostenosis.** Abnormal narrowing of the trachea.

**tracheostoma.** An artificial opening through the neck into the trachea.

**tracheostomy.** Surgical creation of an opening into the trachea through the neck.

**tracheotomy.** Surgical incision into the trachea.

**tracheotomy tube.** A metal tube which is placed in the aperture made from the outside of the neck into the trachea to enable the patient to breathe when he is in danger of asphyxiation due to obstruction in the normal breathing channels.

**trachitis.** See TRACHEITIS.

**trachoma.** A highly contagious virus disease of the eyelids, characterized by small glistening elevations on the conjunctiva and later by severe scarring, contractures, and deformity of the lids. It may lead to blindness.

**trachomatous.** Pertaining to or affected with trachoma.

**trachyphonia.** Hoarseness of the voice.

**tract. 1.** A pathway or course. **2.** A bundle of nerve fibers; any of the nervous pathways of the spinal cord or brain. **3.** A group of parts or organs serving some special purpose, such as the intestinal, respiratory, or genitourinary tracts.

**traction.** The act of drawing or dragging.

**ambulatory traction.** Traction exerted by a walking splint or brace on a fractured limb or inflamed joint while the patient is up and about.

**axis traction.** Traction which is in the axis or direction of a channel, as of the pelvis, through which a body, such as a baby, is to be drawn.

**bed traction.** Any type of traction in which the patient is, of necessity, confined to bed.

**head traction.** Traction exerted upon the head; usually employed in the treatment of neck injuries.

**skeletal traction.** Traction applied to long bones by such means as pins or wires; used in orthopedics.

**weight traction.** Traction exerted by means of a weight connected to a limb to maintain a fractured bone in position during recovery.

**tractotomy.** Surgical cutting of a nerve tract.

**tractus.** A tract.

**tragal.** Relating to the tragus.

**tragalism.** Lust.

**tragophonia, tragophony.** A bleating type of voice.

**tragus. 1.** The small piece of skin and cartilage which projects outwards and slightly over the ear opening; also called *hircus.* **2.** One of the hairs growing at the opening of the ear.

**trait.** Any characteristic, quality, or property of an individual.

**trance. 1.** The hypnotic state resembling sleep. **2.** A form of catalepsy characterized by a prolonged condition of abnormal sleep in which the vital functions are suspended and from which the patient, as a rule, cannot be aroused. Breathing is almost imperceptible and sensation abolished. The onset and reawakening are both very sudden.

**tranquilizer.** Any of several drugs capable of relieving tension, usually without causing depression or extreme drowsiness.

**transection.** Cross section.

**transference.** In psychoanalysis, the revival of forgotten and repressed experiences of childhood which are relived, not as they actually occurred but in relationship to the attending psychoanalyst or doctor. The term is also applied to an intense emotional attachment of the patient to the doctor as a compensation for an inadequate adjustment to reality.

**transfusion.** A transfer of blood into the veins; the introduction of blood, saline solution, or other liquids directly into the blood stream.

**transiliac.** Crossing from one ilium to the other.

**transillumination.** Illumination of an object by transmitted light; illumination of the walls of a cavity by a light which penetrates them; the projection of brilliant light through the substance of a hollow organ, a method sometimes used to reveal fluid in a nasal sinus or to illuminate a hydrocele. In the latter case, if the light transmits, the swelling contains clear fluid, but if it is opaque it contains either a tumor or blood.

**transmigration.** The act of passing across or through anything, such as the passing of the egg cell from the ovary to the womb; the passage of the white blood cells through the walls of the capillaries.

**transmission.** The communication or transfer of anything, especially disease, from one person to another or from one place to another.

**placental transmission.** The conveyance of drugs or disease products through the placental circulation of the mother into her baby.

**transmutation. 1.** The act of changing. **2.** The turning of one substance into another.

*The ancient alchemists always dreamed that one day they would be able to change lead into gold, and history records many incidents of charlatans who claimed to have achieved this. However, it was only with the invention of the atomic pile that the dream has come near to realization, for chemical elements have been altered into other elements, though not lead into gold!*

**transonance.** Transmitted resonance, such as the heart sounds heard through the chest wall.

**transpiration.** The discharge of fluid or gas through the skin; the material thus emitted.

**transplantation.** The transplanting of tissues taken from another body or from another part of the same body.

*In the past the transplantation of organs or tissue from one body to another has proved unsuccessful because the re-*

*cipient body has always rejected strange tissue. Now new techniques are making transplantation possible and already the cornea of an eye from a dead body can be transplanted onto the eye of a live person to restore the sight. Some success has been achieved in transplanting kidneys and the heart from one person to another. In the case of some heart transplants life has been extended more than a year. The enthusiasts even visualize the day when any worn organ can be replaced, and though this is a dream at the moment it seems not beyond the power of practical application in the future.*

**transposition.** Usually refers to a change in the position of internal organs, such as finding an organ situated on the opposite side of the body to normal. Occasionally the heart is found on the opposite side (a condition called dextrocardia), and sometimes also the appendix is found on the left side of the body instead of on the right.

**transudate.** A liquid or other substance produced by transudation.

**transudation.** The passing of fluids through a membrane, especially of blood serum through the walls of the capillaries.

**transurethral.** Refers to any operation performed by passing an instrument down the urethra.

**transvaginal.** Across or through the vagina.

**transverse.** Lying crosswise; at right angles to the long axis of the body.

**transversectomy.** Surgical removal of the transverse process of a vertebra.

**transvesical.** Through the urinary bladder.

**transvestism.** The wearing of clothes belonging to the opposite sex.

**transvestite.** One addicted to transvestism.

**trapezium.** 1. The first bone on the thumb side of the second row of carpal bones of the wrist and hand. 2. A band of fibers in the brain.

**trauma.** Any injury or wound.

**psychic trauma.** An emotional shock leaving a deep psychological impression.

**traumatic.** Pertaining to a wound or injury.

**traumatism.** A state resulting from trauma.

**traumatopathy.** Any disease arising from a wound or injury.

**traumatopnea.** The escape of air through a wound in the chest wall.

**traumatopnoea.** See TRAUMATOPNEA.

**tremble.** To shake or quiver.

**tremor.** An involuntary quivering or shaking.

**tremulous.** Shaking or trembling.

**trench fever.** An acute infection of several days' duration caused by a rickettsial germ and transmitted by the body louse.

**trench mouth.** A disease which affects the gums and the oral mucous membrane and manifests itself by tenderness and bleeding of the gums. The suspected bacteria causing the disorder are also found in the healthy mouth and it is for this reason that trench mouth is thought to be brought on by poor hygiene and nutritional deficiencies.

*Trench mouth derived its name during the First World War when it was prevalent among soldiers in the trenches.*

**Trendelenburg's operation.** An operation in which the long saphenous vein in the thigh is tied, as part of the treatment of varicose veins in the leg.

**Trendelenburg's position.** The patient lies on his back with the operating table tilted so that the head is low. This position enables the surgeon to operate in the lower part of the abdomen, such as on the prostate gland, bladder, or womb, with his field of operation free of coils of intestine, which fall by gravity towards the top of the abdomen when the patient is in this position.

**trepan.** See TREPHINE.

**trepanning.** Boring; using the trephine.

**trephination.** See TREPHINING.

**trephine.** A sawlike surgical instrument for removing a disc of bone or other tissue; to remove with such an instrument either a circular segment of bone from the skull or part of the sclera in order to relieve excessive pressure within these structures.

**trephining.** The operation of using a trephine.

**Treponema.** A genus of germs which cause such diseases as syphilis and yaws.

**treponemicidal.** Destructive of species belonging to the genus *Treponema*.

**tribadism.** Sexual excitement between two women, practiced by friction of the genitals. Also called *lesbianism, sapphism.*

**triceps.** Having three heads, usually applied to a muscle.

**trichangia.** The capillary blood vessels.

**trichangiectasis.** Dilation of the capillary blood vessels.

**trichauxis.** Excessive growth of hair on part or the whole of the body.

**trichiasis.** Ingrowing eyelashes, which irritate the eye.

**trichiniasis.** See TRICHINOSIS.

**trichinophobia.** Neurotic dread of trichinosis.

**trichinosis.** A disease caused by eating half-cooked pork containing the larvae of a small worm which is parasitic in pigs and occasionally in man. The symptoms produced are nausea, giddiness, colic, and fever in the early stages and later there is prostration accompanied by swellings in the muscles, edema of the face, and delirium. The possibility of this disorder is a very good reason for insuring that pork products are thoroughly cooked.

**trichitis.** Inflammation of the hair roots.

**trichobezoar.** A hairball. Some insane patients pull out their own hair and swallow it until their stomach is completely distended by a trichobezoar, or hairball, which has to be removed by a surgical operation.

**trichocardia.** Inflammation of the pericardium with pseudomembranous elevations which resemble hair. Also called *hairy heart.*

**trichocephaliasis.** A disease caused by infestation with threadworms.

**trichoclasia, trichoclasis.** See TRICHORRHEXIS NODOSA.

**trichoepithelioma.** A skin tumor having its origin in the hair roots.

**trichoglossia.** A thickening of the tongue papillae, producing an appearance as if the tongue were covered with hair. Also called *hairy tongue.*

**trichoid.** Like hair.

**tricholith.** A hairy stone.

**trichologia.** Plucking out of the hair; seen in babies and small children and in certain mental disorders.

**trichologist.** One who studies the hair and its diseases; usually a skin specialist in medical practice. However, the title is sometimes adopted by hairdressers in order to invest themselves with a feeling of importance and to impress the public, so that in this context trichologist means no more than a hairdresser with a posh name and little or no real knowledge of diseases.

**trichology.** The study of the hair and its diseases.

**trichomatose.** Matted.

**trichomatosis.** A matted state of the hair.

**trichomatous.** Pertaining to or affected with matted hair.

**trichomonad.** Trichomonas.

**trichomonal.** Relating to the trichomonas.

**Trichomonas.** A genus of ciliate protozoa, a low form of life.

**Trichomonas intestinalis.** A species of *Trichomonas* which attacks the intestines, producing diarrhea and enteritis.

**Trichomonas vaginalis.** A species of *Trichomonas* found in the vagina. It produces a form of white discharge called leucorrhea.

**trichomoniasis.** The state of being attacked by species of the genus *Trichomonas*.

**trichomycosis.** Any disease of the hair caused by a fungus parasite.

**trichonosis, trichonosus, trichopathy.** Any disease of the hair.

**trichophagy, trichophagia.** The habit of eating hair; seen in small children and insane persons. See TRICHOLOGIA.

**trichophobia.** A morbid fear of hair.

**trichophytic.** 1. Pertaining to the trichophyton fungus, a parasite which attacks hair and produces ringworm. 2. Contributing to the growth of hair; an agent that contributes to the growth of hair.

**Trichophyton.** The genus *Trichophyton*, a fungus, of which several species are causative agents for ringworm.

**trichophytosis.** A contagious disease of the skin and hair, occurring mostly in children and due to the invasion of the skin by the fungus *Trichophyton*. It is characterized by circular scaly patches and partial loss of hair. Also called ringworm.

**trichopoliosis.** Greying of the hair.

**trichoptilosis.** Trichorrhexis.

**trichorrhea.** Rapid loss of hair.

**trichorrhexis.** Brittleness of the hair.

**trichorrhexis nodosa.** An atrophic condition of the hair, usually affecting the beard, and characterized by irregular, nodelike thickenings on the hair shaft that are really partial breakages of the hair. The hairs often break, leaving a brushlike end; thus the condition produces a certain amount of alopecia. Also called *trichoclasia, trichoclasis*.

**trichorrhoea.** See TRICHORRHEA.

**trichoschisis.** Splitting of the hairs.

**trichoscopy.** Inspection of the hair.

**trichosis.** Any hair disease.

**Trichosporon.** A genus of fungus which causes trichomycosis.

**trichosporosis.** The disease produced by infestation with the fungus *Trichosporon*.

**trichotillomania.** The neurotic urge to pluck out one's own hair.

**trichromatopsia.** Possessing normal color vision; the power to see all three primary colors.

**trichuriasis.** Infestation of the intestinal tract with a species of threadworm, *Trichuris trichiura*.

**tricipital.** Having three heads; relating to the triceps muscle.

**tricorn.** Three-horned, or having three processes.

**tricornute.** Possessing three hornlike prominences.

**tricrotic.** Having three waves to one pulse beat.

**tricrotism.** The quality of being tricrotic.

**tricuspid.** 1. Having three cusps. 2. Pertaining to the tricuspid valve, a heart valve situated in the opening between the right atrium and the right ventricle.

**trident, tridentate.** Three-toothed or three-pronged.

**trifacial nerve.** The fifth cranial nerve. Also called *trigeminal nerve*.

**trigeminal.** Separating into three sections.

**trigeminal nerve.** The fifth cranial nerve, which divides into three main branches and supplies the face. Also called *trifacial nerve*.

**trigeminal neuralgia.** Pain in the trigeminal nerve. See also NEURALGIA; TIC; TIC DOULOUREUX.

**trigger finger.** 1. A condition in which difficulty is at first experienced in flexing or extending a finger, but in which the movement is later performed, with a sudden click or jerk. 2. The forefinger of the hand that is dominant.

**trigger knee.** A state in which the movement of the knee joint suddenly ceases during flexion or extension and the leg jerks sideways.

**trigonal.** Relating to a trigone.

**trigone.** A triangle.

**trigone of the bladder.** A smooth triangular area situated inside the urinary bladder, just behind the opening of the urethra. It is an especially sensitive area, and irritation of it by inflammation or the presence of a stone sets up a spasm which causes intense pain at the end of the act of passing urine.

**trilabe.** A three-pronged instrument used for removing stones from the bladder.

**trilaminar.** Having three layers.

**trilateral.** Having three sides.

**trilobate.** Having three lobes.

**trilocular.** Having three cells.

**trimensual.** Recurring every three months.

**trimester.** A period of three months; often used in relation to pregnancy.

**trimethylene.** An anesthetic. Also called *cyclopropane*.

**trinitrin.** Glyceryl trinitrate; used in the treatment of angina pectoris.

**trinitroglycerin.** Trinitrin.

**trinucleate.** Having three nuclei.

**tripara.** A woman who has had three pregnancies resulting in three viable children.

**triphasic.** Having three phases or variations.

**triphthemia.** The accumulation of waste products in the blood.

**triplegia.** Paralysis of one arm and leg on one side of the body, together with paralysis of either the arm or leg of the other side.

**triple-X syndrome.** A congenital abnormality associated with mental defects and underdevelopment of the sexual organs; considered to be due to an abnormality of the sex chromosome pattern.

**triradial, triradiate.** Radiating in three directions.

**triskaidekaphobia.** Morbid fear of the number thirteen.

**trismoid.** A form of lockjaw occurring in newborn infants and believed to be caused by pressure on the back of the skull during labor.

**trismus.** Lockjaw, an early symptom of tetanus.

**tristimania.** Depression, melancholia.

**tritanopia.** A defect in a third constituent essential for color vision, such as violet blindness.

**triturable.** Capable of being reduced to a fine powder.

**triturate.** To produce a fine powder.

**trituration.** The process of producing a fine powder.

**trocar.** A surgical instrument consisting of a perforator enclosed within a cannula and used for puncturing a cavity. The perforator is then removed, leaving the cannula within the cavity to drain out fluid.

**trochanter.** One of two bony knobs at the upper end of the femur. The major trochanter is on the outer side, and the minor trochanter is on the inner side of the bone.

**trochanteric.** Relating to a trochanter.

**troche, trochiscus.** A lozenge or medicated tablet.

**trochlea.** Any part or process that acts as a pulley.

**trochlear.** Acting as or pertaining to a pulley; pertaining to the trochlear nerve of the eyeball.

**trochocardia.** Displacement of the heart due to its rotary movement on its own axis.

**trochoid.** Acting as a pulley or pivot.

**troilism.** An abnormal sexual relationship practiced by three persons: either two women and one man, or one woman and two men.

**tromomania.** Delirium tremens.

**tromophonia.** A trembling of the voice.

**trophesial, trophesic.** Pertaining to trophesy.

**trophesy.** Defective nutrition of a part from disorder of the nerves regulating nutrition.

**trophic.** Pertaining to the functions concerned in nutrition, digestion, and assimilation of food.

**trophic centers.** The nerves governing the nutrition of organs.

**trophotaxis.** Cell adjustment in relation to stimuli originating from nutritive materials.

**tropical abscess.** See AMEBIC ABSCESS.

**Trueta method.** A treatment of war wounds used during the Spanish Civil War by Trueta, a Spanish surgeon now in England. Developed from the Winett-Orr closed plaster technique for the treatment of wounds, it is now called the Orr-Trueta method. It consists in immediate removal of all gross contamination and devitalized tissue, including surgical excision of skin along the edges of the wound, which is then filled with gauze and dusted with sulfanilamide powder. A skin-tight plaster bandage is then applied without padding, except for bony prominences. No deep sutures are used, and generally the wound is not re-dressed for at least 21 days. Trueta's original method was without the use of the sulfanilamide powder, or with greatly reduced doses, and included packing with petroleum jelly gauze. It is especially used for the treatment of compound fractures.

**truncal.** Pertaining to the trunk.

**truncated.** Deprived of limbs or accessory parts.

**truncus.** A trunk.

**trunk.** 1. The torso; the main part of the body to which the head and limbs are attached. 2. The main stem of a blood vessel or nerve.

**truss.** Any mechanical apparatus for preventing the recurrence of a rupture that has been reduced.

*It is of great importance that a patient should reduce his rupture and put on his truss before he gets out of bed in the morning, because attempts to put on the truss in the erect position involves a risk of nipping the rupture and causing pain or obstruction.*

**trypanocide.** Any drug or agent destructive of trypanosomes.

**trypanolysis.** The destruction of trypanosomes.

**Trypanosoma.** A type of parasitic protozoan belonging to the genus *Trypanosoma* which infests the blood plasma of both animals and man, producing disease and transmitted by insects.

**Trypanosoma brucei.** A parasite which causes nagana in horses and other domestic animals in tropical Africa.

**Trypanosoma cruzi.** A parasite which causes Chagas' disease in South America and American sleeping sickness.

**Trypanosoma evansi.** A parasite which causes surra in horses and cattle.

**Trypanosoma gambiense.** A parasite which causes African sleeping sickness.

**Trypanosoma hippicum.** A parasite which causes murrina (a form of sleeping sickness) in large domestic animals.

**Trypanosoma rhodesiense.** A parasite which causes East African sleeping sickness.

**trypanosome fever.** Trypanosomiasis or sleeping sickness. See BARBIERO FEVER.

**trypanosomiasis.** Any disease caused by a trypanosoma.

**trypesis.** See TREPHINING.

**trypsin.** An enzyme produced by the pancreas, and which changes proteins into peptones and polypeptides; an enzyme which takes part in the digestive process of proteins.

**trypsinogen.** The substance which produces trypsin; a precursor of trypsin.

**tryptic.** Pertaining to trypsin.

**tryptolytic.** Splitting up or dissolving tryptones.

**tryptone.** Any peptone formed by the action of trypsin.

**tsetse fly.** An insect almost wholly restricted to Africa. This fly carries parasitic protozoa of the genus *Trypanosoma*, the causative agents of sleeping sickness in man and a similar disease, nagana, in cattle.

**tsutsugamushi disease.** A disease caused by parasitic rickettsia and transmitted by the larva of a mite, and endemic in Japan, Sumatra, and New Guinea.

**tuba.** A tube.

**tubal.** Pertaining to a tube.

**tubal pregnancy.** A form of ectopic pregnancy which takes place in the Fallopian tube and not in the womb. It is usually due to obstruction or spasm of the Fallopian tube which will allow the male cell to filter through, but once the fertilized ovum, which is larger, tries to migrate to the womb it is prevented by the obstruction and must grow in that position. By about the eighth week of pregnancy the egg bursts the Fallopian tube, causing a severe hemorrhage requiring emergency surgery.

**tube.** A hollow cylindrical structure.

**air tube.** Any tube of the lung.

**alimentary tube.** The intestinal tract.

**auditory tube.** The canal made up partly of bone and partly of cartilage, connecting the pharynx with the middle ear cavity on each side. Also called *tube, auditiva, pharyngotympanic tube, eustachian tube.* See EUSTACHIAN TUBE, below.

**auricular tube.** The external auditory meatus (the ear opening).

**bronchial tube.** A bronchus (one of the larger air passages within the lungs).

**capillary tube.** A tube with a minute bore.

**cathode tube.** A vacuum tube, frequently with a thin window opposite the cathode, to permit cathode rays to emerge.

**digestive tube.** The intestinal tract; the alimentary tract from mouth to anus.

**drainage tube.** A tube of glass, rubber, or other material, inserted into a wound or cavity to allow the escape of fluids.

**eustachian tube.** The tube leading from the back of the nose to the middle ear. Its purpose is to equalize pressure on both sides of the eardrum, which would otherwise be pushed in by atmospheric pressure and prevented from vibrating, thus making hearing impossible. Also called *otopharyngeal tube, otosalpinx, auditory tube.*

*In infants this tube is almost horizontal, but with growth it gradually becomes more vertical until, in the adult, it is at an angle of 60 degrees. Since infants spend considerable time on their backs, infections such as colds in the back of the nose can quickly run down the eustachian tube and inflame the middle ear, producing earache, purulent discharges through a perforated eardrum, and possibly deafness. Therefore it cannot be too strongly emphasized that all earaches in children are due to an inflamed eardrum and middle ear disease and should always receive medical advice and treatment before the drum is perforated and the ear discharging. Much deafness in adults is caused by badly treated or untreated middle-ear disease in childhood. If a head cold produces catarrh and obstruction of the eustachian tube, the air behind the eardrum is absorbed, and the drum is depressed and fixed. The result is a muffled sense of hearing. An individual suffering with this condition should not fly in an airplane until he has recovered because, when climbing to a height, or descending rapidly to ground level, the alteration in atmospheric pressure may burst the eardrum, causing a bloody discharge from the ear, and intense pain.*

**Fallopian tube.** The tube, named after an Italian anatomist who first described it, which conveys the egg or ovum from the ovary to the uterus. There are two such tubes, one emerging on each side of the top of the uterus and ending in a funnel-shaped area (the infundibulum) at the ovary. Each month an egg erupts from an ovary and by chemical attraction passes into the infundibulum and proceeds into the center of the tube. If a male cell or spermatozoon is present, the egg becomes fertilized and passes down the rest of the tube into the upper portion of the uterus, where it embeds itself into the lining to commence a pregnancy. If the egg is not fertilized it passes out at menstruation. Also called *uterine tube, oviduct.*

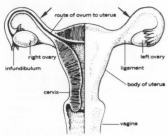

FALLOPIAN TUBE (arrows)

**feeding tube.** A rubber tube inserted into the stomach via either the mouth or the nose, for the purpose of introducing food into the stomach.

**intubation tube.** A tube for insertion into the larynx through the mouth; used in anesthetics.

**nasotracheal tube.** A rubber tube or catheter, inserted into the trachea by way of the nose or mouth.

**roentgen tube.** A vacuum vessel containing a source of electrons and two electrodes, the positive anode and the negative cathode, at a considerable potential difference. The cathode contains the source of electrons, as a hot filament, and the anode is of sturdy construction to withstand the bombardment by the cathode rays. At the anode, the energy of the cathode rays is converted into 98 percent of heat and 2 percent of x-rays. The tube is cooled by passing water through a surrounding jacket.

**Ryle's tube.** A thin rubber tube passed into the stomach and used for giving a test meal.

**Southey's tube.** A small silver tube for subcutaneous drainage.

**stomach tube.** A rubber tube used for irrigation or evacuation of the stomach contents. Also called *stomach pump.*

**tracheotomy tube.** A metal tube for placing in the opening made by a surgical incision into the trachea when there is obstruction to breathing.

**uterine tube.** The Fallopian tube.

**tubectomy.** Surgical excision of a part of the Fallopian tube.

**tubercle. 1.** A small nodule. **2.** A rounded prominence on a bone. **3.** The specific lesion produced by the germ of tuberculosis, consisting of a collection of spherical cells, sometimes including

giant cells, and surrounded by a layer of spindle-shaped cells.

**tubercula.** Tubercules.

**tubercular.** Pertaining to a tubercle. Strictly speaking, the correct adjective is tuberculous. However, both terms are now used synonymously by doctors when referring to tuberculosis infection.

**tuberculated.** Covered with tubercles.

**tuberculid, tuberculide.** Any skin lesion produced by tuberculosis.

**tuberculin.** Material derived from the tubercle bacillus, and used in various forms for the diagnosis of tuberculosis in children and cattle. When injected into the skin tuberculin causes no reaction in a healthy subject, but in an individual already affected with tuberculosis it produces an inflammatory area at the point of the injection.

**tuberculitis.** Inflammation of a tuberculous node or its surrounding area.

**tuberculocele.** Tuberculosis of a testicle.

**tuberculocide.** An agent which destroys the tubercle bacillus.

**tuberculocidin.** A substance derived by treating tuberculin with platinum chloride. It is used in the same way as tuberculin, but is claimed to be free from injurious after-effects sometimes noted with tuberculin treatment.

**tuberculoderma.** A tuberculous skin disease.

**tuberculoid.** Having a similarity to tuberculosis.

**tuberculoma.** A tuberculous swelling.

**tuberculosis.** An infectious disease caused by the bacterium *Myobacterium tuberculosis,* commonly known as the tubercle bacillus. It may effect the lungs, the intestinal tract, the lymphatic glands, the bones, the skin, and the brain. However, more than 90 percent of deaths from tuberculosis in the United States and more than 80 percent in Great Britain are due to tuberculosis of the lungs. It is transmitted from person to person and from animals to man, and it is for this reason that children up to the age of about five years should drink only cow's milk that has been boiled or pasteurized. The germ is contained within a natural envelope which was previously impervious to drugs, but modern drugs can penetrate this envelope and destroy the germ, thus avoiding the necessity for many drastic surgical operations. The symptoms vary according to the site of the lesion, but wasting, loss of strength, anemia, fever, and sweating are among those ordinarily observed. Tuberculosis of the lungs may be insidious, and the first warning may be the sudden onset of a pleural effusion, spitting of blood, or a cough with loss of weight and debility.

Known since time immemorial as phthisis, the name tuberculosis was first introduced by Schönlein in 1834.

**active tuberculosis.** Tuberculosis which is actively progressing.

**acute generalized miliary tuberculosis.** Areas of tuberculosis occurring widely throughout the body due to dissemination by the bloodstream.

**avian tuberculosis.** Tuberculosis affecting birds and which can be transmitted to man.

**bovine tuberculosis.** Tuberculosis affecting cattle and which can be transmitted to man, usually via milk.

**bronchogenic tuberculosis.** Extension of tuberculosis in the lung via the bronchi.

**caseous tuberculosis.** A type of tuberculosis characterized by a cheeselike form of necrosis.

**chronic fibroid tuberculosis.** A slowly spreading lung tuberculosis producing extensive fibrosis in the lung.

**chronic ulcerative tuberculosis.** The most prevalent type of lung tuberculosis, in which ulceration has led to necrosis and the formation of cavities.

**closed tuberculosis.** Tuberculosis in which no tuberculosis germs are present in the sputum, so that the disease cannot be transmitted to another person.

**endogenous tuberculosis.** The spread of tuberculosis to another part or organ from an original site of active disease within the body.

**exogenous tuberculosis.** Tuberculosis which arises from a source outside the body.

**glandular tuberculosis.** Tuberculosis arising in glands, usually in the neck, from bovine tuberculosis.

**hematogenous tuberculosis.** Tuberculosis spread via the bloodstream.

**inactive tuberculosis.** Tuberculosis which is arrested; the areas are covered with scar tissue.

**incipient tuberculosis.** The very earliest stage of tuberculosis infection.

**latent tuberculosis.** Tuberculosis in a dormant phase, which may become active again.

**open tuberculosis.** Tuberculosis in an active phase and infectious for other people.

**pelvic tuberculosis.** Tuberculosis affecting the uterine tubes and other pelvic organs.

**primary tuberculosis.** The initial infection which normally results in healing and the laying down of calcium. This is the "spot on the lung" seen in so many chest x-rays of adults and it indicates that the person has been invaded by the germ (probably in childhood) and has successfully fought and won the battle against the infection.

**pulmonary tuberculosis.** Tuberculosis affecting the lung.

**tuberculotoxin.** A poison produced by the tubercle bacillus.

**tuberculous.** Pertaining to tuberculosis. See also TUBERCULAR.

**tuberosity.** A prominence on a bone.

**tuberous.** Resembling a tuber.

**tuberous sclerosis.** A familial disease in which tumors form on the surfaces of the brain, characterized by mental deterioration and epileptic fits. Congenital tumors of the eye, kidney, and heart muscle may be associated.

**tubo-abdominal.** Pertaining to the Fallopian tube (oviduct) and the abdomen.

**tubo-ovarian.** Pertaining to the Fallopian tube and the ovary.

**tuboperitoneal.** Pertaining to the Fallopian tube and the peritoneum.

**tubular.** Shaped like a tube; relating to a tubule; occurring in a tube.

**tubule.** A small tube.

**tubuli.** The plural of tubulus.

**tubulus.** A tubule.

**tugging.** A pulling sensation.

**tracheal tugging.** A physical sign seen in cases of aneurysm of the aorta. With each heartbeat the trachea is seen to be subjected to a pull.

**tularaemia.** See TULAREMIA.

**tularemia.** An infectious disease transmitted to man by rodents.

**tulle gras.** An open gauze network impregnated with soft paraffin, balsam of Peru, and vegetable oils, and sterilized. It is used as a dressing for wounds, as it does not stick.

**tumefacient.** Causing a swelling.

**tumefaction.** The condition of being swollen; a swelling.

**tumescence.** The state of becoming tumid; a swelling.

**tumid.** Swollen or distended.

**tumidity.** Being swollen or distended.

**tumor.** A swelling; a new growth of cells or tissues characterized by being independent of the laws of growth of the host. It is progressive, of unknown cause, and in malignant form is limited only by the nutrition provided by the host.

**adipose tumor.** A fatty tumor; lipoma.

**benign tumor.** A tumor that grows by expansion, does not exhibit the features of malignant tumors by invading other tissues, and is not likely to recur after removal.

**blood tumor.** A hematoma.

**chromaffin tumor.** A tumor of the sympathetic nervous system, most often discovered in the suprarenal glands, but occasionally in other sites. It is made up of chromaffin cells which have a strong affinity for taking up

chrome salts. This tumor may be accompanied by high blood pressure.

**dermoid tumor.** A dermoid cyst.

**Ewing's tumor.** A true bone tumor usually occurring in the shaft of a long bone, producing a fusiform swelling. It is invasive but does not produce secondary deposits elsewhere in the body, although it is apt to recur.

**fibroid tumor.** Usually a fibromyoma of the womb. This benign tumor may occur within, in the wall, or on the outer surface of the womb, causing symptoms depending on its situation.

**giant-cell tumor.** 1. A tumor of the jaw; also called *epulis*. 2. A tumor occurring at the end of long bones, causing thinning of the compact bone and characterized by the presence of giant cells.

**malignant tumor.** A tumor which invades and destroys surrounding tissues, may produce secondary deposits elsewhere in the body, and is likely to recur after removal.

**Pott's puffy tumor.** A doughy swelling on the scalp due to a collection of pus caused by osteomyelitis of the skull.

**tumour.** See TUMOR.

**tunic, tunica.** A tunic or covering membrane.

**tunnel anaemia.** See TUNNEL ANEMIA.

**tunnel anemia.** A disease due to the infestation of the intestines with a nematode worm; characterized by anemia, digestive upsets, and mental inertia. Also called *hookworm disease, ancylostomiasis*.

**tunnel disease.** See CAISSON DISEASE.

**turbid.** Cloudy.

**turbidity.** Cloudiness.

**turbinal.** Any turbinated bone; any of the three bony protuberances situated inside the nostril on its outer wall.

**turbinated.** Shaped like an inverted cone.

**turbinectomy.** Surgical removal of a nasal turbinate bone.

**turbinotome.** A surgical knife used in turbinotomy.

**turbinotomy.** Surgical incision into a turbinate bone.

**turgescence.** The state of being swollen or distended.

**turgid.** Swollen, congested, distended.

**turgor.** Turgescence.

**Turner's syndrome.** A congenital abnormality characterized by shortness of stature, webbing of the neck (a filling out of the skin from the top of the neck to shoulder area), swelling of the tissues, defective nails, short fingers, and cubitus valgus.

**tussal.** Pertaining to the nature of a cough.

**tussicular.** Relating to a cough.

**tussis.** A cough.

**tussive.** Produced by a cough.

**tutamen.** A shield, protection, or defense.

**twelfth cranial nerve.** The hypoglossal nerve, which gives motor innervation to the tongue.

**twilight sleep.** The production of partial anesthesia by hypodermic administration of morphine and scopolamine during childbirth. In this state the memory of the pain is abolished but not the pain itself.

**twinge.** A sudden sharp pain.

**twins.** Two offspring born of the same pregnancy.

**binovular twins.** Twins resulting from the exceptional release of two eggs from the ovaries, each becoming fertilized at the same time. Unlike uniovular twins, they may be one of each sex. Also called *fraternal twins, dizygotic twins.*

**conjoined twins.** Twins developed from a fertilized egg which has incompletely split into two, resulting in two individuals being joined at some part of their bodies and sometimes even having a part in common. Also called *Siamese twins.*

**fraternal twins.** See BINOVULAR TWINS, above.

**identical twins.** See UNIOVULAR TWINS, below.

**Siamese twins.** See CONJOINED TWINS, above.

**uniovular twins.** Twins resulting from the splitting of a fertilized egg into two parts, each of which develops into a separate individual. These twins are always of the same sex—two boys or two girls. Also called *identical twins, mono-ovular twins, monozygotic twins.*

**twitch.** A sudden jerk.

**twitching.** An irregular spasm.

**tyle, tyloma.** A callus.

**tylosis.** 1. Extreme thickening of the skin of the soles and palms. 2. A type of inflammation of the eyelids in which the edges are thickened and hard.

**tympanectomy.** Surgical removal of the tympanic membrane.

**tympanic.** 1. Relating to the tympanum. 2. Resonant.

**tympanic membrane.** A thin membrane extending across the ear canal separating the outer ear and middle ear. Also called *eardrum.*

**tympanism.** Distension by gas. See TYMPANITES.

**tympanites.** Gross distension of the abdomen due to a collection of gas in the intestines or peritoneal cavity. Also called *meteorism.*

**tympanitic.** Pertaining to tympanites.

**tympanitic abscess.** An abscess containing gas.

**tympanitis.** Inflammation of the eardrum. Also called *otitis media.*

**tympanotomy.** Incision of the eardrum. If the eardrum is distended by fluid or pus, an incision is made into it to allow the fluid to emerge. If the fluid is allowed to burst through, a circular opening is punched out and the eardrum may be permanently perforated, whereas a surgical slit folds together and unites once drainage has been completed. Also called *paracentesis of the eardrum.*

**tympanum.** The middle ear.

**tympany.** 1. Tympanities. 2. A resonant or bell-like percussion note elicited over a cavity.

**type.** 1. A distinguishing mark, emblem, stamp, or symbol. 2. A normal or average example. 3. In pathology, classification of a disease by its distinguishing features.

**typhaemia.** See TYPHEMIA.

**typhemia.** The presence of typhoid bacteria in the blood.

**typhic.** Relating to typhoid fever or to typhus.

**typhinia.** See FAMINE FEVER.

**typhlectasis.** Distension of the cecum.

**typhlectomy.** Surgical removal of the cecum.

**typhlenteritis.** Inflammation of the cecum.

**typhlitis.** 1. Inflammation of the cecum. 2. An old term for appendicitis.

**typhlolithiasis.** The formation of concretions in the cecum.

**typhlology.** The study of blindness.

**typhlomegaly.** Enlargement of the cecum.

**typhlon.** The cecum.

**typhloptosis.** Downward displacement of the cecum.

**typhlorrhaphy.** Suture of the cecum.

**typhlosis.** Blindness.

**typhlostenosis.** Abnormal narrowing of the cecum.

**typhlotomy.** Surgical incision of the cecum.

**typhobacillosis.** Poisoning of the system due to toxins produced by the typhoid germ.

**typhoidal.** Resembling typhoid.

**typhoid fever.** An infectious fever of a septicemic type caused by the germ *Salmonella typhosa*.

**typholysin.** Any agent destructive of the typhoid germ.

**typhomalarial.** Symptomatic of both typhoid and malaria.

**typhomania.** Lethargy accompanied by delirium, such as is seen in typhus and other fevers.

**typhopaludism.** A type of malaria characterized by symptoms of typhoid.

**typhopneumonia.** Pneumonia coexisting with typhoid fever.

**typhose.** Resembling typhoid fever.

**typhosepsis.** Poisoning of the system resulting from typhoid fever.

**typhosis.** The typhoid state.

**typhotoxin.** A deadly poison formed by the typhoid germ.

**typhous.** Pertaining to the nature of typhus.

**typhus fever.** An acute, infectious, louse-borne disease. Also called *epidemic typhus, fleck typhus, jail fever, camp fever.*

**typing of blood.** The procedure whereby the blood group of a patient is determined. See BLOOD: BLOOD GROUPS.

**tyrannism.** Morbid cruelty, of which sadism is one form.

**tyrein.** Coagulated milk casein.

**tyremesis.** The vomiting of caseous material, common among nursing infants.

**tyroid.** Resembling cheese.

**tyroma.** Caseous tumor.

**tyromatosis.** Caseation. Also called *tyrosis.*

**tyrosis.** Tyromatosis.

**tyrotoxicon.** A ptomaine of highly poisonous nature, sometimes occurring in stale milk, cheese, and ice cream. It produces grave symptoms of marked prostration and sometimes death.

**tyrotoxin.** A poison closely resembling curare; a product of bacterial infection of cheese or other milk products.

# U-V

**ula.** The gum; the fleshy structure covering the tooth-bearing border of the jaws. Also called *gingiva.*

**ulaemorrhagia.** See ULEMORRHAGIA.

**ulalgia.** Pain in the gums.

**ulatrophia.** Shrinking of the gums.

**ulcer.** A loss of substance on the surface of the skin or a mucous membrane, often followed by disintegration of other tissues.

**Aden ulcer.** See TROPICAL ULCER, below.

**amputating ulcer.** A penetrating ulcer encircling a part, such as a toe, leading ultimately to the complete loss of that part, such as is seen in yaws.

**Annam ulcer.** See TROPICAL ULCER, below.

**aphthous ulcer.** See CANKER SORE.

**atheromatous ulcer.** An ulcer of the lining of an artery due to breakdown of an atheromatous plaque.

**atonic ulcer.** An ulcer which shows no disposition to heal.

**autochthonous ulcer.** A syphilitic chancre.

**Bahia ulcer.** See LEISHMANIASIS.

**Bauru ulcer.** See LEISHMANIASIS.

**callous ulcer.** An ulcer with little tendency to heal. It occurs most frequently on the legs of middle-aged women and is due to poor circulation and often to a lack of cleanliness. Also called *indolent ulcer.*

**chrome ulcer.** An ulcer due to the action of chrome salts; seen in those who work with such material. Also called *tanner's ulcer.*

**creeping ulcer.** An ulcer which slowly extends and enlarges; the characteristic margin is wavy or serpentlike. Also called *serpiginous ulcer.*

**Curling's ulcer.** A duodenal or gastric ulcer which sometimes follows and is associated with extensive burns of the skin.

**decubitus ulcer.** A bedsore.

**diphtheritic ulcer.** 1. An ulcer associated with the germ of diphtheria. 2. Used loosely to describe any ulcer which has a fibrinous exudate. It occurs as a form of tropical ulcer.

**duodenal ulcer.** A chronic ulcer of the duodenum and more than probably a form of stress disease. It occurs in those of a worrying disposition. The symptom is an upper-abdominal pain coming on after eating food and at first relieved by taking more food. It frequently wakes the patient in the early hours of the night. The pain occurs in cycles, between which the patient can eat what he likes with apparent impunity, but eventually the episodes of pain become more frequent until they are continuous. It is because of these naturally occurring painless intervals that so many claims are made by the makers of proprietary preparations that their product has cured duodenal ulcer. In fact, the ulcer has become painless in spite of the treatment and during the intermission the sufferer has written the enthusiastic letter which is published as advertising material. A corrective note that the writer subsequently had a hemorrhage from the ulcer is, of course, never published. Medical treatment consists of giving antacid medicines, not allowing the patient to go for more than two hours without either having some bland food or a dose of medicine; a dose of olive oil swallowed at bedtime to keep down the formation of acid during the night; sedatives to the nervous system; and psychotherapy to lessen nervous tension. Surgical treatment has changed over the years from bypass operations to partial removal of the stomach and duodenum, and an operation now being tried consists of oversewing the ulcer and cutting the nerve supplying the duodenum. In the United States it is claimed that if the duodenum is frozen solid for several hours, by passing into it tubes which work like a miniature refrigerator, the ulcer will subsequently heal.

**endemic ulcer.** An ulcer occurring in special geographic areas, such as tropical ulcer.

**exuberant ulcer.** An ulcer with an excess of granulation tissue growing from its base.

**Gaboon ulcer.** A type of tropical ulcer closely resembling a syphilitic sore.

**gastric ulcer.** An ulcer affecting the lining of the stomach, having similar characteristics to a duodenal ulcer.

**Hunner's ulcer.** An ulceration of the lining of the urinary bladder.

**indolent ulcer.** An ulcer having little tendency to heal. Also called *callous ulcer.*

**Jacob's ulcer.** A rodent ulcer, especially of the eyelid. See also RODENT ULCER, below.

**Jeddah ulcer.** A form of tropical sore. See TROPICAL SORE, below.

**leprous ulcer.** An ulcer which occurs either in the nose or on the skin due to the breakdown of a cutaneous lesion of leprosy.

**lupoid ulcer.** An ulcer of the skin resembling lupus vulgaris.

**Marjolin's ulcer.** An ulcer due to malignant change in an indolent ulcer or scar, especially a scar resulting from an old burn or an x-ray burn.

**Mozambique ulcer.** See TROPICAL ULCER, below.

**peptic ulcer.** An ulcer of the mucous membrane of the esophagus, stomach, or duodenum caused in part by the action of the acid gastric juice.

**rodent ulcer.** A form of malignant disease with more or less deep penetration, affecting especially the face, neck, and scalp. It is a very slow growth which tends to bleed very readily if touched and thus draws attention to itself before any gross damage is done. It is curable by radium plates or surgical excision.

**serpiginous ulcer.** See CREEPING ULCER, above.

**tanner's ulcer.** An ulcer of the skin of the hands seen in skin tanners. Also called *chrome ulcer.*

**Tashkend ulcer.** A crusted ulcer developing especially on the face and endemic in the region of Tashkend, Asiatic Russia.

**trophic ulcer.** An ulcer due to a disturbance of the nutrition of a part, for instance a varicose ulcer.

**tropical ulcer. 1.** A skin ulcer usually on the lower extremities and prevalent in tropical climates. It may be acute, chronic, or gangrenous. The cause is unknown; also called *Naga sore, Aden ulcer, Annam ulcer, Mozambique ulcer, Yemen ulcer,* and other names of geographical significance. **2.** Cutaneous leishmaniasis.

**varicose ulcer.** A chronic ulcer of the skin due largely to malnutrition of the skin resulting from stagnant venous congestion produced by varicose veins. Also called *leg ulcer.*

**venereal ulcer.** A syphilitic chancre.

**Yemen ulcer.** See TROPICAL ULCER.

**ulceration.** The formation of ulcers.

**ulcerative.** Relating to ulceration or characterized by the presence of ulcers.

**ulcerative colitis.** Ulceration of the lining of the intestines. See COLITIS.

**ulcerous.** Showing ulceration.

**ulcus.** An ulcer.

**ulectomy. 1.** Surgical removal of scar tissue. **2.** Surgical removal of part of the gums.

**ulemorrhagia.** Bleeding from the gums.

**ulerythema.** A skin disease characterized by scar formation.

**uletic. 1.** Relating to scars. **2.** Relating to gums.

**ulitis.** Inflammation of the gums.

**ulna.** The larger and inner of the two bones of the forearm and on the side of the small finger.

**ulnad.** Towards the ulnar bone.

**ulnar.** Relating to the ulnar artery, bone, vein, or nerve in the forearm.

**ulnocarpal.** Relating to the ulna and the carpus.

**ulnoradial.** Relating to the ulna and the radius bones of the forearm.

**ulocarcinoma.** Cancer of the gums.

**ulodermatitis.** Inflammation of the skin accompanied by scar formation.

**uloglossitis.** Combined inflammation of the gums and the tongue.

**uloid.** Resembling a scar; a spot resembling a scar and produced by degeneration.

**uloncus.** A tumor of the gum.

**ulorrhagia.** Bleeding from the gums.

**ulorrhea.** See ULORRHAGIA.

**ulorrhoea.** See ULORRHEA.

**ulosis.** Scarring.

**ulotomy.** Surgical incision of the gum.

**ulotrichous.** Having woolly hair.

**ultramicroscopic.** Too small to be seen under a conventional microscope.

**ultrared.** The same as infrared, the nonluminous heat rays of the spectrum.

**ultraviolet rays.** Light waves lying beyond the violet rays of the spectrum. They cannot be seen by the eye. They are capable of destroying bacteria, are used for their tonic effect, as in ultraviolet light baths, and also for provoking a violent inflammatory reaction in the skin to dry it up in such cases as acne.

**ululation.** Hysterical wailing.

**umbilectomy.** Excision of the umbilicus.

**umbilical.** Pertaining to the umbilicus, its cord, or its blood vessels.

**umbilical cord.** The cordlike structure connecting the fetus to the placenta, via which the mother supplies her unborn baby with blood, oxygen, and food, and receives its waste products.

**umbilicate.** Like the umbilicus.

**umbilicus.** The round depressed scar in the middle of the abdomen, marking the point of entry of the umbilical cord. Also called *navel.*

**unciform.** Hooked or hook-shaped.

**unciform bone.** A hook-shaped bone in the second row of the carpal bones of the wrist. Also called *hamate bone.*

**uncinariasis.** A disease caused by infestation with a nematode worm of the genus *Uncinaria.* Also called *hookworm disease.*

**uncinate.** Hooked.

**uncinatum.** The unciform bone.

**unconscious.** Insensible; in a coma.

**unconsciousness.** The condition of being insensible. See COMA.

**unction.** An ointment; the process of anointing.

**unctious.** Greasy or oily.

**uncus. 1.** A hooklike structure. **2.** A special portion of the brain.

**undinism.** A mental state in which the individual derives sexual excitement from looking at water, urine, or the act of passing urine.

**undulant.** Wavelike, fluctuating.

**undulant fever.** See ABORTUS FEVER.

**undulation.** A wavelike movement.

**undulatory.** Moving in waves.

**unfruitful.** Barren.

**ungual.** Pertaining to a fingernail or toenail.

**unguent, unguentum.** An ointment.

**unguiculate.** Possessing nails or claws.

**unguinal.** Pertaining to a fingernail or toenail.

**unguis.** A fingernail or a toenail.

**uniaxial.** Having one axis.

**unibasal.** Having a single base.

**unicellular.** Having one cell.

**unicorn.** Possessing a single horn.

*In the Middle Ages unicorn horn was highly prized as a form of medical treatment. The horn was supposed to be derived from the mythical animal but was, in reality, nothing more than ivory or goat horn. It was sold at enormous prices and there is a record of one being bought in Germany in the sixteenth century for the equivalent of $75,000. When the dauphin married Catherine de Medici, Pope Clement VII, the bride's uncle, presented Francis I, the bridegroom's father, with a piece of unicorn's horn. It was said to be capable of destroying poison that* *had been mixed with food, and as poisoning was then the commonest way of removing one's enemies, those in exalted positions were always at risk and took elaborate but useless precautions against it. When Elizabeth, daughter of Henry II, had smallpox, Anne de Montmorency sent a piece of unicorn's horn for her treatment. In England its reputation as an antidote for poison lasted until the reign of Charles II, when the Royal Society was requested to investigate the properties of a cup made from alleged unicorn's horn, it being claimed that any poisonous drink put into the cup would have its poison neutralized. The Royal Society reported that the cup was made from rhinoceros horn and was quite useless for the purpose. After this public report the use of any horn as an antidote for poison came under a cloud and henceforth was dropped.*

**unicorn uterus.** A uterus, one side of which is either undeveloped or imperfectly developed.

**unilateral.** Relating to one side only.

**unilobar.** Consisting of one lobe.

**unilocular.** Having only one loculus.

**union.** The joining up of a fractured bone; healing.

**uniovular.** Developed from one ovum.

**uniovular twins.** Twins that have risen from a single fertilized egg. See also TWINS.

**unipara.** A woman who has had one pregnancy resulting in a viable offspring.

**uniparous.** Having given birth to only one child.

**Unna's dermatosis.** Seborrheic eczema. See SEBORRHEA DERMATITIS.

**Unna's paste.** A mixture of zinc oxide, gelatin, and glycerin. It is heated and applied with a brush; when cold it sets to a firm protective substance.

**unofficial.** Applied to a remedy not included in the pharmacopoeia.

**urachal.** Pertaining to the urachus.

**urachus.** The stemlike structure connecting the urinary bladder with the allantois, which is a fetal membrane developing as a prolongation of the yolk sac and contributing to the formation of the umbilical cord and placenta. After birth, the urachus is represented by a fibrous cord, situated between the top of the bladder and the navel.

**uracrasia.** Any disorder of the urine.

**uracratia.** Incontinence of urine.

**uraemia.** See UREMIA.

**uraemic.** See UREMIC.

**uraniscochasma.** Cleft palate. Also called *uranoschisis.*

**uranisconitis.** Inflammation of the palate.

**uraniscoplasty.** Surgical repair of a cleft palate. Also called *uranoplasty.*

**uraniscorrhaphy.** Suture of a cleft palate. Also called *staphylorrhaphy.*

**uraniscus.** The palate.

**uranism.** Homosexuality.

**uranist.** A homosexual.

**uranoplasty.** See URANISCOPLASTY.

**urari.** See CURARE.

**urate.** A salt of uric acid.

**uratic.** Characterized by urates.

**uratoma.** A concretion formed of urates. Also called *tophus.*

**uratosis.** The deposition of crystalline urates in the tissues.

**uraturia.** The presence of excessive quantities of urates in the urine.

**urea.** The chief nitrogenous constituent of urine and the principal end product of the combustion of protein in the body. Also called *carbamide.*

**urea concentration test.** Performed to test the efficiency of the kidney. The patient drinks 100 cubic centimeters of water containing 15 grams of urea. The concentration of the urea in the urine is then measured at the end of one hour and again at the end of two hours.

**ureal.** Pertaining to urea.

**ureameter.** An apparatus for estimating the amount of urea contained in urine. Also called *ureometer.*

**ureapoiesis.** The formation of urea.

**urecchysis.** The leaking of urine from the bladder into the surrounding tissues, as in fractures of the pelvis associated with a torn bladder.

**uredo.** A burning sensation of the skin; urticaria.

**uremia.** The retention in the blood of constituents more normally found in the urine, due to failure of the kidneys to excrete them. It is characterized by headache, giddiness, vomiting, blindness, convulsions, and coma.

**uremic.** Characterized by uremia.

**ureometer.** See UREAMETER.

**uresis.** Passing urine; urination.

**uretal.** Pertaining to a ureter.

**ureter.** The tube that conveys the urine from the kidney to the bladder. It is from 16 to 18 inches long.

**ureteral.** Pertaining to the ureter.

**ureteralgia.** Pain arising in the ureter; usually the result of either a stone or blood clot passing down from the kidney.

**ureterectasis.** Dilation of the ureter.

**ureterectomy.** Surgical removal of the ureter.

**ureteric.** Pertaining to the ureter.

**ureteritis.** Inflammation of the ureter.

**ureterocele.** A dilation of the lower end of the ureter, forming a pouch.

**ureterocervical.** Pertaining to the ureter and the cervix.

**ureterocolostomy.** An operation performed when it is necessary to remove a urinary bladder affected by a grave disease. The ureters are removed from the bladder and implanted into the colon, so that the urine is passed into it. Also called *ureterosigmoidostomy.*

**ureterocystostomy.** Surgical rejoining of a ureter into the bladder.

**ureteroproctostomy.** Surgical transplantation of a ureter from the bladder into the intestine.

**ureterolith.** A stone in a ureter.

**ureterolithiasis.** The presence of stones in the ureter.

**ureterolithotomy.** Surgical opening of a ureter to remove a stone.

**ureteroplasty.** Surgical repair of a ureter.

**ureteropyelitis.** Inflammation of both a ureter and the pelvis of a kidney.

**ureteropyosis.** Inflammation of a ureter accompanied by pus formation.

**ureterorrhagia.** Bleeding from a ureter.

**ureterorrhaphy.** Surgical suturing of a ureter.

**ureterosigmoidostomy.** See URETEROCOLOSTOMY.

**ureterostegnosis.** See URETEROSTENOSIS.

**ureterostenoma.** See URETEROSTENOSIS.

**ureterostenosis.** Constriction of a ureter. Also called *ureterostegnosis, ureterostenoma.*

**ureterostoma.** 1. The opening of the ureter into the bladder. 2. Fistula of the ureter.

**ureterostomy.** An operation to form a fistula into the ureter through which it may discharge urine. Sometimes the ureter is brought through a hole in the skin of the abdomen, the urine being collected in an appliance fitted over the opening.

**ureterotomy.** Surgical opening of a ureter.

**ureteroureterostomy.** Surgical formation of a passage between the ureters or between different parts of the same ureter.

**ureterouterine.** Relating to a ureter and the uterus.

**ureterovaginal.** Relating to a ureter and the vagina.

**ureterovesical.** Relating to a ureter and the bladder.

**urethra.** The canal through which the urine is discharged, extending from the neck of the bladder to the urethral meatus (external opening). In the male, it is divided into the prostatic portion, the membranous portion, and the spongy or penile portion, and is about 9 inches long. The prostate gland surrounds the urethra. In elderly men this gland sometimes enlarges, constricts the urethra, and makes it difficult or impossible to pass urine. The condition can be relieved temporarily by passing a catheter into the bladder, and permanently by surgical removal of the prostate. In the female the urethra is about 1½ inches long.

**urethral.** Pertaining to the urethra.

**urethralgia.** Pain arising in the urethra.

**urethratresia.** A condition of the newborn in which the urethra is blocked and urine cannot be passed.

**urethrectomy.** Surgical removal of part or the whole of the urethra.

**urethremphraxis.** Obstruction in the urethra. Also called *urethrophraxis*.

**urethritis.** Inflammation of the urethra. One cause of urethritis is the venereal disease gonorrhea, which produces a copious discharge of yellow pus from the urethra. Some cases of urethritis are due to nonvenereal germs.

**urethrocele.** A condition usually seen in the female, in which part of the urethra protrudes through its opening.

**urethrocystitis.** Inflammation of the urethra and the bladder.

**urethrodynia.** Pain arising in the urethra.

**urethropenile.** Relating to the penis and the urethra.

**urethroperineal.** Relating to the urethra and the perineum.

**urethrophraxis.** Obstruction of the urethra. Also called *urethremphraxis*.

**urethrophyma.** A tumor of the urethra.

**urethroplasty.** Surgical repair of the urethra.

**urethrorectal.** Relating both to the urethra and the rectum.

**urethrorrhagia.** Bleeding from the urethra.

**urethrorrhaphy.** Surgical suturing or repair of the urethra.

**urethrorrhea.** Any discharge, other than urine, from the urethra.

**urethrorrhoea.** See URETHRORRHEA.

**urethroscope.** A surgical instrument containing a light and lenses for examining the interior of the urethra.

**urethroscopy.** Examination of the interior of the urethra by means of a urethroscope.

**urethrospasm.** Painful spasm of the urethra.

**urethrostenosis.** A stricture of the urethra.

**urethrostomy.** The surgical creation of an opening into the urethra.

**urethrotomy.** Surgical cutting of a stricture of the urethra.

**urethrovaginal.** Relating to both the urethra and the vagina.

**urethrovesical.** Relating to both the urethra and the bladder.

**uretic.** Relating to urine; an agent that promotes the flow of urine.

**uric.** Relating to the urine.

**uric acid.** A normal constituent of the blood and urine, it occurs in man as the end product of the combustion of purine. In gout there is a defect in this process of dealing with uric acid, which results in a high blood level of uric acid and a decreased excretion, with deposits of urates in special areas, the commonest being around the big toe joint.

**uricacidaemia.** See URICACIDEMIA.

**uricacidemia.** An excess of uric acid in the blood; gout.

**uricaciduria.** An excess of uric acid in the urine.

**uricaemia.** See URICEMIA.

**uricemia.** See URICACIDEMIA.

**uricocholia.** The presence of uric acid in the bile.

**uricolysis.** The splitting up of uric acid.

**uricolytic.** Relating to uricolysis.

**uridrosis.** The presence of uric acid or other urinary substances in the sweat.

**urina.** Urine.

**urina cruenta.** Blood-stained urine.

**urina galactodes.** Milky urine.

**urinaemia.** See URINEMIA.

**urinemia.** Uremia.

**urinal.** A vessel for the reception of urine.

**urinalysis.** The chemical analysis of urine.

**urinary.** Relating to urine.

**urinary organs.** Those organs concerned with the production and discharge of urine; that is, the kidneys, the ureters, the urinary bladder, and the urethra.

**urination.** The act of passing urine. Also called *micturition*.

**urine.** The fluid excreted by the kidneys. In health it has an amber color, is slightly acid in reaction, has a faint odor, and a specific gravity of 1.018 to 1.020. The quantity excreted in 24 hours varies with the amount of fluid drunk, but averages between 1000 and 1500 cubic centimeters (3 pints). Other normal constituents of urine are urea, chlorides, sulphates, phosphates, together with organic acids, pigments, and hormones. In disease the most important abnormal constituents present are albumin, sugar, blood, pus, acetone, diacetic acid, fat, tube casts, various cells, and bacteria.

**incontinence of urine.** Inability to hold the urine. Bed-wetting of children and young persons is called *enuresis*.

**residual urine.** The urine remaining in the bladder after urination. This damming back of urine is due to an obstruction pressing on the outlet. In the male it may be due to enlargement of the prostate and in the female due to dropping of the bladder into the vagina, as the result of stretching of the vagina at childbirth.

**suppression of urine.** A term indicating that the kidneys have stopped producing urine.

**urinemia.** See UREMIA.

**uriniferous.** Conveying urine.

**urinogenital.** Pertaining to the urinary and genital organs. Also called *urogenital*.

**urinogenous.** Producing urine.

**urinologist.** A specialist in diseases of the urinary organs. Also called *urologist*.

**urinoma.** A cyst containing urine.

**urinometer.** An instrument for measuring the specific gravity of urine.

**urinometry.** Estimation of the specific gravity of urine with a urinometer.

**urinosanguineous.** Containing both urine and blood.

**urinoscopy.** The examination of urine. Also called *uroscopy*.

**urinous.** Having the characteristics of urine, such as a urinous odor.

**urning.** A male homosexual.

**urnism.** Homosexuality. Also called *uranism*.

**urobilin.** A bile pigment produced by the putrefaction of bilirubin (the red bile pigment) in the gut, and excreted by the kidney into the urine. The principal pigment that colors urine yellow.

**urobilinaemia.** See UROBILINEMIA.

**urobilinemia.** The presence of urobilin in the blood; jaundice.

**urobilinogen.** A chemical which is the precursor of urobilin.

**urobilinuria.** An excess of urobilin in the urine.

**urocele.** A swelling of the scrotum caused by the escape of urine from the bladder.

**urochesia.** The passing of urine through the anus.

**urochrome.** A yellow pigment found in urine.

**uroclepsia.** Unconscious urination.

**urocrisia.** Diagnosis by means of urinary examination and analysis.

**urocrisis.** 1. The critical stage of a disease distinguished by the sudden passage of a large volume of urine. 2. Severe pain occurring in any part of the urinary tract, such as occurs in tabes dorsalis.

**urocyanogen.** A blue pigment found in urine, especially in cases of cholera. See UROCYANOSIS.

**urocyanosis.** Blue discoloration of urine, usually from the presence of excessive amounts of indican, a glucoside, oxidized to indigo blue. Also called *indicanuria*.

**urocyst.** The urinary bladder.

**urocystic.** Relating to the urinary bladder.

**urocystitis.** Inflammation of the urinary bladder. Also called *cystitis*.

**urodialysis.** Suppression of urine.

**urodynia.** Pain that arises with the passage of urine.

**urogenital.** Pertaining to the urinary and genital organs.

**urogenous.** Producing urine.

**urography.** The study of the urinary tract by outlining it with radiopaque dyes.

**urogravimeter.** An instrument for measuring the specific gravity of urine.

**urohaematin.** See UROHEMATIN.

**urohaematonephrosis.** See UROHEMATONEPHROSIS.

**urohaematoporphyrin.** See UROHEMATOPORPHYRIN.

**urohematin.** Altered hematin, derived from the blood, and found in the urine.

**urohematonephrosis.** Dilatation of the kidney with a mixture of blood and urine.

**urohematoporphyrin.** A urinary pigment occasionally found in the urine in certain diseases.

**urolagnia.** Sexual excitement aroused by watching a person pass urine.

**urolith.** A stone found in the urine.

**urolithiasis.** The presence of stones in the urine.

**urologist.** A specialist in disorders of the urinary tract.

**urology.** The study of diseases of the urinary tract.

**urolutein.** A yellow pigment found in urine.

**uromancy.** Prognosis based on the examination of the urine.

**uromelanin.** A black pigment occasionally found in the urine.

**urometer.** An instrument for measuring the specific gravity of the urine.

**uroncus.** A tumor containing urine.

**urophan.** Any substance which, taken into the body, appears in the urine chemically unchanged.

**urophein.** A grey pigment found in the urine.

**uroplania.** Urine discovered elsewhere than in the urinary organs; discharge of urine from an opening other than the normal openings in the urinary tract.

**uropoiesis.** The process of secreting urine.

**uropsammus.** Urinary gravel.

**uropyoureter.** An infected ureter containing pus.

**urorosein.** A rose-colored pigment found in urine.

**urorrhagia.** Excessive passage of urine.

**urorrhea.** Involuntary passage of urine.

**urorrhoea.** See URORRHEA.

**uroschesis.** Retention of urine; inability to pass urine.

**uroscopy.** Examination of urine.

**urosepsis.** A toxic condition caused by the escape of urine into tissues other than the urinary tract.

**uroseptic.** Pertaining to urosepsis.

**urosis.** Any disease of the urinary tract.

**urostealith.** A fatty material found in stones in the urinary tract.

**urotoxic.** Pertaining to poisonous substances found in the urine or being excreted in the urine; pertaining to poisoning by urine or its constituents.

**uroureter.** A distension of the ureter by urine.

**urous.** Having the characteristics of urine.

**urticaria.** A skin condition characterized by intensely itching wheals with elevated, usually white, centers and a surrounding area of red skin (erythema). The wheals appear in crops, are widely distributed over the body surface, tend to disappear in a day or two, and are usually unattended by a general upset of the system. Urticaria is an allergic disorder produced by the development of histamine in the skin in response to an irritant, such as a nettle sting, insect bite, or jellyfish sting. Contact with flannel, recently dyed clothing, or with cheap furs may also start an attack. Certain foods, notably shellfish, tinned fish and meat, pork, pickles, mushrooms, and strawberries may produce urticaria in some people. In others, drugs such as penicillin, quinine, aspirin, and the sulfa drugs may be responsible. The presence of intestinal worms may also provoke an attack, and in many cases there is a notable nervous or psychotic influence. Local relief may be obtained by applying calamine lotion or an antihistamine cream. Internally, relief may be obtained by swallowing ephedrine tablets or one of the antihistamine drugs. Recurring attacks demand extensive and thorough investigation of the person's nervous system and habits to pinpoint the exciting cause of the disorder. Also called *hives, nettle rash.*

**urticarial.** Relating to urticaria.

**ustulation.** Drying by means of heat; scorching.

**ustus.** Burned.

**uteralgia.** Pain arising in the uterus.

**uterectomy.** Surgical removal of the uterus. Also called *hysterectomy.*

**uterine.** Pertaining to the uterus.

**uteritis.** Inflammation of the uterus.

**uteroabdominal.** Pertaining both to the uterus and the abdomen.

**uterocele.** A hernia of the uterus.

**uterocervical.** Pertaining to the uterus and the cervix uteri.

**uterodynia.** Pain arising in the uterus.

**uterofixation.** Surgical fixation of the uterus, usually to the abdominal wall, to prevent it from prolapsing into the vagina or falling backwards into an abnormal position. Also called *hysteropexy.*

**uterogestation.** A normal pregnancy occurring within the uterus.

**uterolith.** A stone in the uterus.

**uteromania.** See NYMPHOMANIA.

**utero-ovarian.** Pertaining to both the uterus and the ovary.

**uteropelvic.** Relating both to the uterus and the pelvic ligaments.

**uteropexy.** See UTEROFIXATION.

**uteroplacental.** Referring both to the uterus and the placenta.

**uteroplasty.** Surgical repair of the uterus.

**uterosacral.** Pertaining both to the uterus and the sacrum.

**uterosclerosis.** Hardening of the uterus from disease.

**uteroscope.** A speculum for examining the uterus.

**uterotomy.** Surgical opening of the uterus, such as is done to remove the baby at cesarian section. Also called *hysterotomy.*

**uterotubal.** Pertaining both to the uterus and the Fallopian tube.

**uterovaginal.** Pertaining both to the uterus and the vagina.

**uterovesical.** Pertaining both to the uterus and the urinary bladder.

**uterus.** The womb. The organ of pregnancy which receives and holds the fertilized egg until it has developed

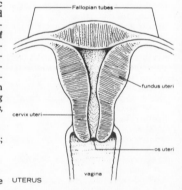

UTERUS

into a full term baby and then, by contracting its muscular walls, expels the baby during the act of parturition. The uterus is a pear-shaped, muscular organ three inches long by two inches wide and one inch thick and is divided into three portions: *the fundus,* the upper and broad portion, from which *the body* gradually narrows to *the cervix* or neck. The orifice, called the *os uteri,* communicates with the vagina. The whole organ is suspended in the pelvis by the broad, round, and uterosacral ligaments. The Fallopian tubes, the canals which convey the eggs from the ovaries to the uterus, enter one on each side of the fundus.

**anteflexion of the uterus.** The normal position of the uterus of being bent forwards.

**fetal uterus.** A uterus which has failed to develop to the size normal for the age of the woman.

**gravid uterus.** A pregnant uterus.

**infantile uterus.** A uterus normally formed but arrested in development. It may be the cause of sterility or repeated abortions. Sometimes the administration of hormones will induce this type of uterus to develop.

**retroflexion of the uterus.** A uterus which is displaced backwards but which has its cervix in the normal position.

**retroversion of the uterus.** Backward displacement of the uterus with forward displacement of the cervix.

**uterus bicornuis.** A uterus divided into two compartments, due to a developmental defect.

**uterus didelphys.** A double uterus. It is possible for a pregnancy to occur in each part.

**uterus masculinus.** A blind vestigial pouch opening into the prostatic part of the urethra. It is the male counterpart of the uterus, hence its name.

**utricle.** A delicate membranous sac communicating with the semicircular canals of the ear.

**prostatic utricle.** See UTERUS: UTERUS MASCULINUS.

**utricular.** Relating to the utricle.

**utriculitis.** Inflammation of the utricle.

**utriculus.** See UTRICLE.

**uvea.** The pigmented part of the eye, including the iris, ciliary body, and the choroid.

**uveal.** Pertaining to the uvea.

**uveitis.** Inflammation of the uvea.

**uveoparotid.** Relating to the uvea and the parotid gland.

**uviformis.** The central layer of the choroid.

**uvula.** The muscular body hanging from the free border at the back of the soft palate.

**uvulaptosis.** A relaxed and pendulous condition of the uvula. Also called *uvuloptosis.*

**uvulectomy.** Surgical removal of the uvula.

**uvulitis.** Inflammation of the uvula.

**uvuloptosis.** See UVULAPTOSIS.

**uvulotomy.** Surgical excision of the uvula.

**vaccigenous.** Cultivating vaccines.

**vaccinal fever.** A feverish reaction that follows vaccination.

**vaccinate.** To inoculate with vaccinia virus.

**vaccination. 1.** Inoculation with the virus of vaccinia to protect against smallpox. **2.** Inoculation with any organism to produce immunity against a given infectious disease.

*Vaccination against smallpox originated in Gloucestershire in 1797, when Dr. Jenner noticed that dairymaids who got sores on their fingers from cowpox sores on the udders of cows developed an immunity to smallpox. Jenner took some matter from a sore on a dairymaid named Sarah Nelmes and with it vaccinated the arm of a boy named James Phipps, who was later exposed to smallpox and found to be immune. Confusion often arises in the public's mind between vaccination and inoculation. However, in recent years it was decided by international agreement that all such measures taken to protect against disease would be called inoculation, therefore vaccination now becomes inoculation against smallpox. Preventive inoculation can now be offered against anthrax, tuberculosis, brucellosis, cholera, diphtheria, whooping cough, the typhoid and paratyphoid group of diseases, rabies, and other diseases, and the list is still growing.*

**vaccine.** A preparation of attenuated or killed microorganisms administered for the prevention or treatment of infectious disease.

**autogenous vaccine.** A vaccine made from a culture of a germ obtained from the patient himself.

**bacterial vaccine.** An emulsion of bacteria, killed, living, or attenuated, used for raising the immunity of a patient suffering from infection by the same germ.

**BCG vaccine.** A vaccine made from cultures of the germ of tuberculosis (bacille Calmette-Guérin). Also called *Calmette's vaccine.*

**heterogeneous vaccine.** A vaccine prepared from germs derived from a source other than the patient himself.

**homologous vaccine.** A vaccine prepared from the patient's own germs.

**mixed vaccine.** A vaccine prepared from more than one type of germ.

**polyvalent vaccine.** A vaccine made from cultures of two or more strains of the same species of bacteria.

**sensitized vaccine.** A vaccine prepared from killed germs, to which has

been added antibody material from the patient.

**stock vaccine.** A vaccine prepared from a standard mixture of various bacteria bred in a laboratory.

**TAB vaccine.** A vaccine prepared against typhoid, paratyphoid A, and paratyphoid B. Also called *triple vaccine for typhoid.*

**vaccinella.** False vaccinia, a secondary skin rash which sometimes follows an attack of cowpox.

**vaccinia.** Cowpox, a contagious disease of cows, characterized by blisters and ulcers of the skin, which usually appear around the teats and the udders. The disease is transmissible to man through handling infected cows and by vaccination. It confers immunity against smallpox.

**vaccinial, vacciniform.** Resembling vaccinia.

**vacciniola.** A skin eruption which occasionally follows vaccinia, having a close resemblance to the rash of smallpox.

**vaccinization.** Thorough vaccination by giving inoculations until the virus produces no reaction. It has been used with some success in the prevention of recurrent herpes labialis.

**vaccinogenous.** Producing vaccine.

**vaccinophobia.** A neurotic dread of being vaccinated.

**vacuolation.** The development or production of vacuoles.

**vacuole.** Any clear space formed in the protoplasm of a living cell.

**vagal.** Relating to the vagus nerve.

**vagal attack.** A condition characterized by a feeling of impending death, shortness of breath, discomfort in the heart, and a sinking sensation, supposed to be due to vasomotor spasm. The vagus nerve carries nerve impulses to the heart, and excessive stimulation of the vagus may result in slowing the heartbeat. In many cases there is a large element of neurosis and emotional instability. Also called *vasovagal attack.*

**vagina. 1.** A sheath. **2.** The canal of membrane and muscle extending from the vulval opening to the cervix of the uterus. It forms the birth canal.

**vaginal. 1.** Pertaining to a sheath. **2.** Pertaining to the vagina.

**vaginalitis.** Inflammation of the covering of the testicle.

**vaginate.** Sheathed.

**vaginectomy. 1.** Surgical removal of the covering of a testis to cure hydrocele. **2.** Surgical removal of the vagina.

**vaginismus.** Painful spasm of the muscular fibers in the walls of the vagina. It occasionally is induced by a fear of either pain or pregnancy, or a feeling of emotional guilt at the sexual act, which may be severe enough to completely prevent sexual intercourse.

**vaginitis.** 1. Inflammation of the vagina. 2. Inflammation of any sheath.

**vaginodynia.** Neuralgic pain in the vagina.

**vaginofixation.** Fixation of the womb to the vaginal peritoneum in the treatment of retroflexion of the womb.

**vaginoperitoneal.** Relating both to the vagina and the peritoneum.

**vaginoplasty.** Surgical repair of the vagina.

**vaginoscope.** An instrument for examining the vagina; a speculum for use in the vagina.

**vaginotomy.** Surgical incision into the vaginal wall. Also called *colpotomy.*

**vaginovesical.** Pertaining to both the vagina and the bladder.

**vagitus.** The cry of an infant.

**vagotomy.** Surgical division of the vagus nerve, sometimes performed in the treatment of duodenal ulcer.

**vagotonia, vagotony.** Irritability of the vagus nerve.

**vagus nerve.** The tenth cranial nerve, a mixed nerve containing both sensory tracts and motor tracts. It supplies the soft palate, pharynx, and larynx and also the nonstriped muscles of the respiratory and alimentary tracts; thus disorders of this nerve have a profound and widespread effect. Also called *pneumogastric nerve.*

**valerian.** A foul-smelling extract from the valerian plant; at one time commonly used in sedative medicines.

**valetudinarian.** An invalid.

**valgus.** A term used to denote a position of turning outwards.

**vallate.** Having a wall or raised edge; cup-shaped.

**vallecula.** Any furrow or depression.

**vallecular.** Pertaining to a vallecula.

**valval.** Pertaining to a valve.

**valvate.** Possessing valves.

**valve.** A device which prevents the reflux of the contents in a vessel, tube, or passage.

VALVE (venous)

**anal valves.** Folds of membrane at the junction of the rectum and anal

canal. Also called *valves of Morgagni, valves of Ball.*

**aortic valve.** A valve at the junction of the aorta and the left ventricle of the heart.

**atrioventricular valves.** Valves between the atria and the ventricles of the heart. Also called *mitral and tricuspid valves.*

**auriculoventricular valves.** See ATRIOVENTRICULAR VALVES, above.

**bicuspid valve.** See MITRAL VALVE.

**ileocecal valve.** A valve at the junction of the terminal ileum and the cecum, which prevents a reflux of the contents of the cecum back into the ileum. Also called *ileocolic valve.*

**mitral valve.** A valve containing two cusps, situated between the left atrium and the left ventricle of the heart. It is commonly affected by rheumatic fever producing mitral stenosis.

**pulmonary valve.** A valve consisting of three cusps, situated between the right ventricle and the pulmonary artery.

**pyloric valve.** A valve situated at the pyloric end of the stomach, which prevents regurgitation of food from the duodenum back into the stomach. This is the valve that becomes enlarged and obstructed in the disorder called pyloric stenosis. See also STENOSIS: PYLORIC STENOSIS.

**tricuspid valve.** A valve having three cusps, situated between the right atrium and the right ventricle of the heart.

**valvotomy.** Surgical cutting of a heart valve to overcome an obstruction to the flow of blood.

**valvula.** A small valve.

**valvulitis.** Inflammation of a valve.

**Van den Bergh's test.** A test used for bilirubin in the blood, to determine, in cases of jaundice, whether there is obstruction to the flow of bile.

**vapors.** An old term for the emotional reaction now called hysteria.

**vapours.** See VAPORS.

**varicella.** See CHICKENPOX.

**varices.** The plural of varix.

**variciform.** Resembling a varix.

**varicocele.** Dilatation of the veins running down each side of the scrotum, forming a soft elastic swelling that feels like a collection of worms under the skin, and more prominent on the left side than the right. It may produce aching of the testicle, which can be relieved by wearing a suspensory bandage or, in extreme cases, by surgery.

**varicocelectomy.** Surgical excision of a varicocele.

**varicose.** Resembling or having the characteristics of a varix.

**varicose veins.** A swollen and knotted condition of the veins, usually of the legs. Each vein has valves which pre-

vent blood stagnating in the vein and the muscular action of the legs forces the blood upwards from the bottom of the leg towards the thigh. If the vein dilates, the valves become incompetent and the entire column of blood from the thigh to the foot falls backwards and stagnates. This results in defective blood supply to the skin, which then breaks down and forms a varicose ulcer. These veins can be dealt with either surgically or, in minor cases, by injection. The reason why varicose veins can be removed without harmful effect on the leg is that there are two sets of veins, one set deep in the leg within the muscles, and the other set just under the skin. If the surface veins, which show and produce the knotted blue cords, are removed, the circulation is maintained by the deep veins. Hemorrhoids are a form of varicose veins of the rectum.

**varicosity.** The condition of being varicosed.

**varicotomy.** Surgical removal of a varicose vein.

**varicula.** A varicosity in the veins of the conjunctival membrane of the eye.

**variola.** Smallpox.

**variolar.** Relating to smallpox.

**variolate.** 1. Characterized by the presence of pustules resembling smallpox. 2. To inoculate with smallpox virus; vaccination.

**variolation.** Vaccination against smallpox, with the unmodified virus.

**varioloid.** A mild form of smallpox seen in persons who either have been vaccinated against smallpox or who have had smallpox but have not acquired complete immunity to the disease. The immunity they possess is sufficiently strong to lessen the virulence of the attack.

**variolous.** Pertaining to smallpox.

**variolovaccine.** Cowpox or smallpox vaccine produced by inoculating a heifer.

**varix.** A swollen or knotted condition of a vein, artery, or lymph vessel; usually refers to a vein. See also VARICOSE VEINS.

**vas.** A vessel.

**vasal.** Vascular; having blood vessels.

**vascular.** Consisting of or having blood vessels.

**vascularity.** The state of having blood vessels; being vascular.

**vascularization.** The act of becoming vascular; having blood vessels.

**vascularize.** To supply with blood vessels.

**vasculitis.** Inflammation of a blood or lymph vessel.

**vasculum.** A small vessel.

**vas deferens.** The excretory duct of the testis.

**vasectomy.** Excision of the vas deferens.

**vasifactive.** Forming new vessels.

**vasiform.** Having the characteristics of a duct or blood vessel.

**vasitis.** Inflammation of the vas deferens.

**vasoconstriction.** Narrowing of the blood vessels, especially the arterioles.

**vasoconstrictive.** Promoting constriction of blood vessels.

**vasoconstrictor. 1.** Causing constriction of blood vessels. **2.** An agent that causes constriction of blood vessels.

**vasodepression.** A depressing effect on the circulation.

**vasodepressor.** Lowering the blood pressure by relaxing the blood vessels.

**vasodilator. 1.** Causing the dilatation of blood vessels. **2.** An agent that causes dilatation of the blood vessels.

**vasofactive, vasoformative.** Forming new blood vessels.

**vaso-inhibitor.** An agent which inhibits vasomotor nerves.

**vaso-inhibitory.** Depressing vasomotor action.

**vasoligation.** A surgical operation in which the vas deferens is tied. If done on both sides it produces sterility.

**vasomotion.** The increase or decrease in the caliber of a blood vessel.

**vasomotor.** Regulating the contraction and expansion of blood vessels (vasoconstriction and vasodilatation).

**vasomotor rhinitis.** Congestion of the nasal mucous membranes which occurs at any period of the year, irrespective of whether or not there are pollens in the air.

**vasomotorial, vasomotory.** Relating to vasomotor function.

**vasoneuropathy.** Any disorder affecting the blood vessels and nerves simultaneously.

**vasoneurosis.** Any disorder of the vasomotor system. Also called *angioneurosis.*

**vasoparesis.** A partial paralysis of the vasomotor nerves.

**vasopressin.** A hormone, produced by the posterior lobe of the pituitary gland in the brain, which has the power to raise blood pressure and increase the movements of the intestines.

**vasorrhaphy.** Suture of the vas deferens.

**vasosection.** Severing of part or the whole of a blood vessel or of the vas deferens.

**vasospasm.** Spasm of the blood vessels.

**vasostimulant.** Stimulant to vasomotor action.

**vasotomy.** Incision of the vas deferens.

**vasotrophic.** Pertaining to the nutrition of the vessels.

**vasovagal attack.** See VAGAL ATTACK.

**V.D.** Abbreviation for venereal disease.

**vection.** The passing of disease germs from the sick to the healthy.

**vector.** An organism, usually an arthropod, which can convey germs from one host to another as, for instance, malaria is conveyed by a type of mosquito.

**vegetation.** Flowery excrescences resembling plants, such as those seen on the heart valves in endocarditis. The term is also applied to papillomas and polyp growths.

**adenoid vegetations.** Enlargement of the adenoids at the back of the nose.

**vegetative.** Possessing the power of growth.

**vehicle.** A liquid or solid substance, generally without medicinal effect itself, used as a medium or carrier for the active ingredient of a medicine.

**vein.** A blood vessel carrying blood from the tissues towards the heart. Veins, like arteries, have three coats (an inner, middle and an outer) but they are not as thick as those of the arteries. Many veins, especially those near the surface, have valves which permit the blood to flow only in one direction. In all veins except the pulmonary vein the blood is dark-colored owing to the lack of oxygen. When a vein is cut the blood oozes out, whereas in a cut artery it spurts out with each beat of the heart.

fat, longitudinal muscle and elastic fibers
circular muscle
endothelium
VEIN

**velamen.** A membrane, covering, or veil.

**velamentum.** A covering membrane.

**velar.** Pertaining to a velum.

**veldt sore.** A disease common in the African desert, but also seen in Australia and Burma. It is characterized by multiple, shallow, chronic, painful ulcers on exposed parts of the body of light-skinned individuals, and usually follows some slight damage, such as an insect bite. Exposure to sunlight is necessary to initiate the disease, and there are usually secondary germ invaders. Also called *Barcoo disease, desert sore, septic sore.*

**vellication.** A twitching or spasm of muscle.

**velosynthesis.** Surgical repair of a cleft soft palate. Also called *staphylorrhaphy.*

**velum.** Any veillike structure.

**vena.** A vein.

**venenation.** A poisoned condition.

**veneniferous.** Conveying poison.

**venenose, venenous.** Poisonous.

**venenosity.** The state of being poisoned.

**venepuncture.** Surgical puncturing of a vein.

**venereal.** Pertaining to or produced by sexual intercourse. The word originates from the Latin for Venus, Goddess of Love.

**venereal diseases.** Diseases such as gonorrhea, syphilis, and chancroid, usually acquired by sexual intercourse with an infected person.

**venereal sore.** See HARD SORE.

**venereologist.** A specialist in the treatment of venereal diseases.

**venereology.** The study of venereal diseases.

**venereophobia.** Morbid fear of being infected with venereal disease.

**venery.** Sexual intercourse.

**venesection.** The taking of blood from a vein. Also called *phlebotomy.*

**venesuture.** The suturing of a vein. Also called *phleborrhaphy.*

**veniplex.** A network of veins.

**venom.** Poison, particularly that secreted by certain snakes, spiders, and insects.

**venomosalivary.** Secreting a poisonous saliva.

**venomous.** Secreting venom; poisonous.

**venosity. 1.** A condition in which there is an excess of venous blood in a part of the body. **2.** Well supplied with blood vessels or venous blood.

**venous.** Relating to the veins.

**venous blood.** The dark type of blood found in the veins.

**venous hum.** The murmur heard on listening over a vein.

**vent.** An outlet, especially the anus.

**venter. 1.** The abdomen. **2.** Any belly-shaped part, such as the contractile portion of a muscle.

**ventrad.** Towards any ventral aspect.

**ventral. 1.** Relating to the abdomen or to any venter. **2.** Denoting a position on the abdominal or lower side of a body.

**ventricle.** A small organized cavity within an organ. Also called *ventriculus.*

**brain ventricles.** Four cavities within the brain, which contain cerebrospinal fluid.

**heart ventricles.** The two lower chambers of the heart. The right ventricle pumps blood through the pulmonary artery to the lungs, and the left ventricle pumps blood through the arteries to the rest of the body.

**ventricular.** Relating to a ventricle.

**ventriculostomy.** A surgical operation in which a temporary opening is made into a ventricle in the brain.

**ventriculus.** 1. A ventricle. 2. The stomach.

**ventricumbent.** Lying with the abdominal surface downwards; prone.

**ventriduct.** To bring or convey towards the ventral aspect.

**ventrifixation.** Surgical suturing of a displaced organ, especially the womb, to the abdominal wall. Also called *ventrofixation, ventrosuspension.*

**ventrimeson.** The middle line on the abdominal surface of the body.

**ventrocystorrhaphy.** Surgical suturing of the bladder or a cyst to the abdominal wall.

**ventrofixation.** See VENTRIFIXATION.

**ventrose.** Having a belly or a bellylike swelling; potbellied.

**ventrosuspension.** See VENTRIFIXATION.

**ventrotomy.** Surgical incision into the abdominal cavity. Also called *celiotomy.*

**venula, venule.** A small vein.

**venular.** Relating to a venula.

**verbigeration.** Babbling of senseless words and phrases.

**vergence.** Movement of the eye; convergence is looking in and divergence is looking out.

**vergetures.** White lines seen on the skin during pregnancy and obesity caused by the skin being stretched. Also called *striae.*

**vermicide.** Any agent which destroys intestinal worms.

**vermicular.** Resembling the appearance of a worm.

**vermiculate.** Resembling a worm.

**vermiculation.** Wormlike movements such as occur in the human intestine. Also called *peristalsis.*

**vermiform.** Worm-shaped.

**vermiform appendix.** A small, blind tube which opens from the cecum. See APPENDIX.

**vermifugal.** Expelling worms.

**vermifuge.** A drug that expels worms.

**vermin.** A collective name for animal parasites.

**verminous.** Infested with vermin; pertaining to vermin.

**vermis.** A worm.

**vernal.** Relating to the spring of the year.

**vernix caseosa.** A cheesy deposit found on the skin of a newborn baby.

**verruca.** A wart.

  **verruca acuminata.** A wartlike growth, usually of venereal origin.

  **verruca carnea.** A soft fleshy wart.

**verruca glabra.** A smooth wart.

**verruca plana.** A small, smooth wart, usually multiple, occurring on the face, neck, back of the hands, wrists, and knees.

**verruca plantaris.** A wart on the sole of the foot.

**verruca senilis.** A flat, greasy wart occurring on the skin of the elderly.

*Warts are probably caused by a virus and can be transferred from one part to another, as can be seen on a child's hand, where a wart on one finger is soon faced by one on an adjoining finger. There are numerous treatments for warts, from surgical removal to destruction with agents such as nitric acid and liquid nitrogen.*

**verruciform.** Wartlike.

**verrucose, verrucous.** Warty; having many warts.

**verrucosis.** A condition characterized by the presence of many warts.

**verruga peruana.** An infectious skin disease occurring in Peru. Also called *Peruvian wart.*

**version.** The act of turning, particularly manual turning of the unborn baby into a position to facilitate delivery.

**abdominal version.** Manipulations made exclusively through the mother's abdominal wall. Also called *external version.*

**bimanual version.** Manipulation by one hand on the abdominal wall and with the other hand in the vagina. Also called *combined version.*

**bipolar version.** Version performed by manipulating both the head and pelvis of the baby.

**cephalic version.** Version performed to ensure that the baby will be born head first.

**combined version.** See BIMANUAL VERSION, above.

**external version.** See ABDOMINAL VERSION, above.

**internal version.** Version performed by introducing the entire hand within the womb.

**pelvic version.** Version performed to bring about a breech presentation.

**podalic version.** Version in which the hand is introduced into the vagina and one or both feet of the baby are brought to the outlet of the vagina.

**spontaneous version.** Version made by the baby itself without artificial assistance. In the early months of pregnancy the baby is constantly altering its position.

**vertebra.** Any one of the 33 bones forming the spinal column. They comprise seven cervical (neck) vertebrae, twelve thoracic or dorsal (chest) vertebrae, five lumbar vertebrae (in the small of the back), five sacral vertebrae, which are fused together to form the sacrum (the rear wall of the pelvis) and four coccygeal, which are fused together to form the coccyx (the vestige of a tail in the human). A typical vertebra consists of a body and an arch, the latter being formed by two pedicles and two laminas. The arch supports seven processes—four articular, two transverse, and one spine.

**vertebral.** Relating to a vertebra.

**vertebrarium.** The spinal column.

**vertebrate.** An animal having a vertebral column.

**vertebrectomy.** Surgical removal of a vertebra.

**vertebrochondral.** Relating to a costal cartilage and a vertebra.

**vertebrocostal.** Relating to vertebra and a rib.

**vertebrosternal.** Relating to a vertebra and the sternum.

**vertex.** The crown of the head.

**vertiginous.** Related to or affected with vertigo.

**vertigo.** An extreme form of giddiness such as a feeling of swaying or unsteadiness. It may be due to psychological causes or to a disease of the blood, brain, ear, eye, or stomach. The condition is sometimes so severe that the patient falls and vomits. Transient attacks of dizziness should not be called vertigo, which is much more severe. A special form of vertigo, called Ménière's disease or Ménière's syndrome, is characterized by tinnitus, deafness, and severe attacks of giddiness that can be precipitated merely by shaking the head from side to side.

**auditory vertigo.** Vertigo due to disease of the ears. Also called *aural vertigo.*

**cerebral vertigo.** Vertigo due to disease of the brain.

**gastric vertigo.** Vertigo due to a disorder of the stomach.

**labyrinthine vertigo.** Vertigo associated with disorders of the labyrinth.

**objective vertigo.** Vertigo in which the individual feels he is standing still while everything else is moving around him.

**subjective vertigo.** Vertigo in which the patient feels that he is spinning round.

**vesica.** The bladder.

**vesica fellea.** The gall bladder.

**vesical.** Relating to the bladder.

**vesicant.** Causing blisters; blistering; a blistering agent.

**vesication.** The formation of a blister.

**vesicatory.** Blistering; a blistering agent.

**vesica urinaria.** The urinary bladder.

**vesicle.** A small bladder, especially a small sac containing liquid; a skin blister, such as is seen in chickenpox.

**vesicoabdominal.** Relating both to the bladder and the abdomen.

**vesicocele.** Hernia of the bladder, a prolapse of the bladder. The condition is mostly seen in women, especially those who have had the supporting muscles in the vagina stretched by several pregnancies. Also called *cystocele.*

**vesicocervical.** Relating both to the bladder and the cervix.

**vesicoprostatic.** Relating both to the prostate gland and the bladder.

**vesicopubic.** Relating to the bladder and the pubes or pubic bone.

**vesicorectal.** Relating both to the bladder and the rectum.

**vesicorenal.** Relating both to the bladder and the kidney.

**vesicospinal.** Relating both to the urinary bladder and the spinal cord.

**vesicotomy.** Surgical incision into the bladder. Also called *cystotomy.*

**vesicoureteral.** Relating to the urinary bladder and the ureter.

**vesicourethral.** Relating both to the bladder and the urethra.

**vesicouterine.** Relating both to the bladder and the uterus.

**vesicovaginal.** Relating both to the bladder and the vagina.

**vesicula.** A vesicle.

**vesicula fellea.** The gall bladder. Also called *vesica fellea.*

**vesicular.** Relating to or composed of vesicles.

**vesicular breathing.** The sound produced by air entering and leaving healthy lungs; the normal sound of breathing heard through the stethoscope.

**vesiculation.** The formation of vesicles.

**vesiculectomy.** Surgical removal of the whole or part of the seminal vesicles.

**vesiculiferous.** Having vesicles.

**vesiculiform.** Shaped like a vesicle.

**vesiculitis.** Inflammation of a vesicle, especially of a seminal vesicle.

**vesiculobronchial.** Refers to the sound heard over the chest when both normal and bronchial breath sounds are heard.

**vesiculopapular.** Pertaining to a skin rash which consists of both vesicles and papules.

**vesiculopustular.** Pertaining to a skin rash consisting of both vesicles and pustules.

**vessel.** Any tube or canal that conveys either blood or lymph.

**vestibular.** Relating to a vestibule.

**vestibule.** A chamber or cavity at the entrance to a canal; an approach.

**vestibulo-urethral.** Relating both to the vestibule of the vulva and the urethra.

**vestibulum.** Any vestibule, but frequently the vestibule of the ear.

**vestige.** A trace or remnant of something formerly present or more fully developed; a rudiment.

**viability.** Ability to live after birth. Refers principally either to premature labors or cesarian operations performed before term. See also BIRTH.

**vibratile, vibration.** Moving to and fro.

**vibratory.** Marked by vibrations.

**vibrissae.** The hairs that grow from inside the nostrils. Also refers to the whiskers of such animals as the cat.

**vicarious.** Taking the place of something else; a habitual discharge occurring in an abnormal situation.

**vicarious menstruation.** Very rarely, groups of cells normally situated in the lining of the womb are found deposited in abnormal situations such as the eye and the lung, and this results in bleeding from these parts during the woman's menstrual period.

**vichy water.** A mildly laxative and antacid mineral water obtained from Vichy, France. It has been used in Europe for the treatment of rheumatic and gouty conditions and for disorders of the liver. These spa waters, although very popular in France, probably have not the slightest effect on the disease process. The benefit of spa treatment is more due, perhaps, to the discipline of having to take proper exercise and a reducing diet than to the medicinal effect of the water.

**vicious union.** The term applied to the faulty joining of a fractured bone. Also called *mal-union.*

**villi.** Minute, elongated projections from the surface of a membrane.

**villiferous.** Bearing villi.

**villose, villous.** Relating to a villus; covered with villi.

**villosity.** The state of having villi.

**villus.** A minute, elongated projection from the surface of a mucous or other membrane. While villi occur in several parts of the body, those most commonly referred to are the intestinal villi, which project into the lumen of the small intestine, each villus containing blood vessels and lacteal vessels through which the digested food passes into the bloodstream. Villi also exist in the placenta and provide the communication between the circulation of the mother and her unborn baby.

**Vincent's angina.** A severe infection occurring inside the mouth. It affects the tonsils and gums and is very contagious; the so-called "trench mouth" of the First World War.

**vinculum.** A ligament.

**vinum.** A solution of medicinal substances dissolved or suspended in wine.

**violinist's cramp.** A neurosis affecting violin players and marked by spasm of the fingers. See also NEUROSIS: OCCUPATIONAL NEUROSIS.

**viper venom.** Venom from Russell's viper; has been used to control bleeding in cases of hemophilia.

**Virchow's disease.** See LEONTIASIS OSSEA.

**viremia.** A condition in which viruses are found in the bloodstream.

**virile.** Characteristic of manhood.

**virilescence.** The acquisition by some women, following the change of life, of characteristics, such as a beard or deepening of the voice, more commonly associated with the male. The development of male characteristics may occur in some endocrine disturbances, such as Cushing's syndrome.

**virilia.** The male sex glands.

**viripotency.** In a female, the characteristic of being old enough to be capable of sexual intercourse.

**virulence.** The disease-producing potential of germs.

**virulent.** Having the nature of a poison; violent in action.

**viruliferous.** Containing or carrying a germ.

**virus.** One of a group of disease-producing microorganisms smaller than the accepted bacterial forms.

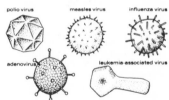

VIRUS (five typical examples)

*Most viruses are too small to be seen by ordinary microscopes, but they were known to exist long before means were found to see them because of the effects they produced. Viruses multiply in the body very much like bacteria, but, unlike bacteria, they have never been cultivated in inanimate culture media, and can only be grown on living cells, such as the embryo of the chick. The best-known virus diseases of man include rabies, poliomyelitis, sleeping sickness, encephalitis, smallpox, chickenpox, shingles, the common cold, influenza, measles, yellow fever, and mumps.*

**vis.** Force or energy.

**vis a tergo. 1.** An impelling force; the force of circumstances. **2.** Force exerted from the back; said of venous blood pressure originating in the bloodstream by the heartbeat.

**vis conservatrix.** The natural resistance to injury or disease.

**vis medicatrix naturae.** Nature's healing power.

**viscera.** The plural of viscus, any one of the organs situated in the chest or abdomen. The term applies particularly to the organs of the abdominal cavity, such as the liver, spleen, kidneys, pancreas, gall bladder, urinary bladder, stomach, and intestines.

**viscerad.** Towards the viscera.

**visceral.** Pertaining to a viscus or viscera.

**visceralgia.** Pain in the viscera or in any organ.

**visceroptosis.** Prolapse; malplacement or dropping of an abdominal organ. Also called *splanchnoptosis.*

**viscid.** Thick, sticky, adhesive.

**viscometer, viscosimeter.** An apparatus for measuring the viscosity of fluids.

**viscosity.** The condition of being viscous. It normally refers to the flow rate of a fluid, that is, its ability to flow fast or slow.

**viscous.** Viscid; pertaining to a viscus.

**viscus.** A large internal organ in one of the body cavities; the singular of viscera.

**vision.** The act of seeing; sight.

**achromatic vision.** Loss of color sense; color blindness.

**binocular vision.** Coordinated use of both eyes; normal vision.

**central vision.** Vision with the macula lutea of the retina.

**chromatic vision.** Color vision.

**double vision.** A vision in which one object is seen as two. The most common type is due to a derangement of the muscle balance of the two eyes, as a result of which the images of an object are thrown upon nonidentical points of the retina of the eye. It may be the result of a divergent squint in which the image of the right eye appears upon the left side and that of the left eye upon the right side. It may occur as evidence of serious brain disease. Also called *diplopia.*

**night vision.** The ability of the eye to see in dim light. Poor night vision may be due to an inherent defect of the retina of the eye, due to vitamin deficiencies, or to excessive exposure of the eye to sunlight.

**scotopic vision.** Perception of shape and form without recognition of color, as occurs in dim light.

**solid vision.** The perception of depth of objects obtained by binocular vision and which is denied to those with only one eye. Also called *stereoscopic vision.*

**tunnel vision.** The extremely contracted visual field characteristic of hysteria.

**visual.** Relating to vision.

**visual acuity.** The degree of eyesight present in a patient.

**visual adaptation.** The ability of the eyes to adjust themselves to changed conditions of light. To do this, the pupil opens in the dark and closes down to a small hole under the effect of strong light.

**visual field.** The area of space visible to the fixed eye.

**visual purple.** An organic pigment of the retina which is bleached to yellow by light. It is a protein closely related to vitamin A. Also called *erythropsin, rhodopsin.*

**visuo–auditory.** Pertaining to sight and hearing.

**vital capacity.** The volume of air that can be breathed out from the lungs after a complete respiration.

**vital center.** The brain center which controls breathing.

**vital statistics.** Statistics of births, deaths, marriages, and diseases.

**vitals.** Those organs essential to life.

**vitamin.** One of a group of organic compounds present in minute quantities in natural foodstuffs. They are essential for the normal growth and maintenance of life since the body is unable to synthesize them for itself. They are effective in small amounts. Vitamins do not furnish energy, but are essential for the transformation of energy and for the regulation of metabolism. When first discovered, vitamins were thought to be chemicals called amines and hence were called vital amines, which was later shortened to vitamins.

**vitamin A.** A vitamin necessary for maintenance of normal development of skin and visual acuity. Deficiency of vitamin A leads to wasting of skin cells, an increased susceptibility to attack by germs, and may also be responsible for night blindness. It is found in fish liver oil, milk fat, and many pigmented vegetables. It is probably also associated with normal development and growth.

**vitamin B.** Originally thought to be a single vitamin, vitamin B is now known to comprise several different vitamins and is usually referred to as the vitamin B complex, which includes vitamin $B_1$ (thiamine), vitamin $B_2$ (riboflavin), vitamin $B_6$ (niacin and pyridoxine), and many other substances. The vitamin B complex is found in high concentration in yeast, liver, whole-grain cereals, milk, glan-

dular organs, eggs, certain leafy vegetables, malt, and wheat germ. Vitamin $B_1$ is necessary for normal digestion of carbohydrates, for the maintenance of normal appetite, for the proper functioning of muscular tissues, reproduction, and lactation. Deficiency of this vitamin leads to nerve disorders and heart failure, and total lack of it causes beriberi. Vitamin $B_2$ is necessary for protection against pellagra. Vitamin $B_{12}$ is used in the treatment of pernicious anemia.

**vitamin C.** Ascorbic acid. This vitamin is found in cabbage, lettuce, lemons, oranges, pineapple, raspberries, spinach, and tomatoes. Vitamin C has been produced artificially. It is necessary for the maintenance of health in teeth, bones, and walls of blood vessels. Deficiency leads to scurvy, which is characterized by hemorrhages in various parts of the body. See also ASCORBIC ACID.

**vitamin D.** This vitamin is found in cod liver oil and milk, and lack of it in the diet, especially in growing children, results in rickets.

**vitamin E.** This vitamin is found in wheat germ oil, cottonseed oil, corn oil, lettuce, alfalfa, and beef liver. In animals, at least, a deficiency of it results in sterility. Recent studies indicate vitamin E's importance in maintaining a healthy heart.

*Vitamins and babies.* Small babies need extra supplements of vitamins A, D, and C, at least until they are on a completely mixed diet, and these can be supplied by either cod liver oil or halibut liver oil mixed with orange juice or rose hip syrup. Breast-fed babies should receive their vitamins from the mother's milk, but it is not always safe to rely on this source and extra vitamins should be given separately from the breast feeds. Bottle-fed babies should also receive their vitamins separately and not have them included in the milk feed. Once the child is on an adequate mixed diet of milk, butter, fruit, and vegetables, he will obtain from his food all the vitamins he can possibly use and any additions will be surplus to requirements and excreted either in the feces or in the urine. The vast quantities of cod liver oil and malt administered to protesting children in the past served little purpose except to impress the mother with her determination to rear a healthy child. Harmful effects have been reported from excessive intake of vitamin A and D.

**vitiligo.** Piebald skin; a skin disorder marked by a loss of the natural pigment in patches, leaving white areas. Also called *leukoderma.*

**vitium.** A defect.

**vitodynamic.** Relating to vital forces.

**vitreous.** Glasslike.

**vitreous chamber.** The part of the eyeball situated behind the lens.

**vitreous humor.** The transparent jellylike substance which fills the vitreous chamber of the eye.

**vitriol.** Any crystalline sulfate.

**vitrum.** Glass.

**viviparous.** Bringing forth live offspring, as opposed to laying an egg which has to be hatched.

**vocal cords.** Two chords situated within the larynx and controlled by muscles which open and close to produce alterations in sound and the voice.

**void.** To evacuate, especially the evacuation of urine and feces.

**vola.** A concave surface.

**vola manus.** The hollow of the hand or palm.

**vola pedis.** The hollow of the foot.

**volar.** Pertaining to the palm or sole.

**volition.** The will to act.

**volitional.** Relating to the will.

**Volkmann's deformity.** Congenital dislocation of the ankle.

**Volkmann's ischemic contracture.** Shrinkage of the muscles in a limb due to their blood supply being cut off by an overtight splint or bandage. When a splint or a bandage is used to secure a fracture, unless great care is taken, the tissues react to the injury and swell. This cuts off the blood supply in the limb and results in tremendous scarring, which may cause permanent disability. The parts below a splint or bandage should therefore, be constantly observed to ensure that the circulation has not been cut off. If the lower parts become congested or blue, the splint or bandage should be loosened and reapplied.

**Volkmann's spoon.** A sharp surgical spoon used for scraping.

**volsella.** A forceps with a hook at the end of each blade. Also called *vulsella, vulsellum.*

**Voltolini's disease.** Acute inflammation of the internal ear.

**voluntary.** Controlled by the will.

**volvulus.** A twisting of the bowel upon itself so as to cause obstruction, occurring most frequently in the sigmoid colon.

**vomer.** The thin plate of bone forming the back part of the nasal septum.

**vomerine.** Relating to the vomer.

**vomit.** 1. To eject the contents of the stomach. 2. The substance vomited.

**vomiting.** The forcible ejection of the contents of the stomach through the mouth.

**coffee-ground vomiting.** Vomiting from the stomach of partially digested blood which has the appearance of ground coffee.

**cyclic or cyclical vomiting.** Vomiting recurring at regular intervals. The average age of onset is from three to seven years, though it can occur as late as eleven years. The attacks tend to spontaneous cure at puberty but some patients develop migraine. There is usually a marked family history of migraine or of bilious attacks in the parents. It is generally agreed that in these children the nervous system is unstable, and this combined with a deficient digestion of carbohydrate may account for the condition. In the main these children require more rest, attention to their nervous condition, with an increase of carbohydrates, and a decrease of fat in their diet. An old-fashioned but useful treatment for these children is to give them unlimited quantities of barley sugar to eat. They often also require a sedative to placate nervous excitement and instability. Also called *period vomiting, bilious attacks.*

**fecal vomiting.** Vomiting due to intestinal obstruction. It commences with normal stomach contents, then becomes bilious and, if not relieved, even the presence of feces is apparent.

**period vomiting.** See CYCLIC VOMITING, above.

**pernicious vomiting.** Vomiting sometimes seen in pregnancy, and so excessive as to threaten the life of the mother.

**projectile vomiting.** A form in which the vomit is suddenly and forcibly projected from the mouth, usually without preceding nausea. It is observed in some diseases of the brain and in pyloric stenosis of babies.

**vomitory.** Any agent acting as an emetic.

**vomiturition.** Repeated ineffectual efforts at vomiting; retching.

**vomitus.** That which is vomited.

**vonulo.** A lung disease characterized by considerable pain; occurring in West Africa.

**Voronoff's operation.** The famous rejuvenation operation of transplanting the testicles of an ape into a human.

**vulcanization.** A process of imparting greater elasticity, durability, and hardness to rubber by heating it with sulfur. The rubber gloves used by the housewife to protect her hands contain quite an element of sulfur which may produce a dermatitis. Therefore those women who have skin sensitive to detergents and other agents used in the kitchen, should wear cotton or nylon gloves under the rubber gloves.

**vulnerability.** Susceptible to injury or infection.

**vulnerary.** Pertaining to the healing of wounds or an agent that promotes the healing of wounds.

**vulnerate.** To wound.

**vulnus.** A wound.

**Vulpian's atrophy.** Progressive wasting of the muscles of the shoulder and upper arm.

**vulsella, vulsellum.** See VOLSELLA.

**vulva.** The external genital organs at the opening of the vagina, consisting of the labia minora and the labia majora.

**vulvar.** Relating to the vulva.

**vulvectomy.** Surgical removal of the vulva.

**vulvismus.** See VAGINISMUS.

**vulvitis.** Inflammation of the vulva.

**vulvopathy.** Any disease of the vulva.

**vulvo-uterine.** Pertaining to both the vulva and the uterus.

**vulvovaginal.** Relating to the vulva and the vagina.

**vulvovaginitis.** Inflammation of the vulva and the vagina.

# W-X-Y-Z

**Wagstaffe's fracture.** A fracture of the ankle which results in the foot being rotated inwards.

**wallerian degeneration.** The wasting away of a nerve after it has been cut.

**Walther's canal.** The duct of the sublingual salivary gland.

**wandering abscess.** An abscess which burrows in the tissues and erupts at a point distant from its origin. Also called *hypostatic abscess.*

**wandering cell.** A leukocyte.

**wandering organ.** An organ which gets out of its normal position from losing its attachment or tethering position.

**Warren-Tay-Sachs disease.** See TAY-SACHS DISEASE.

**wart.** A raised growth of the skin produced by a virus. See VERRUCA.

**Wassermann reaction.** A blood test for syphilis.

**Waterhouse-Friderichsen syndrome.** A disease characterized by meningococcal septicemia and meningitis and associated with bleeding into the suprarenal glands. The syndrome is more common in infants than adults. The syndrome is only occasionally diagnosed during life, but is suggested by symptoms of cyanosis, collapse, and fall in blood pressure in a patient suffering from meningococcal meningitis.

**wax.** 1. The material of the bees' honeycomb. 2. Ear wax.

**waxing.** 1. Increasing in size. 2. Applying a coating of wax.

**waxy degeneration.** See AMYLOID DEGENERATION.

**weasand.** An old term for the trachea.

**weaver's bottom.** Chronic bursitis of the tuber ischii. It is caused by prolonged sitting on hard surfaces irritating the two bones (the tuber ischii) in the buttocks, and as a sequel the bursae over the bones become swollen and painful, making sitting impossible. The condition was formerly common among handloom weavers, who sat on hard benches, and basket weavers, who sat cross-legged on the floor.

**Weber's syndrome.** A condition characterized by paralysis of the third cranial nerve on the same side of the brain as the lesion, accompanied by paralysis of the arm and leg on the opposite side. Also called *syndrome of the cerebral peduncle.*

**Weber's test.** A hearing test in which the vibrations from a tuning fork, placed on the forehead of a normal person, are referred to the midline and heard equally in both ears. In middle ear deafness of one side, the sound is heard in the diseased ear. In deafness due to disease of the auditory nerve on one side, the sound is heard better in the normal ear.

**Wegner's disease.** Separation of the epiphyses of long bones in congenital syphilis.

**Weil's disease.** See LEPTOSPIROSIS.

**Weinberg's test.** A blood test for the presence of a hydatid cyst or hydatid disease.

**Weingarten's syndrome.** A condition commonly found in India and Ceylon in which there is an increase of eosinophils in the blood associated with asthma and bronchitis. In some cases there is an association ascribed to infestation of the bronchi by parasitic mites. Also called *Löffler's syndrome.*

**Weir-Mitchell's disease.** See ERYTHROMELALGIA.

**Weiss's sign.** A muscular contraction of the face following light tapping over the facial muscles; seen in tetany.

**wen.** An old name for a sebaceous cyst.

**Werdnig-Hoffmann paralysis.** A type of progressive muscular atrophy.

**Werlhof's disease.** See PURPURA: HEMORRHAGIC PURPURA.

**Wernicke-Mann type.** A form of spastic hemiplegia.

**Wernicke's aphasia.** Loss or impairment of the capacity to use words correctly. Sometimes the words are uttered fluently but inappropriately, as a form of jargon. Also called *cortical sensory aphasia.*

**Wernicke's disease.** A form of acute hemorrhagic polioencephalitis (inflammation of the grey matter of the brain associated with bleeding).

**Wernicke's sign.** An eye sign which occurs in cases where there is blindness in one half of the visual field. If a light is shone on the blind half there is no pupil reaction, but if shone on the good half the pupil contracts, indicating that the disease process is situated in front of the geniculate bodies of the brain.

**Wernicke's syndrome.** Loss of memory and other symptoms associated with senility. Also called *presbyophrenia.*

**Wertheim's operation.** An operation performed to remove the whole of the womb and as much surrounding tissue as possible.

**wet dream.** See POLLUTION: NOCTURNAL POLLUTION.

**Wharton's duct.** The duct of the salivary gland situated below the lower jaw and which conveys saliva to the mouth.

**wheal.** A blister on the skin produced by urticaria, the stroke of a whip, or an insect bite.

**Wheelhouse's operation.** Surgical division of a stricture of the urethra.

**whelk.** An old term for a wheal or pimple.

**whey.** The liquid separating from curd when milk is clotted.

**whipworm.** A parasitic worm found in the human intestines.

**whisky nose.** See RHINOPHYMA.

**Whitehead's operation.** 1. An operation for the removal of hemorrhoids. 2. An operation for removing the tongue.

**white leg.** See PHLEGMASIA ALBA DOLENS.

**white pox.** A disease resembling chickenpox and occurring in Brazil.

**whites.** A popular name for leukorrhea.

**white-spot disease.** A condition characterized by circumscribed patches of hard skin on the neck and upper part of the trunk. Also called *morphea guttata.*

**whitlow.** An old general term for any abscess type of inflammation occurring at the end of a finger or toe. Also called *felon, paronychia.*

**whooping cough.** An acute specific fever of high infectivity most frequently seen in children, characterized by catarrh of the respiratory tract and by paroxysmal cough, which may or may not be associated with the inspiratory laryngeal spasm which produces the distinctive "whoop." Also called *pertussis.*

*Whooping cough has been so much modified by preventive inoculation that a classical example is now seldom seen. The usual picture is of upper-respiratory catarrh with a paroxysmal cough that is worse at night. If these conditions occur during a known local epidemic of the disease the diagnosis is practically certain. The incubation period is about two weeks, after which the disease develops in three stages: a catarrhal, a paroxysmal, and a convalescent stage. During the catarrhal stage the patient may run a temperature and have what appears to be a heavy catarrhal cold, except that the cough is more troublesome and signs of bronchitis on the chest are absent. This stage lasts for one or two weeks, after which there is a tendency for the cough to become paroxysmal, with greater severity at night, giving rise to suffusion of the face and sometimes retching or vomiting. The paroxysmal stage is unmistakable. A brief, deep inspiration is followed by a rapid succession of short coughs, with the mouth open and the tongue protruding, which are continued until the chest is almost emptied of air. The face becomes livid, the eyes fill with tears, the eyeballs protrude, the skin is bathed in sweat, and the child appears about to suffocate. Relief is suddenly afforded by relaxation of the spasm and the occurrence of a long-drawn crowing inspiration, the whoop, which refills the lungs with air. This stage may last from two to ten weeks, after which convalescence begins.*

**Whytt's disease.** Acute hydrocephalus caused by tuberculosis meningitis. See also HYDROCEPHALUS.

**Wichmann's asthma.** See LARYNGISMUS STRIDULUS.

**Widal-Abrami disease.** Acquired hemolytic jaundice. See also JAUNDICE.

**Widal's reaction.** A blood test for typhoid fever.

**Wilde's cone of light.** A cone of reflected light seen on the eardrum during examination.

**Wilkinson's ointment.** Compound sulfur ointment.

**Willan's lepra.** See PSORIASIS.

**Willett forceps.** Midwifery forceps designed for applying scalp traction during childbirth.

**Williamson's sign.** A sign sometimes seen in pneumothorax or pleural effusion, in which there is diminished blood pressure in the leg compared with the arm of the same side.

**Willis' circle.** A circle of arteries situated at the base of the brain at the back of the skull. Occasionally in an apparently healthy young adult a weakness in one of these arteries causes a sudden hemorrhage which can kill in an instant. Typically, the patient is seized with a violent headache referred to the back of the skull, which steadily gets worse until he becomes unconscious. It is a form of subarachnoid hemorrhage. See also SUB-ARACHNOID.

**Wilms' tumor.** A malignant tumor of the kidney observed in early childhood.

**Wilms' tumour.** See WILMS' TUMOR.

**Wilson's disease.** 1. A rare progressive disease of the nervous system named after the neurologist S. A. K. Wilson; also called *progressive lenticular degeneration;* see LENTICULAR: PROGRESSIVE LENTICULAR DEGENERATION. 2. A disease named after the dermatologist W. J. E. Wilson, being an inflammatory reaction of the skin characterized by shedding of its surface. This condition sometimes follows the administration of certain drugs, such as the sulfonamides, and poisoning by such substances as arsenic; also called *exfoliative dermatitis.*

**windpipe.** The trachea.

**wine spot.** A nevus.

**wintergreen.** Methyl salicylate; used as a liniment, or as an ointment in combination with menthol, for the relief of fibrositis, rheumatism, lumbago, arthritis, and the like.

**Wirsung's duct.** The duct conveying enzymes from the pancreas to the duodenum. Also called *pancreatic duct.*

**wisdom tooth.** The last double tooth on each side of each jaw. See TOOTH.

**witch hazel.** An astringent derived from a shrub of the genus *Hamamelis.*

**witch's milk.** The milky fluid sometimes found issuing from the breasts of newborn babies. See also BREAST.

**Wolff-Parkinson-White syndrome.** A form of premature excitation of the ventricles of the heart, which may be permanent, transient, or paroxysmal. The heart is usually normal and the condition is only diagnosed by means of the electrocardiograph.

**womb.** The uterus.

**wool fat.** Anhydrous lanolin.

**woolsorters' disease.** See ANTHRAX.

**word blindness.** Inability to understand written or printed words.

**word deafness.** Inability, though sounds are heard, to understand the spoken word due to disease of the auditory center.

**word salad.** A jumble of meaningless words used by some patients suffering from a psychosis, especially schizophrenia.

**Woulfe's bottle.** A bottle used for passing gas through a liquid.

**wound.** An injury brought about through disruption by physical means of the continuity of the body's external or internal surfaces.

**abrasion wound.** A wound in which the surface of the skin is scraped.

**contused wound.** A wound produced by a blunt instrument usually without breaking the skin.

**gunshot wound.** A wound made by a projectile from a gun.

**incised wound.** A wound caused by a cutting instrument.

**lacerated wound.** A wound in which the tissues are torn.

**open wound.** A wound having a free, gaping, external opening.

**penetrating wound.** A wound that pierces the walls of a cavity or enters an internal organ.

**puncture wound.** A wound made by a pointed instrument.

**W.R.** Abbreviation for Wassermann reaction, a blood test for syphilis.

**wrist.** The part connecting the forearm and the hand, consisting of eight carpal bones and their ligaments. Also called *carpus.*

**wristdrop.** Inability to bend the hand backwards due to paralysis of the extensor muscles. It is characteristic of lead poisoning but may occur in other ailments.

**writer's cramp.** Painful spasms of the fingers on attempting to write. See NEUROSIS: OCCUPATIONAL NEUROSIS.

**wryneck.** See TORTICOLLIS.

**xanthaemia.** See XANTHEMIA.

**xanthelasma.** See XANTHOMA.

**xanthemia.** Yellow pigments in the blood.

**xanthine.** A yellow nitrogenous compound found in body tissues and fluids.

**xanthinuria.** The presence of xanthine in the urine.

**xanthochroia.** Yellow staining of the skin.

**xanthochromatic.** Having a yellow color.

**xanthochromia.** Any yellowish discoloration, as of the skin or spinal fluid.

**xanthochroous.** Having a yellow skin.

**xanthocyanopsia, xanthocyanopsy.** A form of color vision in which the individual is able to see yellow and blue but not red or green.

**xanthoderma, xanthodermia.** A yellow color of the skin.

**xanthodontous.** Having yellow teeth.

**xanthokyanopy.** See XANTHOCYANOPSIA.

**xanthoma.** A disorder characterized by the presence of yellow nodules on the skin, and due to a disturbance of lipoid metabolism. Also called *xanthelasma.*

**xanthomatosis.** A disorder of lipoid metabolism characterized by excessive deposits of lipoids in the body. A generic name for a group of diseases which include Hand-Schüller-Christian's disease of children, Gaucher's disease, and Niemann-Pick's disease.

**xanthomatous.** Pertaining to xanthoma.

**xanthomyeloma.** See XANTHOSARCOMA.

**xanthopathy.** Any disease characterized by yellow pigmentation of the skin.

**xanthophane.** A yellow pigment found in the retina.

**xanthopsia.** Yellow-colored vision. A symptom that may occur in jaundice, picric acid poisoning, and santonin poisoning.

**xanthopsin.** Visual yellow. It develops from the action of light on rhodopsin.

**xanthosarcoma.** A malignant disease attacking fascial planes (fibrous tissue coverings of organs and muscles) and tendon sheaths. Also called *xanthomyeloma.*

**xanthosis.** A yellow coloration of the skin, seen sometimes in cases of cancer.

**xanthous.** Yellow or yellowish.

**xanthuria.** Excessive xanthine in the urine.

**X-chromosome.** A chromosome associated with sex determination. See CHROMOSOME; SEX; SEX DETERMINATION.

**xenogenesis.** The production of children unlike the parents.

**xenogenous.** Caused by a foreign body.

**xenomenia.** See VICARIOUS MENSTRUATION.

**xenoparasite.** An organism normally not parasitic, which gains entry into a host and causes disease because of the host's lowered resistance.

**xenophobia.** A neurotic dread of strangers.

**xenophonia.** An alteration in the tone or quality of the voice.

**xenophthalmia.** Traumatic conjunctivitis.

**Xenopus.** A genus of amphibians. A South African toad used for performing pregnancy tests belongs to this genus.

**xeransis.** A drying up; a gradual loss of moisture.

**xerantic.** Causing a drying up.

**xerasis.** An old term for a disease of the hair, characterized by excessive dryness and cessation of growth.

**xerocollyrium.** An eye ointment.

**xeroderma, xerodermia.** Dry skin; a disease characterized by dry, harsh, scaly, discolored skin, which rubs off as a dust. Also called *ichthyosis.*

**xeroderma pigmentosum.** A rare skin disease beginning in childhood and characterized by the presence of pigmented spots, atrophy, and contraction, so that the child's skin resembles that of a very old person. It is worse in those areas exposed to the sun and is made worse by it. Patients cannot bear bright light on the eyes, and parts of the skin become wartlike and thickened, some developing into malignant growths. The disease has a familial tendency and is eventually fatal. Also called *Kaposi's disease.*

**xeroma.** See XEROPHTHALMIA.

**xeromenia.** A condition in which all the bodily changes of menstruation occur but without the loss of blood.

**xeronosus.** An abnormally dry state of the skin.

**xerophagy, xerophagia.** Eating dry food.

**xerophthalmia.** A dry thickened condition of the conjunctiva and cornea. It may be the result of chronic inflammation, a disease of the tear-producing apparatus, or vitamin A deficiency. Also called *xeroma, xerophthalmus.*

**xerosis.** Excessive dryness of the skin, or conjunctiva.

**xerostoma, xerostomia.** Excessive dryness of the mouth resulting from diminished salivary secretions.

**xerotic.** Characterized by dryness.

**xerotripsis.** Dry friction.

**xiphicostal.** Pertaining to the xiphoid cartilage at the lower end of the breastbone and the ribs.

**xiphisternal.** Pertaining to the xiphisternum.

**xiphisternum.** The xiphoid cartilage at the lower end of the sternum.

**xiphocostal.** See XIPHICOSTAL.

**xiphodynia.** Pain in the xiphoid cartilage at the lower end of the sternum.

**xiphoid.** Sword-shaped.

**xiphoiditis.** Inflammation of the xiphoid cartilage at the lower end of the sternum.

**x-rays.** Electromagnetic radiations produced by passing a high-voltage electric current through a Coolidge tube—that is, a vacuum tube with a cathode consisting of a spiral filament of incandescent tungsten and an anode of massive tungsten. The rays so produced are similar to the gamma rays emitted by radioactive substances. X-rays can penetrate tissues and are used both for taking photographs of the internal structures of the body and for the treatment of some skin conditions and deep-lying growths. Also called *roentgen rays.*

*X-rays, like many other important discoveries, were discovered accidentally. On November 8th, 1895, at Wurzburg University in Germany, Wilhelm Roentgen was working in a darkened room passing electricity through a Crookes tube (a glass vacuum tube) shielded by black paper, when he discovered that rays from the tube were passing through the covering and making fluorescent a piece of paper that had been coated with barium platinocyanide. Further research revealed that these rays, which Roentgen called x-rays, could pass through many substances and even fog a photographic plate.*

**yawning.** An involuntary gaping open of the mouth, often accompanied by involuntary stretching of the muscles and accompanied by a deep inspiration. It usually occurs during the drowsy state produced by fatigue or boredom and is a prelude to sleep. Many people find it almost impossible not to yawn when they see someone else doing so, even if not particularly tired or bored themselves. Yawning occurs mostly when a person is sitting at rest in a warm, comfortable atmosphere.

**yaws.** A contagious disease caused by the spirochete *Treponema pertenue,* and occurring in hot climates. It is characterized by the formation of raspberrylike swellings on the face, hands, feet, and external genitals. These run together to form masses or they may form pustules or ulcers. There is a close similarity between yaws and syphilis since they are both caused by related microorganisms, but yaws is not a veneral disease. Also called *frambesia tropica, pian, parangi* (Ceylon), *bubas* (Brazil), *coco* (Fiji).

**Y-chromosome.** See CHROMOSOME; SEX; SEX DETERMINATION.

**yeast.** The common name of a group of fungi, most of which belong to the genus *Saccharomyces.* Yeasts are of economic importance since they are used as leavening for bread, for initiating alcoholic fermentation, and medicinally as a source of B-complex vitamin. Some yeasts are pathogenic to man.

**yelk.** Yolk.

**yellow fever.** An acute infectious disease of tropical and subtropical regions caused by a virus disseminated by a particular type of mosquito. The incubation period varies from a few hours to several days, and the disease begins with a chill and pain in the head, back, and limbs. The temperature rises rapidly up to 105°, when vomiting starts. There is constipation; the urine is scanty and contains albumin. A remission follows, after which, in severe cases, the temperature rises again to its original height, jaundice develops, and the vomit becomes dark from the presence of blood. The disease is often fatal, and is of immense concern to countries like India, which, though harboring the type of mosquito that spreads yellow fever, has not so far become contaminated by the germ. In these days of rapid movement, air travelers who have come from or passed through a yellow fever belt are not allowed to land in nonyellow fever areas unless they have received an inoculation against this very virulent disease.

**y-ligament.** The iliofemoral ligament situated in the region of the hip joint.

**yogurt, yohourt.** A preparation of curdled milk, fermented by bacteria of the genus *Lactobacillus.*

**yoke bone.** The cheek bone.

**yolk.** The yellow part of an egg suspended in the white portion or albumen; the material in the egg or ovum that furnishes food in the early stages of the developing embryo.

**Young-Helmholtz theory.** A theory which attempts to explain how color vision is obtained in the human eye: three sets of retinal fibers are said to be responsible for the colors red, green, and violet.

**Young's rule.** A method of determining the correct dose of drugs for children. The age of the child is divided by the age of the child plus twelve. This gives the fraction of the adult dose suitable for the child.

**Zambesi fever.** A nonmalarial fever occurring in indigents of the Zambesi Valley of southern Africa.

**Zambesi ulcer.** An ulcer found on the leg or foot of natives of the Zambesi Valley of southern Africa. It is caused by the larva of a fly which penetrates the skin.

**zeismus.** A skin disease attributed to the overuse of maize in the diet. Also called *zeism.*

**zelotypia.** A morbid zeal in any undertaking, occupation, or effort.

**zoanthropy.** A type of insanity in which the patient believes he has become an animal.

**zoic.** Pertaining to animal life.

**zonaesthesia.** See ZONESTHESIA.

**zonesthesia.** A sensation like that produced by a tight girdle encircling the waist. Also called *girdle pain.*

**zooerastia.** Sexual intercourse with an animal.

**zoogamy.** The sexual reproduction of animals; mating.

**zoogenesis.** The generation of animal forms.

**zoogenous.** Giving birth to live young.

**zoogeny.** The study of the reproduction and development of animal forms; the study of the evolution of animals.

**zooid.** 1. Resembling an animal. 2. One individual in a united colony of animals, as in certain corals.

**zoology.** The study of animal life.

**zoonoses.** Diseases common to man and animals. They include the following: *Bacterial diseases.* Anthrax, brucellosis, leptospirosis, pasteurellosis, salmonella, staphylococcal and streptococcal infections, and tuberculosis.

*Fungal infections.* Ringworm. *Protozoal infections.* Toxoplasmosis. *Parasitic infections.* Worms, hydatid disease, fleas, lice, mange, and scabies.

**zoophilism.** The love of animals, usually immoderate love of certain animals; antivivisectionism.

**zoophobia.** Morbid fear of animals.

**zoophyte.** An invertebrate animal that superficially resembles a plant, such as the sponges.

**zooplasty.** Surgical transplantation of tissues from a lower animal to man.

**zoopsia.** The hallucinations of seeing animals, such as pink elephants, which commonly occurs in delirium tremens of alcohol poisoning.

**zoster.** See HERPES ZOSTER.

**zosteriform.** Resembling herpes zoster.

**zwitterion.** An ion which carries both positive and negative charges.

**zygal.** Yoked; having the form of a yoke.

**zygapophysis.** An articular process of a vertebra.

**zygoma.** The arch formed by the union of the temporal bone and the zygomatic bone; the cheek bone.

**zygomatic.** Relating to the zygoma.

**zygote.** A cell formed by the union of two gametes, as an egg and sperm; a fertilized egg; the organism produced from a cell formed by the union of two gametes.

**zymad.** The organism causing a zymotic disease.

**zymase.** An enzyme; an ingredient of yeast which brings about alcoholic fermentation.

**zymasis.** Extraction of the active ingredient of yeast by hydraulic pressure.

**zyme.** 1. An enzyme. 2. Any agent that produces a zymotic disease.

**zymic.** Pertaining to ferments.

**zymocyte.** Any organism causing fermentation.

**zymogen.** An inactive substance that is capable of being converted into an active enzyme; a proenzyme.

**zymogenic.** Causing fermentation; relating to or producing a zymogen.

**zymoid.** A poison from decaying tissues; resembling a ferment.

**zymology.** The science of fermentation.

**zymolysis.** Fermentation or digestion produced by an enzyme.

**zymolytic.** Pertaining to zymolysis.

**zymophyte.** A bacterium which causes fermentation.

**zymose.** An enzyme catalyzing cane sugar. Also called *invertin, invertase, sucrase.*

**zymosis.** 1. The process of fermentation. 2. The development of zymotic disease; any infectious or contagious disease.

**zymotic.** 1. Relating to fermentation. 2. A general term for any infective or contagious disease.

# Recommended Weights in Pounds for Women

*(without clothing)*

| Height ft. in. | Small Frame | Medium Frame | Large Frame |
|---|---|---|---|
| 4  8 (142 cm) | 88-94 (39.9-42.6 kg) | 92-103 (41.7-46.7 kg) | 100-115 (45.4-52.2 kg) |
| 4  9 (145 cm) | 90-97 (40.8-44.0 kg) | 94-106 (42.6-48.1 kg) | 102-118 (46.3-53.5 kg) |
| 4  10 (147 cm) | 92-100 (41.7-45.4 kg) | 97-109 (44.0-49.4 kg) | 105-121 (47.6-54.9 kg) |
| 4  11 (150 cm) | 95-103 (43.1-46.7 kg) | 100-112 (45.4-50.8 kg) | 108-124 (49.0-56.2 kg) |
| 5  0 (152 cm) | 98-106 (44.5-48.1 kg) | 103-115 (46.7-52.2 kg) | 111-127 (50.3-57.6 kg) |
| 5  1 (155 cm) | 101-109 (45.8-49.4 kg) | 106-118 (48.1-53.5 kg) | 114-130 (51.7-59.0 kg) |
| 5  2 (157 cm) | 104-112 (47.2-50.8 kg) | 109-122 (49.4-55.3 kg) | 117-134 (53.1-60.8 kg) |
| 5  3 (160 cm) | 107-115 (48.5-52.2 kg) | 112-126 (50.8-57.1 kg) | 121-138 (54.9-62.6 kg) |
| 5  4 (163 cm) | 110-119 (49.9-54.0 kg) | 116-131 (52.6-59.4 kg) | 125-142 (56.7-64.4 kg) |
| 5  5 (165 cm) | 114-123 (51.7-55.8 kg) | 120-135 (54.4-61.2 kg) | 129-146 (58.5-66.2 kg) |
| 5  6 (168 cm) | 118-127 (53.5-57.6 kg) | 124-139 (56.2-63.1 kg) | 133-150 (60.3-68.0 kg) |
| 5  7 (170 cm) | 122-131 (55.3-59.4 kg) | 128-143 (58.1-64.9 kg) | 137-154 (62.1-69.9 kg) |
| 5  8 (173 cm) | 126-136 (57.2-61.7 kg) | 132-147 (59.9-66.7 kg) | 141-159 (64.0-72.1 kg) |
| 5  9 (175 cm) | 130-140 (59.0-63.5 kg) | 136-151 (61.7-68.5 kg) | 145-164 (65.8-74.4 kg) |
| 5  10 (178 cm) | 134-144 (60.8-65.3 kg) | 140-155 (63.5-70.3 kg) | 149-169 (67.6-76.7 kg) |

# Recommended Weights in Pounds for Men

*(without clothing)*

| Height ft. in. | Small Frame | Medium Frame | Large Frame |
|---|---|---|---|
| 5  1 (155 cm) | 106-114 (48.1-51.7 kg) | 112-123 (50.8-55.8 kg) | 120-135 (54.4-61.2 kg) |
| 5  2 (157 cm) | 109-117 (49.4-53.1 kg) | 115-127 (52.2-57.6 kg) | 123-138 (55.8-62.6 kg) |
| 5  3 (160 cm) | 112-120 (50.8-54.4 kg) | 118-130 (53.5-59.0 kg) | 126-142 (57.1-64.4 kg) |
| 5  4 (163 cm) | 115-123 (52.2-55.8 kg) | 121-133 (54.9-60.3 kg) | 129-146 (58.5-66.2 kg) |
| 5  5 (165 cm) | 118-127 (53.5-57.6 kg) | 124-137 (56.2-62.1 kg) | 132-150 (59.9-68.0 kg) |
| 5  6 (168 cm) | 122-131 (55.3-59.4 kg) | 128-141 (58.1-64.0 kg) | 136-155 (61.7-70.3 kg) |
| 5  7 (170 cm) | 126-135 (57.1-61.2 kg) | 132-146 (59.9-66.2 kg) | 141-160 (64.0-72.6 kg) |
| 5  8 (173 cm) | 130-139 (59.0-63.1 kg) | 136-150 (61.7-68.0 kg) | 145-164 (65.8-74.4 kg) |
| 5  9 (175 cm) | 134-144 (60.8-65.3 kg) | 140-154 (63.5-69.9 kg) | 149-168 (67.6-76.2 kg) |
| 5  10 (178 cm) | 138-148 (62.6-67.1 kg) | 144-159 (65.3-72.1 kg) | 153-173 (69.4-78.5 kg) |
| 5  11 (180 cm) | 142-152 (64.4-69.0 kg) | 148-164 (67.1-74.4 kg) | 158-178 (71.7-80.7 kg) |
| 6  0 (183 cm) | 146-156 (66.2-70.8 kg) | 152-169 (69.0-76.7 kg) | 162-183 (73.5-83.0 kg) |
| 6  1 (185 cm) | 150-161 (68.0-73.0 kg) | 156-174 (70.8-79.0 kg) | 167-188 (75.8-85.3 kg) |
| 6  2 (188 cm) | 154-165 (69.9-74.8 kg) | 161-179 (73.0-81.2 kg) | 172-193 (78.0-87.5 kg) |
| 6  3 (190 cm) | 158-169 (71.7-76.7 kg) | 166-184 (75.3-83.5 kg) | 176-198 (79.8-89.8 kg) |